Breast Imaging
A Correlative Atlas

Thieme

Breast Imaging
A Correlative Atlas

Beverly E. Hashimoto, M.D. , F.A.C.R.
Section Head, Ultrasoud
Virginia Mason Medical Center
Seattle, Washington

Donald Bauermeister, M.D.
Chief of Pathology
Virginia Mason Medical Center
Seattle, Washington

and

Clinical Professor, Pathology
University of Washington
Seattle, Washington

Thieme
New York · Stuttgart

Thieme Medical Publishers, Inc.
333 Seventh Ave.
New York, NY 10001

Editor: Felicity Edge
Editorial Assistant: Diane Sardini
Director, Production and Manufacturing: Anne Vinnicombe
Production Editor: Becky Dille
Marketing Director: Phyllis Gold
Sales Manager: Ross Lumpkin
Chief Financial Officer: Peter van Woerden
President: Brian D. Scanlan
Compositor: Primustype
Printer: Maple-Vail Book Manufacturing Group

Library of Congress Cataloging-in-Publication Data
Hashimoto, Beverly.
Breast imaging : a correlative atlas / Beverly Hashimoto, Donald Bauermeister.
p. ; cm.
ISBN 1-58890-109-2 (TMP : alk. paper)--ISBN 3131319518 (GTV : alk. paper)
1. Breast--Imaging--Atlases. 2. Breast--Diseases--Diagnosis--Atlases. I. Bauermeister, Donald E. II. Title.
[DNLM: 1. Mammography--Atlases. 2. Mammography--Case Report. 3. Breast Diseases--diagnosis--Atlases. 4. Breast Diseases--diagnosis--Case Report 5. Ultrasonography, Mammary--Atlases. 6. Ultrasonography, Mammary--Case Report. WP 17 H3475b 2003]
RG493.5.D52 H37 2003
618.1'90754—dc21 2002070341

Printed in the United States of America

5 4 3 2 1

TMP ISBN 1-58890-109-2
GTV ISBN 3 13 131951 8

Table of Contents

Explanation of Tables of Contents

This book has two tables of contents. The book is primarily organized according to the first table of contents, Pattern Approach to Mammography. By using this table of contents, one is able to identify the histologic entities that create specific mammographic findings. However, for those who want to study the lesions that produce sonographic abnormalities, there is a second table of contents, Pattern Approach to Breast Sonography. This table of contents cross-references clinical cases that illustrate specific sonographic findings.

Pattern Approach to Breast Imaging

Pattern Approach to Breast Sonography

Foreword

In the modern world of medical pedagogy, the practitioner must become a perpetual student. Through seminars, journals, meetings, day-to-day conversations with colleagues, and the wonderful new world of the Internet, today's radiologist is constantly challenged by an ever-expanding world of knowledge. The immense volume of complex information does not alter the need to quickly apply this information in daily casework. The textbook remains an integral part of this knowledge base. However, modern textbooks no longer can be simple repositories of information. Such texts are impractical considering the pace of modern medicine and the seemingly ever-increasing caseload. Current reality mandates that textbooks serve as a practical "desk reference," a tool that helps to rapidly answer questions as they arise in one's daily casework. This textbook, *Correlative Atlas of Breast Imaging*, meets this need brilliantly. It is timely, clearly written, excellently illustrated, and has the simplicity and brevity necessary to serve as a useful desk reference.

This textbook is well organized for the practicing radiologist who usually employs mammography primarily, and then uses sonography or other modalities to answer questions either raised or not addressed by the mammogram. Dr. Hashimoto organizes her textbook by mammographic findings and then effectively illustrates the pathologic entity. Each chapter carries the clinician radiologist through an analysis according to the specific mammographic abnormality.

This text documents the integral importance of sonography in breast imaging. Breast imaging now requires a multidisciplinary approach. The use of all modalities, as discussed in the text, must be brought to bear on the clinical problems encountered in the individual case. Increasing importance is being placed on the proposition that breast imagers not only attempt to find as many breast cancers as technically possible, but to find them without subjecting ten women to needless breast biopsies for every cancer detected. The surest means to this end is the appropriate application of alternative technologies to film mammography.

I first met Dr. Beverly Hashimoto as a resident in Radiology at the University of California, San Francisco. I was very pleased when she accepted a fellowship in diagnostic sonography under my direction. She showed herself to be a student of extraordinary talent and to have an admirable dedication of purpose. I believed she was well suited to a typical academic post at a university. Instead she opted to join the prestigious Virginia Mason Clinic. Beverly helped to teach me that an inquisitive mind could flourish anywhere. Many university academicians would envy her academic pursuits, publications, and national prominence. The responsibility to advance radiological imaging lies not only in academia but in private practices as well. I am most proud of my students who have achieved significant academic success in a non-university setting.

Although magnetic resonance imaging is likely to have an increasing impact on solving breast imaging problems as time goes on, currently sonography has the greatest ancillary benefit to film mammography. Breast sonography has a somewhat checkered past. In the early- to mid-1980s, there was a strong push by several equipment developers to produce an automated, whole-breast, sonographic imaging device. Shortly after achieving success, claims of great ability in the detection of breast cancer began to appear. However, the data ultimately indicated the automated, whole-breast, sonographic imaging was not on a par with radiographic mammography. The experience left a bad taste in the mouths of many sonologists and mammographers. This episode undoubtedly retarded the growth and acceptance of sonographic breast imaging. However, to their credit, a small cadre of dedicated researchers took up the task of developing sonography in breast imaging for more than deciding whether a mass was cystic or not. Dr. Hashimoto figures prominently in this group of dedicated researchers. This book is the culmination of her years of excellent work in this medical arena.

Roy A. Filly, MD
Professor of Radiology, of Surgery, and of Obstetrics, Gynecology and Reproductive Sciences
Chief, Section of Diagnostic Sonography
University of California, San Francisco

Preface

This book is targeted for breast imagers who want to improve their interpretative skills by learning a method to analyze and integrate mammographic and sonographic findings. This method is based on developing familiarity with specific mammographic and sonographic image patterns. After a radiologist is familiar with these patterns, the imager can approach both mammographic and sonographic lesions in a systematic manner and reach a logical assessment. To facilitate this process, imaging sections 3–10 of this book are devoted to providing visual examples of these mammographic and sonographic patterns. Because most breast problems initially present with a mammographic examination, the sections are organized by specific mammographic findings according to the primary table of contents (Pattern Approach to Breast Imaging). Each mammographic pattern is illustrated by a variety of benign and malignant entities. Furthermore, the introduction of each section schematically illustrates the clinical approach to analyzing the mammographic abnormality.

The second goal of this book is to emphasize the multidisciplinary nature of breast imaging. This multidisciplinary approach is emphasized by the secondary table of contents (Pattern Approach to Breast Sonography) that organizes the individual cases into sonographic patterns. Furthermore, the cases in this book include other imaging modalities such as magnetic resonance and various nuclear medicine techniques. The utility of these modalities is discussed in the context of common clinical problems that are illustrated in the individual imaging cases.

Sonographic examination of the breast has become more important in breast imaging. As equipment improves, imagers are able to see lesions that previously were not visible sonographically. This improved detection not only enhances one's confidence in finding malignancies earlier, but also in identifying benign lesions. However, the potentially important contribution of sonography is greatly hindered by inadequate equipment, suboptimal imaging technique, and inconsistent operator training. The third purpose of this book is to demonstrate the importance of high-resolution sonography in breast imaging. Several cases show images of the same lesion with both with high- and low-resolution equipment. These cases also demonstrate the importance of utilizing high contrast, post-processing techniques in the detection of benign and malignant entities. Hopefully, this book will enhance the sonographic skills of breast imagers by encouraging the use of high quality, high-resolution equipment and optimal technique. Furthermore, by reviewing the sonographic appearance of the numerous breast abnormalities presented in this book, one can broaden one's visual sonographic experience.

The final objective of this book is to provide an atlas of a wide variety of pathologic entities within the breast. This book includes both unusual mammographic and sonographic appearances of common pathologies as well as examples of rare breast abnormalities. By grouping the pathologies within mammographic imaging patterns, one can use this book as a base for developing differential diagnoses.

In summary, I hope this book is used both as a quick reference guide to review the schematic work-up of a particular mammographic finding as well as a more detailed reference to study methods to optimize sonographic technique and integrate alternative imaging modalities.

Beverly E. Hashimoto

Acknowledgments

I could not have completed this book without the help of Jennifer Sonntag. Her enthusiastic effort allowed me to keep on schedule and her creative ideas solved many unanticipated logistical problems. I am also indebted to Lynn Wiitala who supported me at the beginning of this project and helped organize the patient data and imaging. Dr. Donald Bauermeister contributed pathology expertise for this project. Our conversations cross correlating specific cases have greatly improved my ability to understand the imaging appearance of benign and malignant lesions. The contributors, Drs. Kramer, Lee, and Morgan, have not only written part of the material in this book, but also have helped choose images and edit text. I am also grateful for the radiologists at Virginia Mason Medical Center. They have unselfishly shared their clinical and technical expertise. I especially appreciate the magnetic resonance imaging advice from Dr. Larry Holder and the administrative support from my department chiefs during this project: Drs. Michael Morishima and Lucy Glenn.

My sanity was saved by Morris Ferensen from Virginia Mason Medical Photography who answered all my imaging questions and processed the sonographic images. Nancy Honssinger created all the schematic diagrams.

A special acknowledgment goes to the technical and support personnel of the John H. Walker Center for Diagnostic Imaging at Virginia Mason Medical Center. Although I am indebted to everyone in the film room, I want to express individual thanks to Scott Borman, Michael Whiting, Alice Wirth, Jon Komatsu, Mary Ann Fernandez, Linda O'Connell, and Melissa Park. I am also lucky to be associated with wonderful imaging technologists including sonographers Shannon Boswell, Karen Adler, Irina Askerova, Becky Brickson, Stacy Buck, Shelly Carlisle, Chris Chapman, Danielle Ashour, Nancy Honssinger, Lisa Levan, Lori Lewis, Suzy Murray Dirks, Lynette Passey, Gisele Sodell, Jeff Thiel, Terri Jarvi, Jane Nova, Selwyn Pacleb; mammography technologists Mary Anne Madsen, Diana Pearsall, Darlene Fanus, Lori Carrier, Kay Molenaar, Barbara Zaragoza; general radiology technologist Heather Lyon; radiology administrative director John Eusek; and manager Vicki Wiitala.

Medical librarians Ann Robertson and Jan Gallagher kept me up-to-date on the literature and found difficult foreign or old references. Maggie Womack was vital in obtaining pathology material for all the patients in the book.

At Thieme Publishers, Jane Pennington initially provided guidance in the development of this project and is responsible for getting this project started. Diane Sardini, Felicity Edge, and Becky Dille have patiently provided support and advice in the completion of the project.

I also want to thank Drs. Roy Filly and Peter Callen. You have taught me the importance of approaching clinical questions in a creative yet systematic manner.

Finally, I am particularly grateful for the constant emotional support from my family: parents Doris and Ben, sister Claire, husband Vincent, and children Ben, Dean and Elissa. Without your cheerleading, I could never have attempted this project.

To Doris and Claire Hashimoto for your positive spirit and courage in facing breast cancer.

List of Contributors

Donald Bauermeister, M.D.
Department of Pathology
Virginia Mason Medical Center
Seattle, Washington

Beverly E. Hashimoto, M.D., F.A.C.R.
Section Head, Ultrasound
Virginia Mason Medical Center
Seattle, Washington

Dawna J. Kramer, M.D.
Deputy Chief, Radiology
Virginia Mason Medical Center
Seattle, Washington

Marie E. Lee, M.D., F.A. C.R.
Section Head, Nuclear Medicine
Virginia Mason Medical Center
Seattle, Washington

Gail N. Morgan, M.D.
Section Head, Eastside Satellite Radiology Clinics
Virginia Mason Medical Center
Seattle, Washington

Section I

Approach to Mammographic Analysis

Chapter 1

General Overview

There are three critical factors that lead to identifying mammographic abnormalities: production of high-quality images, perception of a lesion, and characterization of the finding. A team of people is needed to produce high-quality mammograms. The radiologist and the technologist should constantly be evaluating images for film contrast, exposure parameters, patient position, and image processing. Furthermore, a radiation physicist should work with the technologists to monitor equipment performance.

Perception of mammographic abnormality is the first step in identifying a breast malignancy. Perception is aided by a systematic review of the mammographic examination. Consistent systematic review of the mammogram is critical in avoiding perceptual errors. Tabar and Dean's *Teaching Atlas of Mammography* has an excellent explanation of a horizontal and vertical masking technique that facilitates identification of abnormal mammographic asymmetries. Masking entails physically covering portions of the film so that only small corresponding regions of the two breasts are visible. In a busy practice, this technique may not be practical, but one can develop the ability to visually mask by focusing on a small area of the breast and comparing it to the equivalent area on the contralateral side. My personal method involves this latter technique. I visually horizontally mask all breast views and then perform a second focused review of the axilla and the subareolar regions (Fig. 1-1).

During the review of the mammographic examination, one may identify asymmetries or calcifications. One should classify the asymmetry as a density or architectural distortion. The densities should be further analyzed and subdivided into either masses or asymmetric densities. Using the following methods, the breast imager then analyzes the lesion and assigns an assessment category according to the American College of Radiology Breast Imaging Reporting and Data System (BI-RADS). These assessment categories are the following:

- Category 0—Need additional imaging evaluation. This evaluation may include additional mammographic views (e.g., spot compression) or other imaging modalities (e.g., ultrasound).
- Category 1—Negative. The breasts are normal.
- Category 2—Benign finding. The mammogram is normal, but there is a finding that the interpreter wishes to describe.
- Category 3—Probably benign finding. Short-interval follow-up suggested. The finding has a high probability of being benign and is not expected to change in appearance. In this book, I generally assume that the patient will be reimaged about 6 months after this assessment is made.
- Category 4—Suspicious abnormality. Biopsy should be considered. The radiologist has enough concern about the lesion that biopsy is being recommended.
- Category 5—Highly suggestive of malignancy. Appropriate action should be taken.

Patterns of Mammographic Abnormality

After finding an asymmetry, the breast imager should classify the finding into one of four patterns: mass, asymmetric density, calcifications, and architectural distortion.

Masses

If a density is identified, then the radiologist should first clarify if the density is a mass or a focal asymmetric density. A mass is a density that has a consistent shape when imaged at different angles and with different patient positions. If one concludes that the lesion is a mass, then one should determine whether the shape of the mass is circumscribed or irregular. Circumscribed masses are round, oval, or lobulated (see Section 3). Circumscribed masses are commonly benign. Only 1.4% of well-defined circumscribed masses are malignant. As there are many benign lesions in this category, diagnostic evaluation should be directed to

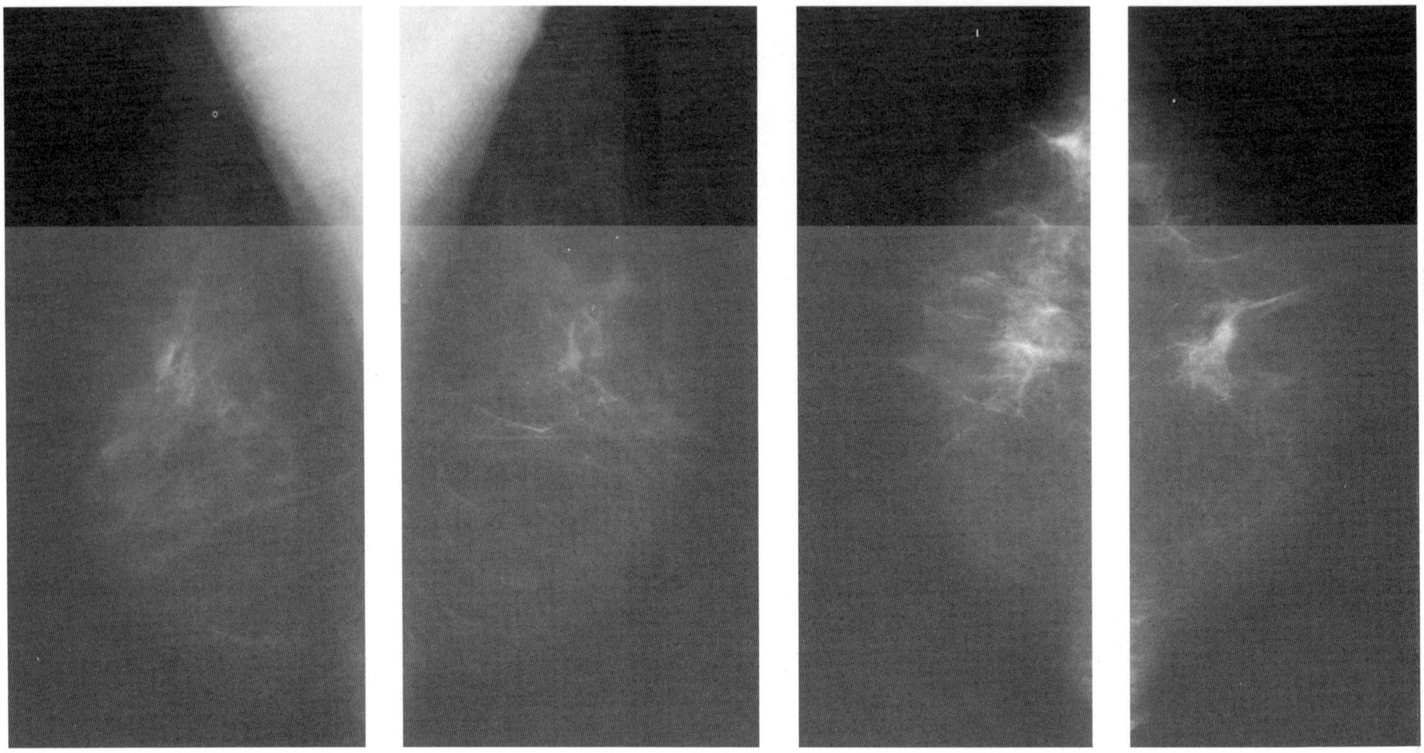

A

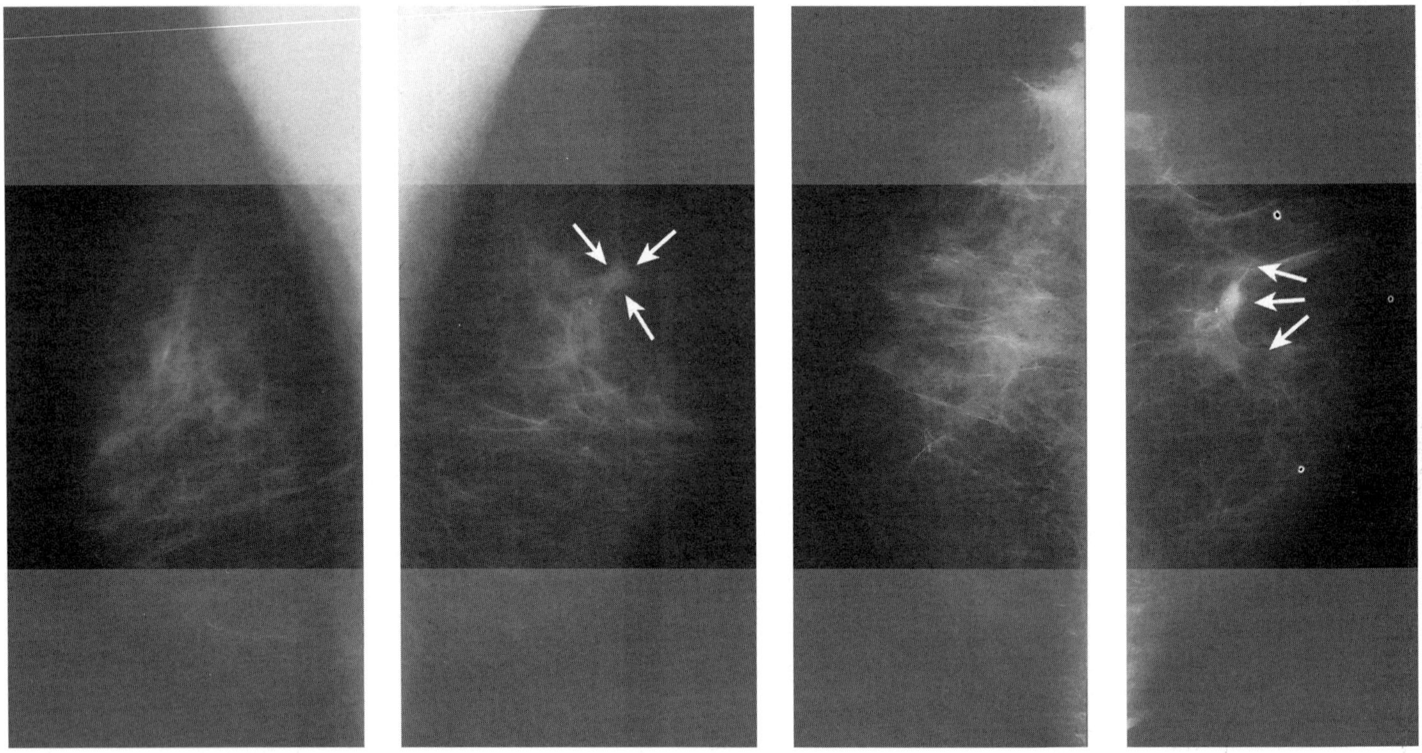

B

Figure 1–1. (*A–C*). *Systematic method to review mammograms. Horizontal examination: Initially, one should focus on a small region in the superior section of the right film and then compare it to the comparable left side. One should then proceed inferiorly in the mammogram and continue this process. In this case, there is trabecular thickening and architectural distortion at the 12:00 position of the left breast (arrows). This lesion is an infiltrating ductal carcinoma.* (*D*). *Systematic method to review mammograms (axillary and subareolar examination). After the hori-*

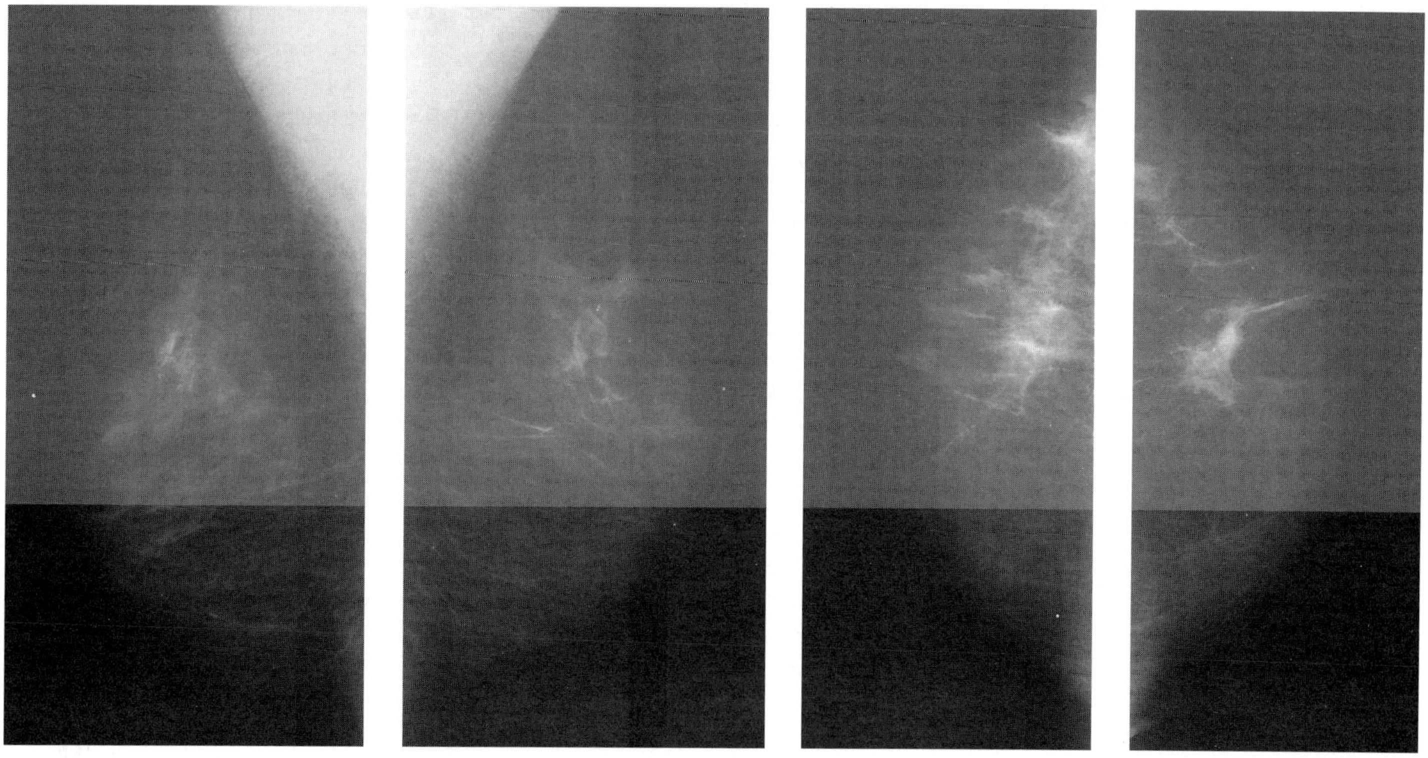

C

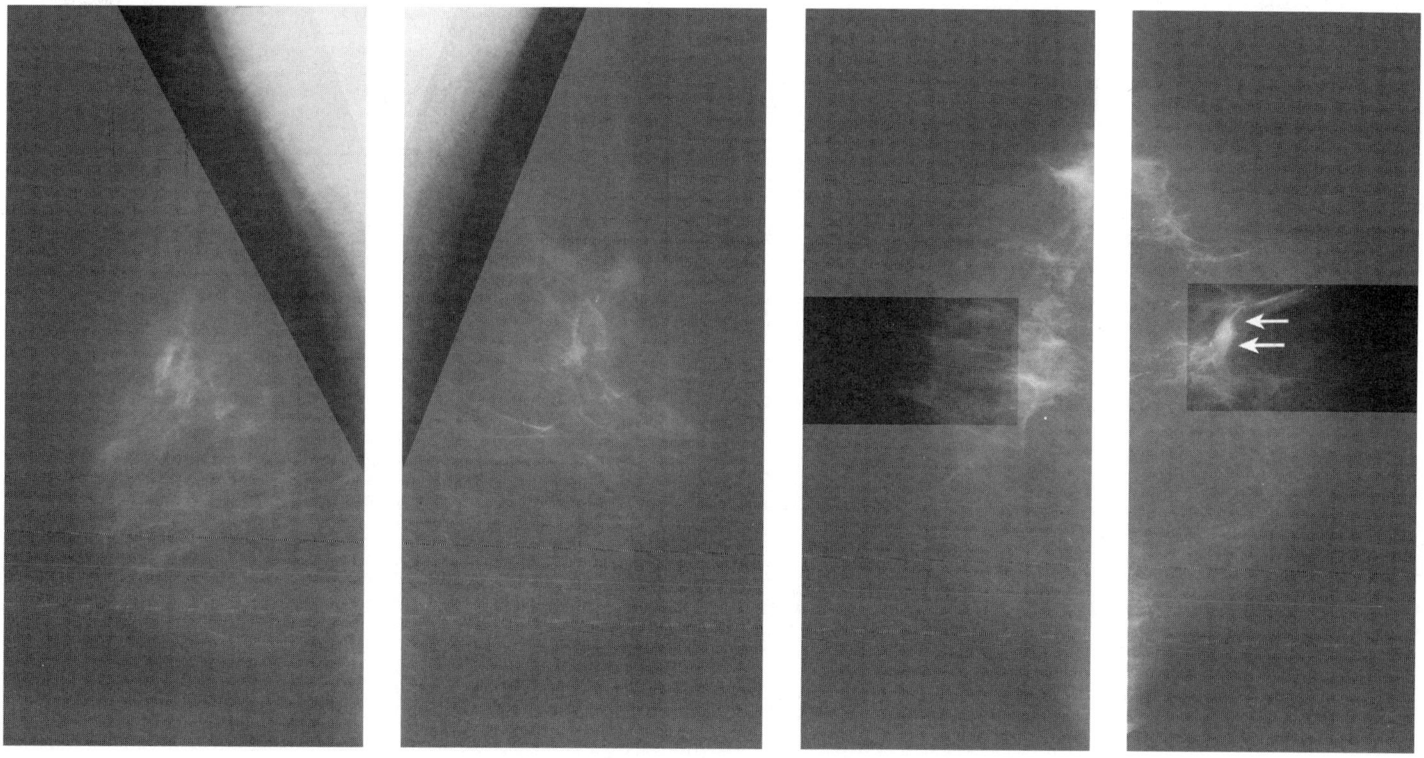

D

zontal examination, one should study the axillary and subareolar regions of each breast and compare each area to the contralateral side. The axillary region is important because the upper outer quadrant contains the highest percentage of breast cancers. Extra attention to the subareolar region is worthwhile as this area exhibits a complex architecture consisting of numerous ductal lines. Subareolar architectural distortion is commonly difficult to identify.

excluding many of these benign lesions from being biopsied. The first step is to analyze the density of the mass. If the mass contains fat, then the abnormality is benign (Category 2) and does not require biopsy. If the mass has a density equal or greater than parenchyma, then further examination is necessary. The next step is to examine the margins of the mass. If the margins are sharp or obscured by the surrounding parenchyma, then the mass should be examined sonographically. If the mass clearly has ill-defined or spiculated borders, then biopsy is indicated (Category 4 or Category 5). This biopsy may be performed sonographically as almost all of these lesions are sonographically visible, particularly if they are larger than 4 to 5 mm.

As noted earlier, circumscribed mammographic masses that have well-defined or obscured margins should be examined sonographically. Of these masses, sonographically identified cysts are obviously benign (Category 2). If the mass is well-defined and uniformly hyperechoic to fat, it is probably benign (Category 3). The mass is also probably benign (Category 3) if it has all of the following characteristics: (1) shape: round, oval, or one or two large lobulations; (2) margin: well defined with hyperechoic thin capsule; (3) echogenicity: uniformly hypoechoic; (4) size: 1 cm or smaller.

If the margin is extremely well defined but does not have a hyperechoic capsule, I also assess it as probably benign (Category 3). To characterize whether a margin is well defined one must have high-quality, high-resolution, and high-frequency (≥10 MHz) equipment. Furthermore, the entire margin must be well defined and clearly visible (Fig. 1–2). Finally, there should not be any other associated abnormality such as sonographic architectural distortion. In this situation, I am also assuming that I have seen the patient only once and there is no evidence of growth. If the lesion has been identified on earlier imaging exams and has grown in size or if it is larger than 1 cm, then I will recommend biopsy (Category 4).

The reason for biopsing large or growing well-defined lesions is that some of the masses in this category will be malignant. As long as a malignancy is small, it has a good prognosis since the probability of metastasis is low. However, to have a good prognosis, it is best for the patient to be Stage 1 (primary tumor smaller than 2 cm) at the time of diagnosis. Short-interval follow-up of a small (<1 cm) well-circumscribed mass that has a low probability of malignancy is a reasonable method to avoid unnecessary biopsies.

If the mass has any other sonographic characteristics, then it is Category 4 or Category 5. Examples of these lesions include: (1) solid masses within cysts, (2) masses that have any other shape or that are microlobulated, (3) lesions that exhibit heterogeneous echogenicity or that present as a focal area of intense shadowing, (4) tumors with either completely or partially ill-defined margins, (5) masses associated with other sonographic abnormalities such as architectural distortion.

Masses with microlobulations or other shapes that cannot be classified as circumscribed should be considered irregular in shape (see Section 4). Although benign etiologies may produce an irregular mammographic mass, all mammographically irregular masses should be pathologically examined unless the lesion is a benign scar. Scars resulting from previous surgery may appear similar to malignancies. A careful patient history with a map of the scar is necessary to correlate the mammographic abnormality with the clinical information. If this information is insufficient, previous films commonly document either stability or reduction of the lesion density and size. Occasionally, sonography may be necessary to differentiate scar from malignancy. In these cases, sonography may confidently exclude malignancy if only hyperechoic architectural distortion is present without mass. Furthermore, sonographically scars change in appearance with different transducer positions. Even if there is a wide area of severe shadowing in one view, the orthogonal view will demonstrate only a thin line of architectural distortion characteristic of scar. Because scar attenuates high-frequency more than low-frequency ultrasound, commonly low-frequency sonography is more effective in characterizing scar (see Case 178, Section 9).

Besides scar, other benign entities produce irregular masses. These lesions include fat necrosis, sclerosing adenosis, focal fibrosis, hematoma, abscess, and benign neoplasms such as fibroadenomas or papillary lesions. However, unless the patient has a clinical history or symptoms suggesting recent trauma, surgery, or infection, these lesions cannot be differentiated from malignancy and should be biopsied. When clinical information suggests that a hematoma or abscess may be responsible for the mammographic abnormality, then sonography is useful to identify these processes.

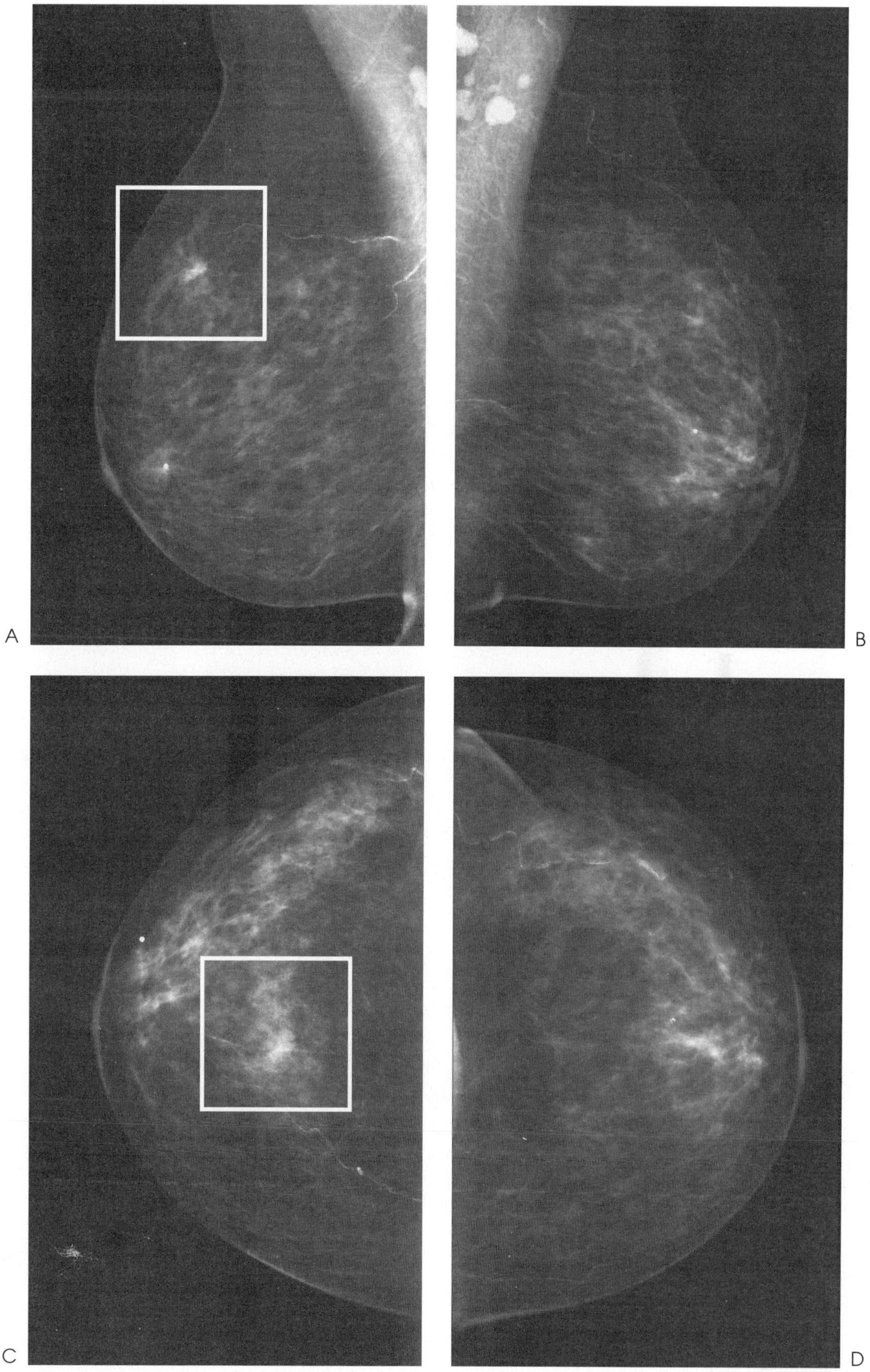

Figure 1-2. *(A). Right MLO digital mammogram. (B). Left MLO digital mammogram. (C). Right CC digital mammogram. (D). Left CC digital mammogram.*

Figure 1-2 continued on next page ▷

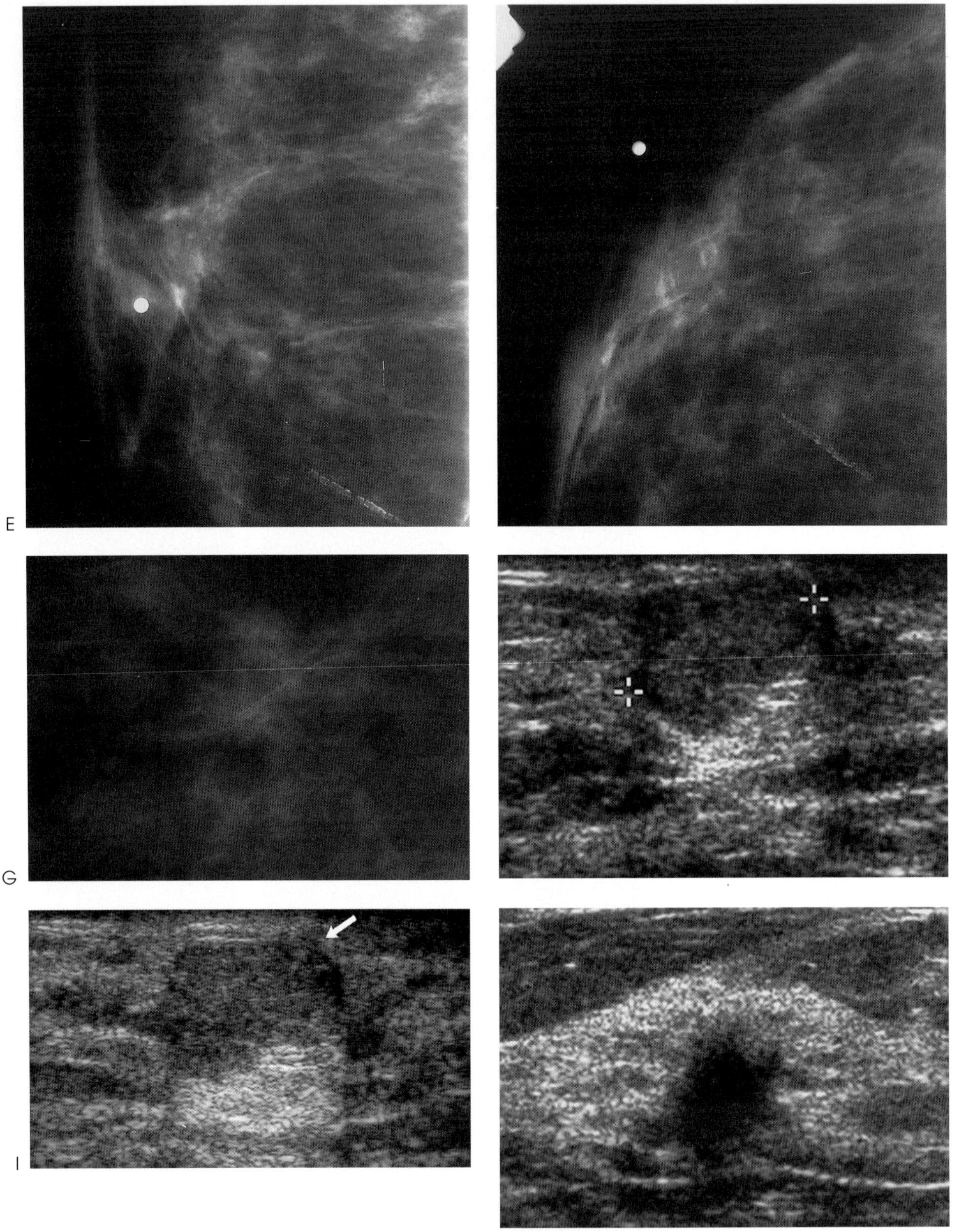

Figure 1–2. (continued from previous page) *(E). Right MLO spot magnification mammogram. (F). Right CC spot magnification mammogram. (G). Right MLO spot magnification mammogram. (A–G). There is a palpable right breast mass that is labeled with a radiopaque dot at the 3:00 location near the nipple. The mass is not well delineated on either the screening or the spot magnification views (E,F). In the right upper outer quadrant in the middle third of the breast (square), there is an irregular mass that is confirmed on the spot magnification view (G). (H). Right antiradial breast sonogram: The palpable mass corresponds to a well-defined oval hypoechoic mass. On this view, the mass appears probably benign. (I). Right antiradial breast sonogram: This is the same mass as Figure 1–2H, but in a slightly different position. Subtle irregularity of the margin (arrow) is present. These features change the assessment so that the lesion is suspicious. This mass is infiltrating mucinous carcinoma. (J). Right antiradial breast sonogram: This hypoechoic irregular mass corresponds to the irregular mammographic mass (G). This mass is infiltrating ductal carcinoma.*

Finally, radial scars also produce irregular masses. The mammographic characteristics of radial scars include: (1) change in appearance from one mammographic projection to another; (2) no dense central mass; (3) the radiating lines are long and thin; (4) the radiating structures are commonly dominated by radiolucent linear lines; (5) no skin thickening; (6) very little palpable abnormality. Although radial scars may be differentiated from malignancy, radial scars are commonly associated with malignant neoplasms and, therefore, should be excised.

Asymmetric Densities

Analysis of an asymmetric density should start with a close evaluation of the entire mammographic examination. It is important to initially define if the asymmetric density diffusely involves a large area of the breast or a small area (see Section 6). If the density is diffuse, then the skin should be carefully examined. If the density is only due to increased fibroglandular tissue, then a physiologic or pharmacologic etiology may be responsible. Heterogeneous or extremely dense parenchymal composition is more common in younger premenopausal women, but is also common in older women, especially those with fibrocystic changes. Medications such as estrogen replacement therapy sometimes increase the overall mammographic parenchymal density.

If skin thickening is present then the etiologies include axillary lymphatic obstruction, lymphatic spread of breast cancer, inflammation, and systemic fluid overload. Axillary lymphatic drainage may be blocked by ipsilateral breast cancer metastases or hematologic malignancies (e.g., lymphomas). Lymphatic spread of breast cancer to the contralateral breast will block lymphatic channels and produce lymphedema. Inflammation and abscess will thicken the skin and produce increased density, particularly around the areola. In this situation, the axillary portion of the breast is relatively spared. Finally, any condition that produces systemic fluid overload such as heart failure or renal failure will produce breast lymphedema.

If the asymmetric density involves a small area, then one should carefully examine the area to determine if the density represents a mass, normal asymmetric fibroglandular tissue, or overlap of normal parenchymal tissue. A focal asymmetric density is a density that cannot be reliably identified on more than one view. If the density is only visible on the craniocaudal (CC)view, a 90 degree mediolateral (ML) may demonstrate the mass better than the mediolateral oblique (MLO) view. Spot compression of a density may clarify the shape of the mass, but sometimes malignancies such as lobular carcinoma may compress and blend into the normal breast parenchymal background. For small or less-dense lesions, consider using rolled or oblique views to confirm the presence of the mass (Fig. 1-3). Normal fibroglandular tissue will blend into the adjacent tissue with oblique views. The tissue will have the same internal curvilinear pattern as the rest of the breast. Furthermore, the tissue will not exhibit any architectural distortion. If one cannot distinguish between a mass and normal fibroglandular tissue, then sonography may be useful. However, to adequately perform this differentiation, one must have high resolution and frequency, be familiar with the normal sonographic appearance of breast parenchyma, and be comfortable with cross correlating mammography with sonography (see Section 2). If the woman is high risk for malignancy and high-frequency sonography is negative or unavailable, then magnetic resonance is a reasonable method to clarify the etiology of a worrisome asymmetric density.

Calcifications

There are a wide variety of breast calcifications (see Section 5). Analysis of calcifications should start with excluding calcifications that are characteristic for benign lesions. If the calcification does not fit in these obviously benign categories, then the shape of the calcification should be analyzed and placed into patterns that can be related to American College of Radiology BI-RADS assessment categories.

Calcifications or densities simulating calcifications that may be excluded from further workup include technical artifacts, substances on the skin (e.g., lotions, deodorants), and calcifications that are pathognomonic for benign entities. Processor artifacts and dirty screens may produce tiny dots or irregularities that are confused for calcifications. These artifacts are generally whiter than calcifications and have unusual shapes. Constant evaluation of processing is critical to avoid these problems. Materials on the skin may also initially ap-

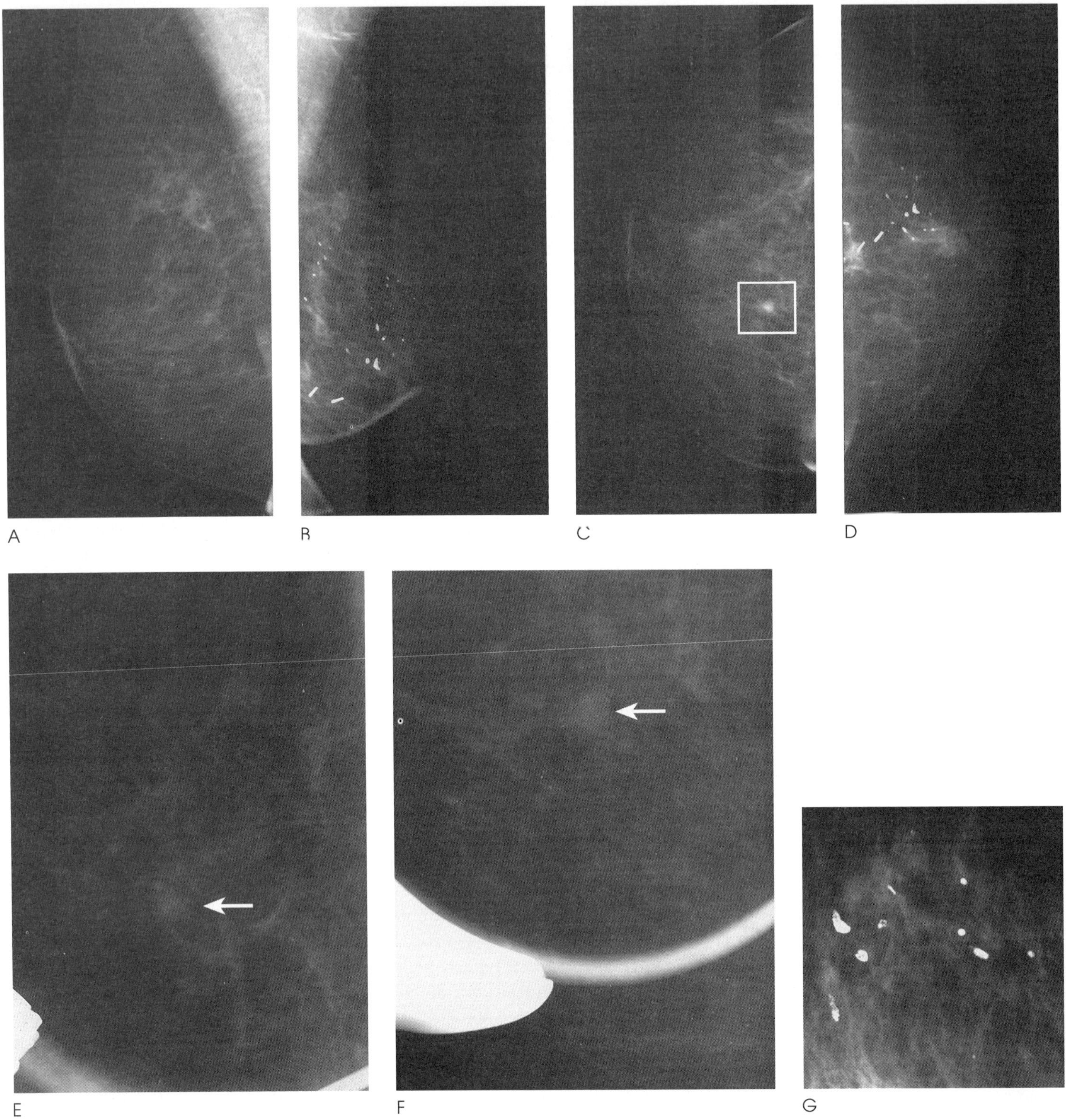

Figure 1–3. (A). Right MLO digital mammogram. (B). Left MLO digital mammogram. (C). Right CC digital mammogram. (D). Left CC digital mammogram. (E). Right MLO spot compression mammogram (arrow points to mass). (F). Right CC spot compression mammogram. (G). Left LM digital mammogram (close-up). (A–G). The patient has had left lumpectomy and radiation therapy 7 years ago. The left breast demonstrates stable scarring and benign calcifications from fat necrosis (see 3B,D,G). In the right breast there is an asymmetric density (square) that is initially visible only on the CC view. However, spot compression views (E–F) demonstrate that it is an ill-defined mass (arrow). This mass is infiltrating ductal carcinoma.

pear as calcifications. However, these densities are unusual in configuration and are commonly located in the axilla. Thorough cleansing of the skin prior to reevaluation generally removes these particles. Educating patients to avoid using these materials prior to mammography will also reduce encountering this problem. Certain calcifications are pathognomonic for benign entities. These include oil cyst, dermal, vascular, secretory, and milk of calcium calcifications (Figs. 1–3B,D,G). By reviewing these characteristic calcifications in texts or teaching files, one can confidently identify these benign calcifications.

If calcifications or densities are not included in the above categories, then further analysis is necessary. The first characteristic to examine is size. If the calcifications are large, then they are benign. Malignant calcifications are generally smaller than 0.5 mm. The smallest thickness or diameter of a benign calcification is more than 1 to 2 mm. These large calcifications may be confidently excluded from further evaluation.

If the calcification is small, then one should study the shape of the calcification. The shape of calcifications should be categorized into four patterns: (1) round or punctate, (2) amorphous or indistinct, (3) heterogeneous or pleomorphic, and (4) fine linear, branching, or casting calcifications. If the calcifications are round or punctate, then one should determine whether they are clustered or scattered. If they are scattered, then they are benign (Category 2). If they are clustered but have been stable for 3 years, then they are benign (Category 2). If they are new or on a baseline mammogram, then they are probably benign (Category 3) and should be followed by 6-month examinations for a total of 1 year and then yearly evaluations for a total of 3 years. If these calcifications change into a more suspicious shape or increase in number, then biopsy is warranted (Category 4). The reason that new clustered punctate calcifications should be followed is that occasionally, ductal carcinoma may present with punctate clustered calcifications. These calcifications may represent either a variant of the malignant amorphous pattern (see below) or cancerization of lobules (Section 5, Cases 83, 86).

If the calcifications are amorphous in shape, they should be biopsied (Category 4). Amorphous calcifications are commonly round, but they are hazy in appearance and do not have sharp, smooth edges. Malignant amorphous calcifications are generally clustered, but occasionally these calcifications may cover a larger area such as a segment or quadrant of the breast. Malignant amorphous calcifications are the result of superimposition of numerous tiny calcifications within the mucin secreted by cells of ductal carcinoma in situ. Sometimes, amorphous calcifications may overlap in appearance with the round, punctate pattern. Very early, tiny amorphous calcifications may appear punctate. If they are initially misidentified, this error would be discovered as long as the calcifications are closely followed.

Heterogeneous or pleomorphic calcifications are irregular in shape. Furthermore, they also vary in size and density (Fig. 1–4). These calcifications have also been described as resembling "crushed stones" or "granulated sugar." The larger calcifications are commonly larger than amorphous calcifications, but they are still smaller than 0.5 mm in size. Malignant heterogeneous calcifications generally present in a cluster unless the patient presents with advanced disease. These calcifications are commonly the result of necrosis from intermediate- or lower-grade ductal carcinoma in situ. Therefore, heterogeneous calcifications should be biopsied (Category 4).

Like heterogeneous calcifications, fine linear and branching calcifications are irregular calcifications that vary in size and density. However, unlike heterogeneous calcifications, these calcifications form thin, irregular lines that occasionally branch. These calcifications are generally clustered, but extensive disease will present with a segmental distribution. These calcifications should be biopsied (Category 4). High-grade ductal carcinoma in situ produces extensive calcified necrosis that fills the ducts. The configuration and alignment of these calcifications mirror the intraductal spread of malignancy. When a large number of these calcifications are present, they are extremely suspicious, and in those cases, assessment of these calcifications may be upgraded to Category 5.

Architectural Distortion

Generally, mammographers easily recognize asymmetric densities or calcifications unless these findings are small or partially obscured by normal fibroglandular tissue. However, perception of architectural distortion is more difficult since parenchymal patterns vary with different individuals. Perception and characterization of architectural distortion are aided by recognizing normal parenchymal anatomy. The breast parenchymal pattern consists of

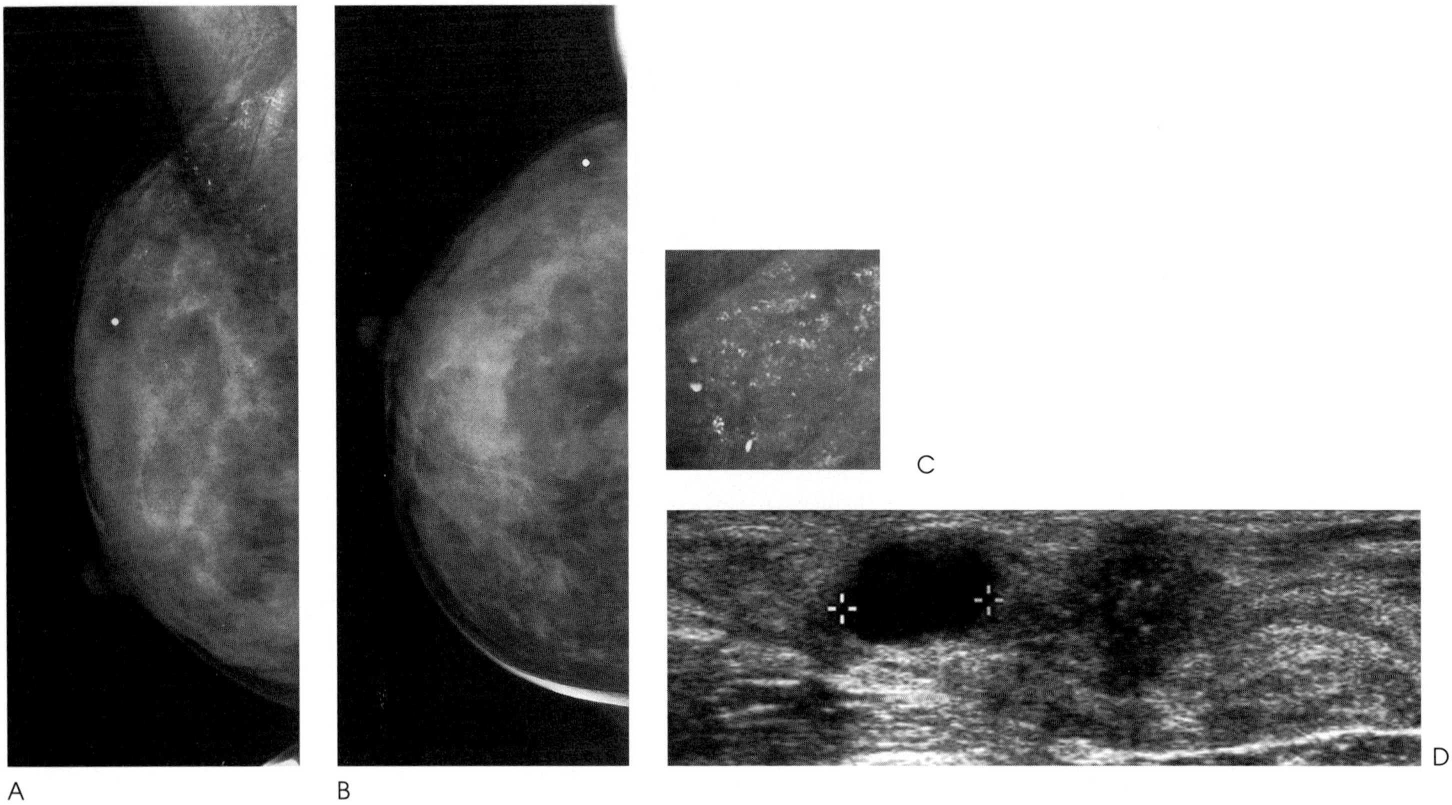

Figure 1-4. (A). Right MLO digital mammogram. (B). Right CC digital mammogram. (C). Right MLO digital mammogram (close-up). (A–C). In the upper outer quadrant of the right breast, there is a palpable lump that is labeled with a radiopaque dot. Just distal to the dot are extensive heterogeneous calcifications. (D). Right antiradial breast sonogram: The palpable mass corresponds to a combination of a cyst and a spiculated hypoechoic mass with punctate calcifications. Mastectomy specimen shows that this sonographic mass and the mammographic calcifications are mixed infiltrating lobular and ductal carcinoma with an extensive intraductal component.

thin, curvilinear lines that are directed toward the nipple. This radiating pattern is only broken by blood vessels. Adjacent to the subcutaneous fat, the Cooper's ligaments form a scalloped parenchymal edge. The parenchymal edge generally thins out into the axilla and chest wall. These areas commonly form ill-defined curvilinear, feathery borders in patients with scattered or heterogeneously dense breasts. In patients with extremely dense breasts, these borders tend to be well defined. However, the contours are still curvilinear. With heterogeneously dense and extremely dense breasts, the superior corner of the MLO view and the medial and lateral corners of the CC view are also generally curvilinear or rounded.

Architectural distortion may either be central or peripheral (see Section 7). Central distortion results when the ductal and trabecular lines deviate from the nipple. This distortion is commonly due to a spiculated lesion producing straight lines that point to the center of the abnormality. Commonly, these abnormal spiculations are thicker than normal trabecular lines (Fig. 1–5).

Abnormalities that affect the edge of the parenchyma cause peripheral architectural distortion. Lesions may cause retraction, flattening, straightening, or bulging of the parenchymal contours (Fig. 1–6). When the density in the superior parenchymal edge of the MLO view is affected, it may form a sharp triangular corner. Although some women normally have sharply angulated parenchymal corners, if there is asymmetry between the corners or if there has been a change in configuration, then one should search for a subtle spiculated lesion (Fig. 1–7). Retraction of the posterior edge of the parenchyma has been labeled the "tent sign" as the retraction produces a biconvex V-shaped border resembling the peak of a tent (Fig. 1–8).

When architectural distortion is present, the breast imager should perform additional mammographic views to identify a mass. Spot compression views may demonstrate a spiculated mass. Oblique views may clarify the location of architectural distortion that is initially visible only on one view. Magnification views may be useful to identify associated malignant calcifications.

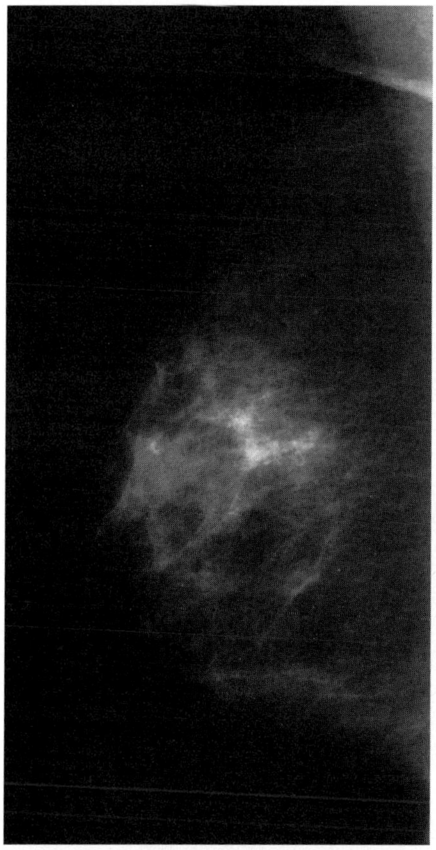

A

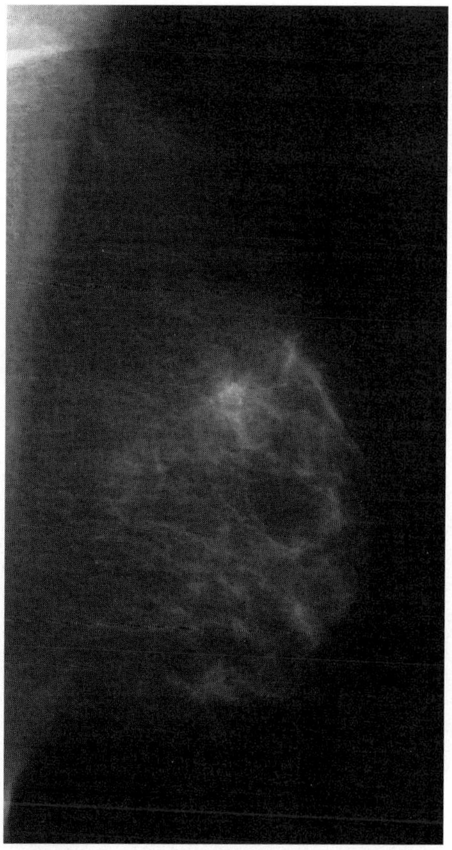

B

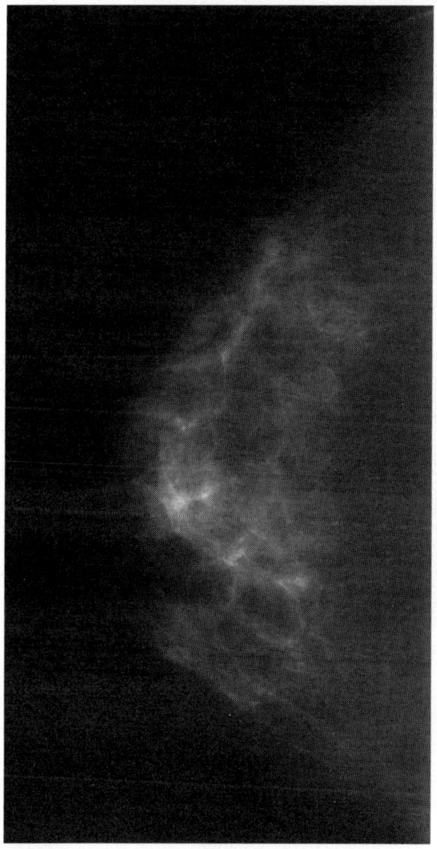

C

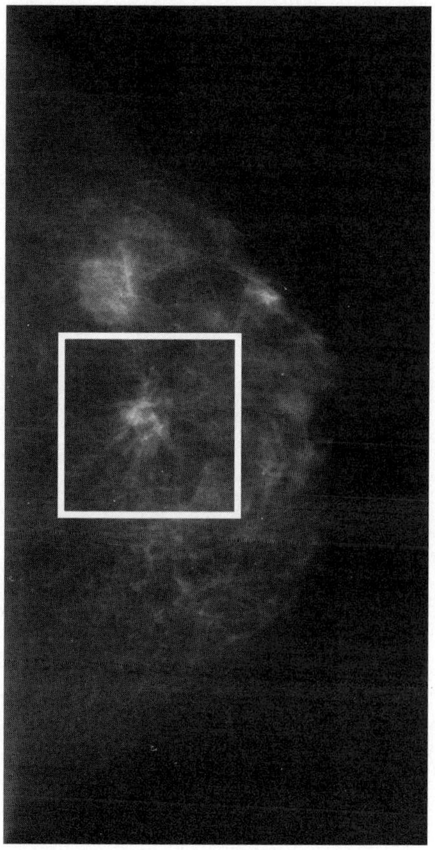

D

Figure 1-5. *(A). Right MLO mammogram. (B). Left MLO mammogram. (C). Right CC mammogram. (D). Left CC mammogram. (E). Left CC spot compression mammogram. (A–E). Central architectural distortion: In the left CC view (D) there is an area of focal architectural distortion (square). The lesion corresponds to the asymmetric density in the superior breast on the MLO view. This architectural distortion is due to a tumor consisting of lobular and infiltrating ductal carcinoma.*

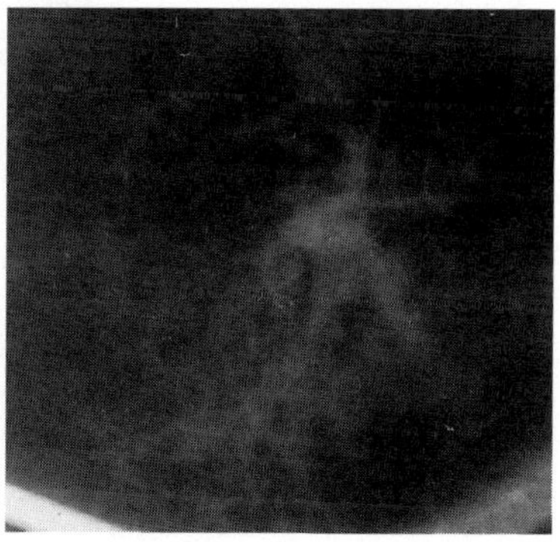

E

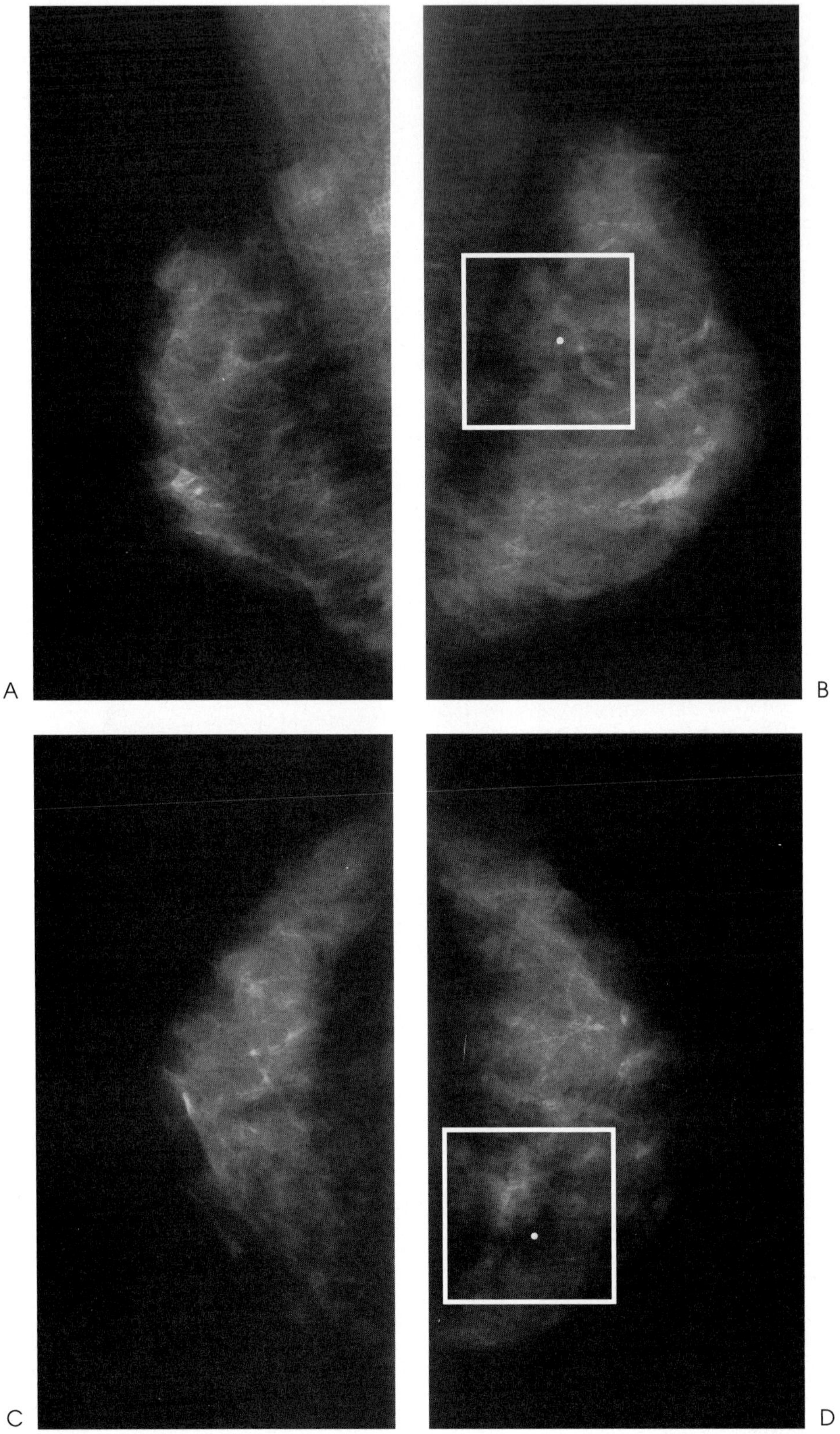

Figure 1-6. *(A). Right MLO mammogram. (B). Left MLO mammogram. (C). Right CC mammogram. (D). Left CC mammogram. (A–D). Peripheral architectural distortion: A lobulated mass extends outside the posterior border of the fibroglandular border (square). This mass corresponds to an infiltrating ductal tumor.*

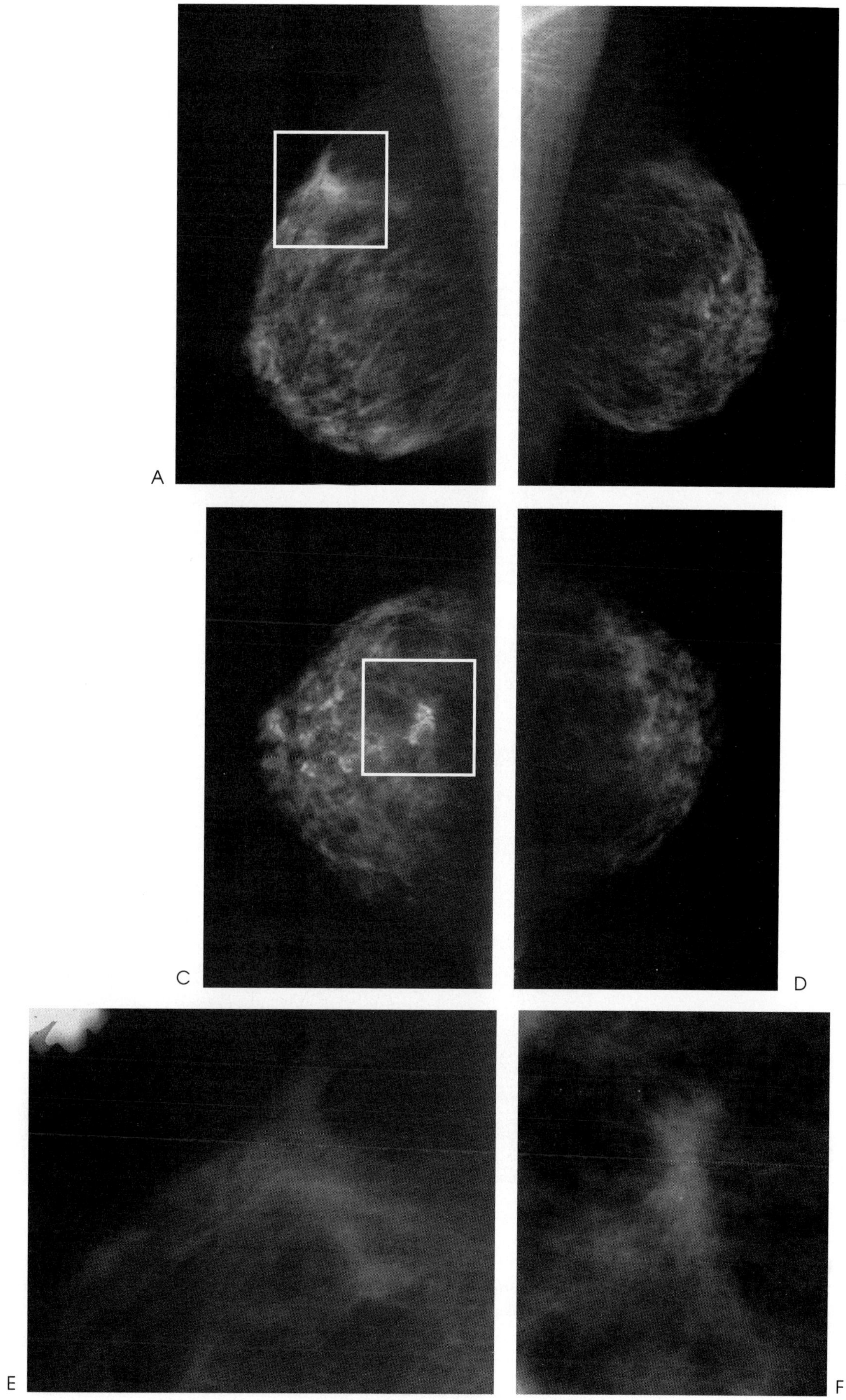

Figure 1–7. (A). Right MLO mammogram. (B). Left MLO mammogram.(C). Right CC mammogram. (D). Left CC mammogram. (E). Right MLO spot magnification mammogram. (F). Right CC spot magnification mammogram. (A–F). Superior peripheral architectural distortion: An irregular mass (marked by a square) at 12:00 produces a sharp angulation of the superior parenchymal corner in the right MLO view (A). This mass represents tubular carcinoma.

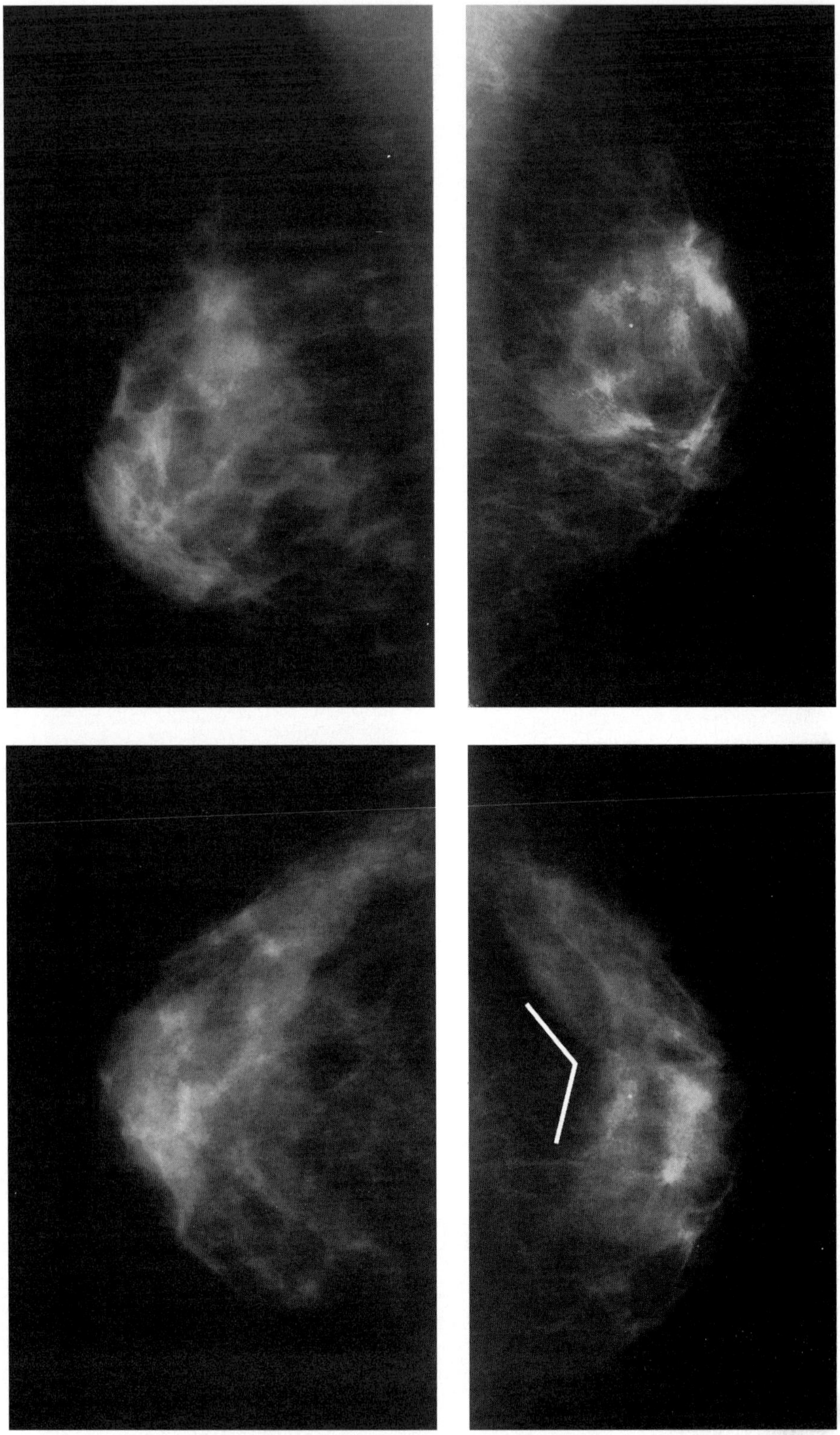

Figure 1–8. (A). Right MLO mammogram. (B). Left MLO mammogram. (C). Right CC mammogram. (D). Left CC mammogram. (E). Left MLO spot magnification mammogram. (F). Left CC spot magnification mammogram. (A–F). Posterior peripheral architectural distortion (tent sign): In the left CC view (D), the posterior parenchymal border exhibits retraction (marked with a V).

Figure 1–8 continued on next page ▷

Causes of architectural distortion include focal fibrosis, sclerosing adenosis, fat necrosis, scar, radial scar, and malignancy. One identifies surgical scars and fat necrosis by correlating regions of previous surgery or trauma with the architectural distortion. Radial scars usually have thin spiculations and a radiolucent center. Neoplasms usually produce architectural distortion that is evident on two orthogonal views and is associated with a dense central mass. Occasionally, malignancies demonstrate very little central density. There-

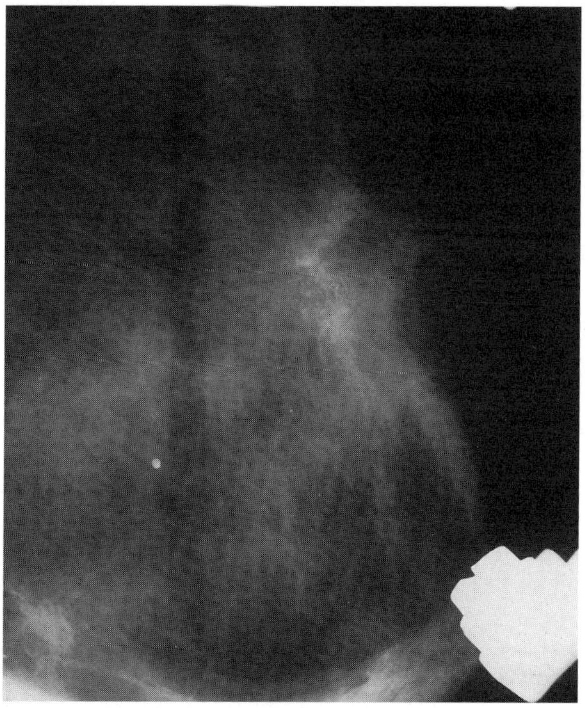
E

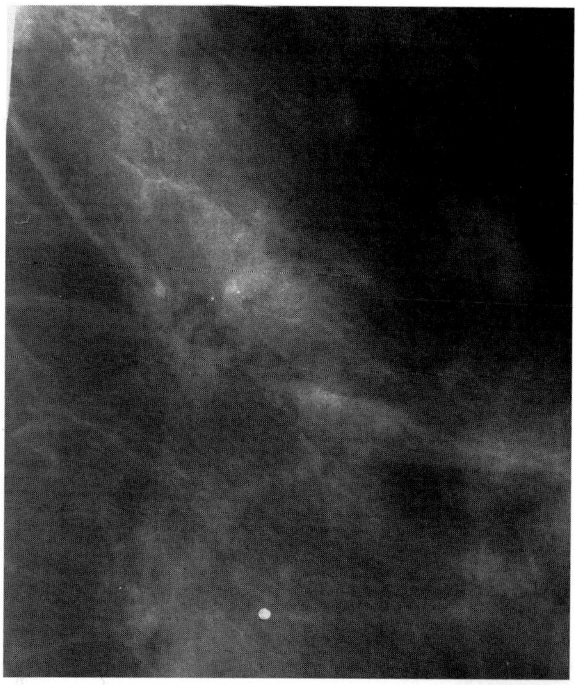
F

Figure 1-8. (continued from previous page) *Spot magnification view demonstrates that the architectural distortion is associated with amorphous calcifications (F). Although the abnormality is difficult to identify in the left MLO view (B), left spot magnification locates the lesion with microcalcifications in the superior breast (E). The mass is an infiltrating ductal carcinoma.*

fore, if architectural distortion is not due to a surgical scar, then it should be biopsied (Category 4).

If the lesion is small or the breast composition is dense, the architectural distortion may only be visible on one view. In these cases, sonography may be useful to demonstrate a mass and localize biopsy. Sonographically, normal fibroglandular tissue and fibrosis will be uniformly hyperechoic. Fat necrosis may either be heterogeneous or hyperechoic echogenicity. Both surgical and radial scars strongly attenuate the sonographic beam so shadowing may be the predominant feature. If heavy shadowing is present, a lower-frequency examination may penetrate the scar and demonstrate no mass. However, in some cases, surgical scars cannot be differentiated from neoplasms and biopsy is necessary. If radial scar is suspected, then excision is necessary. Using high-frequency sonography, malignant masses are either hypoechoic or heterogeneous echogenicity. Sonographic architectural distortion is common. This distortion may appear as hyperechoic haze or spiculations radiating from the tumor. Cooper's ligaments and the anterior fascial line may be distorted.

Sonography may miss a malignant lesion for several reasons. The sonographic examination may miss small masses. However, usually if the neoplasm has created mammographic architectural distortion, there is enough desmoplasia or direct tumor extension for sonographic detection. Therefore, commonly the reasons for error are because the location of the neoplasm is missed or the examiner does not recognize the mass. Reasons for missing the location or not recognizing the mass include examiner inexperience and poor sonographic technique. Since the mammographic findings may be subtle, this sonographic application requires that the examiner be highly skilled in breast sonography. One should be able to cross correlate mammographic and sonographic landmarks to find the lesion.

Even if the examiner is experienced, poor technique or equipment may prevent the imager from identifying masses. Masses are difficult to identify with lower-frequency transducers (<10 MHz). Lower frequencies commonly penetrate masses better than higher frequencies so there is little shadowing and the masses appear hyperechoic. The hyperechoic tumors blend into the surrounding hyperechoic parenchyma. Furthermore, lower frequencies have poorer resolution so the indirect signs of malignancy such as spiculations or distortion of Cooper's ligaments are not visible. Although generally higher frequencies are better than lower frequencies, high-frequency examination also has pitfalls. If the frequency is too high, there may be excessive shadowing. A shadowing malignancy may be hidden by the shadows produced by surrounding fibroglandular tissue. One should use a frequency that allows one to visualize the chest wall. Normal fibroglandular parenchyma will be hyperechoic, but a malignancy will be shadowing, hypoechoic, or heterogeneous echogencity.

Even if one initially does not see a suspicious mass, one may use mammographic and sonographic landmarks (see Section 2) and identify the suspicious breast tissue. The imager may then increase the sonographic frequency and perform a targeted evaluation of the spot to find a subtle mass. If a mass is not discovered, then the sonographic examination should demonstrate the etiology of the mammographic architectural distortion. If the sonographic examination does not clarify the cause of architectural distortion, then the lesion should be classified as Category 4, suspicious, and should be biopsied.

Section II

Sonographic Technique and Cross-Correlation with Mammography

Chapter 2

The main applications of ultrasound are identification of a palpable breast lump and clarification of a confusing mammographic finding. In the past, a common reason that sonographic applications were limited was that the ultrasound examiner could not cross correlate the physical examination or mammographic findings with the sonographic information. This inability to cross correlate the ultrasound examination with the physical examination or mammographic asymmetry is frustrating and leads to long, sonographic examinations. In order to develop the ability to cross correlate sonography with mammography, one should have optimal sonographic equipment and technique, be able to palpate breast masses, be familiar with normal mammographic and sonographic breast anatomy, recognize mammographic and sonographic signs of malignancy, and apply anatomic knowledge to sonographic scanning.

Ultrasound Equipment and Technique

Equipment

In the past, breast ultrasound has required the least sophisticated equipment because there were few sonographic breast applications and these applications required only simple equipment. However, if one wishes not only to have a high rate of localizing solid masses as well as an optimal image to characterize the mass, then one needs a sophisticated machine. In this book, when I refer to high frequency, I am generally referring to imaging with frequencies equal or greater than 10 MHz. To have maximal flexibility, one should have a machine that has linear transducers with frequencies ranging from 7 to 15 MHz.

High frequency is important as many breast structures are small. An important aspect of the technical advancement of mammography is the improvement of spatial resolution. Because of high mammographic resolution, mammographers are identifying smaller and subtler abnormalities. To be an effective adjunctive test, high sonographic spatial resolution is needed to clarify these subtle findings. Because normal breast structures such as ducts and terminal duct lobular units are small, high spatial resolution allows the ultrasound examiner to quickly recognize normal breast architecture and identify small malignant masses in the ductal system.

Besides being able to identify smaller malignancies, high spatial resolution improves the sonographic image so one can better characterize masses. This improved image is similar to the visual effect experienced by a nearsighted person who starts wearing glasses. The image is sharper, and subtle or smaller details are clearer (Fig. 2–1; also see Section 4 Case 57). For breast malignancies, the most important information produced by high-frequency ultrasound is the improved ability to see the margin of the mass and identify secondary signs of malignancy such as spiculation or architectural distortion. Occasionally, one can trace the path of the malignancy through the ductal system and identify the extent of the disease better than mammography (see Section 10, Cases 200 and 201).

Imaging Techniques

Besides the availability of high-frequency transducers, sophisticated ultrasound machines have more technical factors that can be manipulated to improve imaging quality. For breast ultrasound, an important factor in image quality is being able to obtain excellent contrast resolution. The reason contrast resolution is important is that one must be able to distinguish a variety of masses from the background parenchyma. When the breast is fatty, focal masses such as complex cysts, lymph nodes, fibroadenomas, and cancers may be difficult to identify. When the breast is dense, fat necrosis and surgical or radial scars may be hard to locate. Many factors can improve contrast resolution. High spatial resolution produced by high-frequency imaging improves contrast resolution because the assignment of gray shades is more precise. Reducing the dynamic range may improve contrast resolution as this method exaggerates differences between the gray shades of structures. A variety of proprietary postprocessing programs improve contrast resolution by enhancement of specified gray sha-

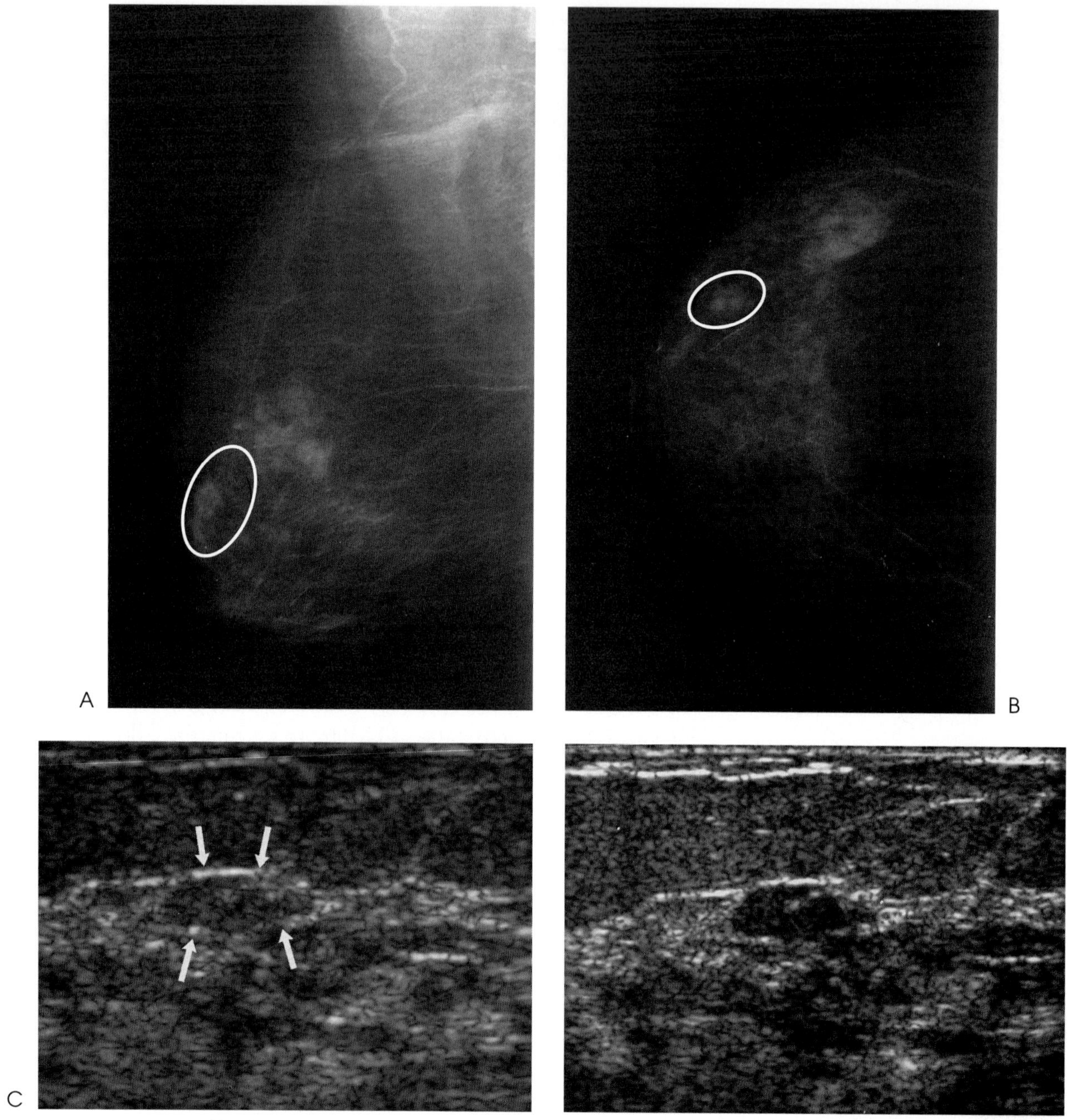

Figure 2–1. *(A). Right MLO mammogram. (B). Right CC mammogram. (A,B). In the upper outer right breast there is a lobulated density (circled). (C). Right radial breast sonogram: A 5 MHz transducer does not clearly demonstrate the lobulated mass (arrows). The inadequate size and contrast resolution results in poor definition of the mass. (D). Right radial breast sonogram: An 8 MHz transducer improves the definition of the mass. This result allows an observer to confidently localize this mass. This mass is a fibroadenoma.*

des on a point-by-point basis. One type of proprietary postprocessing program improves contrast resolution by enhancement of specified gray shades on a region-by-region basis. One should consult the manufacturer of one's equipment to learn which imaging techniques are available (Fig. 2–2; also see Section 3 Case 18).

Besides adjusting image contrast, one should be aware of software methods to optimize resolution. These methods include increasing the line density of the image, increasing the persistence, and adjusting the focal zones. The main disadvantage of these methods is a slower frame rate. If one is merely characterizing a lesion, a slower frame rate may not be a problem. However, the slower frame rate may be disconcerting with real-time imaging of interventional procedures.

Color or power Doppler is a useful method to quickly assess vascularity. Breast vascularity is low, so one should be aware of methods to optimize the color or power Doppler. Generally, this means that one is using a color or power Doppler frequency slightly lower than

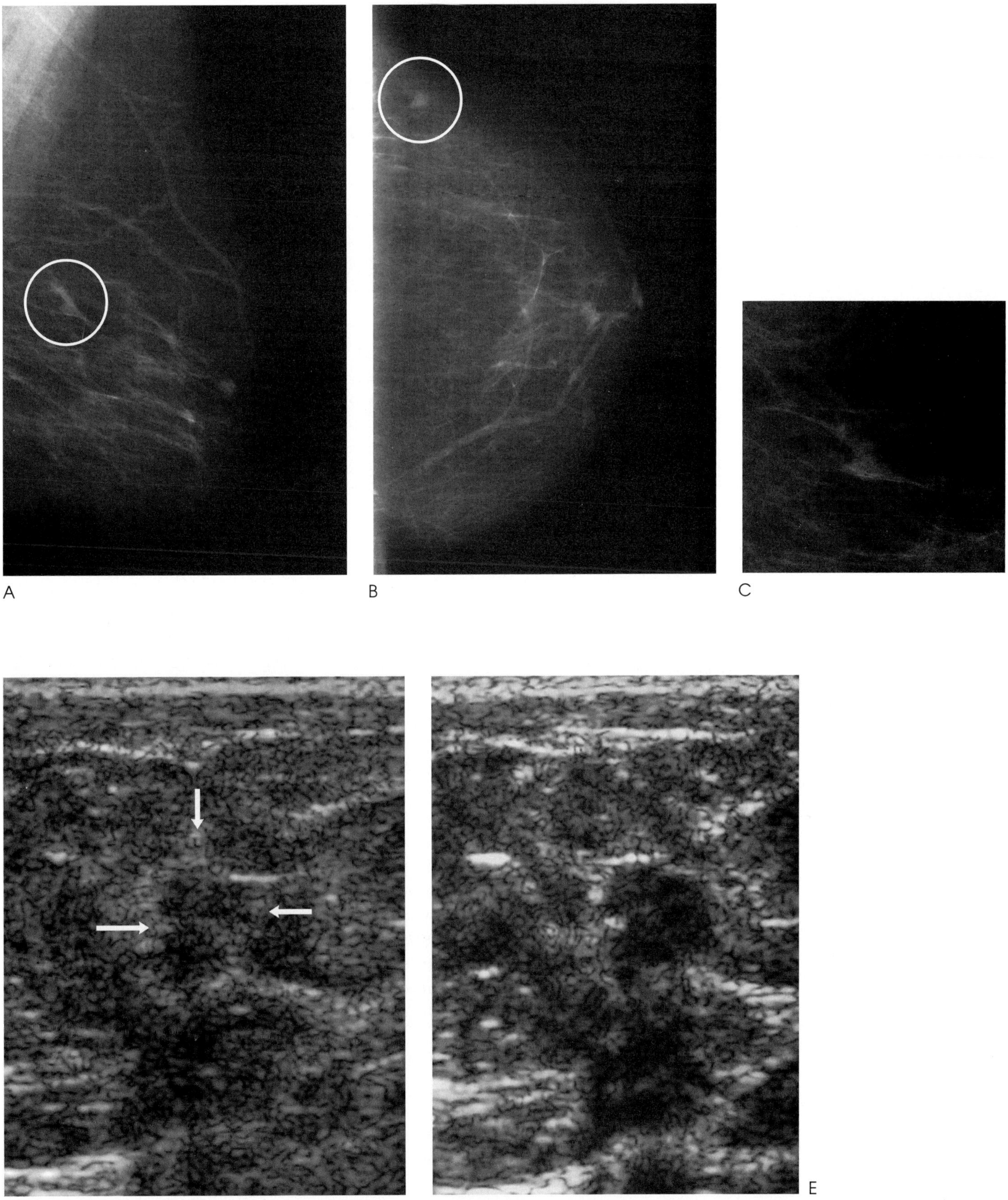

Figure 2–2. *(A). Left MLO mammogram. (B). Left CC mammogram. (C). Left MLO spot magnification mammogram. (A–C). In the left upper outer quadrant, there is a small irregular mass (circle). (D). Left antiradial (8 MHz) breast sonogram: Sonographic examination of the mammographic mass with a low-contrast technique poorly demonstrates the mass (arrows). The hypoechogenicity of the mass blends into the surrounding fat. (E). Left antiradial (8 MHz) breast sonogram: Sonographic examination of the same location as Figure 2–2D with high-contrast technique greatly improves the conspicuity of the mass. This mass is a mucinous carcinoma.*

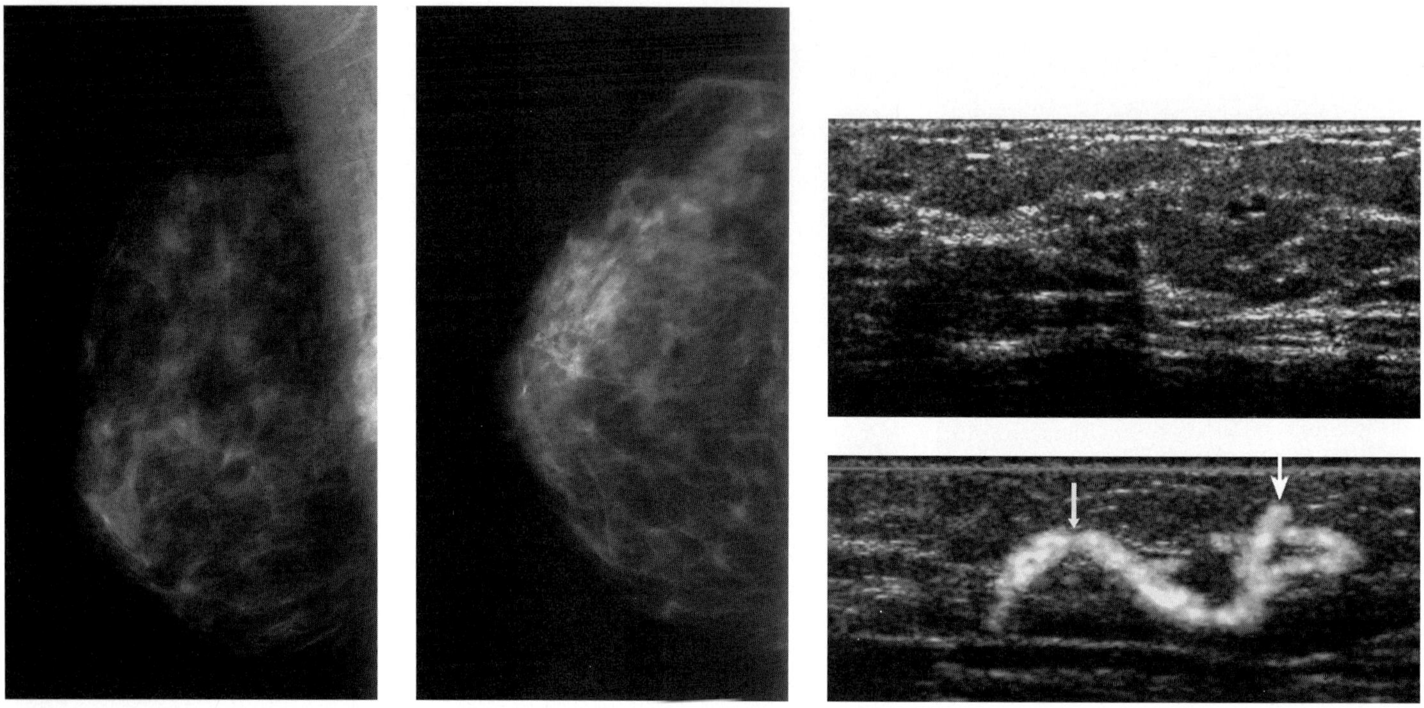

Figure 2–3. *(A). Right MLO mammogram. (B). Right CC mammogram. (A,B). The patient and the breast surgeon have identified some small palpable lumps at the 9:00 position of the right breast. The lumps are arranged in a linear pattern. The left breast has similar lumps that are less conspicuous. Bilateral mammograms are normal. (C). Right radial breast sonogram: Gray scale sonographic examination of the palpable lumps shows normal tissue. (D). Right radial breast sonogram: Color Doppler examination of the palpable lumps demonstrates that the lumps are due to the lateral blood vessels of the breast. Each lump corresponds to the superficial curve of the blood vessel (arrows) (see Color Plate 2–3 D).*

the gray scale frequency and the focal zone adjusted at the correct depth. The filter and scale should be low. The Doppler gain is optimized by initially increasing the gain until the entire screen is filled with color and then by slowly reducing the gain until the color appears only within pulsating vascular structures. If no color is detected using these methods, then the sample volume size should be increased. Increasing the sample volume size reduces color resolution. The color may "bleed" and be demonstrated outside of the vessel walls. Color or power Doppler is useful to delineate vessels or highly vascular structures such as arteriovenous malformations. This Doppler technique is also useful to clarify whether a hypoechoic or anechoic mass is cystic or solid (Fig. 2–3; also see Section 3 Case 32).

Dynamic clips are useful to document vascularity and to demonstrate the spatial relationship of multiple lesions. Dynamic clips are the ideal method to show color flow in pseudoaneurysms or intravenous contrast enhancement of solid masses. Until high-resolution three-dimensional (3-D) imaging is universally available, dynamic clips are an excellent way to demonstrate the relationship of multiple cysts to a solid mass or to show debris or calcifications moving within a complex cyst.

Wide field of view compound imaging is sometimes useful to document larger masses or the relationship of multiple masses in the same plane. The wider field of view provides observers with more landmarks so cross correlation with mammography and magnetic resonance imaging (MRI) may be easier.

Newer sonographic techniques that may have more applications in the future include 3-D imaging and harmonic imaging. Like compound imaging, 3-D imaging may produce a wide field of view that would be similar to a mammogram or magnetic resonance image. In the future, 3-D imaging may also allow surgeons and patients to better appreciate the location and size of sonographic findings and facilitate surgical planning.

Harmonic imaging may improve image resolution and increase both gray scale and color Doppler sensitivity for intravenous sonographic contrast agents. These contrast agents may improve both vascular and gray scale characterization of masses.

Approach to a Palpable Mass

In many breast centers, palpable masses are the most common reason for a breast sonogram. Therefore, it is important that sonographic breast imagers learn how to palpate breasts. Usually, the patient will be able to identify the palpable lump. When the patient locates the lump, the breast imager should confirm the presence of the lump by palpating the area identified by the patient. Even if the lump is obvious, the imager should scan the lump and reconfirm the location of the lump by moving a finger into the scan plane. If the imager cannot detect the lump or if the patient is not sure of the exact location of the lump, then palpation of the entire quadrant is useful. By palpating a larger area, one is able to detect asymmetries within the region. Finally, if palpating the quadrant isn't helpful, then one may palpate the comparable area in the opposite breast. Commonly, the parenchymal pattern of patients is symmetric, so the physical exam is also symmetric. By palpating the corresponding contralateral quadrant, one may detect abnormal asymmetries. This technique is particularly useful with malignancies that are commonly difficult to feel such as lobular carcinoma.

Cross Correlation of Sonographic and Mammographic Image

To accurately, efficiently, and confidently sonographically identify a mammographic abnormality, the personnel who perform the breast sonographic examination should be familiar with mammographic imaging. Furthermore, the ultrasound examiner should be able to review the mammogram and identify internal landmarks that can be cross correlated with the ultrasound. Finally, by confirming the mammographic landmarks sonographically, the examiner should be able to pinpoint the location of the mammographic abnormality in the breast with ultrasound and consequently be able to explain the etiology of the puzzling mammographic finding.

Unfortunately, sometimes the ultrasound examiner does not attempt to closely cross correlate anatomically the ultrasound examination with the mammogram. In some cases, the examiner does not attempt to correlate the exams because he or she does not routinely interpret mammograms and is uncomfortable reviewing mammograms. However, more common reasons for lack of close cross correlation include the following: (1) The sonographic image has a small field of view compared with the mammographic global field of view. (2) The patient position for an ultrasound examination is completely different than the position for the mammographic examination. Therefore, the position of a breast mass for these exams appears extremely different. (3) Even if one places the patient in the same position, the difference in technology between ultrasound and mammography creates different orientations of tissue visualization. (4) Unlike other organs, the breast does not have a uniform or constant normal anatomy. The breasts of different individuals have different breast architecture. Furthermore, some individuals have a right breast that exhibits a pattern different from the left breast. Finally, the breasts of many individuals change with age.

As a result of the reasons stated above, ultrasound examiners commonly ignore internal breast anatomic landmarks and estimate the location of the mammographic abnormality using external landmarks. The most commonly used systems are the "o'clock" method and the quadrant method. The o'clock method views the breast as a circular clock with the nipple in the center of the circle: 12:00 is directly above the nipple; 3:00 is to the left of the nipple; 6:00 is below the nipple; 9:00 is to the right of the nipple. The quadrant method divides the breast into four parts or quadrants. These quadrants are defined by drawing a horizontal and a vertical line through the nipple. The quadrants label four regions of the breast: upper outer quadrant, upper inner quadrant, lower outer quadrant, and lower inner quadrant.

There are several problems with using external anatomic landmarks for locating mammographic abnormalities: (1) Mammographic estimation of location is not accurate and may be difficult to determine if the abnormality is only on one view; (2) The change in patient position between the mammogram and the ultrasound commonly results in changes in the relative position of internal breast structures compared to external landmarks; (3) The external breast position of a handheld transducer does not correlate to a specific internal imaging position.

Estimating location on a mammogram is commonly inaccurate as the standard mammographic views are the craniocaudal (horizontal) and mediolateral oblique views. The greatest source of error is related to the mediolateral oblique view because this view is not oriented 90 degrees to the craniocaudal view. Furthermore, this view's long axis angle varies with the anatomy of the patient. For example, a mass that is deep to the nipple on the craniocaudal view and directly above the nipple in the mediolateral oblique view may be identified as being located at 12:00 but may actually be located between 11:30 and 9:30.

Even if the location of a lesion is accurately identified by the mammogram, the relative position of this lesion may change when the patient changes position for the ultrasound. Usually, the mammogram is performed in the upright position and the ultrasound in the supine position. Because the breast is a flexible structure, the breast changes its shape from one position to the other. In the upright position the position of the breast drops due to gravity. Whereas in the supine position, the breast flattens against the chest wall. Compared with other external landmarks, the nipple may be lower in the upright position compared with the supine position. Therefore, a lesion above the nipple in the upright position may shift to the same level as the nipple in the supine position. For example a 10:00 lesion in the upright position may become a 9:00 lesion in the supine position. The larger the breast, the greater the movement of the breast.

Finally, the external position of the handheld transducer does not necessarily correlate with the internal position of the lesion. Even if a linear transducer is used, the examiner commonly uses a variety of angles and hand pressures to optimally visualize the abnormality. Even slight angulation will produce a discrepancy between the position of the sonographic transducer and the actual position of the lesion. Furthermore, transducer pressure may cause the lesion to shift position relative to the nipple. Both of these factors may produce a discrepancy between the mammographic position and the sonographic position.

Because external landmarks are not reliable in cross correlating mammographic/sonographic abnormalities, one should use internal landmarks. However, one must use a technique that addresses the problems listed earlier: (1) limited sonographic field of view compared with mammography, (2) differences between mammographic and sonographic patient position and technical orientation, and (3) nonuniformity of breast anatomy both between individuals and within the same individual.

By using internal breast anatomic landmarks, one immediately addresses the first two problems. If one identifies location by the internal anatomy of an organ, then relating the position of a focal abnormality from the limited sonographic field of view to a wide field of view modality is not a problem. Furthermore, unlike external landmarks, internal landmarks do not shift with body position. For example, in the abdomen, one is commonly challenged with the problem of sonographically deciding whether a small liver lesion previously identified on a computed tomography (CT) scan is cystic or solid. Even though the CT scan is a wide field of view modality, experienced examiners easily sonographically localize the position of the CT lesion. These examiners are able to confidently localize the lesion because they relate the lesion to the internal anatomy of the liver as displayed on CT and then sonographically find the same hepatic location using the same internal hepatic landmarks. Furthermore, this process of anatomic cross correlation would not be different even if the patient were lying prone because unlike external landmarks, internal anatomic landmarks do not change relative to each other.

Even though internal landmarks solve the problems of limited sonographic field of view and positional changes, many examiners are inhibited from using internal breast landmarks as there is great anatomic variation between different breasts. However, whenever one performs a breast sonogram to identify a mammographic abnormality, one should always have the corresponding mammogram. The mammogram provides an anatomic map to the patient's breast. If one is able to cross correlate mammographic structures with sonographic structures, then one may use the mammogram as a sonographic guide to locating the lesion. Therefore, ideally the sonographic examiner should be able to sonographically interpret the mammographic image.

To systematically cross correlate sonography with mammography, one should be familiar with normal breast anatomy. There are seven main sonographically different structures in the breast and chest wall of the average normal 45-year-old woman. These structures from superficial to deep are the following (Fig. 2–4):

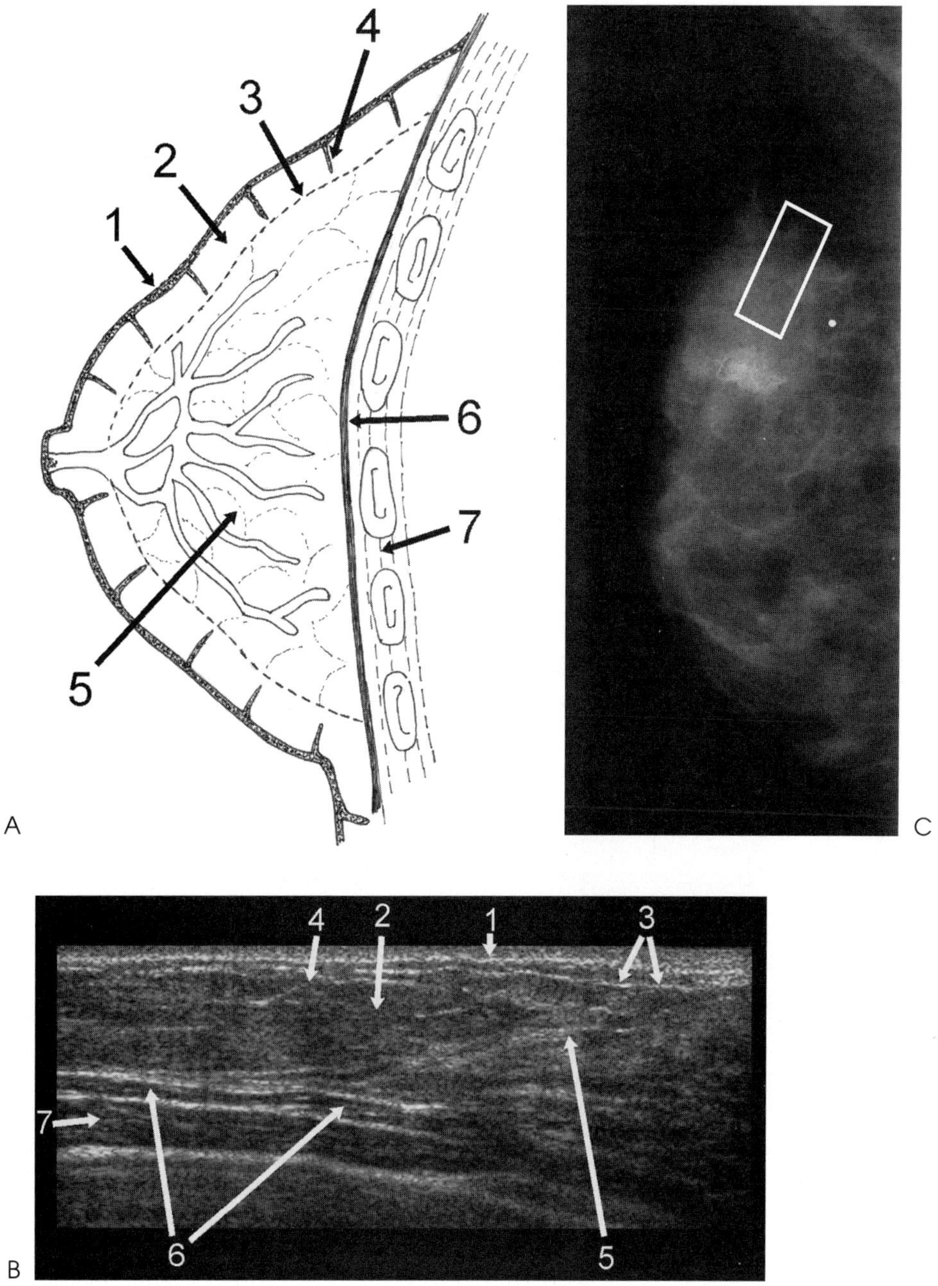

Figure 2–4. *(A). A schematic diagram showing the normal structures of the breast: skin (1), subcutaneous fatty layer (2), superficial fascia (3), Cooper's ligaments (4), glandular tissue (5), anterior chest wall muscles (6), chest wall (7). (B). Radial breast sonogram (10:00 position): Sonographic image demonstrates the normal anatomic structures of the breast: skin (1), subcutaneous fatty layer (2), superficial fascia (3), Cooper's ligaments (4), glandular tissue (5), anterior chest wall muscles (6), chest wall (7). (C). Right MLO mammogram: This is the mammogram of the patient whose sonogram is seen in Figure 2–2B. In the upper outer quadrant, the sonographic image corresponds to the outer edge of the patient's fibroglandular density. Box denotes location of transducer.*

1. Skin: The skin is a hyperechoic 3 mm layer on the surface of the breast.
2. Subcutaneous fatty layer: This structure lies under the skin and appears as an anterior hypoechoic layer of tissue, which tends to thicken at the periphery of the breast and is more prominent in the medial portion of the breast.
3. Superficial fascia: The superficial and deep layers of the fascia envelop the breast. The superficial layer is an undulating hyperechoic line within the subcutaneous fat that parallels the skin. The deep layer is an hyperechoic line within the retromammary fat that parallels the anterior chest wall muscles.
4. Cooper's ligaments: The ligaments are curved hyperechoic lines within the subcutaneous fat, which extend from the superficial fascia to the deeper adjacent tissue.
5. Glandular tissue: Normal glandular tissue consists of hyperechoic glandular lobes that are in a radial arrangement around the nipple. Each lobe is in the shape of a prolate ellipse and is surrounded anteriorly by the subcutaneous fat and posteriorly by the retromammary fat. Within the lobes, main ducts originate from the nipple and end in a series of terminal duct lobular units.
6. Anterior chest wall muscles: This layer is formed by the pectoralis minor and major muscles and appears as a hypoechoic solid layer posterior to the retromammary fat.

7. Chest wall: This structure consists of ribs connected by intercostal muscles and covered on the deep surface by pleura.

Most of these anatomic structures are also generally identifiable mammographically.

Rules of Cross Correlation

Once one is familiar with normal sonographic and mammographic breast anatomy, one will be able to anatomically cross correlate the two modalities. If one is not familiar with cross correlation of these modalities, one should not be intimidated by the task of cross correlating sonographic and mammographic structures. A simple way to start is to remember two basic imaging rules. The first rule is that the background breast tissue appearance is similar on the two modalities. This means that normal fibroglandular parenchyma is white (or dense) on mammography and white (or hyperechoic) on sonography. Furthermore, fat appears dark (or lucent) on mammography and dark (or hypoechoic) on sonography (Fig. 2–5). The main exception to this rule is the presence of dilated ducts that are sonographically dark (hypoechoic) and mammographically white (dense). When the breast tissue is filled with dilated ducts such as in ductal ectasias, the breast tissue appears white (dense) on mammography but has numerous linear dark structures (dilated ducts) on sonography.

When one is aware of the appearance of breast tissue with the two modalities, then when one reviews a mammogram one should be able to predict the sonographic appearance of the breast. For example, a mammographically fatty, lucent breast will be sonographically hypoechoic. Conversely, a mammographically dense breast usually sonographically exhibits diffusely hyperechoic fibroglandular parenchyma.

Generally, the breasts of most women are not completely dense or lucent. This system of pattern recognition is even more valuable in these breasts. When a breast has a mixture of tissues, these tissues form unique mammographic structural patterns that may be sonographically reproduced. For example, commonly the mammogram exhibits dense parenchymal tissue primarily in the upper outer quadrant. Sonographically, one can also outline this tissue by noticing the junction between the hyperechoic parenchyma and the adjacent hypoechoic fat. Furthermore, if the medial aspect of the mammogram is lucent, then the corresponding sonographic examination should display hypoechoic fat.

The second cross correlation imaging rule is that most focal breast masses have dissimilar appearances on the two modalities. For example, lymph nodes, cysts, and fibroadenomas appear white (dense) on mammography but dark (hypoechoic) on sonography. Neoplasms appear white (dense) on mammography but dark (hypoechoic or heterogeneous echogenicity) on sonography. The main common exceptions to this rule are benign scars, radial scars, and occasionally fat necrosis. These lesions are sonographically hyperechoic (white).

If one is familiar with mammographic and sonographic appearance of breast structures, then one will be able to sonographically localize a focal mammographic abnormality using internal anatomic landmarks. The steps that I use when faced with an anatomically difficult breast problem are the following:

1. Review the mammogram and identify the abnormality. Notice the parenchymal pattern between the nipple and the lesion. Also study the pattern of the breast tissue surrounding the abnormality. Estimate the general location of the abnormality (i.e., quadrant and finger breadths from nipple).
2. Place the transducer with one edge at the nipple and sonographically examine the breast in a radial orientation. Look for the same parenchymal patterns that one noticed on the mammogram. When one recognizes the parenchymal landmarks that surround the abnormality, sonographically focus the examination in this area.
3. Sonographically characterize the lesion (Fig. 2–6). Utilizing this method, one would first approach finding the mass in Figure 2–6 by noting the general mammographic location of the lesion near the left 9:00 position. The irregular mass is surrounded by fatty density but linked to the subareolar density by linear densities (Fig. 2–6A–C). One would initially place the transducer near the nipple and confirm the presence of dense (hyperechoic) subareolar tissue. In the inner breast one would extend the transducer away from the nipple following the strands of hyperechoic tissue that extend farthest away from the nipple. This "trail" of hyperechoic tissue will lead to the hypoechoic shadowing mass (Fig. 2–6D) that corresponds to the mammographic mass.

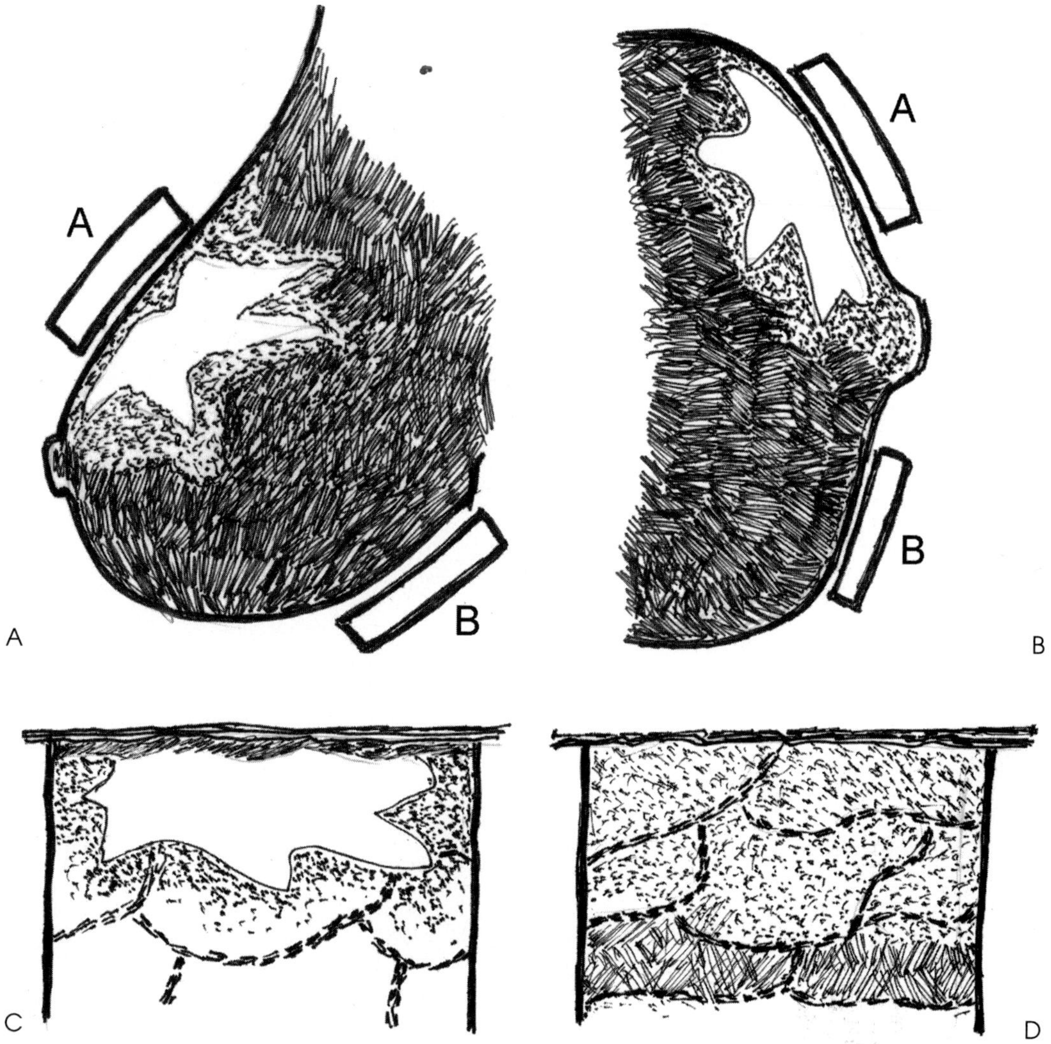

Figure 2–5. These schematic diagrams illustrate the anatomic cross correlation between mammography and sonography. In this patient, transducer A is positioned over the dense fibroglandular tissue in the upper outer quadrant. Sonographically, this tissue is hyperechoic (C). Transducer B demonstrates the fatty parenchyma in the inferior inner quadrant that is sonographically hypoechoic (D). (A). Schematic image of an MLO mammogram show two transducers, labeled A and B. (B). Schematic image of a CC mammogram showing position of transducers A and B. (C). Schematic image of breast sonogram that corresponds to tissue imaged by transducer A. (D). Schematic image of breast sonogram that corresponds to tissue imaged by transducer B.

This method is particularly useful when the mammographic abnormality is not easily visualized. Section 6 Case 120 demonstrates an asymmetric density that is only visible in one mammographic view. In this case, the abnormal density is at the distal border of the fibroglandular density. Therefore, to find this type of lesion, one should start near the nipple and confirm the presence of diffuse hyperechoic fibroglandular tissue. One should then move the transducer toward the outer breast until one visualizes fatty hypoechoic tissue. Then, one should only scan the border between the hyperechoic and hypoechoic tissue. One will then discover the hypoechoic malignant mass.

When evaluating the location of a lesion from the mammogram, internal parenchymal landmarks one should notice include: (1) location of the edge of the parenchyma—many lesions are at the border of the fibroglandular (white) tissue and the fat (dark); (2) configuration of fibroglandular tissue—lesion may be linked to the largest area of this tissue; (3) adjacent masses—mammogram may demonstrate another mass next to the questionable lesion. By cross correlating these mammographic landmarks on the breast sonogram, one will be more successful in identifying mammographic lesions (Fig. 2–7).

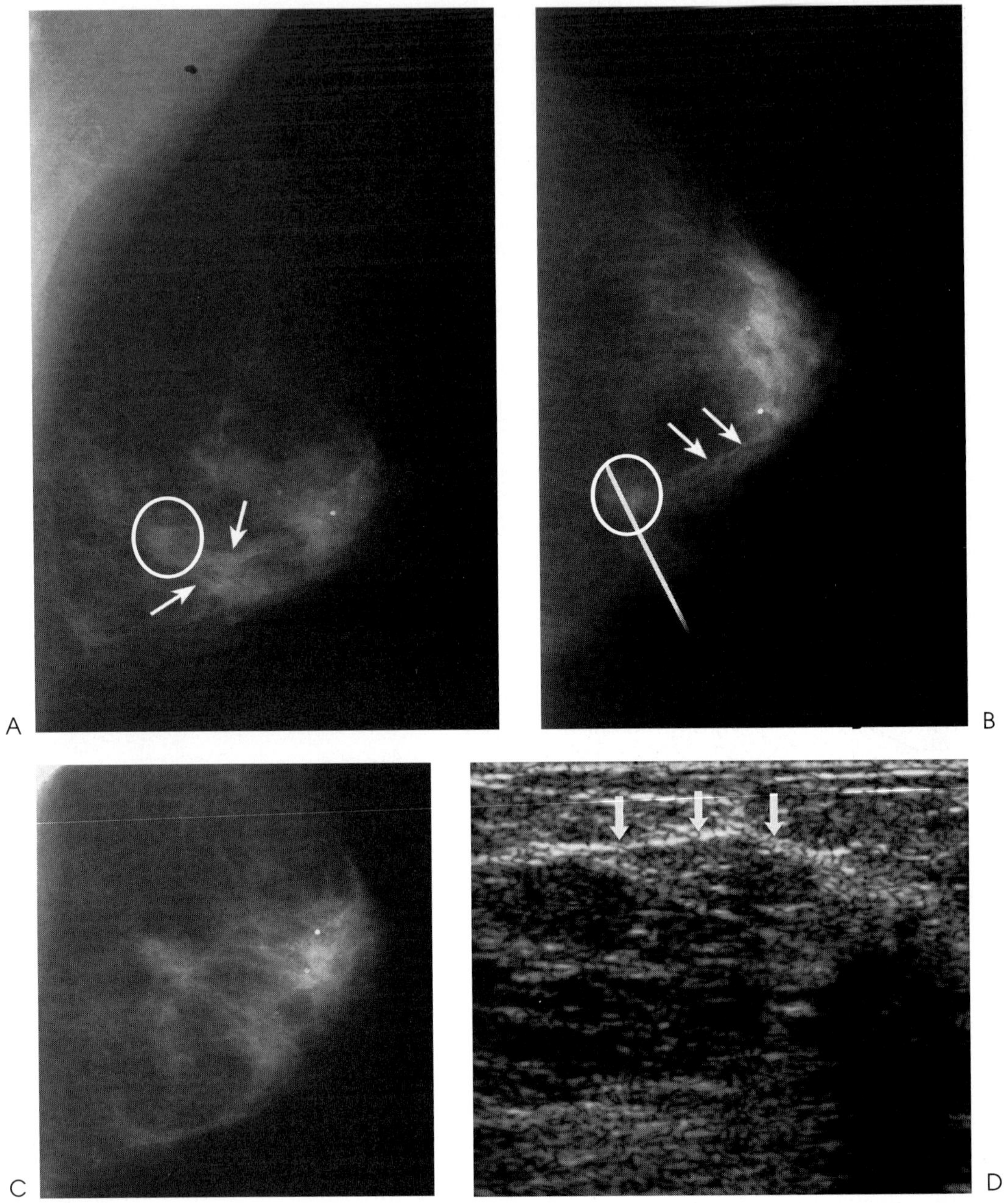

Figure 2–6. Figure 6A. (A). Left MLO mammogram. (B). Left CC mammogram. (C). Left LM spot compression mammogram. (A–C). At the 9:00 position of the left breast, there is an irregular mass (circle). This mass is primarily surrounded by fatty density but is linked with dense spiculations (arrows) to the main subareolar fibroglandular density. (D). Left radial breast sonogram: The mammographic irregular density corresponds to a heavily shadowing focal mass. These mammographic spiculations correspond to the hyperechoic curvilinear tissue (arrows). This mass is infiltrating ductal carcinoma.

Special Sonographic Problems

Shadowing

One difficulty in cross correlating mammography with sonography is sonographic shadowing. Shadowing is confusing. It is a nonspecific finding because it is associated with both benign and malignant entities. Shadowing is particularly a problem for those who use high-frequency equipment as all tissues more readily attenuate high frequencies and, therefore, shadowing is more frequent. To analyze shadowing, one should (1) be familiar with the etiologies of shadowing; (2) if the shadow hides the lesion, reduce or eliminate the shadow; (3) characterize the tissue that causes the shadow.

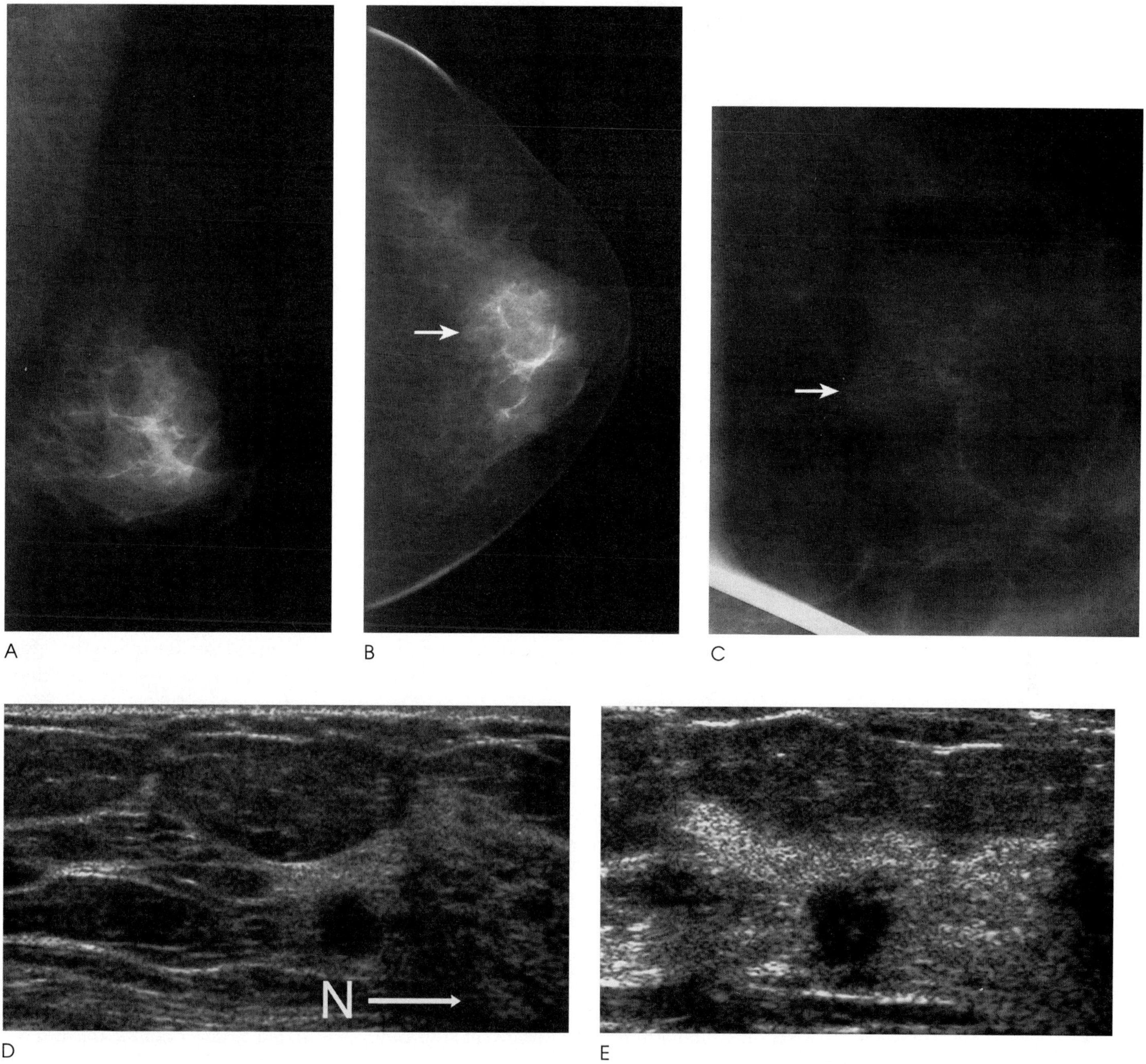

Figure 2–7. *(A). Left MLO digital mammogram. (B). Left CC digital mammogram. (C). Left CC spot magnification mammogram. (A–C). A partially obscured oval density (arrow) is visible in the central area of the CC view. This density is not visible on the MLO view. In the CC view, the density is at the distal edge of the fibroglandular density. (D). Left radial breast sonogram: A hypoechoic mass is present at the 12:00 position of the breast. In this view, the parenchymal anatomy matches the mammographic anatomy of the CC view. On the side closest to the nipple, the tissue is white fibroglandular parenchyma. On the side away from the nipple, the tissue is hypoechoic fat. N, arrow points toward direction of nipple. (E). Left antiradial breast sonogram: The antiradial view demonstrates irregularity of the margins of the mass. This mass is a mixed infiltrating ductal and lobular carcinoma.*

The etiologies of shadowing can be divided into two main categories: (1) reflection and (2) absorption. Reflection of sound is affected by two factors: (1) acoustic impedance and (2) angle of incidence. Acoustic impedance is a fundamental property of matter and is related to the density of the material and the speed of sound in the material. A portion of a sound wave is reflected whenever the wave strikes an interface between two substances with different acoustic impedances. This principle is the basis for diagnostic sonography. The reflected sound is received by the ultrasound machine and transformed into visual information. The amount of reflection is dependent upon the difference in acoustic impedance between the substances. If the difference is great, then a large percentage of the sound wave is reflected. Acoustic impedance differences between most tissues within the breast such as fat and fibroglandular tissue are very small, so generally less than 1% of the sound wave is reflected. However, air and bone have acoustic impedances that are very different from breast tissue. When the sound wave strikes a rib, about 90% of the sound is reflected and when the wave strikes the lung over 99% of the wave is reflected.

The second factor that affects the amount of reflected sound is the angle of incidence or the angle at which the sound strikes an object. The closer the sound beam is to a right angle (or perpendicular to the surface of the object), the less the reflection. The proportion of reflected sound increases with decreasing angles. When the sound beam strikes the object at an extremely acute angle (i.e., critical angle), all of the sound is reflected. This phenomenon is evident when sound hits the side of a curved mass such as a cyst. In this situation, the reflected sound produces thin shadows at the edges of the cyst.

Besides reflection, shadowing is caused by absorption. Absorption is the conversion of sound into heat. A shadow results if the material completely absorbs the sound beam. In the body, absorption is directly proportional to transducer frequency. Therefore, absorption is double for 14 MHz compared with 7 MHz. This increased absorption is the main reason that high frequency is associated with more shadowing than lower-frequency sonography.

Upon encountering a confusing shadow, a breast imager should initially judge whether the shadow is due to reflection or absorption. After making this decision, one should eliminate or reduce the shadow. If the shadow is due to reflection, then the shadow is either due to the acoustic impedance of the material or due to the angle of the sound beam. If the shadowing is due to acoustic impedance, the imager cannot eliminate the shadow, but the imager would have a short list of materials that would produce this shadowing (i.e., air, bone, metal). However, if the shadow is due to the angle of the sound beam, then changing the position of the transducer can eliminate the shadow. Many structures within the breast are curved and create this type of shadow. Pseudomasses may be created by several of these shadows that are close together. To distinguish a true mass from an artifactual one, an imager should routinely study the mass from multiple transducer angles (Figs. 2–8 and 2–9).

If the shadow results from absorption, then one should decrease the frequency of the transducer. This technique is useful to better characterize lesions associated with severe shadowing. Both benign and malignant masses appear as areas of focal shadowing. By lowering the transducer frequency, one may reduce or eliminate the shadowing and be able to visualize the lesion causing the shadow. This technique is useful to differentiate scars or highly absorbing fibroglandular tissue from masses. With lower frequency, no mass will be evident with scars or fibroglandular tissue. The main problem associated with this technique is that lower-frequency imaging still has the disadvantages of relatively poor resolution and contrast. One may miss masses because they may blend into the surrounding fibroglandular tissue. Margins and architectural distortion are poorly defined. To avoid missing masses, one should have a high degree of suspicion. One should closely examine the area for

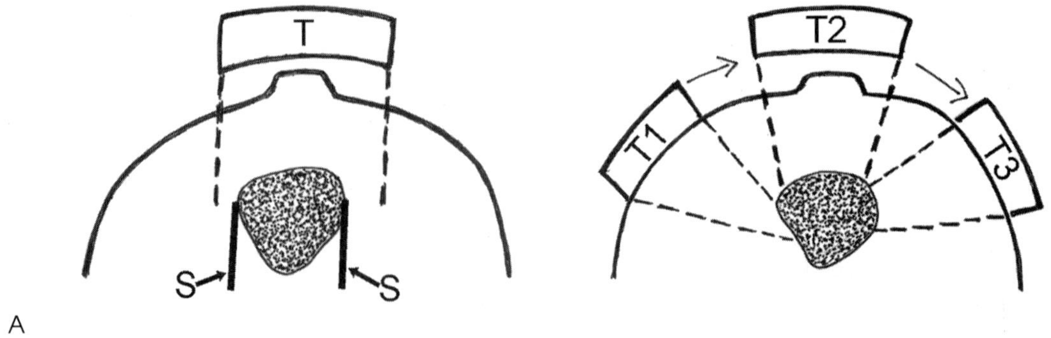

Figure 2–8. (A). Schematic of breast sonogram: When a transducer (T) is positioned over a curved object, the sound at the edges of the object is reflected so shadowing (S) is produced at the edges of the mass. (B). Schematic of breast sonogram: When the transducer (T1–T3) is repositioned around the curved object, shadowing is reduced.

subtle inhomogeneity of architecture and echogenicity. (See Section 3 Cases 12 and 30 and Section 4 Case 47.)

Even after lowering the frequency, shadowing sometimes persists. In this situation, one should first attempt to discover whether the shadowing is caused by a mass or results from the patient's dense fibroglandular tissue. To differentiate shadowing from these sources, one should compare the region of interest with normal fibroglandular tissue of the same breast or the opposite breast. Most women have symmetric fibroglandular tissue. Therefore, if the region of interest is in the right upper outer quadrant, then one should compare this area with the left upper outer quadrant. Or if the patient's mammogram is completely white, then one may compare the region of interest with another area of the same breast. If the normal fibroglandular tissue does not shadow, then one should be suspicious that the shadowing represents an active process. If the patient's normal fibroglandular tissue shadows, then one should try to use a lower frequency in which the fibroglandular tissue appears hyperechoic. One may then use this new lower frequency to evaluate the region of interest.

Finally, if shadowing persists, one should evaluate the appearance of the shadow. Is it focal? Does it persist consistently in multiple angles? Masses that shadow have borders. Therefore, if the shadow has edges that define a focal area, then the shadowing should be considered suspicious for a mass.

Architectural Distortion and Focal Asymmetric Density

Mammographic architectural distortion and asymmetric density are difficult problems to sonographically correlate. When these findings are present without a mass, they are extremely subtle and commonly only visible in one mammographic view. Because obvious architectural distortion or asymmetry may generally be well characterized with mammography alone, sonography is most valuable when the mammographic findings are uncertain. Therefore, if one utilizes sonography for this purpose, one should only use high-resolution equipment and be experienced in cross correlating cases.

The principles for cross correlating architectural distortion and focal asymmetric density are the same as for a mass. One should match the internal sonographic landmarks to the mammogram. If the area of architectural distortion or focal asymmetry is dark sonographically, then one must suspect a mass (Fig. 2–10). Otherwise, the area will appear to be white fibroglandular tissue.

Generally, the sonographic findings are complementary to the mammographic information, so one is more confident about the final recommendation. However, occasionally, the sonographic and mammographic findings are discordant. In this case, if one of the modalities has information indicating malignancy, then one should recommend biopsy of the abnormality (American College of Radiology Breast Imaging Reporting and Data System Categories 4 and 5).

A

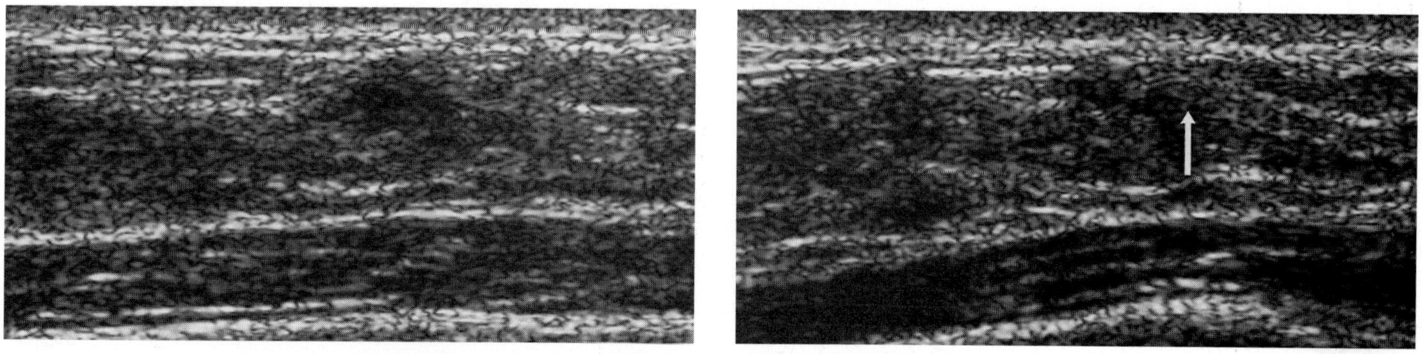

B

Figure 2–9. (A). This 35-year-old woman presents with a palpable lump. Sonographically, the lump has been found to be an ill-defined hypoechoic mass. The mass is considered suspicious and biopsy is recommended. The patient returns 2 days later for the biopsy. When the patient returns, the original hypoechoic area is identified (A), but by slightly changing the angle of the transducer, the hypoechoic area disappears (B). The hypoechoic "mass" represents unusual shadowing from a Cooper's ligament attachment. This attachment is also the etiology of the small superficial palpable lump. (A). Left radial breast sonogram of hypoechoic "mass." (B). Left radial breast sonogram of same area as Figure 2–9A: Pressure on the transducer has slightly changed the incident sonographic angle. Cooper's ligament attachment (arrow).

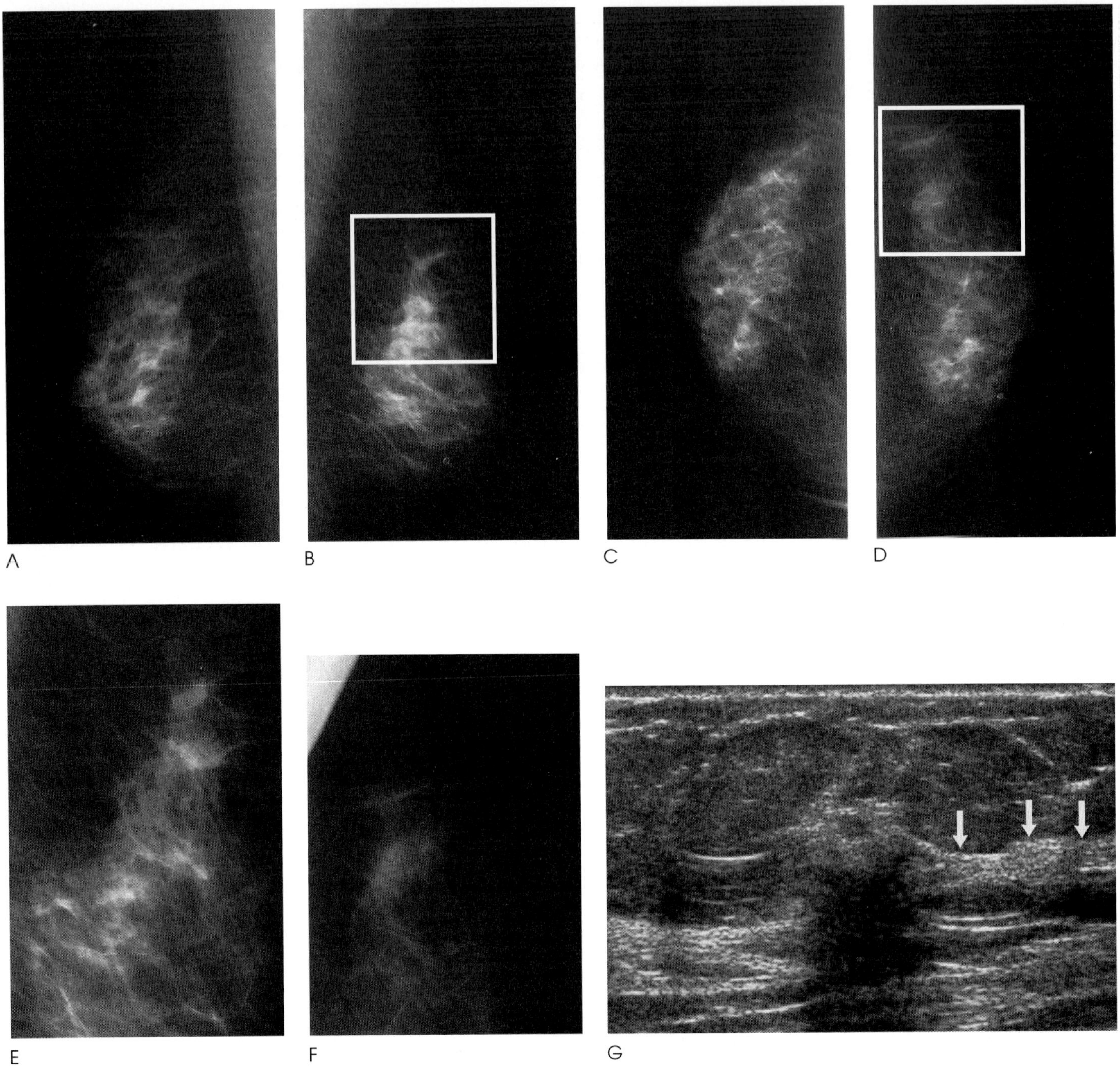

Figure 2–10. *(A). Right MLO mammogram. (B). Left MLO mammogram. (C). Right CC mammogram. (D). Left CC mammogram. (E). Left MLO spot compression mammogram. (F). Left CC spot compression mammogram. (A–F). Subtle architectural distortion (square) is present in the left upper outer quadrant. The architectural distortion blends into the normal central white fibroglandular density. (G). Left radial breast sonogram: Sonographic examination of the left upper outer quadrant demonstrates that the architectural distortion corresponds to an irregular hypoechoic mass with shadowing. The mass is connected to hyperechoic tissue (arrows) that corresponds to the central mammographic fibroglandular density. The mass is a lobular carcinoma.*

Section III

Circumscribed Masses

This is a schematic diagram of the diagnostic approach to mammographic circumscribed masses. For further discussion, see Chapter 1.

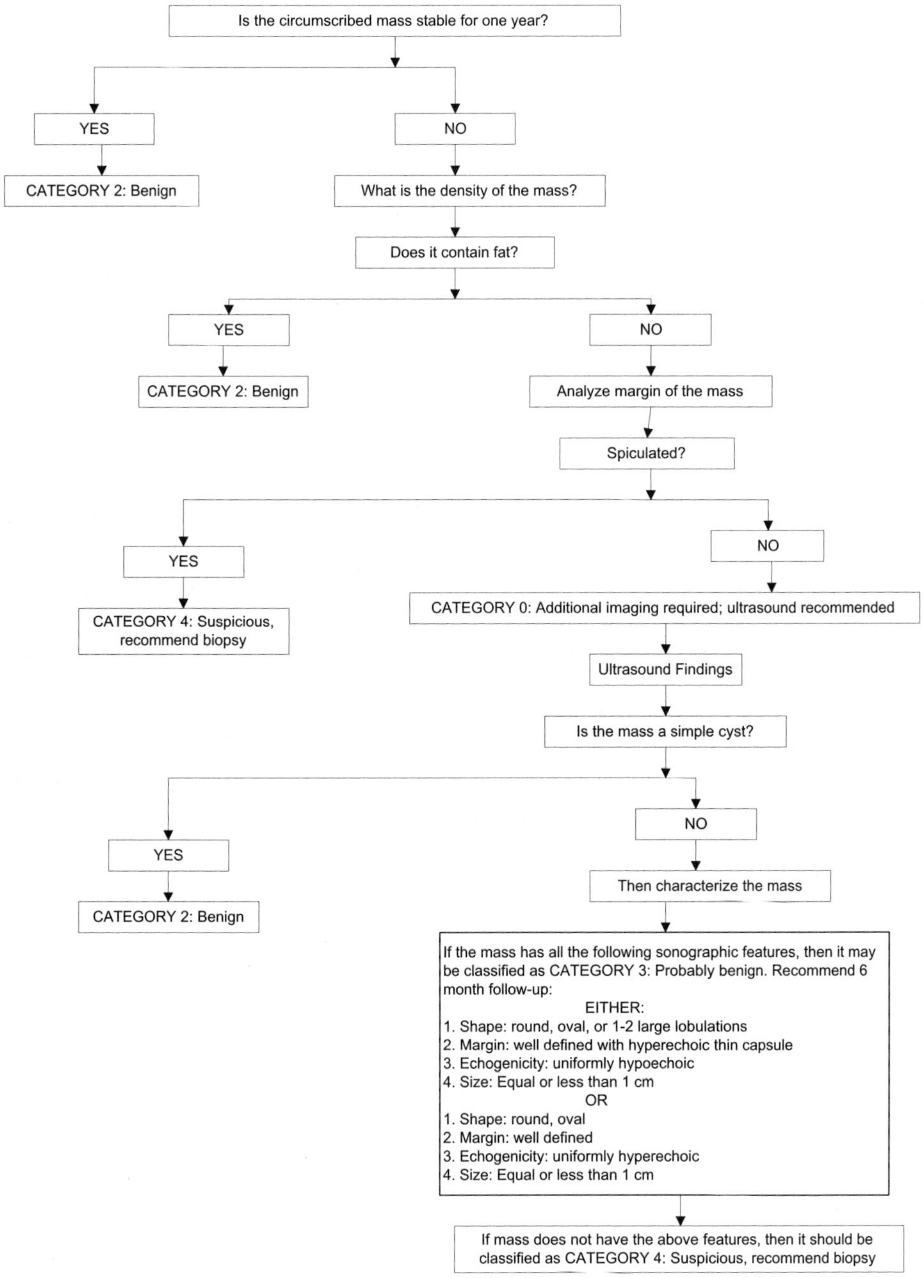

Case 1

Case History

A 39-year-old woman has just stopped breast-feeding her 10-month-old infant and now finds a new breast lump.

Physical Examination

- left breast: 3 cm lump in the upper outer quadrant
- right breast: normal exam

Mammogram

Mass (Fig. 1–1)

- margin: circumscribed
- shape: oval
- density: fat-containing

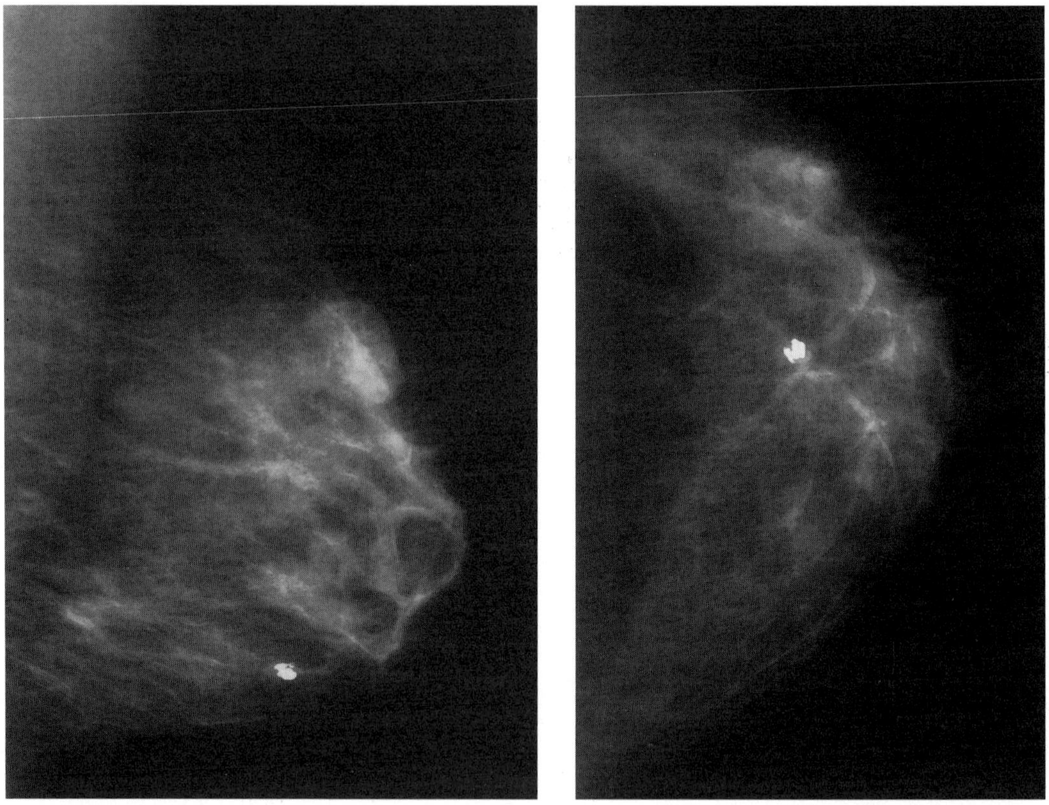

A B

Figure 1–1. In the upper outer quadrant of the left breast, there is a well-defined oval mass. (A). Left mediolateral oblique (MLO) mammogram. (B). Left craniocaudal (CC) mammogram.

Ultrasound

Frequency

- 10 MHz

Mass

- margin: well defined
- echogenicity: isoechoic
- retrotumoral acoustic appearance: single edge shadowing
- shape: ellipsoid (Fig. 1–2)

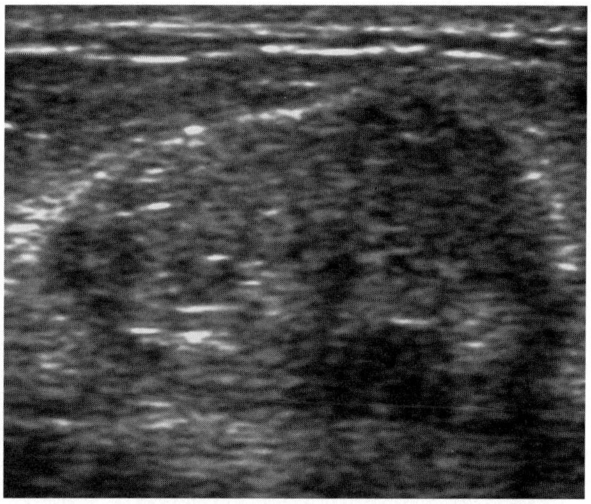

Figure 1–2. Left radial breast sonogram: The mammographic mass identified in Figure 1–1 corresponds to a well-defined mass with heterogeneous echogenicity. Milky fluid was aspirated from this mass.

Pathology

- galactocele

Management

- BI-RADS Assessment Category 2, benign finding

Pearls and Pitfalls

1. Galactoceles are benign milk-filled cysts. This lesion is generally discovered either during or shortly after lactation. Mammographically, galactoceles are well defined, oval, and may appear completely fat density, heterogeneous density, or equal density to glandular parenchyma.
2. Sonographically, galactoceles are hypoechoic, isoechoic, or heterogeneous in echogenicity. Fluid debris levels may be present.

Suggested Readings

1. Salvador R, Salvador M, Jimenez JA, et al. Galactocele of the breast: radiologic and ultrasonographic findings. *Br J Radiol* 1990;63:140–142.
2. Jackson VP, Jahan R, Fu YS. Benign breast lesions. In: Bassett LW, Jackson VP, Jahan R, Fu YS, Gold RH, eds. *Diagnosis of Diseases of the Breast.* Philadelphia: WB Saunders Company; 1997:357–443.

Case 2

Case History

A 39-year-old woman with new left breast lump. Left breast sonography is initially performed. As a result of the sonogram, a mammogram has been done.

Physical Examination

- left breast: 5 cm palpable lump in the upper inner quadrant
- right breast: normal exam

Mammogram

Mass (Fig. 2–1)

- margin: circumscribed
- shape: oval
- density: fat-containing

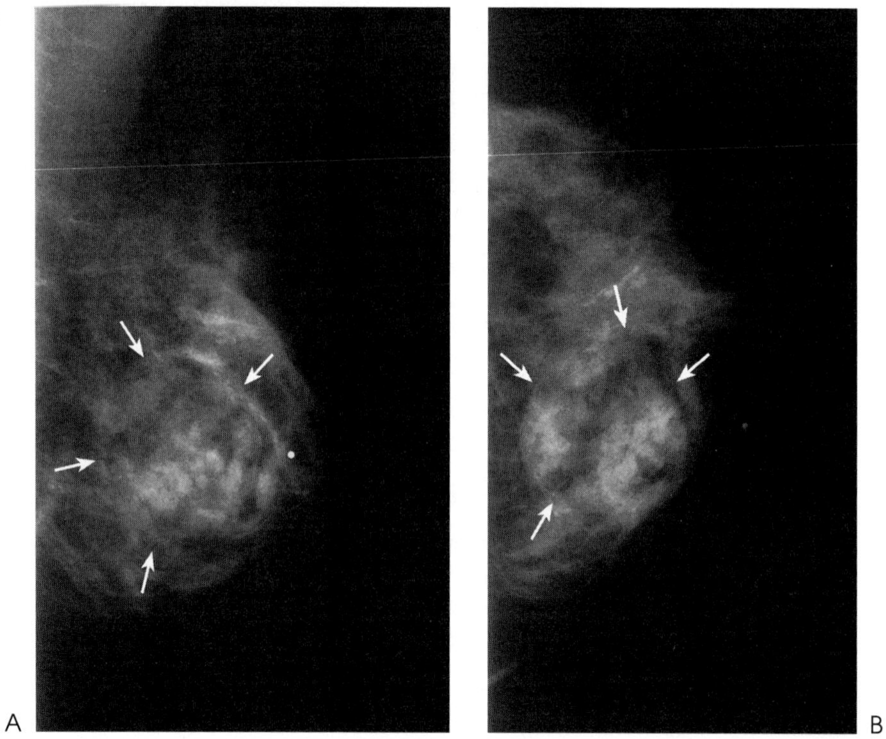

Figure 2–1. At the 9:00 position of the left breast, there is a well-defined oval fat-containing mass with heterogeneous density (arrows). (A). Left MLO mammogram. (B). Left CC mammogram.

Ultrasound

Frequency

- 10 MHz

Mass

- margin: well defined
- echogenicity: heterogeneous
- retrotumoral acoustic appearance: no shadowing
- shape: ellipsoid (Fig. 2–2)

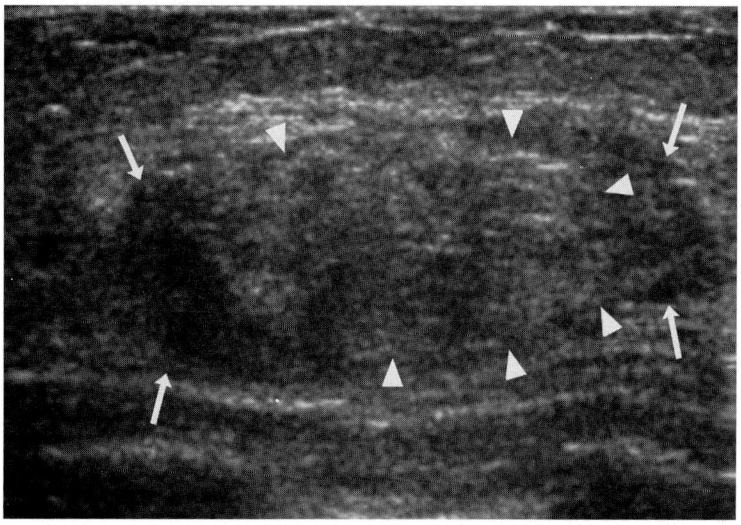

Figure 2–2. Left radial breast sonogram: The palpable lump corresponds to a well-defined, oval, solid mass of heterogeneous echogenicity. The peripheral portion of this mass is isoechoic to fat (arrows) and the central portion is hyperechoic (arrowheads). This mass corresponds to the lesion identified in Figure 2–1.

Pathology

- hamartoma

Management

- BI-RADS Assessment Category 2, benign finding

Pearls and Pitfalls

1. Hamartoma is a benign tumor that consists of mature tissues normally present in the breast. However, usually one element dominates the mass. Mammographically, the mass is well defined but the density of the mass varies with its composition. If the mass does not have much fat, then it may be completely radiopaque. However, if the mass is a mixture of fat and other soft tissues, then it will be mixed density as in this case. If the mass is completely radiopaque, then the differential diagnosis is fibroadenoma, cyst, or carcinoma. If the mass has mixed density, then the mammogram is diagnostic of hamartoma.
2. Sonographically, hamartoma has a variety of appearances. The individual components of the tumor should sonographically match their corresponding normal elements within the breast. The fatty component is isoechoic to fat and the fibroglandular elements are hyperechoic to fat.

Suggested Readings

1. Adler DD, Jeffries DO, Helvie Mak. Sonographic features of breast hamartomas. *J Ultrasound Med* 1990;9:85–90.
2. Altermatt HJ, Gebbers J-O, Laissue J-A. Multiple hamaratomas presenting as discrete breast mass. *Can Assoc Radiol J* 1992;43:218–220.
3. Anderson I, Hildell J, Linell F, et al. Mammary hamartomas. *Acta Radiol* 1979;20:712–720.
4. Beatty SM, Orel SG, McCarthy DM, et al. Breast hamartomas: MR appearance. *Breast Dis* 1995;8:275–281.
5. Crothers JG, Bjkutler NF, Fortt RW, et al. Fibroadenolipoma of the breast. *Br J Radiol* 1985;58:191–202.
6. Evers K, Yeh I-T, Troupin RH, et al. Mammary hamartomas. The importance of radiologic-pathologic correlation. *Breast Dis* 1992;5:35–43.

Case 3

Case History

A 69-year-old woman with a right breast lump.

Physical Examination

- right breast: a 3 cm flat, mobile mass extends from the 1:00 to the 4:00 positions
- left breast: normal exam

Mammogram

Mass (Fig. 3–1)

- margin: circumscribed
- shape: oval
- density: fat-containing

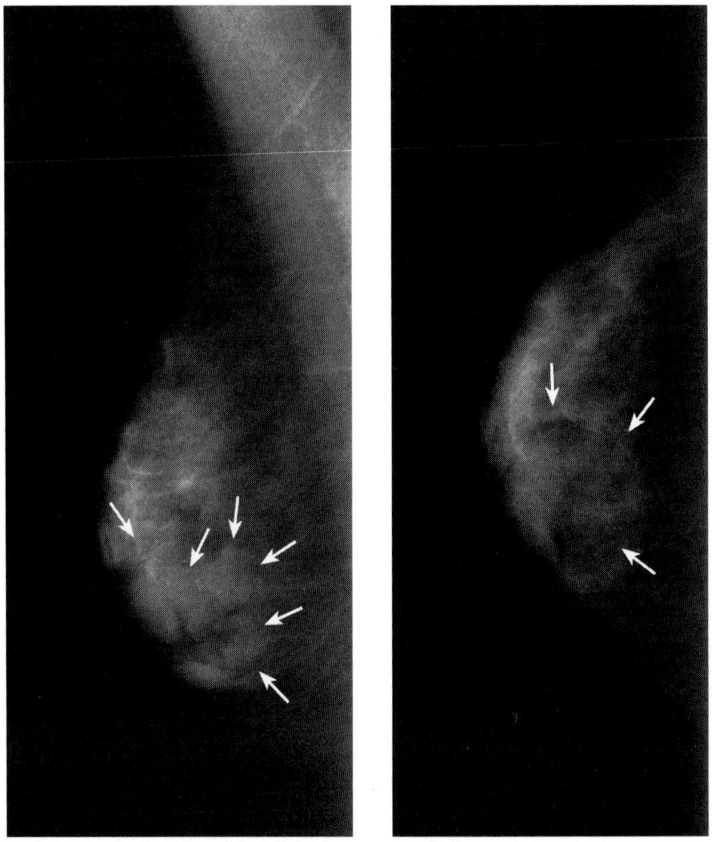

A B

Figure 3–1. In the right inner inferior breast there is a circumscribed mass containing fat (arrows). The mass is partially obscured by the surrounding breast parenchymal density. (A). Right MLO mammogram. (B). Right CC mammogram.

Ultrasound

Frequency

- 13 MHz

Mass

- margin: well defined
- echogenicity: heterogeneous
- retrotumoral acoustic appearance: no shadowing
- shape: ellipsoid (Fig. 3–2)

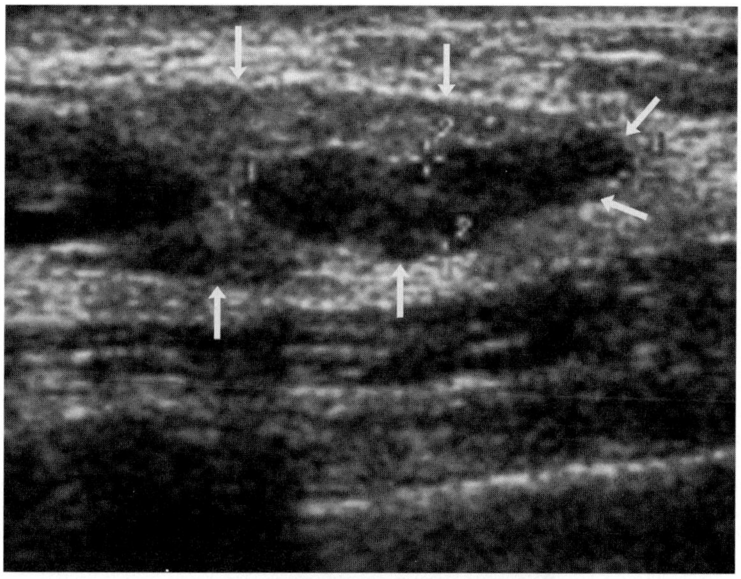

Figure 3–2. Right radial breast sonogram: The palpable lump corresponds to a well-defined mass of heterogeneous echogenicity. The appearance of this mass is confusing because within the mass are multiple focal fatty areas (isoechoic with fat), which are mistaken as individual masses and are measured separately. (Electronic caliper markers measure one fatty area.) The actual mass is a combination of the fatty masses and the more hyperechoic fibroglandular tissues (arrows).

Pathology

- hamartoma

Management

- BI-RADS Assessment Category 2, benign finding

Pearls and Pitfalls

In the literature, hamartomas have also been designated as fibroadenolipomas and adenolipomas. Hamartomas have been reported in patients with a mean age in the late 30s to early 40s. Clinically, the hamartoma may present as a palpable mass, an incidental finding on mammography, or sometimes as tenderness. Rarely a patient presents with nipple inversion or discharge. If the mammogram is performed first, the lesion can be confidently identified if it contains fat. Generally, this mass is not removed. However, in a series in which the tumor was removed, it has been reported to recur in up to 8% of patients.

Suggested Readings

1. Helvie Mak, Adler DD, Rebner M, et al. Breast hamartoma: variable mammographic appearance. *Radiology* 1989;170:417–421.
2. Hessler C, Schnyder P, Ozzello L. Hamartoma of the breast: diagnostic observations of 16 cases. *Radiology* 1978;126:95–98.
3. Jackson FL, Lalani Z, Swallow J. Adenolipoma of the breast. *J Can Assoc Radiol* 1988;39:288–289.

Case 4

Case History

A 73-year-old professional violinist presents for a screening mammogram. She has a history of a soft mass in the upper outer left breast for more than 20 years.

Physical Examination

- left breast: very soft area of asymmetry in the upper outer quadrant
- right breast: normal exam

Mammogram

Mass

- margin: circumscribed
- shape: round
- density: fat-containing

Associated Findings

- completely fatty encapsulated mass in the upper outer quadrant of the left breast (Fig. 4–1)

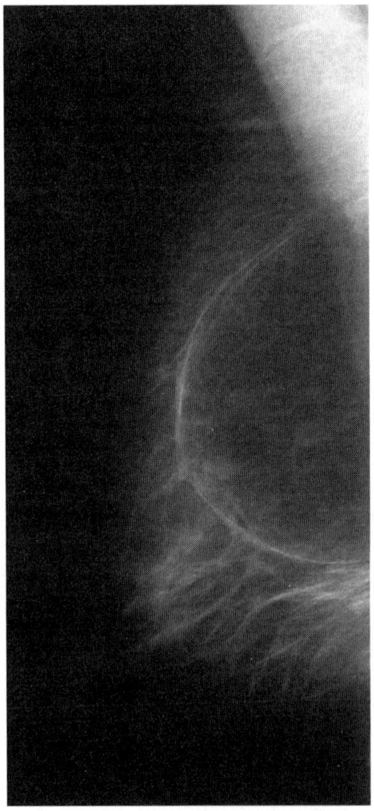

Figure 4–1. Right MLO mammogram: There is a large, well-defined radiolucent lipoma. The small nodule that projects in the center of the mass is a lymph node located just medial to the lipoma on the CC view.

Ultrasound

Frequency

- 11.5 MHz

Mass

- margin: well defined
- echogenicity: isoechoic
- retrotumoral acoustic appearance: no shadowing
- shape: ellipsoid (Figs. 4-2 and 4-3)

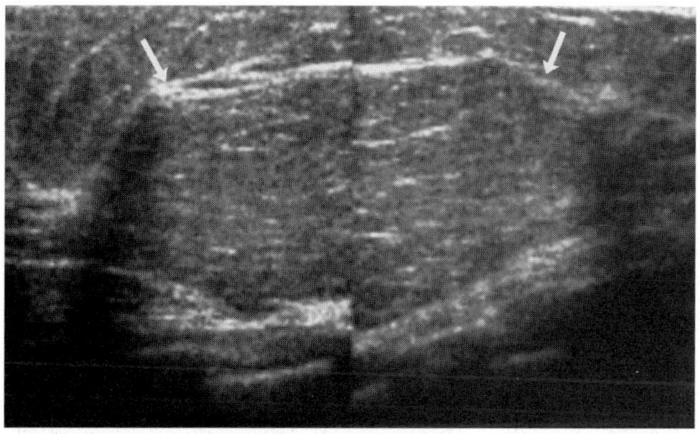

Figure 4-2. Left radial breast sonogram: Combined images of the upper outer quadrant show the margins of the lipoma (arrows). The mass created by the lipoma pushes the thin hyperechoic parenchymal lines (representing lobular regression) superiorly.

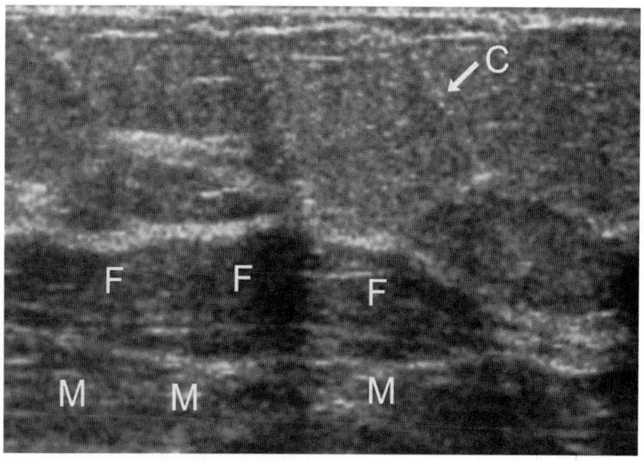

Figure 4-3. Left radial breast sonogram: Sonogram is in a normal portion of the same breast as Figure 4-2. This image is intended to demonstrate the normal architecture of the fatty breast parenchyma. F, fatty breast parenchyma; C, Cooper's ligaments; M, chest wall muscle.

Pathology

- lipoma

Management

- BI-RADS Assessment Category 2, benign finding

Pearls and Pitfalls

1. Mammographic fat-containing masses are benign so sonographic examination is generally not necessary. However, occasionally, a patient is referred for sonography for a palpable fatty mass that has not been mammographically characterized. In these cases it is important to be familiar with the sonographic appearance of fatty masses and recommend mammography to confirm the benign identity of the mass.
2. Sonographically, lipomas are generally oval and well defined. They are hypoechoic, isoechoic, hyperechoic, or heterogeneous in echogenicity. In a fatty breast, isoechoic tumors are sometimes difficult to identify. However, this case emphasizes that lipomas do not have the same internal architecture as normal fatty parenchyma. The echogenic lines within the lipoma do not follow a normal pattern of lobular regression.

Suggested Readings

1. Fornage BD, Tassin GB. Sonographic appearance of superficial soft tissue lipomas. *J Clin Ultrasound* 1991;19:215–220.

Case 5

Case History

A 73-year-old woman presents for screening mammogram.

Physical Examination

- normal exam

Mammogram

Mass (Fig. 5–1)

- margin: circumscribed
- shape: oval
- density: fat-containing

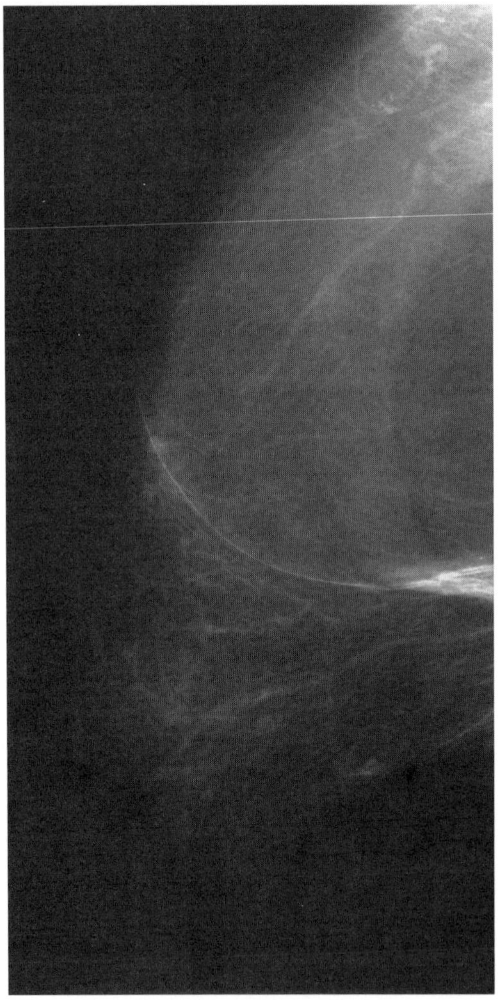

A

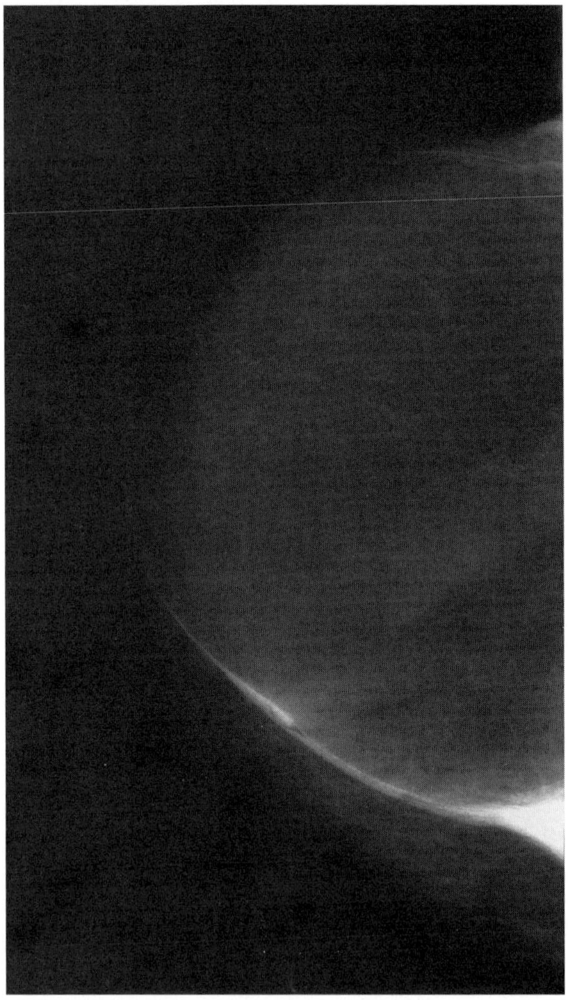

B

Figure 5–1. The right breast is dominated by a fat density mass. This mammographic appearance is diagnostic of a lipoma. (A). Right MLO mammogram. (B). Right CC mammogram.

Pathology

- lipoma

Management

- BI-RADS Assessment Category 2, benign finding

Pearls and Pitfalls

Lipomas are common benign breast masses. The average age of presentation is in the late 40s or early 50s. Generally, these tumors are unilateral. In 3% of cases, bilateral lipomas are present. Histologically, these tumors are composed of mature lipocytes surrounded by a capsule.

Suggested Readings

1. Tavassoli FA. Mesenchymal lesions. In: Tavassoli FA, Fattaneh A, eds. *Pathology of the Breast.* 2nd ed. Stamford: Appleton and Lange; 1999:675–729.

Case 6

Case History

A 48-year-old woman, status post lumpectomy 16 months ago. She now has a small palpable lump in her lumpectomy site. She is initially studied sonographically. Upon discovery of a sonographic nodule, mammographic examination has been performed.

Physical Examination

- left breast: 8 mm lump at the 6:00 position within the scar of her lumpectomy site
- right breast: normal exam

Mammogram

Mass (Fig. 6–1)

- margin: circumscribed
- shape: oval
- density: fat-containing

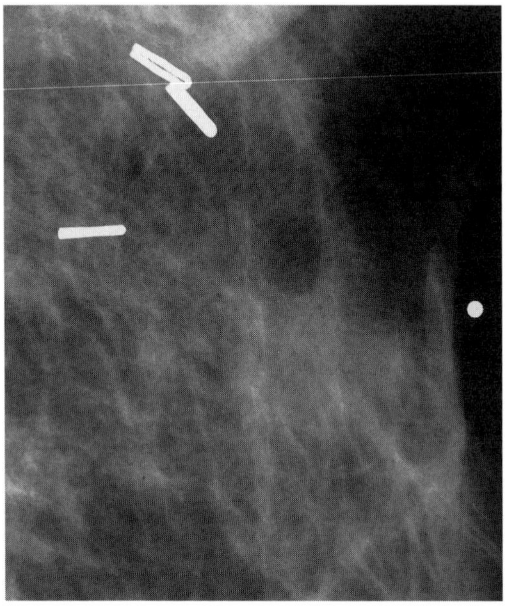

Figure 6–1. Left MLO magnification spot mammogram: In the region of the patient's lumpectomy site there is an oval radiolucent nodule.

Ultrasound

Frequency

- 13 MHz

Mass

- margin: well defined
- echogenicity: hypoechoic
- retrotumoral acoustic appearance: no shadowing
- shape: ellipsoid (Fig. 6–2)

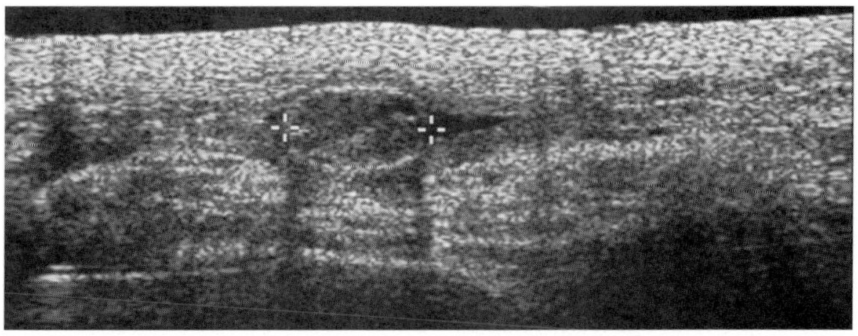

Figure 6–2. Left antiradial breast sonogram: A well-defined oval nodule corresponds to the palpable lump and the oval mammographic lucency. The nodule has a thin hyperechoic rim and a hypoechoic center.

Pathology

- oil cyst

Management

- BI-RADS Assessment Category 2, benign finding

Pearls and Pitfalls

The ultrasound nodule is consistent with either an organizing hematoma or an oil cyst. However, the mammographic fat density of the nodule is diagnostic of an oil cyst.

Suggested Readings

1. Tohno D, Cosgrove DO, Sloane JP. Benign processes—trauma and iatrogenic conditions. In: Tohno D, Cosgrove DO, Sloane JP, eds. *Ultrasound Diagnosis of Breast Diseases.* New York: Churchill Livingston; 1996:139–155.

Case 7

Case History

A 54-year-old woman is status post replacement of a left breast implant and now has a new mass on her screening mammogram.

Physical Examination

- normal exam

Mammogram

Mass (Fig. 7–1)

- margin: circumscribed
- shape: oval
- density: fat-containing

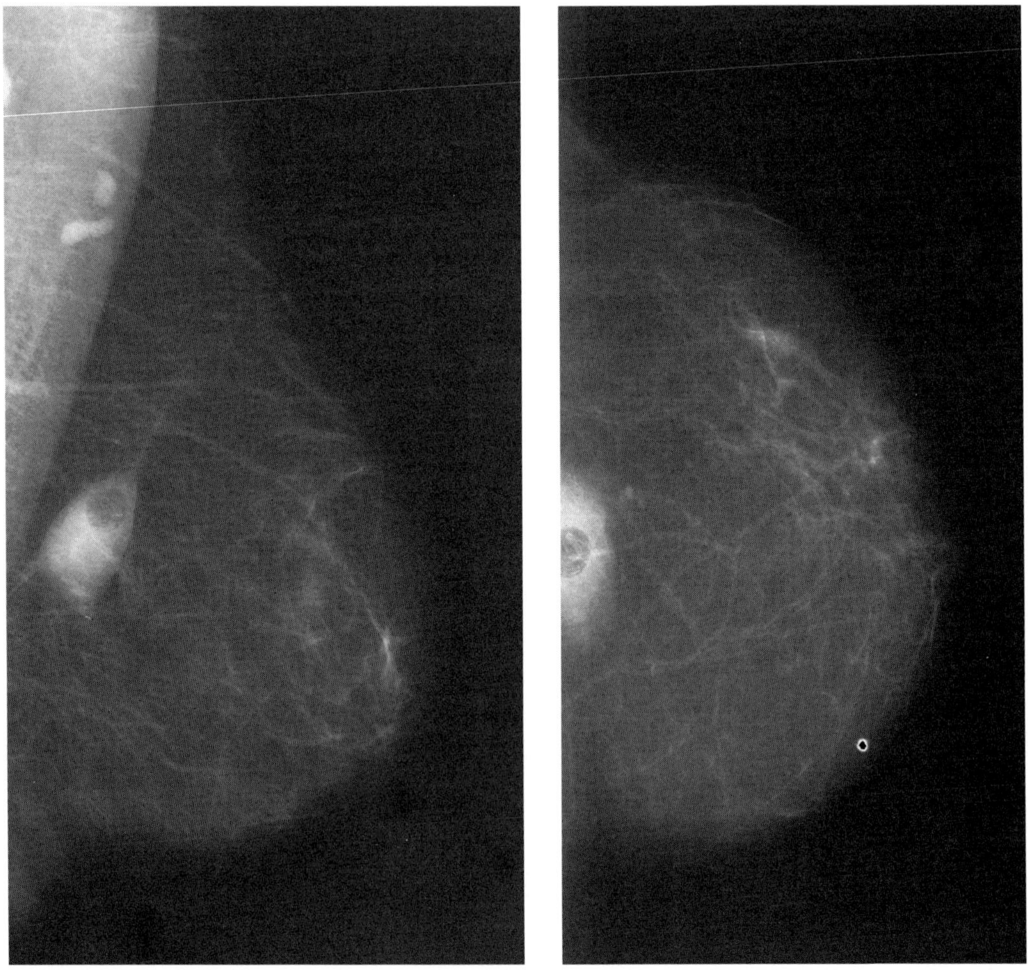

A B

Figure 7–1. Deep to the nipple in the posterior third of the left breast is a well-defined oval mass that contains a round lucent mass. (A). Left MLO mammogram. (B). Left CC mammogram.

Ultrasound

Frequency

- 7.5 MHz

Mass

- margin: well defined
- echogenicity: heterogeneous
- retrotumoral acoustic appearance: enhanced acoustic transmission
- shape: ellipsoid (Fig. 7–2)

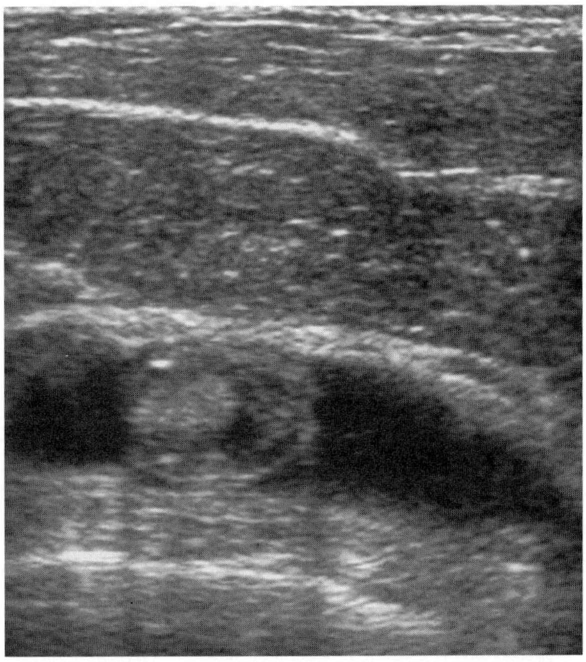

Figure 7–2. Left transverse breast sonogram: The mass identified in Figure 7–1 corresponds to an anechoic fluid-filled cyst that contains a round heterogeneous mass, which represents the lucent mammographic mass. In real time this heterogeneous mass moves with changes in patient position and floats to the top of the fluid.

Pathology

- oil cyst

Management

- BI-RADS Assessment Category 2, benign finding

Pearls and Pitfalls

1. The mammographic mass corresponds to an oil cyst that is floating within a water density cyst. The oil cyst represents fat necrosis that resulted from removal of the previous implant.
2. Sonographically, oil cysts are generally round or oval, hypoechoic, isoechoic, heterogeneous, or less commonly hyperechoic compared with fat. When the oil cyst is not calcified, sound transmission is generally increased or unchanged. As in this case, the identity of the oil cyst is clarified by the mammogram.

Suggested Readings

1. Heywang-Kobrunner SH, Schreer I, Dershaw DD. Post-traumatic, post-surgical and post-therapeutic changes. In: Heywang-Kobrunner SH, Schreer I, Dershaw DD. *Diagnostic Breast Imaging*. New York: Thieme; 1997:280–316.

Case 8

Case History

A 68-year-old woman presents with a new mass on her left screening mammogram.

Physical Examination

- normal exam

Mammogram

Mass (Fig. 8–1)

- margin: circumscribed
- shape: oval
- density: equal density

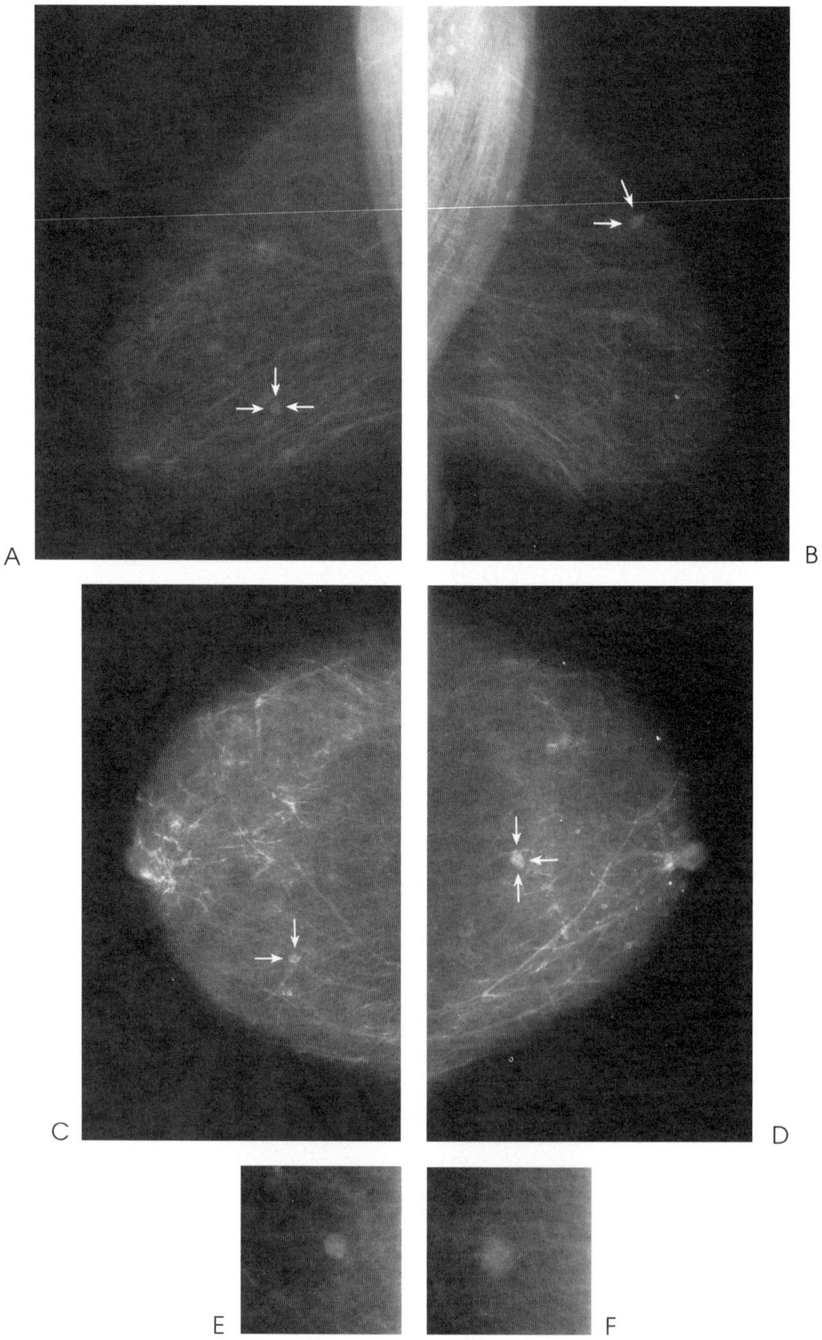

Figure 8–1. At the 12:00 position of the left breast and the 3:00 position of the right breast there are two oval masses (arrows). The spot compression views demonstrate that the margins of the right mass are well defined and the margins of the left mass are ill defined. (A). Right MLO mammogram. (B). Left MLO mammogram. (C). Right CC mammogram. (D). Left CC mammogram. (E). Right CC spot compression mammogram. (F). Left CC spot compression mammogram.

Ultrasound

Frequency

- 10 MHz

Mass

- margin: ill defined
- echogenicity: hyperechoic
- retrotumoral acoustic appearance: no shadowing
- shape: ellipsoid (Figs. 8–2 and 8–3)

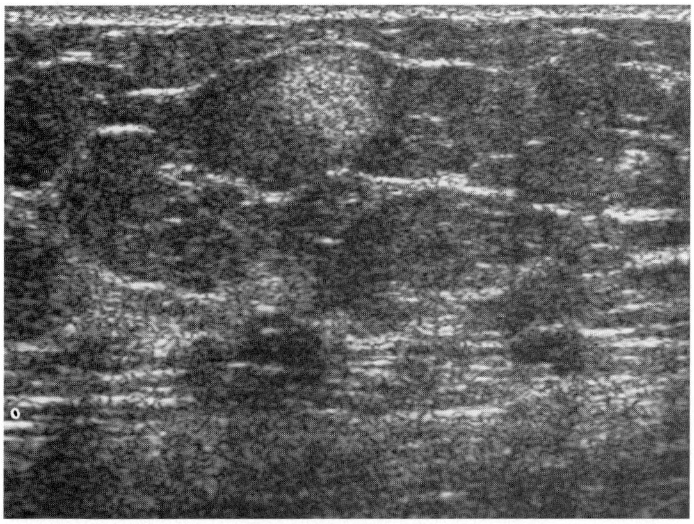

Figure 8–2. Right radial breast sonogram: The right mammographic mass identified in Figure 8–1 corresponds to an oval well-defined hyperechoic mass.

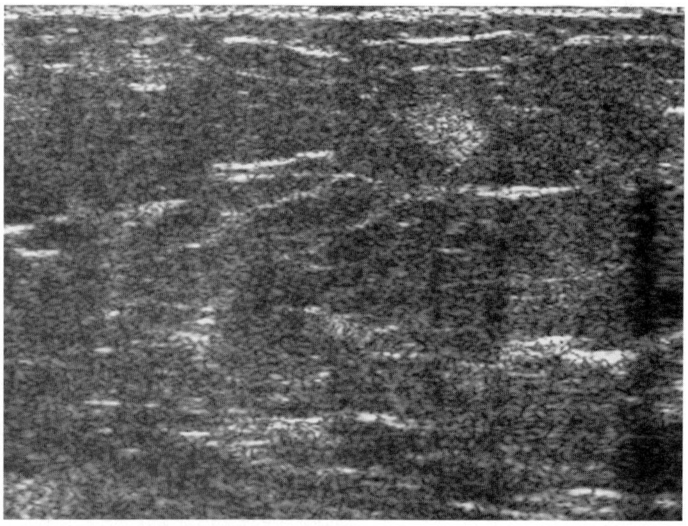

Figure 8–3. Left radial breast sonogram: The left mammographic mass identified in Figure 8–1 corresponds to a hyperechoic mass similar to the right breast mass.

Pathology

- angiolipoma

Management

- BI-RADS Assessment Category 4, suspicious; biopsy should be considered

Pearls and Pitfalls

1. Uniformly hyperechoic sonographic masses are generally benign, but the Category 4 (suspicious) assessment is based upon the information that the masses are new and the left mass is mildly ill defined mammographically.
2. Clinically, angiolipomas resemble lipomas. Over 75% of patients are older than 50 years. Angiolipomas in other sites of the body generally are associated with pain. However, breast angiolipomas are generally painless. Microscopically, the mass consists of mature lipocytes associated with an extensive vascular network. Microthrombi are a prominent feature of the lesion. This mass is benign and does not recur.

Suggested Readings

1. Brown RW, Bhathal PS, Scott PR. Multiple bilateral angiolipomas of the breast. *Aust NZ J Surg* 1982;52:614–616.
2. Fleishman JS, Schwartz RA. Angiolipoma presenting as a breast mass. *Ariz Med* 1980;37:403–404.
3. Sibala JL, Chang CH, Lin F, et al. Computer tomography of angiolipoma of the breast. *AJR* 1980;134:840–841.

Case 9

Case History

A 43-year-old woman presents for screening mammogram.

Physical Examination

- bilateral lumpy breasts; no new lumps

Mammogram

Mass (Fig. 9–1)

- margin: circumscribed
- shape: oval
- density: equal density

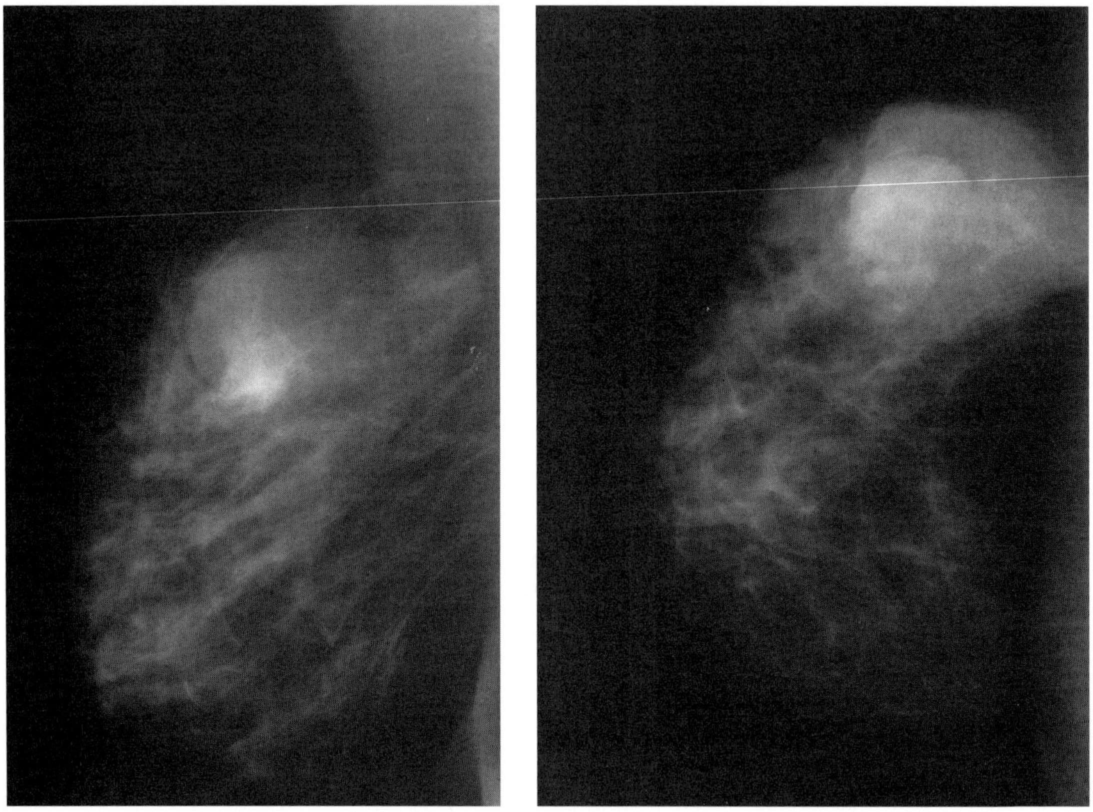

A B

Figure 9–1. In the upper outer quadrant of the right breast there is an oval mass. Part of its margin is obscured by surrounding dense tissue and part of the margin is associated with a lucent halo. (A). Right MLO mammogram. (B). Right CC mammogram.

Ultrasound

Frequency

- 10 MHz

Mass

- margin: well defined
- echogenicity: anechoic
- retrotumoral acoustic appearance: increased acoustic transmission
- shape: ellipsoid (Fig. 9–2)

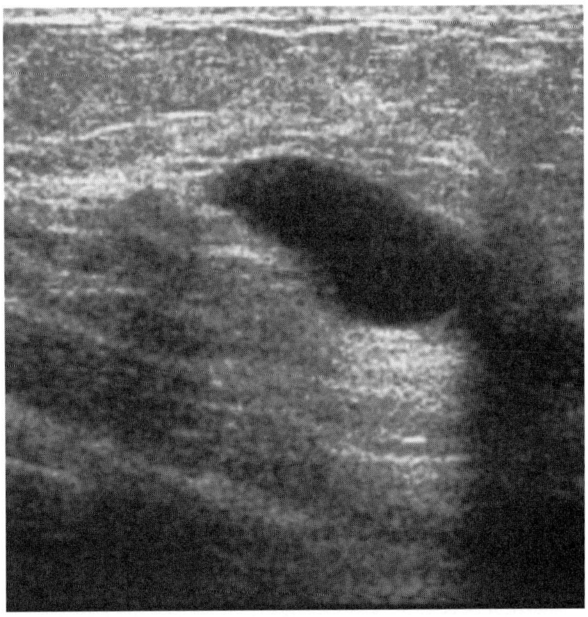

Figure 9–2. Right radial breast sonogram: The mass identified in Figure 9–1 corresponds to a simple cyst. The fluid collection is anechoic with increased acoustic transmission.

Pathology

- cyst

Management

- BI-RADS Assessment Category 2, benign finding

Pearls and Pitfalls

1. Cysts are a component of fibrocystic change. This entity is considered a physiologic developmental process in which there is cystic dilatation of the terminal duct/lobular units. As a result of this origin, the cysts are lined either with epithelial-myoepithelial cells or by metaplastic apocrine cells.
2. Sonography is an excellent method to identify cysts and has been shown to accurately identify cysts in 96 to 100% of cases. As long as the wall of the cyst is well defined, thin, and hyperechoic, small moving particles within a cyst are generally not clinically significant.

Suggested Readings

1. Azzopardi JGK. *Problems in Breast Pathology.* Philadelphia: WB Saunders; 1979:57–72.
2. Murad TM, von Haam E. The ultrastructure of fibrocystic disease of the breast. *Cancer* 1968;22:587–600.
3. Tavassoli FA. Benign lesions. In: Tavassoli FA, Fattaneh A, eds. *Pathology of the Breast.* 2nd ed. Stamford: Appleton and Lange; 1999:115–204.
4. Hilton SVW, Leopold GR, Olson LK, Willson SA. Realtime breast sonography: application in 300 consecutive patients. *AJR* 1988;150:789–790.
5. Jellins J, Kossoff G, Reeve TS. Detection and classification of liquid-filed masses in the breast by gray scale echography. *Radiology* 1977;125:205–212.
6. Sickles EA, Filly RA, Callen PW. Benign breast lesions: ultrasound detection and diagnosis. *Radiology* 1984;151:467–470.

Case 10

Case History

A 51-year-old woman presents for screening mammogram.

Physical Examination

- normal exam

Mammogram

Mass (Fig. 10–1)

- margin: circumscribed
- shape: oval
- density: equal density

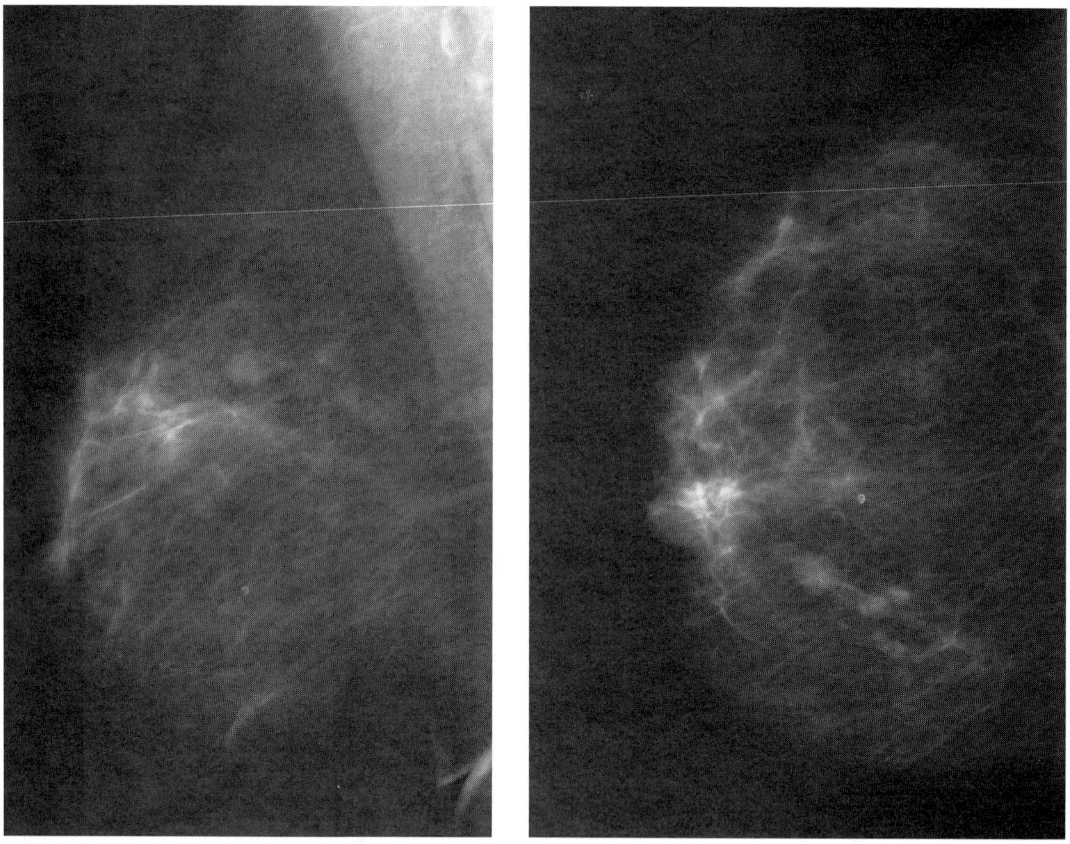

Figure 10–1. In the upper inner quadrant of the right breast, there are two dominant well-defined oval masses. (A). Right MLO mammogram. (B). Right CC mammogram.

Ultrasound

Frequency

- 11.5 MHz

Mass

- margin: well defined
- echogenicity: anechoic
- retrotumoral acoustic appearance: increased acoustic transmission
- shape: ellipsoid (Fig. 10–2)

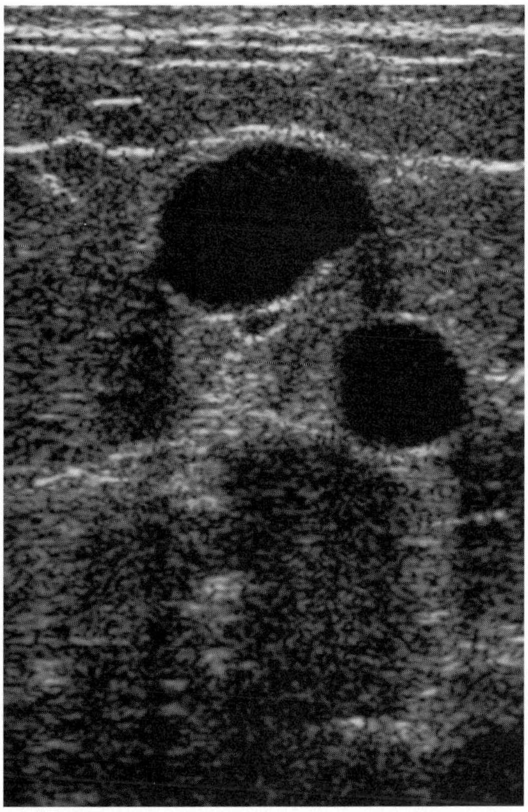

Figure 10–2. Right transverse breast sonogram: The two mammographic masses correspond to two cysts. The fluid collections are anechoic; have well-defined, thin, hyperechoic walls; and have increased acoustic transmission.

Pathology

- cysts

Management

- BI-RADS Assessment Category 2, benign finding

Pearls and Pitfalls

Cysts are a component of fibrocystic change. This process has been identified clinically in about one third of women between 20 and 45 years of age. Autopsy studies have found about 54% of normal breasts have histologic evidence of cystic changes.

Suggested Readings

1. Frantz VK, Pickren JW, Melcher GE, et al. Incidence of chronic cystic disease in so called "normal breasts." A study based on 225 postmortem examinations. *Cancer* 1951;4:762–783.
2. Jones BM, Bradbeber JW. The presentation and progress of macroscopic breast cysts. *Br J Surg* 1980;67:669–671.
3. Leis HP, Kwon CS. Fibrocystic disease of the breast. *J Reprod Med* 1979;22:291–296.
4. Leis HP Jr. Fibrocystic disease of the breast. *J Med Assoc Alabama* 1962;32:97–104.
5. Love SM, Gelman RS, Silen W. Fibrocystic "disease" of the breast—a non-disease. *N Engl J Med* 1982;307:1010–1014.

Case 11

Case History

A 48-year-old woman presents for screening mammogram.

Physical Examination

- no new breast lumps; both breasts normally lumpy

Mammogram

Mass (Fig. 11–1)

- margin: circumscribed
- shape: oval
- density: equal density

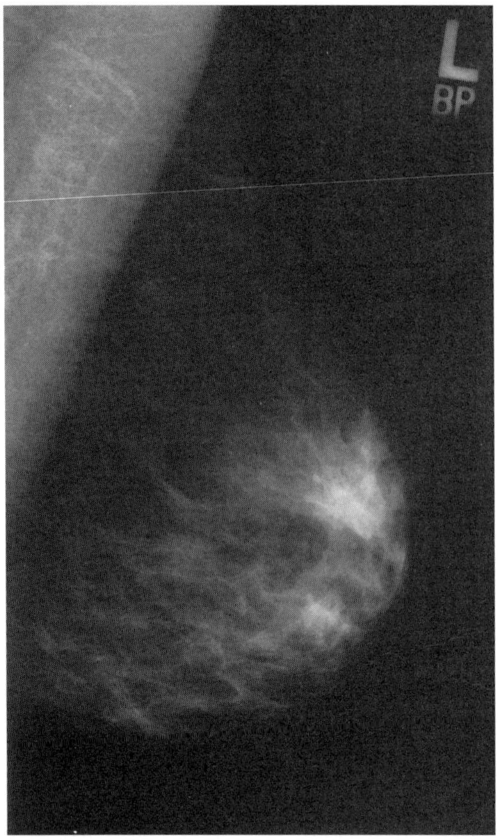
A

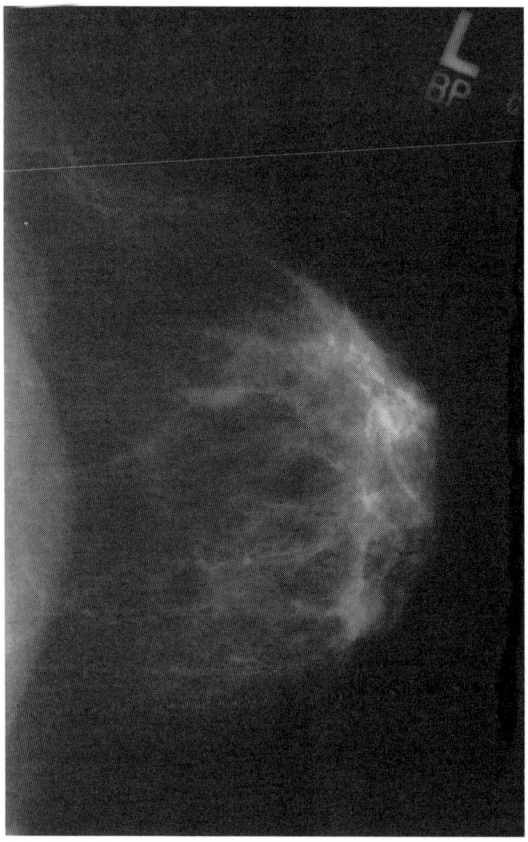
B

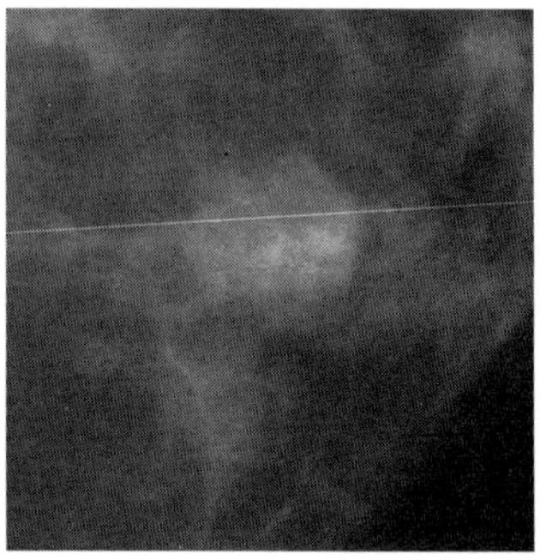
C

Figure 11–1. In the left inferior inner quadrant, there is a circumscribed mass. This mass was new compared to previous exams. (A). Left MLO mammogram. (B). Left CC mammogram. (C). Left CC spot compression mammogram.

Ultrasound

Frequency

- 7.5 MHz

Mass

- margin: well defined
- echogenicity: heterogeneous
- retrotumoral acoustic appearance: bilateral edge shadowing
- shape: ellipsoid (Fig. 11–2)

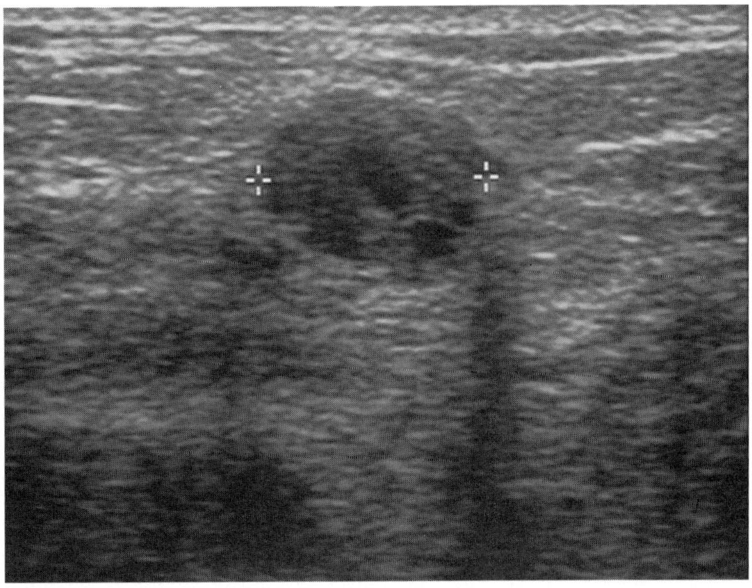

Figure 11–2. Left longitudinal breast sonogram: The mammographic mass corresponds to a well-defined sonographic mass that is predominantly isoechoic to fat with a few anechoic oval lucencies within it. This mass was biopsied and found to be a complex benign cyst.

Pathology

- cyst

Management

- BI-RADS Assessment Category 4, suspicious; biopsy should be considered

Pearls and Pitfalls

Sonography usually is successful in identifying benign cysts. However, occasionally, cysts exhibit internal echoes. These echoes may be caused by poor sonographic technique (e.g., gain settings too high), artifact (e.g., reverberation), proteinaceous debris, hemorrhage, infected debris, or cholesterol crystals. If the material completely moves, then the cyst is probably benign. However, if the material does not move, then an intracystic mass should be considered. In these cases, either aspiration or biopsy should be performed to identify intracystic tumors; 75% of solid intracystic masses are benign (mostly papillomas), 20% malignant, and 5% are phyllodes tumors.

Suggested Readings

1. Khaleghian R. Breast cysts: pitfalls in sonographic diagnosis. *Australas Radiol* 1993;37:192–194.
2. Sohn C, Blohmer J-U, Hamper UM. Fibrocystic changes and breast cysts. In: Sohn C, Blohmer J-U, Hamper UM, eds. *Breast Ultrasound.* New York: Thieme; 1999:75–90.
3. Stavros AT, Dennis MA. The ultrasound of breast pathology. In: Parker SH, Jobe WE, eds. *Percutaneous Breast Biopsy.* New York: Raven Press; 1993:111–127.

Case 12

Case History

A 32-year-old woman presents with a new left breast lump. She is diabetic and has been insulin dependent since childhood.

Physical Examination

- left breast: large hard mass at the 3:00 position
- right breast: normal exam

Mammogram

Mass (Fig. 12–1)

- margin: circumscribed
- shape: oval
- density: high density

Figure 12–1. In the 3:00 to 4:00 position of the left breast, there is a circumscribed oval mass that corresponds to the palpable mass designated by the metallic marker. (A). Left MLO mammogram. (B). Left CC mammogram.

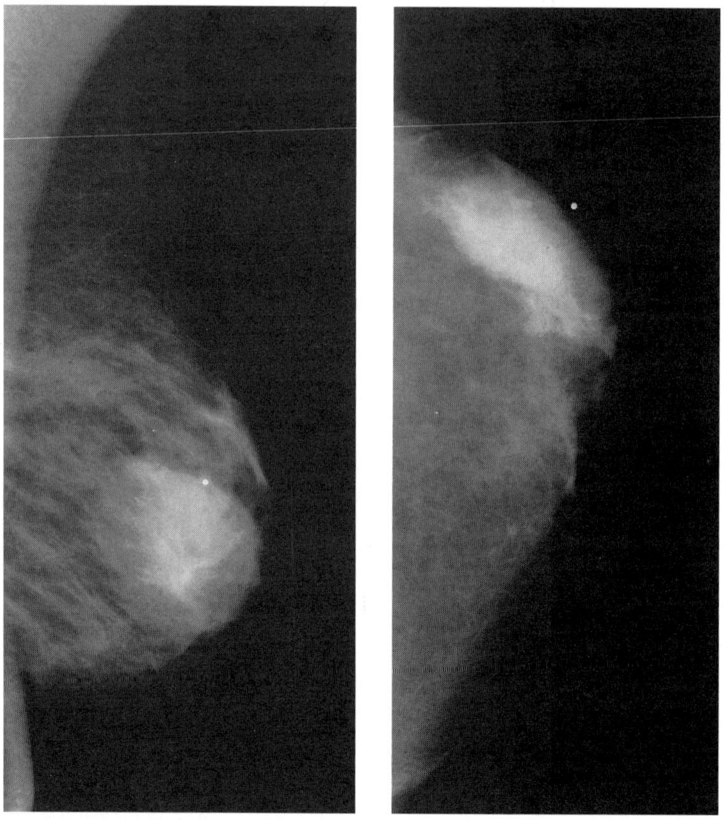

A B

Ultrasound

Low Frequency

Frequency

- 8 MHz

Mass

- margin: ill defined
- echogenicity: hypoechoic
- retrotumoral acoustic appearance: severe shadowing, mass completely obscured
- shape: irregular (Fig. 12–2)

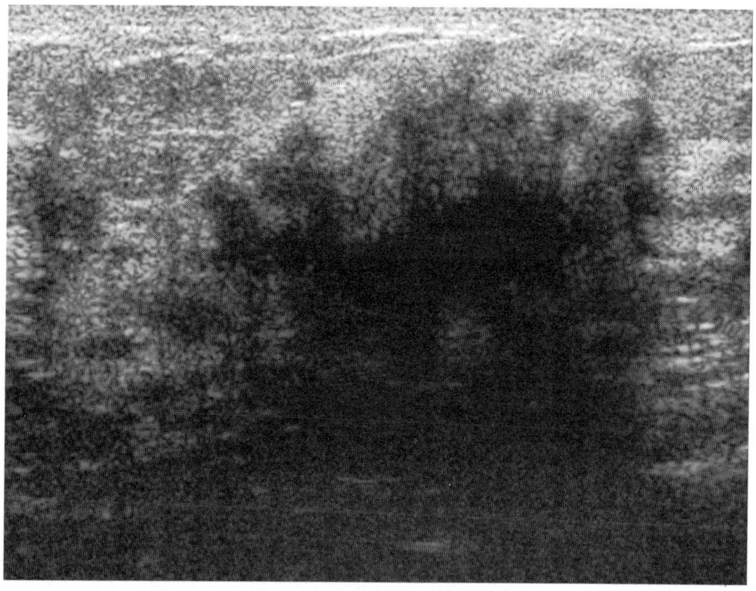

Figure 12–2. Left radial breast sonogram: Examination of the same mass as Figure 12–3 demonstrates that as the frequency decreases, the mass attenuates the sound less so the internal details of the mass becomes more apparent. The mass has a predominantly hyperechoic periphery with multiple linear lucencies centrally.

High Frequency

Frequency

- 13 MHz

Associated Findings

Lower frequency is more informative than high frequency for masses that severely attenuate sound because the internal architecture of the shadowing lesion is better displayed with the lower frequency. (See Fig. 12–3.)

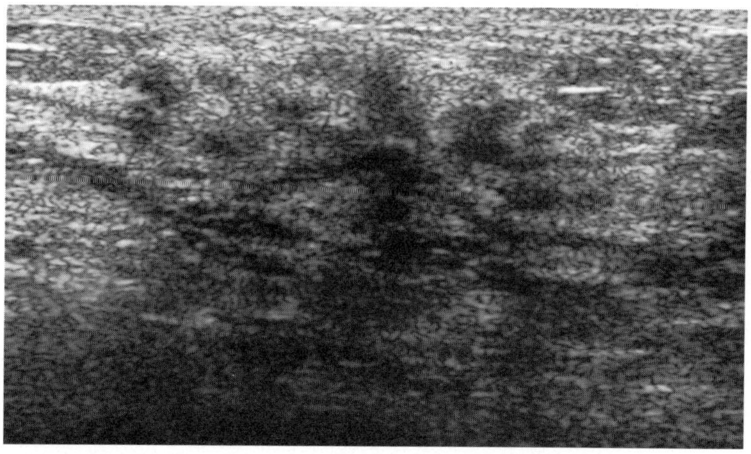

Figure 12–3. Left radial breast sonogram: With high frequency, the palpable mass attenuates the sound so only a heavily shadowing area is evident.

Pathology

- diabetic mastopathy

Management

- BI-RADS Assessment Category 4, suspicious; biopsy should be considered

Pearls and Pitfalls

1. Occasionally diabetes will affect the breast causing diabetic mastopathy. Microscopically, diabetic mastopathy consists of perivasculitis, keloid-like fibrosis, and ductitis and/or lobulitis. Clinically, this abnormality presents as a hard breast mass. The palpable mass cannot be distinguished from malignancy. However, this presentation in a young woman who has had long-term insulin dependence should be a strong clue to the diagnosis.
2. The mammographic findings of diabetic mastopathy include a diffusely dense breast, asymmetric focal density, an irregular mass, and less commonly a circumscribed mass.
3. Sonographically, the fibrosis strongly attenuates sound, so usually only shadowing is evident. With very low frequencies, the internal architecture of the mass is identified.

Suggested Readings

1. Boullu S, Andrac L, Piana L, Darmon P, Dutour A, Oliver C. Diabetic mastopathy, complication of type 1 diabetes mellitus: report of two cases and a review of the literature. *Diabete Metab* 1998;24:448–454.
2. Byrd BF, Hartmann WH, Graham LS, Hoble HH. Mastopathy in insulin-dependent diabetics. *Ann Surg* 1987;205:529–532.
3. Hunfeld KP, Bassler R. Lymphocytic mastitis and fibrosis of the breast in long-standing insulin-dependent diabetics. *Gen Diagn Pathol* 1997;143:49–58.
4. Pluchinotta AM, Talenti E, Lodovichetti G, Tiso E, Biral M. Diabetic fibrous breast disease: a clinical entity that mimics cancer. *Eur J Surg Oncol* 1995;21:207–209.
5. Seidman JD, Schnaper LA, Phillips LE. Mastopathy in insulin-requiring diabetes mellitus. *Hum Pathol* 1994;25:819–824.

Case 13

Case History

A 40-year-old woman presents with a palpable left breast lump.

Physical Examination

- left breast: palpable lump in left lateral breast
- right breast: normal exam

Mammogram

Mass (Fig. 13–1)

- margin: well defined
- shape: oval
- density: equal

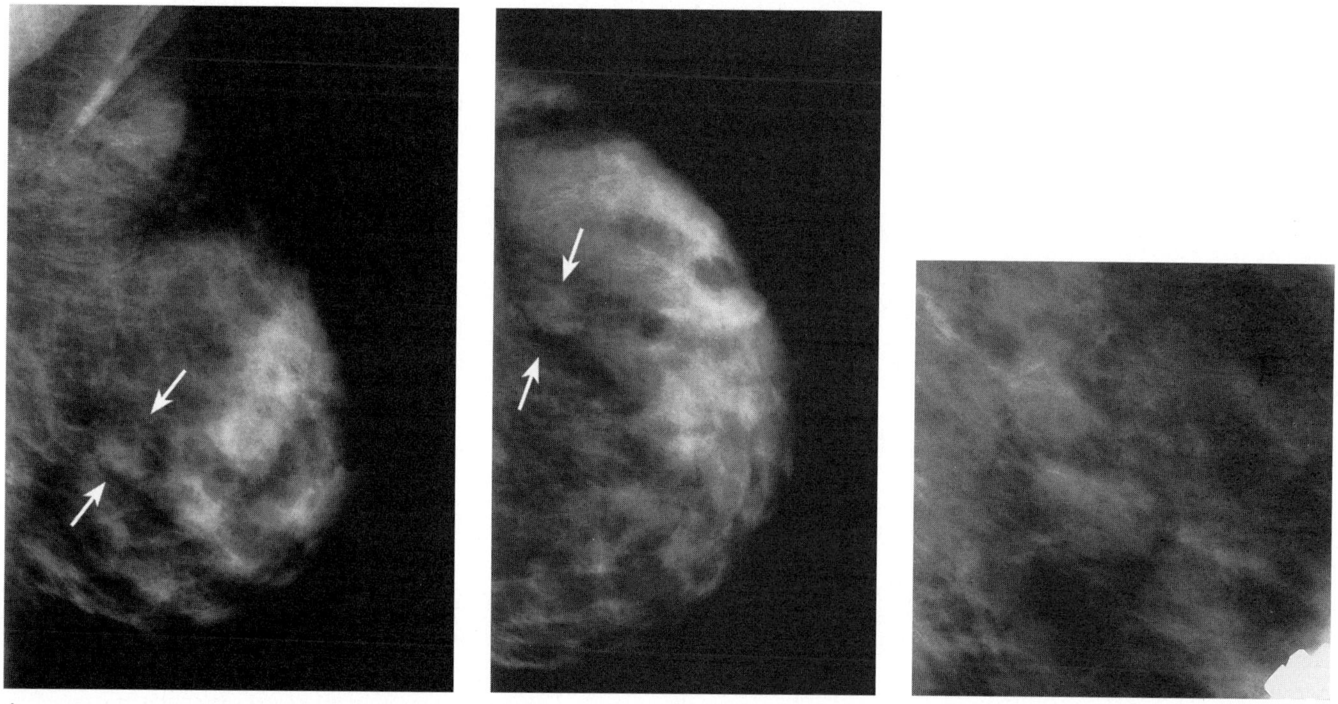

A B C

Figure 13–1. At the 3:00 position of the left breast, there is an oval mass (arrows). The spot compression view demonstrates that the mass has well-defined margins and a lucent halo around part of the border. (A). Left MLO mammogram. (B). Left CC mammogram. (C). Left MLO spot compression mammogram.

Ultrasound

Frequency

- 10 MHz

Mass

- margin: well defined
- echogenicity: hypoechoic
- retrotumoral acoustic appearance: no shadowing
- shape: oval (Fig. 13–2)

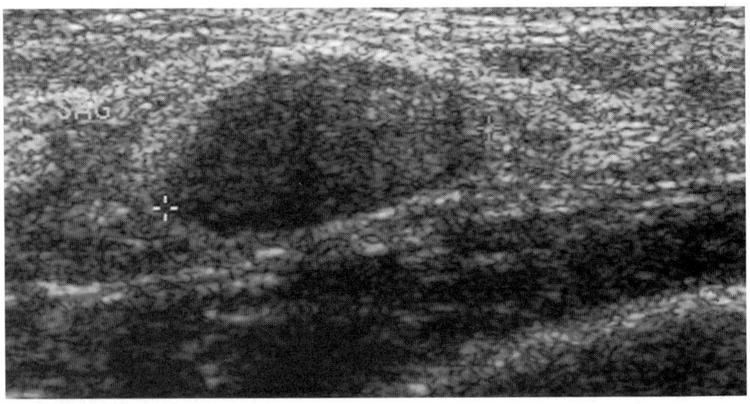

Figure 13–2. Left radial breast sonogram: The oval mammographic density identified in Figure 13–1 corresponds to a well-defined hypoechoic solid mass.

Pathology

- Fibroadenoma

Management

- BI-RADS Assessment Category 3, probably benign; short-interval follow-up

Pearls and Pitfalls

Sonographically, if the mass has a well-defined margin, hyperechoic thin capsule, and no shadowing and is also homogeneously hypoechoic, then the chances of malignancy are very low (<5%). Since this mass represents a new palpable lump that has not been identified previously, we chose short-term follow-up to assess growth rate and stability of appearance. However, the patient chose to biopsy this lesion.

Suggested Readings

1. Cole-Beuglet C, Skoriano RZ, Kurtz AB, Goldberg BB. Fibroadenoma of the breast: sonomammographically correlated with pathology in 122 patients. *AJR* 1983;140:369–375.
2. Fornage BD, Lorigan JB, Andry E. Fibroadenoma of the breast: sonographic appearance. *Radiology* 1989;172:671–675.
3. Jackson VP, Rothschild PA, Kreipke DL, et al. The spectrum of sonographic findings of fibroadenoma of the breast. *Invest Radiol* 1986;21:34–40.
4. Stavros AT, Thickman D, Rapp CL, Dennis MA, Parker SH, Sisney GA. Solid breast nodules: use of sonography to distinguish between benign and malignant lesions. *Radiology* 1995;196:123–134.

Case 14

Case History

A 48-year-old woman presents with a new palpable right lump.

Physical Examination

- right breast: palpable lump at the 10:00 position
- left breast: normal exam

Mammogram

Mass (Fig. 14–1)

- margin: obscured
- shape: oval
- density: equal density

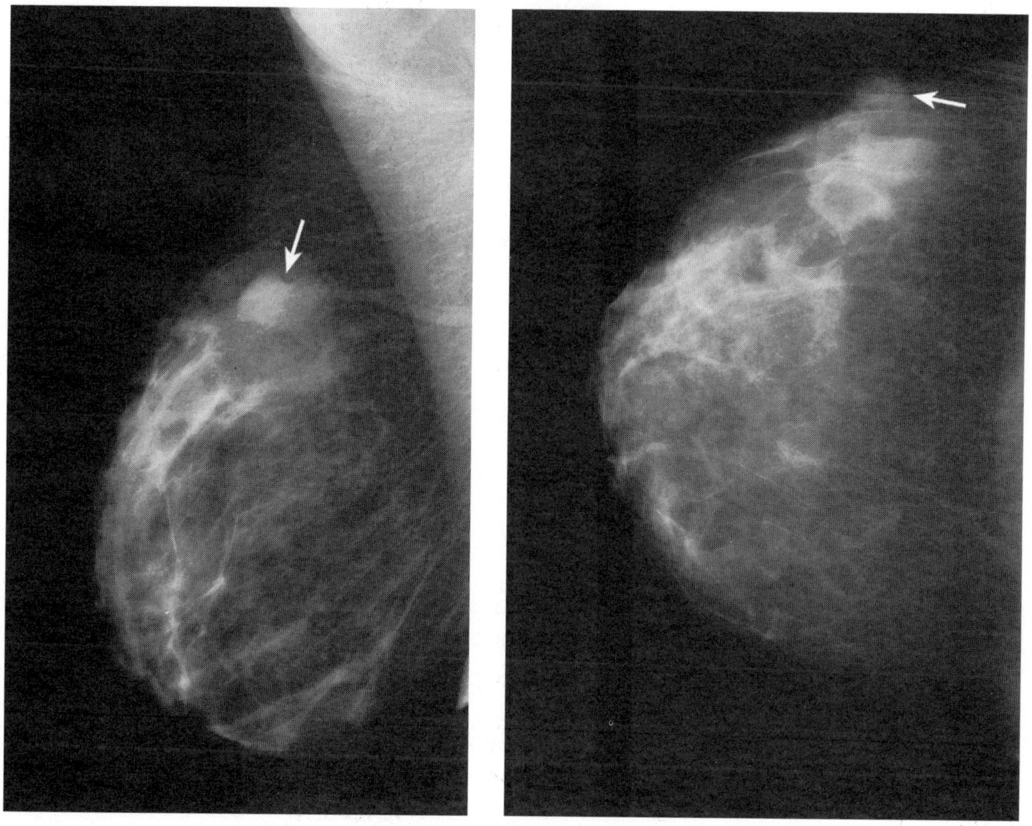

A B

Figure 14–1. In the right upper outer quadrant, there is an oval mass (arrow) with obscured margins, which corresponds to the palpable lump demarcated with a metallic marker. (A). Right MLO mammogram. (B). Right CC mammogram.

Ultrasound

Frequency

- 13 MHz

Mass

- margin: well defined
- echogenicity: hypoechoic
- retrotumoral acoustic appearance: single edge shadowing
- shape: lobulated (Fig. 14–2)

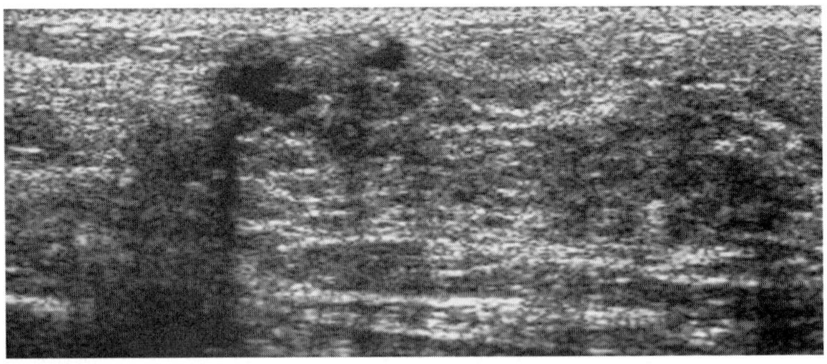

Figure 14–2. Right antiradial breast sonogram: At the 10:00 position, there is a hypoechoic, lobulated mass that corresponds to the mass identified in Figure 14–1.

Pathology

- fibrocystic changes
- stromal hyalization, microscopic cysts, and apocrine metaplasia

Management

- BI-RADS Assessment Category 4, suspicious; biopsy should be considered

Pearls and Pitfalls

1. In retrospect, the sonographic appearance of the mass correlates well with the histology as small cysts are evident within the lesion.
2. Fibrocystic changes generally cause symptoms in premenopausal women. About 75% of affected women are in the fourth or fifth decade. Three clinical stages have been described. Initially, women note premenstrual breast swelling or pain. Later, they develop breast lumps. Finally, the period of breast tenderness becomes continuous throughout the menstrual cycle. After menopause, the symptoms wane. Although at autopsy 25% of women have fibrocystic changes, only 10% of women older than 60 years have symptoms.

Suggested Readings

1. Leis HP, Kwon CS. Fibrocystic disease of the breast. *J Reprod Med* 1979;22:291–296.
2. Tavassoli FA. Benign lesions. In: Tavasolli FA, Fattaneh A, eds. *Pathology of the Breast.* 2nd ed. Stamford: Appleton and Lange; 1999:115–204.
3. Vorherr H. Fibrocystic breast disease: pathophysiology, pathomorphology, clinical picture and management. *Am J Obstet Gynecol* 1986;154:161–179.

Case 15

Case History

A 65-year-old woman presents for her first mammogram.

Physical Examination

- normal exam

Mammogram

Mass (Fig. 15–1)

- margin: circumscribed
- shape: oval
- density: equal density

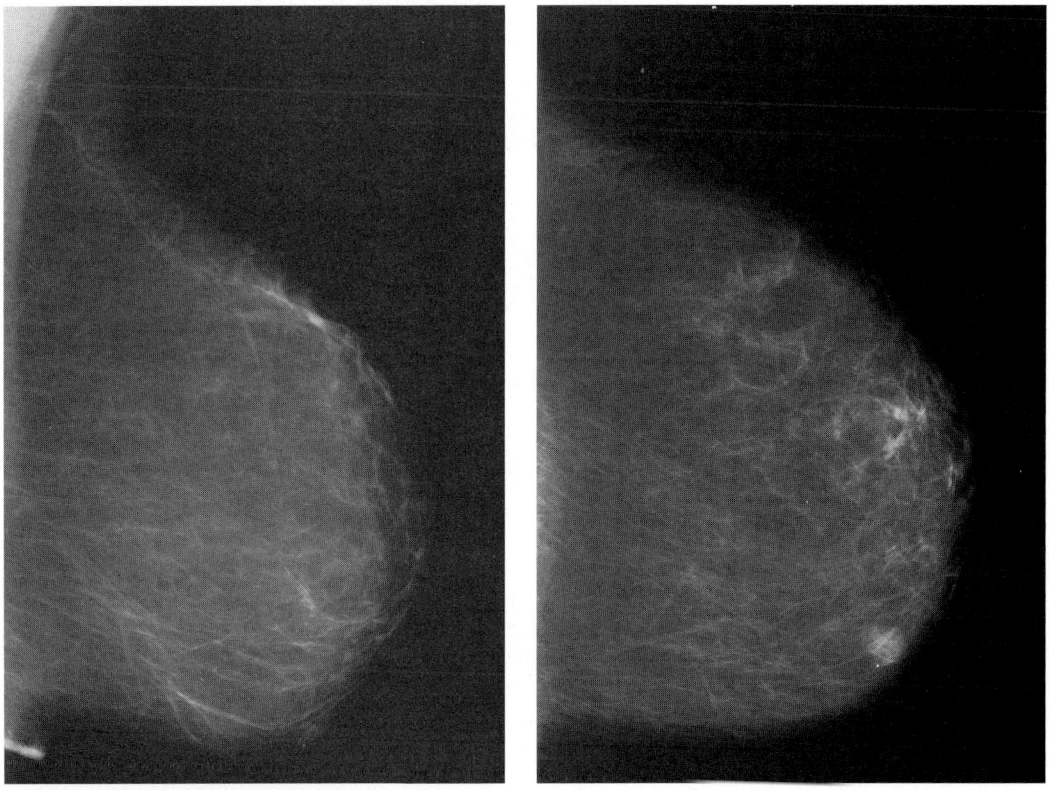

A B

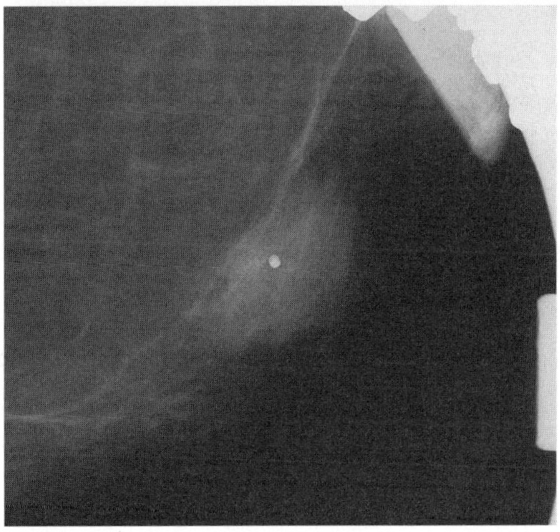

C

Figure 15–1. *In the inferior medial left breast, there is an oval mass with a single round calcification. The spot compression view suggests that the margins are ill defined. (A). Left MLO mammogram. (B). Left CC mammogram. (C). Left MLO spot compression mammogram.*

Ultrasound

Frequency

- 7.5 MHz

Mass

- margin: well defined
- echogenicity: heterogeneous
- retrotumoral acoustic appearance: posterior shadowing distal to mass
- shape: ellipsoid (Fig. 15-2)

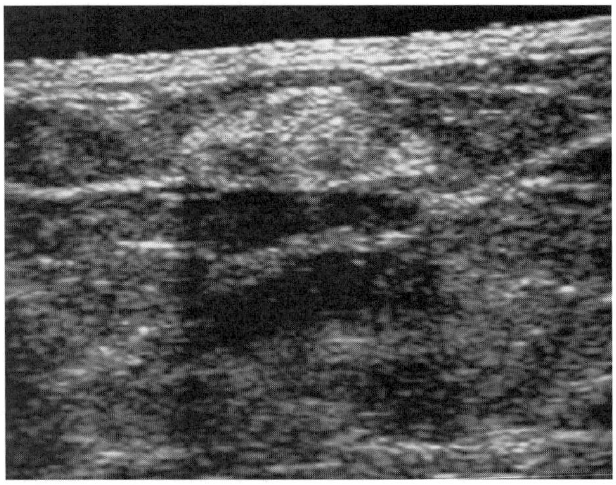

Figure 15-2. Left radial breast sonogram: At the 8:00 position of the left breast there is a well-defined oval mass of heterogeneous (predominantly hyperechoic) echogenicity.

Pathology

- fibrocystic change
- hyalin sclerosis (fibrosis)

Management

- BI-RADS Assessment Category 4, suspicious; biopsy should be considered

Pearls and Pitfalls

1. The recommendation for biopsy is based on the mildly ill-defined mammographic margins and the mildly heterogeneous sonographic echogenicity.
2. When fibrocystic changes produce a circumscribed mammographic mass, the sonographic findings correspond to either a cyst or a focal solid mass. The sonographic appearance of a solid mass is variable and biopsy is generally required. The sonographic fibrocystic masses may be either well or ill defined. They may be hyperechoic, hypoechoic, or heterogeneous echogenicity.

Suggested Readings

1. Love SM, Gelman RS, Silen W. Fibrocystic "disease" of the breast—a non-disease. *N Engl J Med* 1982;307:1010-1014.
2. Teboul M, Halliwell M. *Atlas of Ultrasound and Ductal Echography of the Breast.* 2nd ed. Cambridge: Blackwell Science; 1996:106-110, 180-185.
3. Tohno D, Cosgrove DO, Sloane JP. Benign breast change. In: Tohno D, Cosgrove DO, Sloane JP, eds. *Ultrasound Diagnosis of Breast Diseases.* New York: Churchill Livingston;

Case 16

Case History

A 53-year-old woman presents with a new area of bruising in the right upper breast. She does not remember any trauma. She feels a lump under the bruise.

Physical Examination

- right breast: ecchymosis associated with a palpable nodule in the upper breast at approximately 12:00
- left breast: normal exam

Mammogram

Mass (Fig. 16–1)

- margin: circumscribed
- shape: lobular
- density: equal density

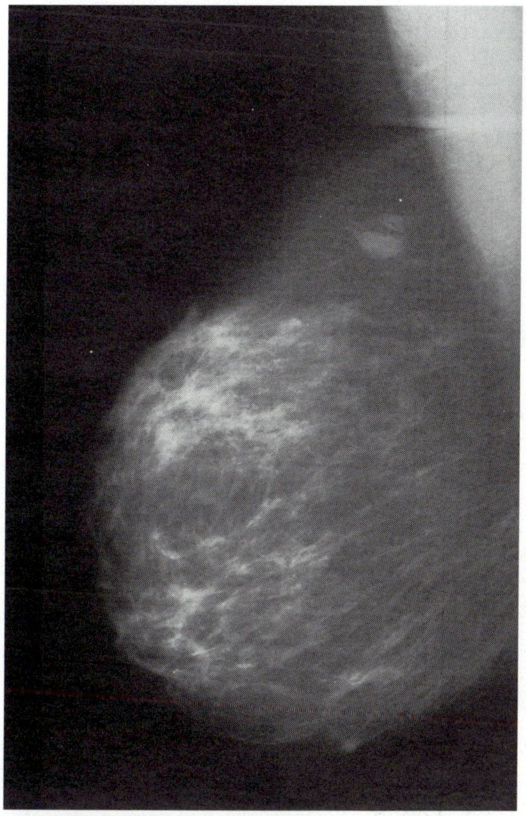
A

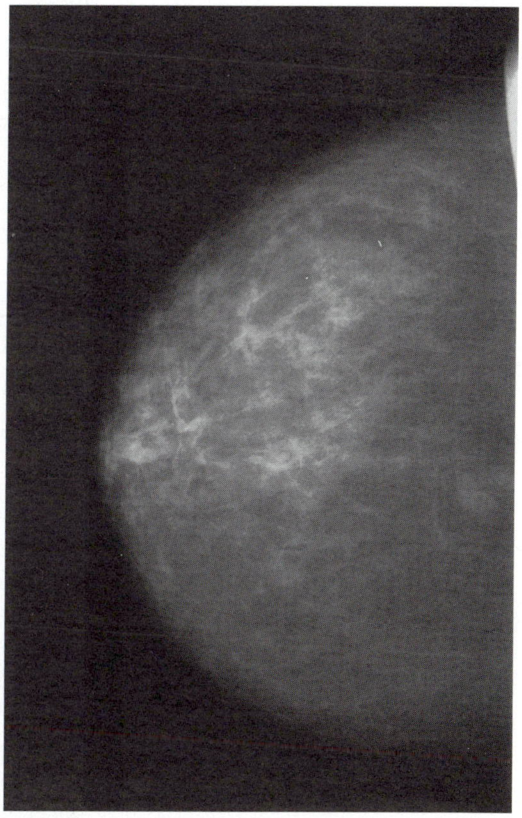
B

C

Figure 16–1. At the 12:00 position of the right breast, there is a lobulated density. (A). Right MLO mammogram. (B). Right CC mammogram. (C). Right CC spot compression mammogram.

Ultrasound

Frequency

- 7 MHz

Mass

- margin: well defined
- echogenicity: heterogeneous
- retrotumoral acoustic appearance: bilateral edge shadowing
- shape: ellipsoid (Figs. 16–2 and 16–3)

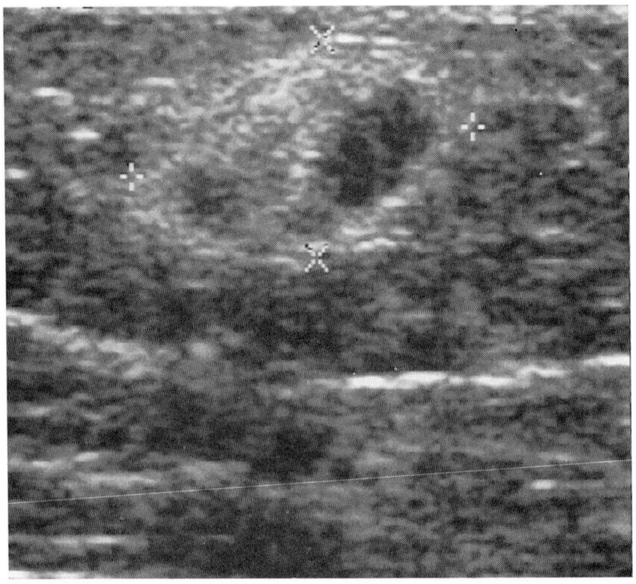

Figure 16–2. Right radial breast sonogram: The mammographic density identified in Figure 16–1 corresponds to an oval mass of heterogeneous echogenicity with a hyperechoic rim.

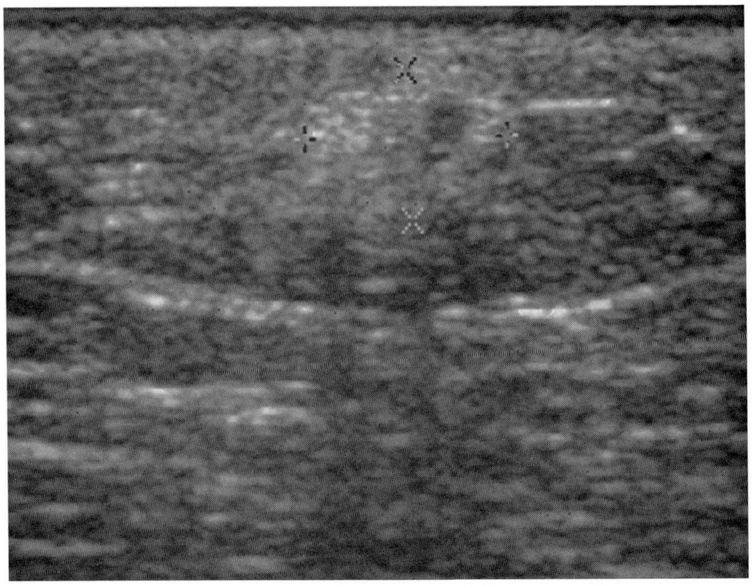

Figure 16–3. Right radial breast sonogram: One month after the sonogram performed in Figure 16–2, the sonographic mass is smaller and has changed in appearance to an oval, predominantly hyperechoic mass. This change in size and appearance is consistent with a healing hematoma.

Pathology

- hematoma

Management

- BI-RADS Assessment Category 3, probably benign; short-interval follow-up

Pearls and Pitfalls

1. Mammographically, acute hematomas are ill-defined or, less frequently, well-defined masses. As the hematoma resolves, a seroma or oil cyst may form, producing a well-defined round or oval mass. Finally, as the hematoma becomes fibrotic, the scar produces an irregular density or architectural distortion. The diagnosis of a breast hematoma rarely requires imaging, since there is usually a clear history of trauma or surgery. In this case, a mammogram 2 years later demonstrates complete resolution of the hematoma.
2. Sonographically, hematomas are uniformly hypochoic or mixed echogenicity. They should demonstrate no internal flow with color Doppler and should decrease in size on subsequent exams.

Suggested Readings

1. Harlow CL, Schackmuth EM, Bregma PS, Zeligman BE, Coffin CT. Sonographic detection of hematomas and fluid after imaging guided core breast biopsy. *J Ultrasound Med* 1994;13:877–882.
2. Stigers KB, King JG, Davey DD, Stelling CB. Abnormalities of the breast caused by biopsy: spectrum of mammographic findings. *AJR* 1991;156:287–291.

Case 17

Case History

A 67-year-old woman presents with an enlarging left breast mass.

Physical Examination

- left breast: multiple stable lumps; enlarging mass cannot be palpated
- right breast: normal exam

Mammogram

Mass (Fig. 17–1)

- margin: obscured
- shape: oval
- density: equal density

Figure 17–1. In the left upper outer quadrant, there is an oval mass (arrows) with obscured margins. The radiopaque circle and dot markers denote a skin lesion in the upper inner breast. (A). Left MLO mammogram. (B). Left CC mammogram. (C). Left MLO spot compression mammogram.

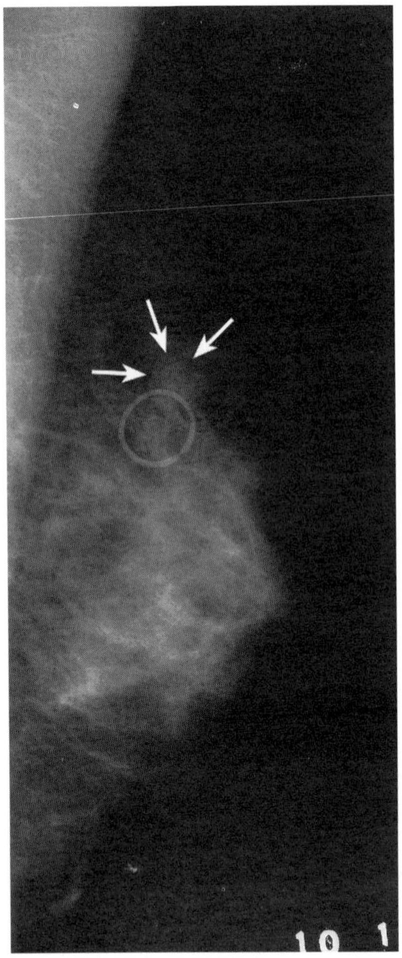

A

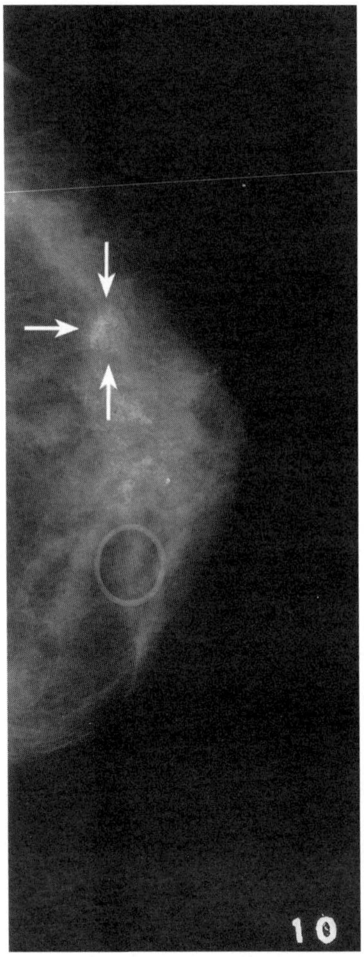

B

C

Ultrasound

Frequency

- 13 MHz

Mass

- margin: well defined
- echogenicity: hypoechoic
- retrotumoral acoustic appearance: single edge shadowing
- shape: lobulated (Fig. 17–2)

A 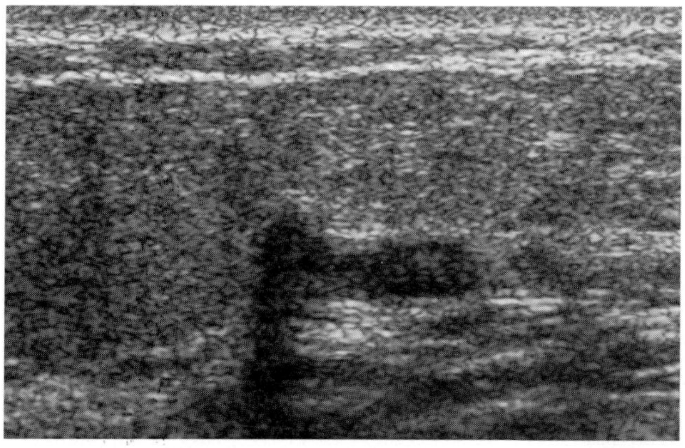 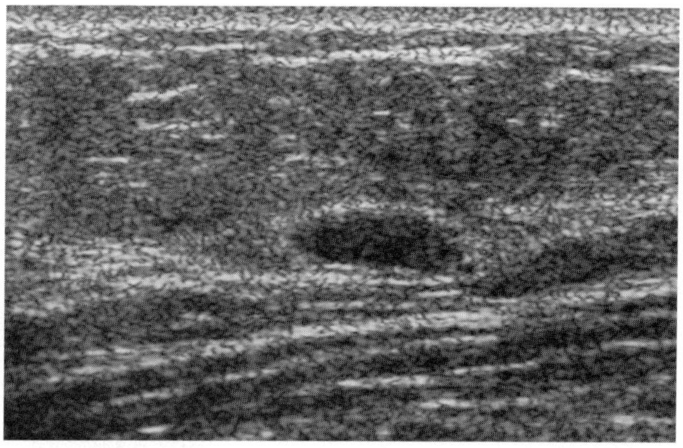 B

Figure 17–2. The mammographic mass identified in Figure 17–1 corresponds sonographically to a well-defined lobulated hypoechoic mass. (A). Left radial breast sonogram. (B). Left antiradial breast sonogram.

Pathology

- leiomyoma

Management

- BI-RADS Assessment Category 4, suspicious; biopsy should be considered

Pearls and Pitfalls

Leiomyomas (smooth muscle) of the breast are extremely rare. They originate from the nipple, subareolar region, or within the breast parenchyma. They present as well-defined solid masses. In this case, the management assessment is based upon the progressive growth of the lesion and the inability to mammographically display well-defined margins.

Suggested Readings

1. Diaz-Arias AA, Jurt MA, Loy TS, et al. Leiomyoma of the breast. *Hum Pathol* 1989;20:396–399.
2. Nascimento AE, Rosen PP, Karas M, et al. Leiomyoma of the nipple. *Am J Surg Pathol* 1979;3:151–154.
3. Tavassoli FA. Mesenchymal lesions. In: Tavassolli FA, Fattaneh A, eds. *Pathology of the Breast.* 2nd ed. Stamford: Appleton and Lange; 1999:675–729.

Case 18

Case History

A 48-year-old woman presents for screening mammogram.

Physical Examination

- normal exam

Mammogram

Mass (Fig. 18–1)

- margin: circumscribed
- shape: oval
- density: equal density

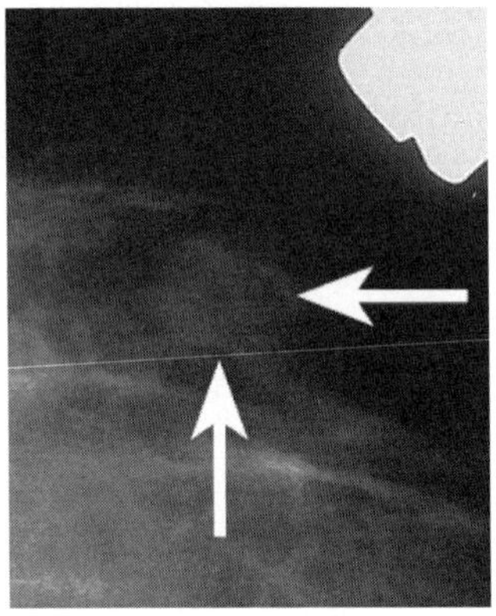

Figure 18–1. Left CC spot compression mammogram: In the outer breast there is an oval mass (arrows).

Ultrasound

Low Frequency

Frequency

- 7.5 MHz

Mass

- margin: well defined
- echogenicity: heterogeneous
- retrotumoral acoustic appearance: single edge shadowing
- shape: ellipsoid (Fig. 18–2)

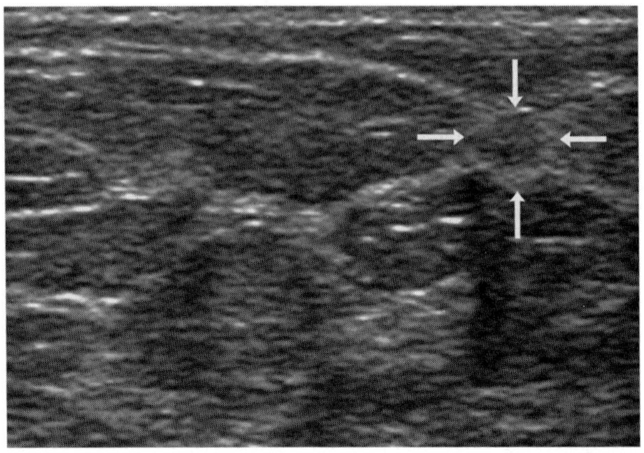

Figure 18–2. Left radial breast sonogram: Using a lower-frequency transducer, the mass (arrows) is difficult to identify.

High Frequency

Frequency

- 11.5 MHz

Associated Findings

In this case, a benign mass is originally missed with the the lower-frequency examination. The mass is missed for two reasons: (1) the echogenicity of the mass matches the surrounding tissues because the dynamic range of the imaging program is too high, and (2) the internal architecture of the mass cannot be resolved due to poor resolution from the lower frequency. The higher-frequency study not only localizes the mammographic mass but also clearly identifies the benign nature of the mass. (See Figs. 18-3 and 18-4.)

Pathology

- lymph node

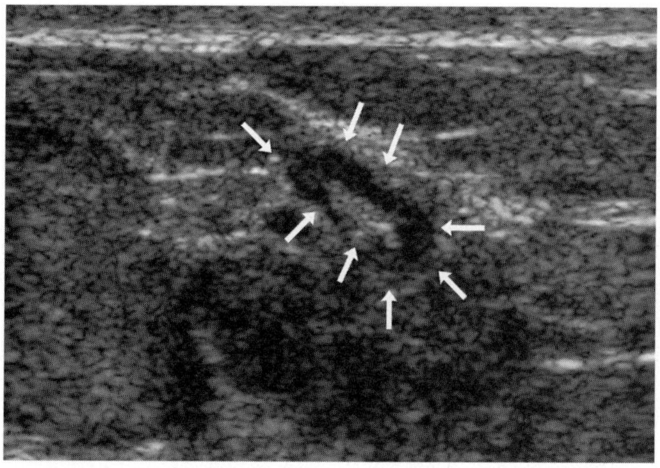

Figure 18-3. Left antiradial breast sonogram: Higher-frequency examination of the same area as Figure 18-2 demonstrates that the mammographic mass is a normal lymph node (arrows).

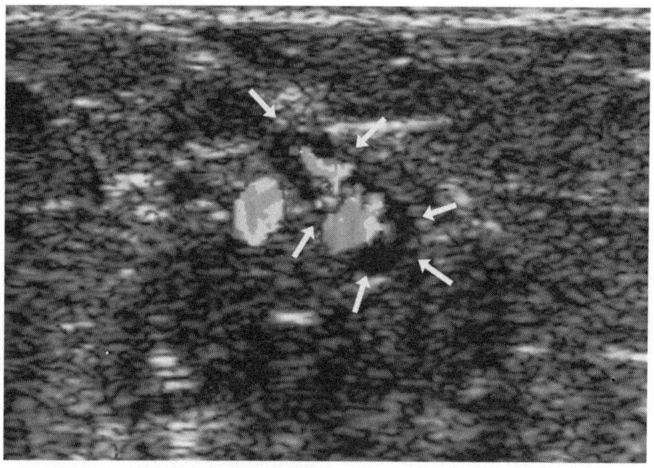

Figure 18-4. Left antiradial color Doppler breast sonogram: Color flow high-frequency images confirm the normal pattern of blood flow through the center of the lymph node (arrows) (see Color Plate 18–4).

Management

- BI-RADS Assessment Category 2, benign finding

Pearls and Pitfalls

Masses may be missed with lower-frequency sonography because the lower resolution provides fewer visual clues to characterize masses. In this case, the hyperechoic center of the lymph node could not be identified with the lower frequency.

Suggested Readings

1. Leucht D, Madjar H. Axillary, supraclavicular and infraclavicular lymph nodes. In: Leucht D, ed. *Teaching Atlas of Breast Ultrasound.* New York: Thieme; 1996:181–188.
2. Sohn C, Blohmer J-U, Hamper UM. Sonography of the axilla. In: Sohn C, Blohmer J-U, Hamper UM, eds. *Breast Ultrasound.* New York: Thieme; 1999, 94–97.

Case 19

Case History

A 53-year-old woman presents for screening mammogram.

Physical Examination

- normal exam

Mammogram

Mass (Fig. 19–1)

- margin: indistinct
- shape: oval
- density: equal density

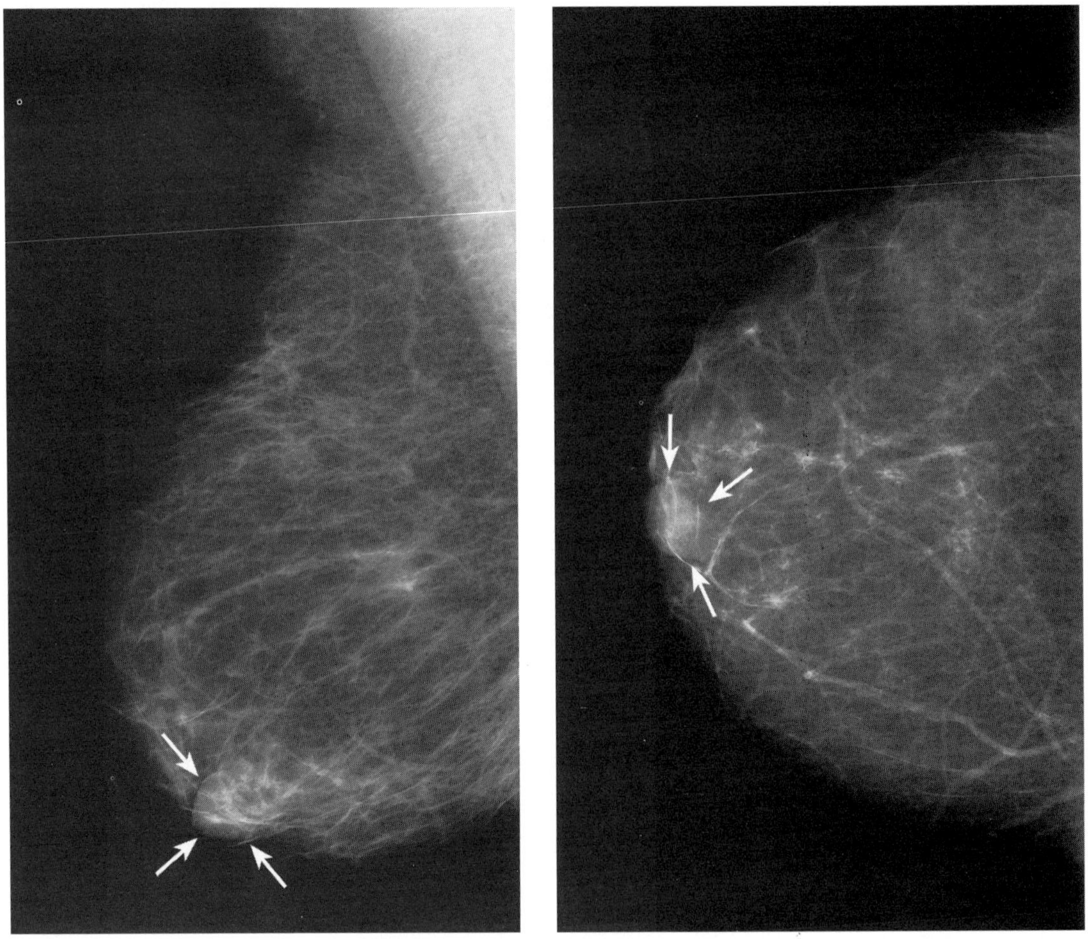

A B

Figure 19–1. *In the subareolar region, there is an oval density (arrows). (A). Right MLO mammogram. (B). Right CC mammogram.*

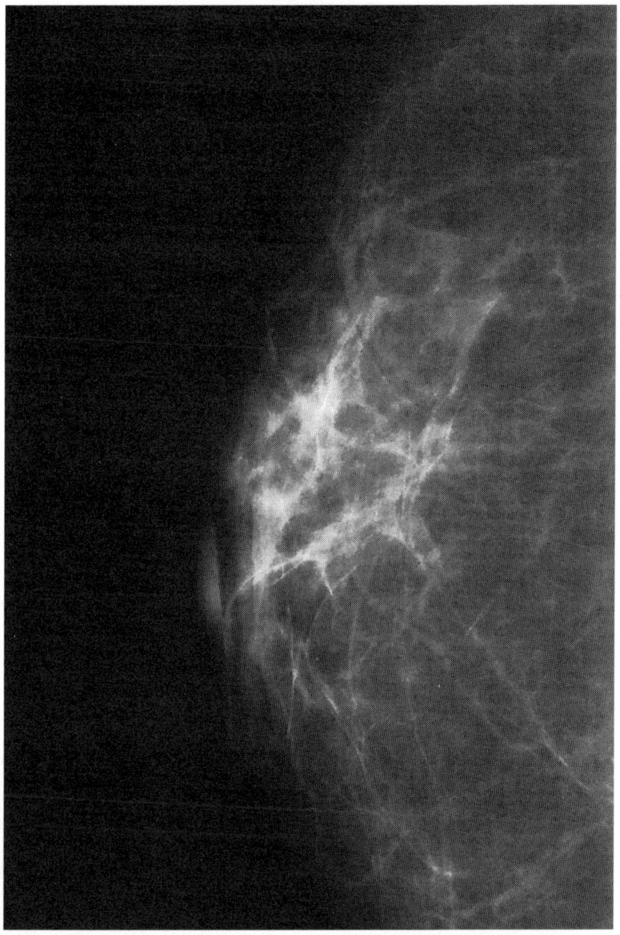

Figure 19–2. Right CC nipple profile mammogram: The oval density corresponds to the nipple.

Pathology

- nipple

Management

- BI-RADS Assessment Category 2, benign finding

Pearls and Pitfalls

If the nipple is inverted or the breast is asymmetric, the nipple may be difficult to place in profile on the routine screening views. Besides being a requirement for good technique, placing the nipple in profile eliminates the mistake of confusing the nipple for an intramammary mass and optimizes the evaluation of the subareolar region. This visualization is necessary to exclude malignant causes for nipple displacement. A nipple profile view may be necessary to image the subareolar area.

Suggested Readings

1. American College of Radiology Committee on Quality Assurance in Mammography. *Mammography Quality Control Manual.* Reston: ACR; 1999:23–112.
2. Bassett LW, Hirbawi IA, DeBruhl N, Hayes MK. Mammographic positioning: evaluation from the view box. *Radiology* 1993;188:803–806.

Case 20

Case History

A 64-year-old woman presents with multiple right breast masses.

Physical Examination

- right breast: 3 cm mass extending from 11.00 to 12:00 (this mass has increased in size since her last exam 1 year ago); stable 3 cm mass at 9:30
- left breast: normal exam

Mammogram

Mass (Fig. 20–1)

- margin: circumscribed
- shape: round
- density: equal density

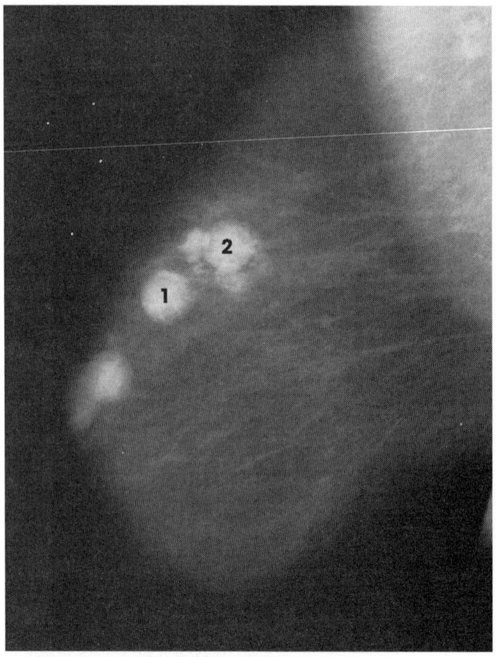

A

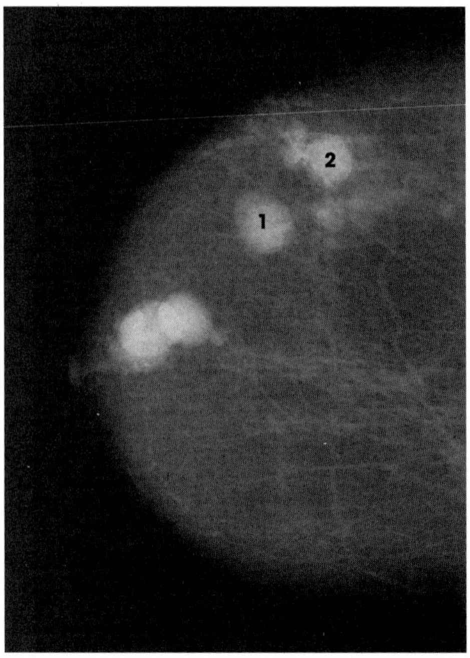

B

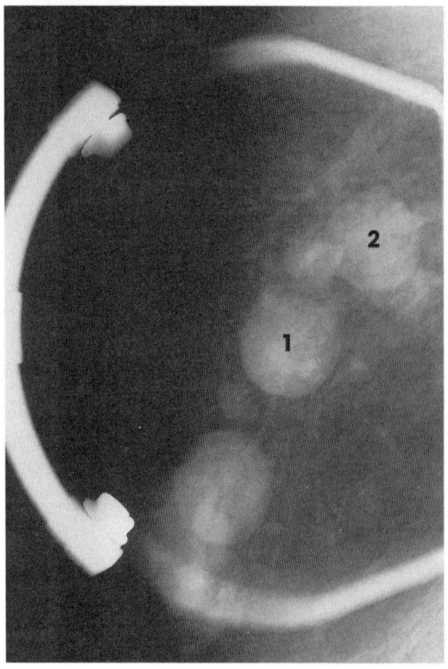

C

Figure 20–1. Multiple well-defined round masses are present in the upper inner quadrant as well as above the nipple at the 12:00 position. Since previous exam, two masses labeled 1and 2 have increased in size. (A). Right MLO mammogram. (B). Right CC mammogram. (C). Right MLO spot magnification compression mammogram.

Ultrasound

Frequency

- 10 MHz

Mass

- margin: well defined
- echogenicity: hypoechoic
- retrotumoral acoustic appearance: increased acoustic transmission
- 0 shape: ellipsoid (Figs. 20–2 and 20–3)

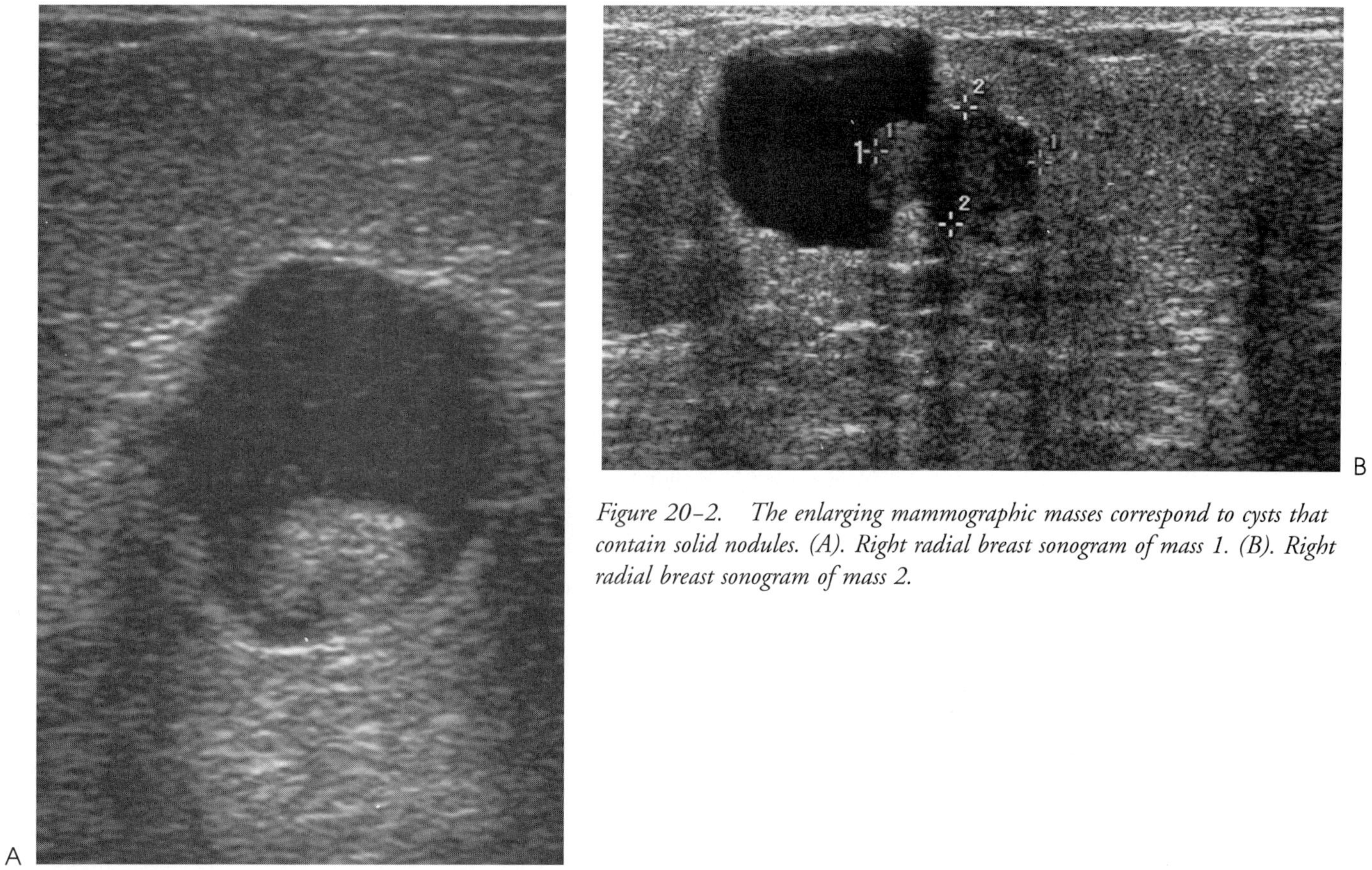

Figure 20–2. *The enlarging mammographic masses correspond to cysts that contain solid nodules. (A). Right radial breast sonogram of mass 1. (B). Right radial breast sonogram of mass 2.*

Other Modalities (Fig. 20–3)

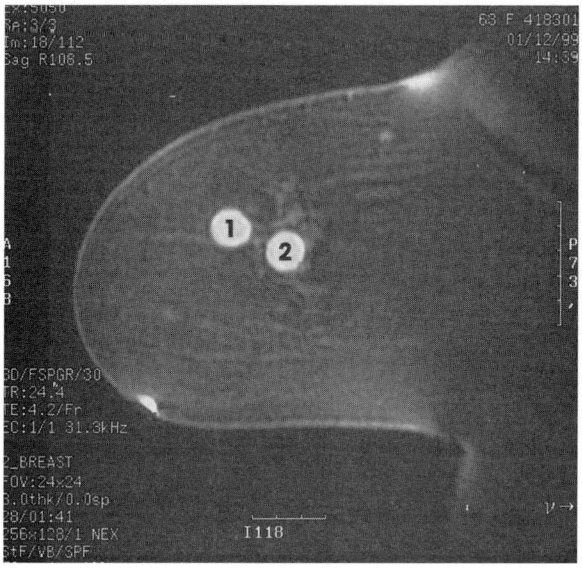

Figure 20–3. *Right dynamic bolus three-dimensional (3-D) volume gradient breast magnetic resonance imaging (MRI): There is enhancement of the solid tissue component of the intracystic masses in the upper outer quadrant. MRI-labeled masses 1 and 2 correspond to the mammographic masses 1 and 2.*

Pathology

- papilloma

Management

- BI-RADS Assessment Category 4, suspicious; biopsy should be considered

Pearls and Pitfalls

1. Papillary lesions represent fewer than 10% of benign breast biopsies. The most common benign papillary lesion is the papilloma. Solitary papillomas are generally central, mammographically occult, and associated with nipple discharge. Multiple papillomas are usually peripheral and are asymptomatic.
2. The most common mammographic findings are circumscribed noncalcified masses or clustered calcifications. Less commonly, these lesions produce asymmetric densities, dilated ducts, and architectural distortion.
3. Sonographically, papillomas are solid, hypoechoic, oval, or lobulated masses. The mass may be within a cyst or a dilated duct. When identified within a cyst, the solid mass protrudes into the cyst or is a thickened area of the cyst wall. When present within a dilated duct, the tumor presents as solid material filling the contour of the duct.

Suggested Readings

1. Liberman L, Bracero N, Vuolo MA, et al. Percutaneous large-core biopsy of papillary breast lesions. *AJR* 1999;172:331–337.
2. Merchant TE, Kievit HC, Beijerink D, van der Putte SC, de Graaf PW. MRI appearance of multiple papilloma of the breast. *Breast Cancer Res Treat* 1991;19:63–67.
3. Woods ER, Helvie MA, Ikeda DM, Mandell SH, Chapel KL, Adler DD. Solitary breast papilloma: comparison of mammographic, galactographic and pathologic findings. *AJR* 1992;159:487–491.

Case 21

Case History

A 58-year-old woman presents with a new density on her screening mammogram.

Physical Examination

- right breast: inflamed obstructed follicle in the medial inferior breast
- left breast: normal exam

Mammogram

Mass (Fig. 21–1)

- margin: circumscribed
- shape: oval
- density: equal density

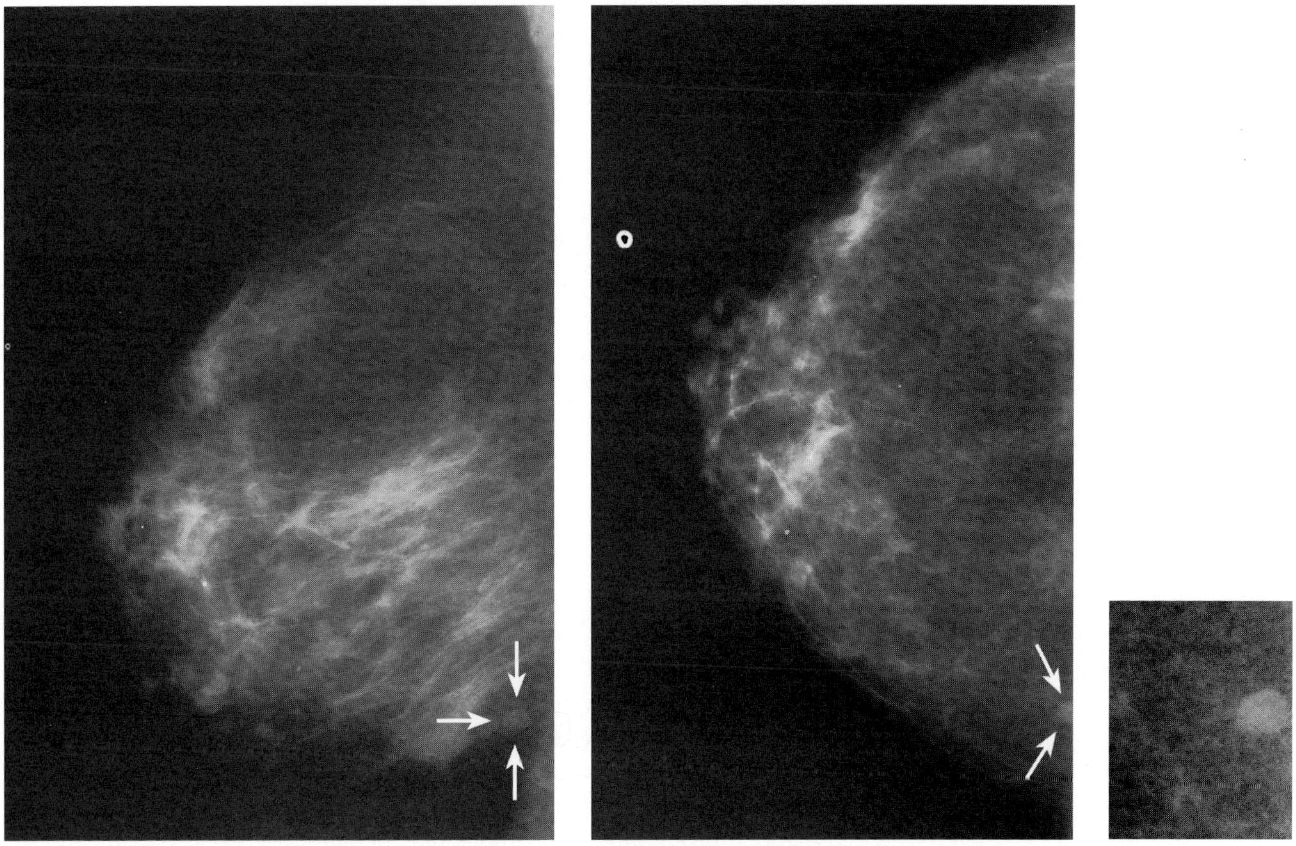

A B C

Figure 21–1. In the right medial inferior breast, there is a well-defined oval density (arrows). (A). Right MLO mammogram. (B). Right CC mammogram. (C). Right CC spot compression mammogram.

Ultrasound

Frequency

- 13.5 MHz

Mass

- margin: well defined
- echogenicity: hypoechoic
- retrotumoral acoustic appearance: enhanced acoustic transmission
- shape: ellipsoid (Fig. 21–2)

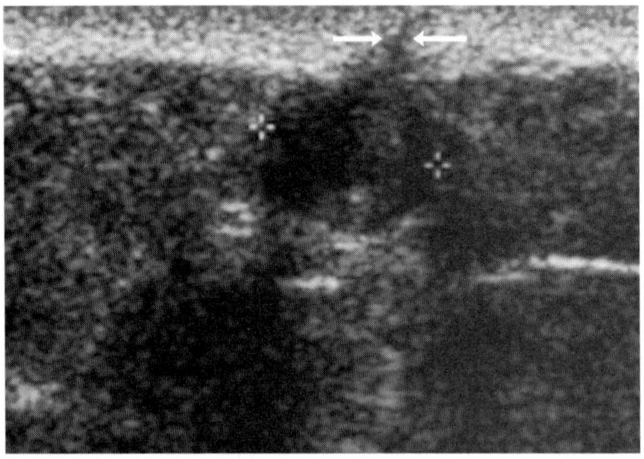

Figure 21–2. Right radial breast sonogram: In the right medial inferior breast there is a complex hypoechoic fluid collection, which corresponds to the mammographic density identified in Figure 21–1. This fluid collection is connected to a thin hypoechoic line, which is the follicular duct extending through the skin (arrows).

Pathology

- sebaceous cyst

Management

- BI-RADS Assessment Category 2, benign finding

Pearls and Pitfalls

Sebaceous cysts and epidermal inclusion cysts appear as well-defined intramammary masses. Sebaceous cysts are retention cysts that originate within sebaceous glands. Epidermal inclusion cysts result from a variety of etiologies. Epidermal inclusion cysts arise within obstructed hair follicles or within embryonic lines of closure. This lesion is also caused by traumatic implantation or squamous metaplasia of the sweat ducts. Sebaceous cysts and epidermal inclusion cysts are most commonly around the areola or in the inferior breast. The best technique to identify these lesions is to place a skin marker on the mass prior to mammographic imaging.

Suggested Readings

1. De Paredes ES. Well defined masses. In: De Paredes ES, ed. *Atlas of Film Screen Mammography*. 2nd ed. Baltimore: Williams and Wilkins; 1992:131–232.
2. Jackson VP, Jahan R, Fu YS. Benign breast lesions. In: Bassett LW, Jackson VP, Jahan R, Fu YS, Gold RH, eds. *Diagnosis of Diseases of the Breast*. Philadelphia: WB Saunders Company; 1997:357–443.
3. Martin JE. *Atlas of Mammography*. Baltimore: Williams and Wilkins; 1982.

Case 22

Case History

A 71-year-old woman presents for a screening mammogram.

Physical Examination

- right breast: seborrheic keratosis on the superior inner breast (marked with round skin marker)
- left breast: normal exam

Mammogram

Mass (Fig. 22–1)

- margin: circumscribed
- shape: lobular
- density: equal density

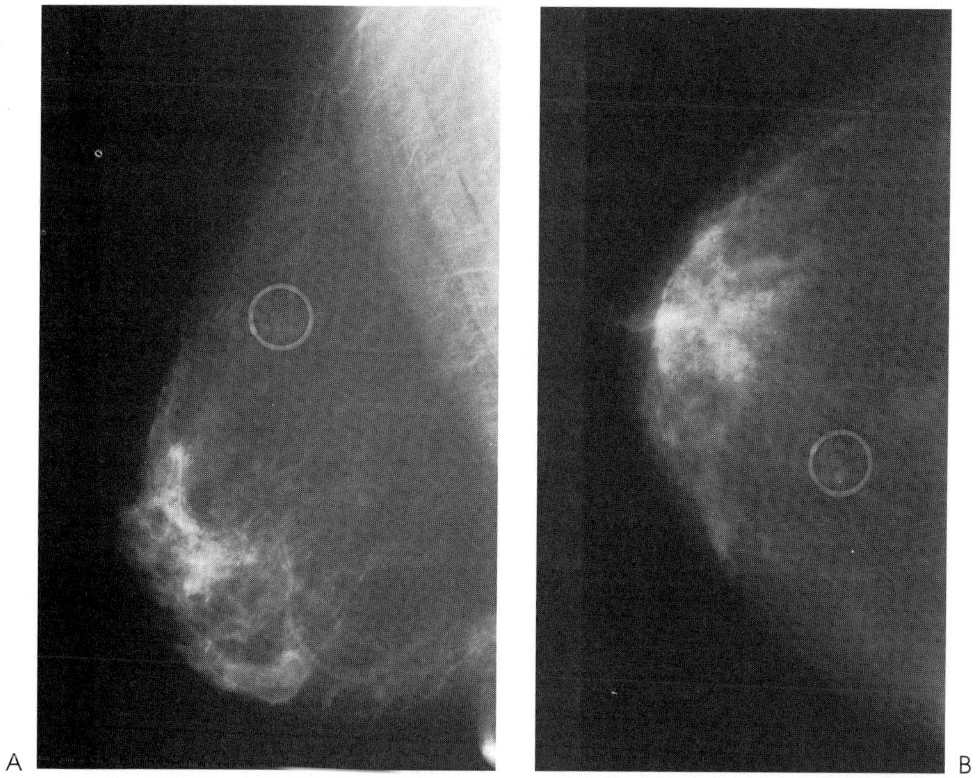

Figure 22–1. In the upper inner right breast, the skin marker is associated with a lesion that consists of multiple oval densities surrounded by lucent lines. (A). Right MLO mammogram. (B). Right CC mammogram.

Pathology

- seborrheic keratosis

Management

- BI-RADS Assessment Category 2, benign finding

Pearls and Pitfalls

Moles, warts, skin tags, and seborrheic keratosis may produce mammographic densities when they are thick or rise above the skin. Because most of the mass is surrounded by air, they are well circumscribed and surrounded by a lucent halo. The seborrheic keratosis illustrated in this case consists of multiple verrucous skin masses that are individually separated by the air in the crevices of the lesion. This radiographic appearance is characteristic of this skin lesion and makes this abnormality easily distinguishable from intramammary masses.

Suggested Readings

1. De Paredes ES. Well defined masses. In: De Paredes ES, ed. *Atlas of Film Screen Mammography.* 2nd ed. Baltimore: Williams and Wilkins; 1992:131–232.
2. Egan RL. Radiographic skin changes. In: Egan RL. *Breast Imaging: Diagnosis and Morphology of Breast Diseases.* Philadelphia: WB Saunders; 1988:344–364.

Case 23

Case History

A 59-year-old woman presents for her screening mammogram.

Physical Examination

- right breast: pedunculated mole in the upper outer breast; otherwise negative exam
- left breast: normal exam

Mammogram

Mass (Figs. 23-1 and 23-2)

- margin: circumscribed
- shape: oval
- density: equal density

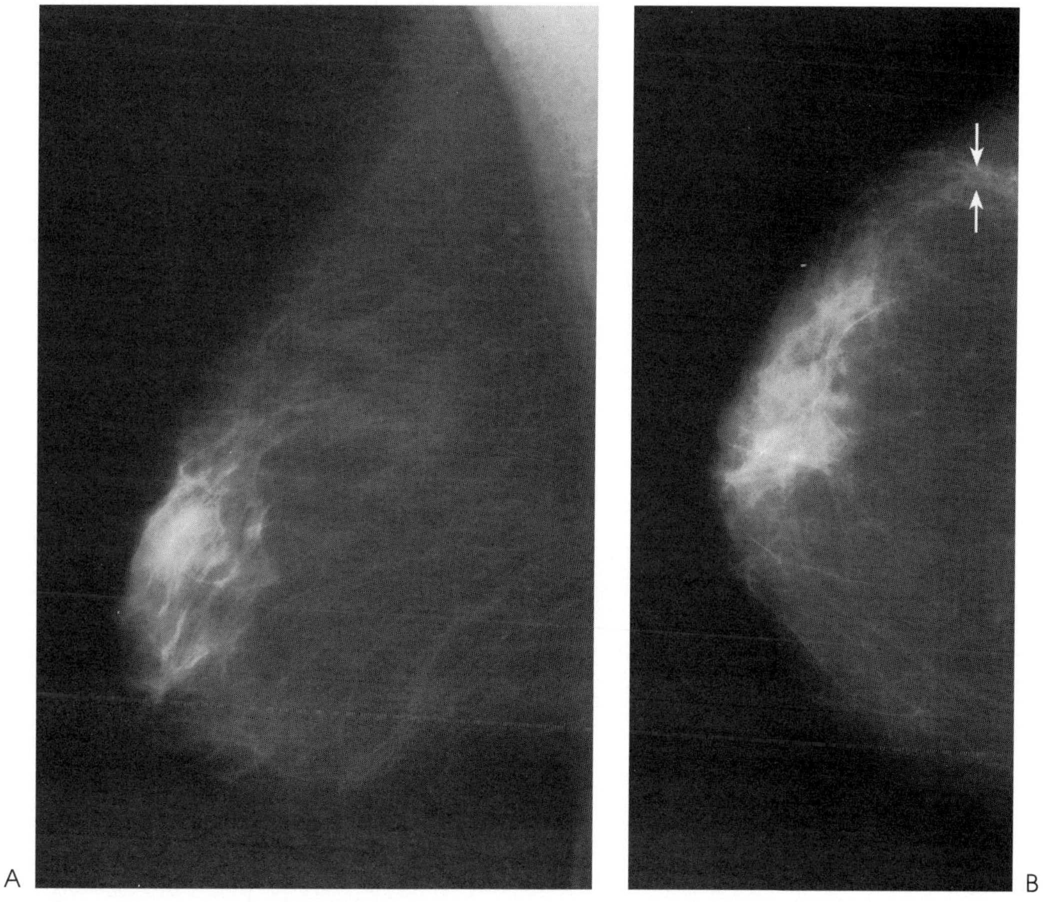

Figure 23-1. In the screening mammogram, the well-defined oval density (arrows) in the right outer breast (only visible on the CC view) is more prominent than in earlier examinations. (A). Right MLO mammogram. (B). Right CC mammogram.

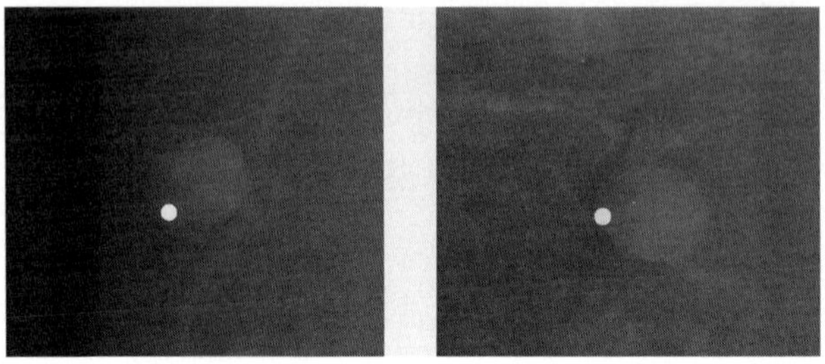

A B

Figure 23–2. When the spot compression views are obtained, a mole is identified in the upper outer breast and is marked with a metallic marker. (A). Right MLO spot compression mammogram. (B). Right CC spot compression mammogram.

Pathology

- mole

Management

- BI-RADS Assessment Category 2, benign finding

Pearls and Pitfalls

When thick skin moles are not marked, they may be mistaken for intramammary masses. These lesions generally have a lucent halo because they are outlined by air. The portion of the mass that attaches to the skin may be indistinct. A metallic skin marker generally clarifies the etiology of the mammographic density. If there is still a question whether the skin mass corresponds to the mammographic density, then tangential views may be performed.

Suggested Readings

1. Kopans DB. Analyzing the mammogram. In: Kopans DB. *Breast Imaging.* 2nd ed. Philadelphia: Lippincott-Raven; 1998:247–350.

Case 24

Case History

A 40-year-old woman presents for her screening mammogram.

Physical Examination

- normal exam

Mammogram

Mass (Fig. 24-1)

- margin: circumscribed
- shape: oval
- density: equal density

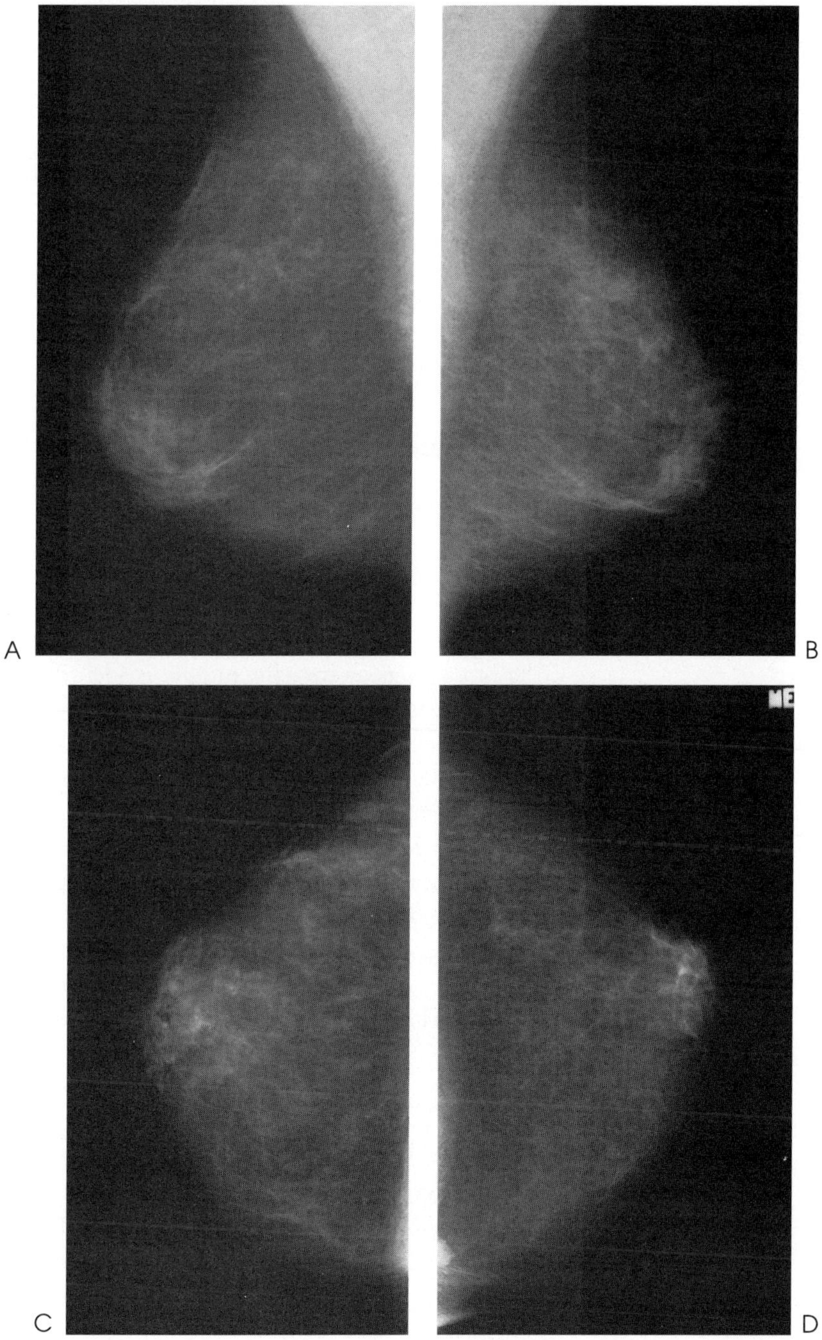

Figure 24-1. In the medial left breast on the CC view, there is a semicircular density. In the medial aspect of the right breast in the CC view, there is a broad triangular density. (A). Right MLO mammogram. (B). Left MLO mammogram. (C). Right CC mammogram. (D). Left CC mammogram.

Ultrasound

Frequency

- 11.5 MHz

Mass

- margin: well defined
- echogenicity: hypoechoic
- retrotumoral acoustic appearance: no shadowing
- shape: ellipsoid (Fig. 24–2)

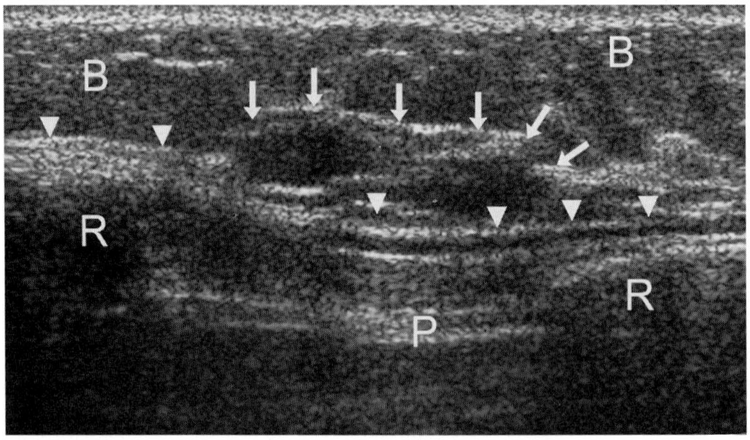

Figure 24–2. Left oblique parasternal breast sonogram: In the medial breast, the sternalis (arrows) is superficial to the pectoralis major muscle (arrowheads). R, rib; P, pleura; B, fatty breast tissue.

Pathology

- sternalis muscle

Management

- BI-RADS Assessment Category 2, benign finding

Pearls and Pitfalls

1. The mammographic density in the medial breast corresponds to the sternalis muscle. In 6% of cadavers, a sternalis muscle is identified either unilaterally or bilaterally. This muscle arises from the superior sternum (near the attachment of the sternocleidomastoid muscle) and lies superficial to the medial aspect of the pectoralis major and then attaches to the inferior sternum. This muscle has no functional purpose. Mammographically, this muscle may appear as a round, triangular, or flame-shaped density associated with the medial breast.
2. If one wishes to confirm that the mammographic density represents the sternalis muscle, then sonography is useful. Sonographically, the sternalis is hypoechoic or isoechoic with breast fat. Sonographic frequencies greater than 10 MHz are useful to better display intramuscular detail. When the transducer is parallel to the long axis of the sternum, one images the long axis of the muscle. The short axis view is perpendicular to the axis of the sternum.

Suggested Readings

1. Bradley FM, Hoover HC, Holka CA, et al. The sternalis muscle: an unusual normal finding seen on mammography. *AJR* 1996;166:33–36.
2. Grant JCB. *An Atlas of Anatomy*. 6th ed. Baltimore: Williams and Wilkins; 1972:27.
3. Kopans DB. Anatomy, histology, physiology, and pathology. In: Kopans DB. *Breast Imaging*. 2nd ed. Philadelphia: Lippincott-Raven; 1998:3–27.

Case 25

Case History

A 44-year-old woman presents for screening mammogram.

Physical Examination

- normal exam

Mammogram

Mass (Fig. 25-1)

- margin: circumscribed
- shape: oval
- density: equal density

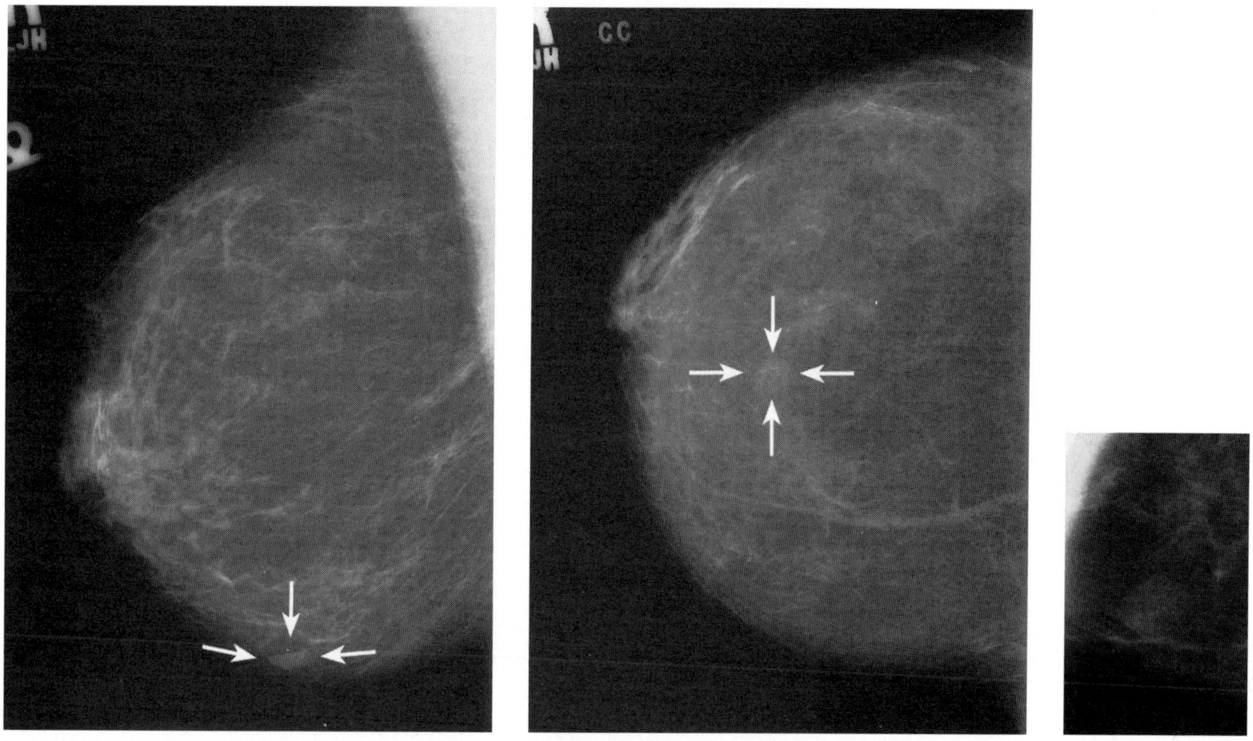

A B C

Figure 25-1. At the 6:00 position of the right breast there is an oval mass (arrows). (A). Right MLO mammogram. (B). Right CC mammogram. (C). Right MLO spot compression mammogram.

Ultrasound

Frequency

- 11.5 MHz

Mass

- margin: well defined
- echogenicity: hypoechoic
- retrotumoral acoustic appearance: no shadowing
- shape: ellipsoid (Fig. 25-2)

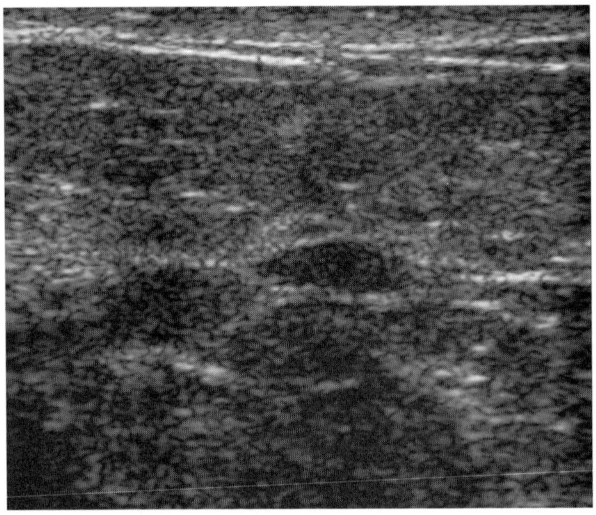

Figure 25-2. Right radial breast sonogram: At the 6:00 position, there is a well-defined hypoechoic mass. This mass was not identifiable with a lower frequency (7 MHz).

Pathology

- venous hemangioma

Management

- BI-RADS Assessment Category 3, probably benign; short-term follow-up

Pearls and Pitfalls

1. The benign vascular masses larger than 5 mm are cavernous, capillary, juvenile, and venous hemangiomas.
2. Mammographically, hemangiomas appear well defined and lobulated. Sonographically, they are well defined, hypoechoic masses that are either oval or lobulated in shape.

Suggested Readings

1. Madding GF, Hershberger LR. Hemangioma of the breast. *Surgery* 1949;26:685-687.
2. Perugini G, Bkonini G, Giardina C, et al. Cavernous hemangioma of the pectoralis muscle mimicking a breast tumor. *AJR* 1994;162:1321-1322.
3. Rosen PP, Tozefezy MA, Boram LH. Vascular tumors of the breast. IV. The venous hemangioma. *Am J Surg Pathol* 1985;9:659-665.

Case 26

Case History

A 69-year-old woman presents for screening mammogram.

Physical Examination

- normal exam

Mammogram

Mass (Fig. 26–1)

- margin: indistinct
- shape: oval
- density: equal density

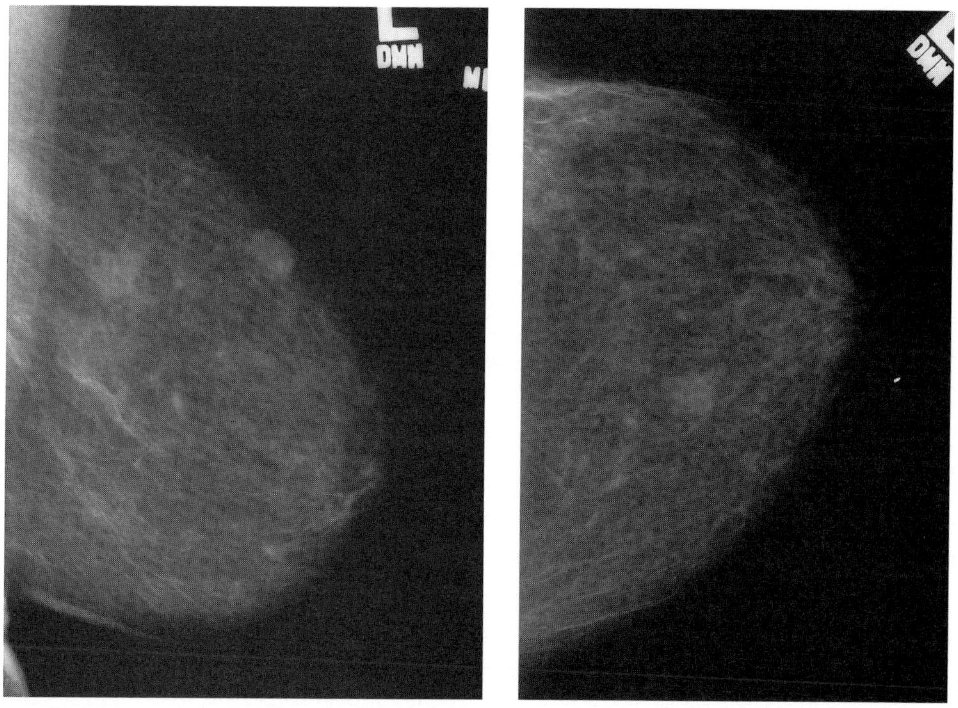

A B

Figure 26–1. In the 1:00 position of the left breast, there is an oval mass that is new since the patient's previous screening mammogram. The margins are well defined in the MLO view but indistinct in the CC view. (A). Left MLO mammogram. (B). Left CC mammogram.

Ultrasound

Frequency

- 13 MHz

Mass

- margin: well defined, microlobulated
- echogenicity: hypoechoic
- retrotumoral acoustic appearance: bilateral edge shadowing
- shape: ellipsoid (Fig. 26–2)

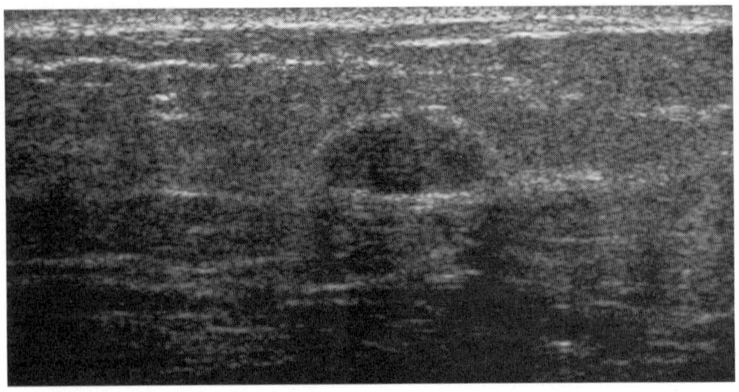

A

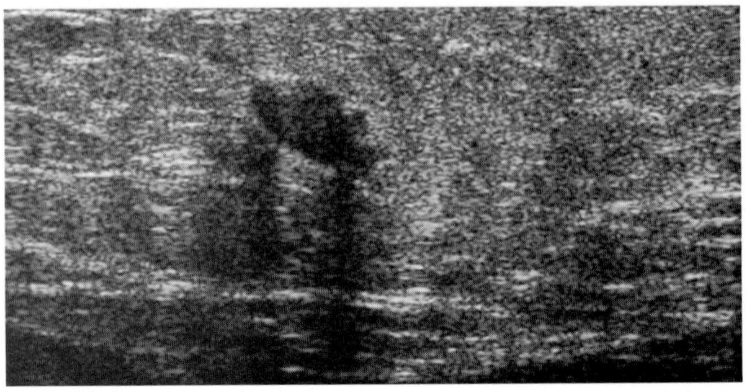

B

Figure 26–2. Although the mass identified in Figure 26–1 is predominantly oval and well defined sonographically (A), a small region of the mass is irregular and lobulated in configuration (B). (A). Left radial breast sonogram. (B). Left antiradial breast sonogram.

Pathology

- pseudoangiomatous stromal hyperplasia

Management

- BI-RADS Assessment Category 4, suspicious; biopsy should be considered

Pearls and Pitfalls

1. Pseudoangiomatous stromal hyperplasia (PASH) is collagenous stromal proliferation associated with diffuse short, tubular spaces lined with spindle cells. This abnormality is present in 23% of all breast specimens and about 50% of male breast specimens. Although this abnomality is not malignant, it may recur after excision.
2. In about half of the cases, PASH presents clinically as a palpable breast lump.
3. Mammographically, PASH most commonly appears as a well-defined circumscribed mass.
4. Sonographically, this entity is a well-circumscribed, oval or round, hypoechoic solid mass.

Suggested Readings

1. Badve S, Sloane JP. Pseudoangiomatous hyperplasia of male breast. *Histopathology* 1995;26:463–466.
2. Cohen MA, Morris EA, Rosen PP, Dershaw DD, Liberman L, Abramson AF. Pseudoangiomatous stromal hyperplasia: mammographic, sonographic, and clinical patterns. *Radiology* 1996;198:117–120.
3. Ibrahim RE, Schiotto CG, Weidner N. Pseudoangiomatous hyperplasia of mammary stroma. Some observations regarding its clinicopathologic spectrum. *Cancer* 1989;63:1154–1160.
4. Ortiz-Rey JA, Alvarez AK, Valbuena L, et al. Pseudoangiomatous hyperplasia of mammary stroma. *Breast Dis* 1995;8:295–299.
5. Polger MR, Denison CM, Lester S, Meyer JE. Pseudoangiomatous stromal hyperplasia: mammographic and sonographic appearances. *AJR* 1996;166:349–352.
6. Tavassoli FA. Vascular lesions. In: Tavassoli FA. *Pathology of the Breast.* 2nd ed. Stamford: Appleton and Lange; 1999:633–673.

Case 27

Case History

A 64-year-old woman presents with left breast pain.

Physical Examination

- left breast: tenderness in the upper outer quadrant associated with mild nodularity
- right breast: normal exam

Mammogram

Mass (Fig. 27–1)

- margin: obscured
- shape: oval
- density: equal density

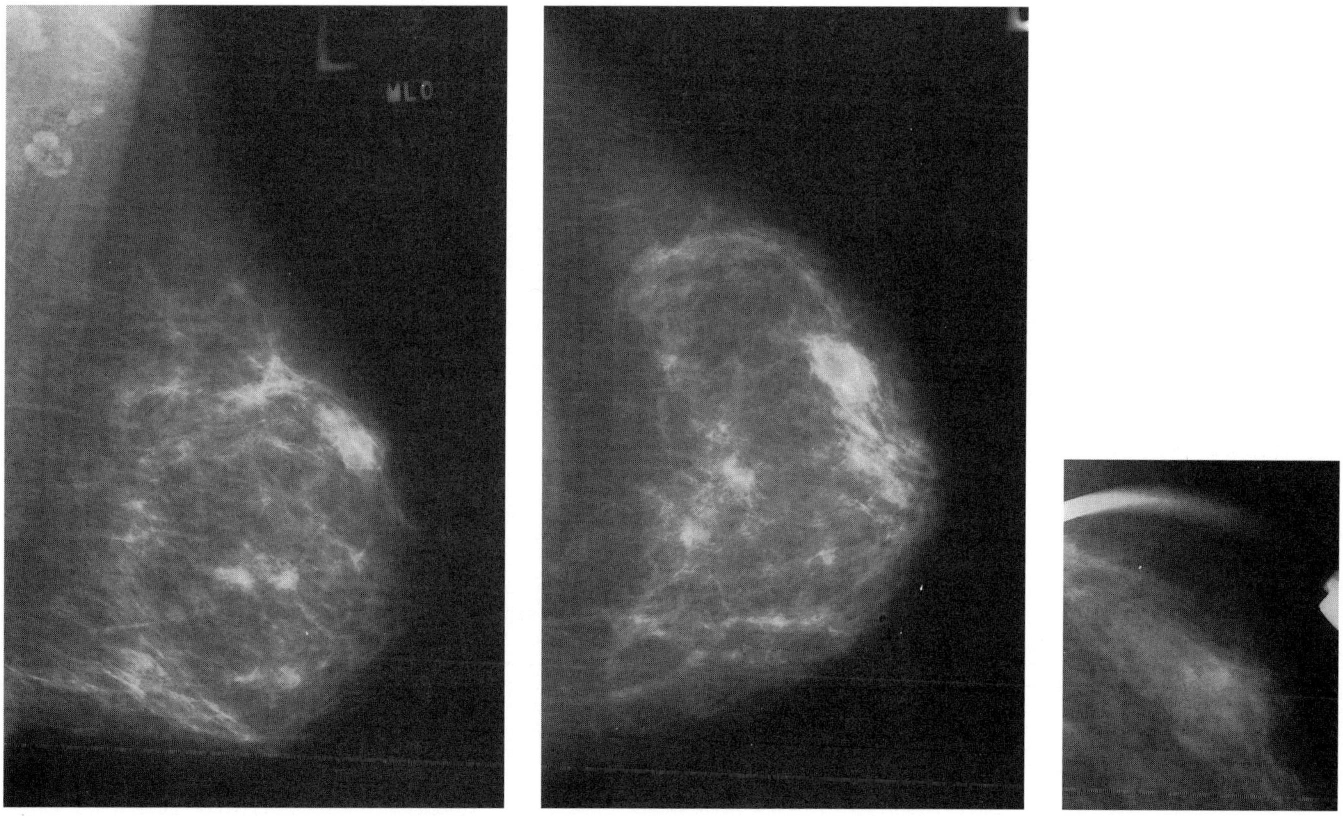

A B C

Figure 27–1. In the left upper outer quadrant, there is an oval mass with ill-defined and obscured margins. (A). Left MLO mammogram. (B). Left CC mammogram. (C). Left MLO spot compression mammogram.

Ultrasound

Frequency

- 7.5 MHz

Mass

- margin: well defined
- echogenicity: hypoechoic
- retrotumoral acoustic appearance: no shadowing
- shape: lobulated (Fig. 27–2)

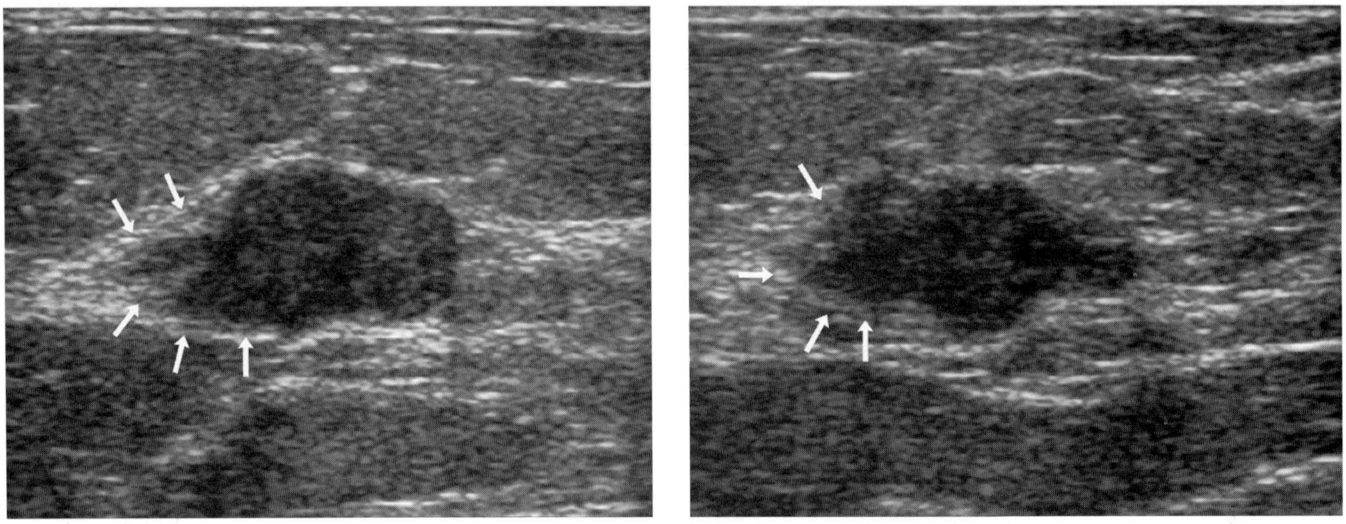

A B

Figure 27-2. In the left upper outer quadrant, the patient's tenderness is centered on a hypoechoic, predominantly lobulated mass. Although most of the margins are well defined, portions of the mass are ill defined and irregular (arrows). (A). Left longitudinal breast sonogram. (B). Left transverse breast sonogram.

Pathology

- adenoid cystic carcinoma

Management

- BI-RADS Assessment Category 4, suspicious; biopsy should be considered

Pearls and Pitfalls

1. Adenoid cystic carcinoma represents less than 1% of breast cancers. It commonly presents as a tender palpable mass.
2. Mammographically, this tumor tends to appear circumscribed oval or lobulated. Less commonly, it may appear as an ill-defined mass or focal asymmetric density. Calcifications occasionally are present.
3. Sonographically, the mass is hypoechoic or heterogeneous echogenicity and lobulated in shape. Portions of the margins are irregular or ill defined. Posterior acoustic shadowing may be present.
4. Generally, this tumor has an excellent prognosis. It rarely metastasizes, but may recur even after mastectomy.

Suggested Readings

1. Bourke AG, Metcalf C, Wylie EJ. Mammographic features of adenoid cystic carcinoma. *Australas Radiol* 1994;38:324–325.
2. Dinkel HP, Clees M, Gassel AM. Role of sonography in detection recurrence in adenoid cystic carcinoma of the breast. *AJR* 1999;173:497 [letter].
3. Santamaria G, Velasco M, Zanon G, et al. Adenoid cystic carcinoma of the breast: mammographic appearance and pathologic correlation. *AJR* 1998;171:1679–1683.

Case 28

Case History

A 72-year-old woman presents with a new left breast lump.

Physical Examination

- left breast: ill-defined firm lump in the upper inner breast
- right breast: normal exam

Mammogram

Mass (Fig. 28–1)

- margin: indistinct
- shape: oval
- density: equal density

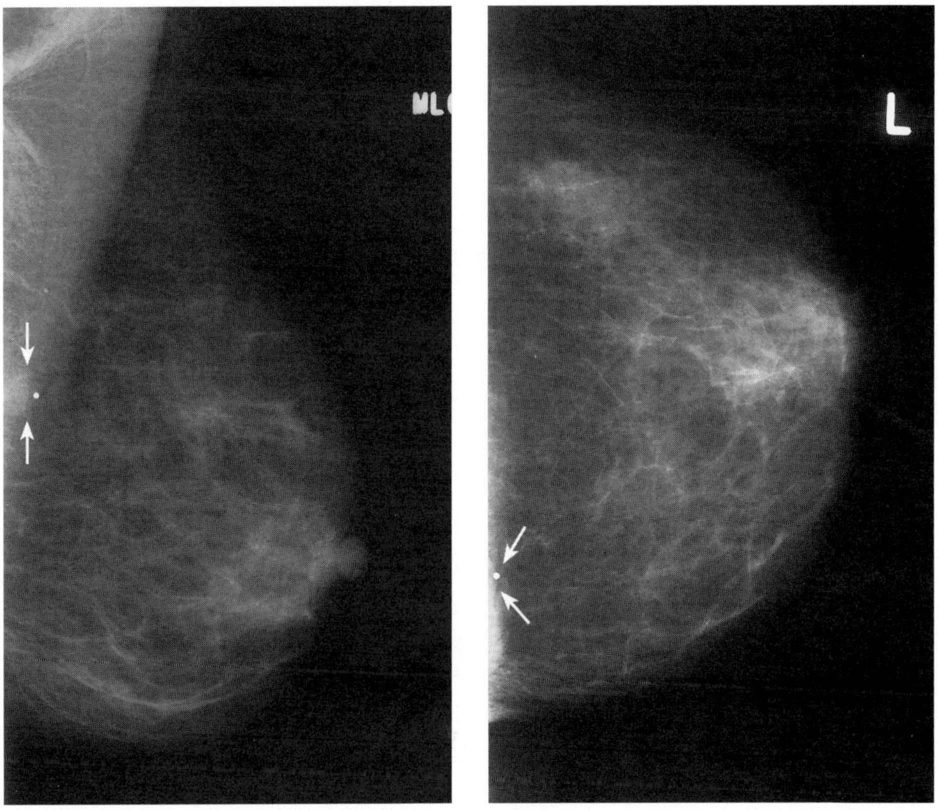

A B

Figure 28–1. In the upper inner breast there is an oval density associated with a metallic marker indicating that the mass is palpable. (A). Left MLO mammogram. (B). Left CC mammogram.

Ultrasound

Frequency

- 7 MHz

Mass

- margin: ill defined
- echogenicity: hypoechoic
- retrotumoral acoustic appearance: no shadowing
- shape: ellipsoid (Fig. 28–2)

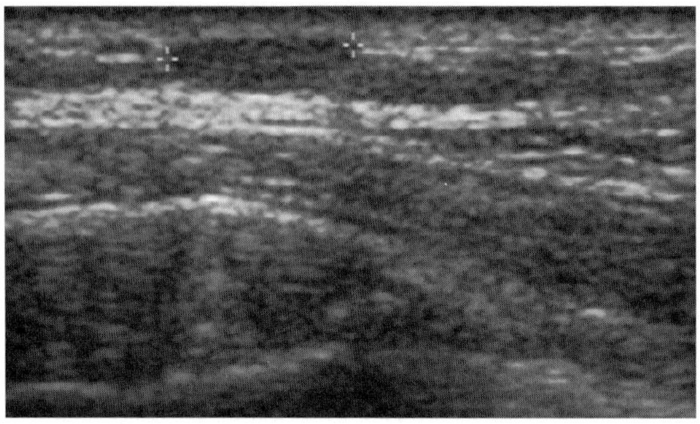

Figure 28–2. Left longitudinal breast sonogram: The palpable lump corresponds to an ill-defined hypoechoic solid superficial oval mass.

Pathology

- angiosarcoma

Management

- BI-RADS Assessment Category 4, suspicious; biopsy should be considered

Pearls and Pitfalls

1. Angiosarcoma represents less than 0.05% of primary breast tumors. Mammographically, this lesion generally presents as a mass with ill-defined borders without spiculations. Microcalcifications are rarely associated with this tumor. Commonly, this neoplasm is not detected mammographically. One paper reports that one third of 29 breast angiosarcomas are missed mammographically.
2. Sonographically, the mass is oval or lobulated, has well-defined or ill-defined margins, and is hypoechoic or heterogeneous in echogenicity.
3. Magnetic resonance demonstrates a mass with low signal intensity on T1-weighted images, high signal on T2-weighted images, and exhibits gadolinium contrast enhancement.
4. Clinically, patients with angiosarcomas have a poor prognosis. One review of the literature reports that 87 patients had a 3-year survival rate of 14%.

Suggested Readings

1. Chen KTK, Kirkegaard D, Bocian J. Angiosarcoma of the breast. *Cancer* 1980;46:368–371.
2. Grant EG, Holt RW, Chun B, Richardson JD, Orson LW, Cigtay OS. Angiosarcoma of the breast: sonographic, xeromammographic, and pathologic appearance. *AJR* 1983;141:691–692.
3. Liberman L, Dershaw DD, Kaufman RJ, et al. Angiosarcoma of the breast. *Radiology* 1992;183:649–654.
4. Molitor JL, Llombart A, Guinebretiere JM, et al. Angiosarcoma of the breast. Apropos of 2 cases. *Bull Cancer* 1997;84:218–222.

Case 29

Case History

A 63-year-old woman presents with a new right breast lump.

Physical Examination

- right breast: palpable lump in the upper inner quadrant
- left breast: normal exam

Mammogram

Mass (Fig. 29–1)

- margin: spiculated
- shape: oval
- density: high density

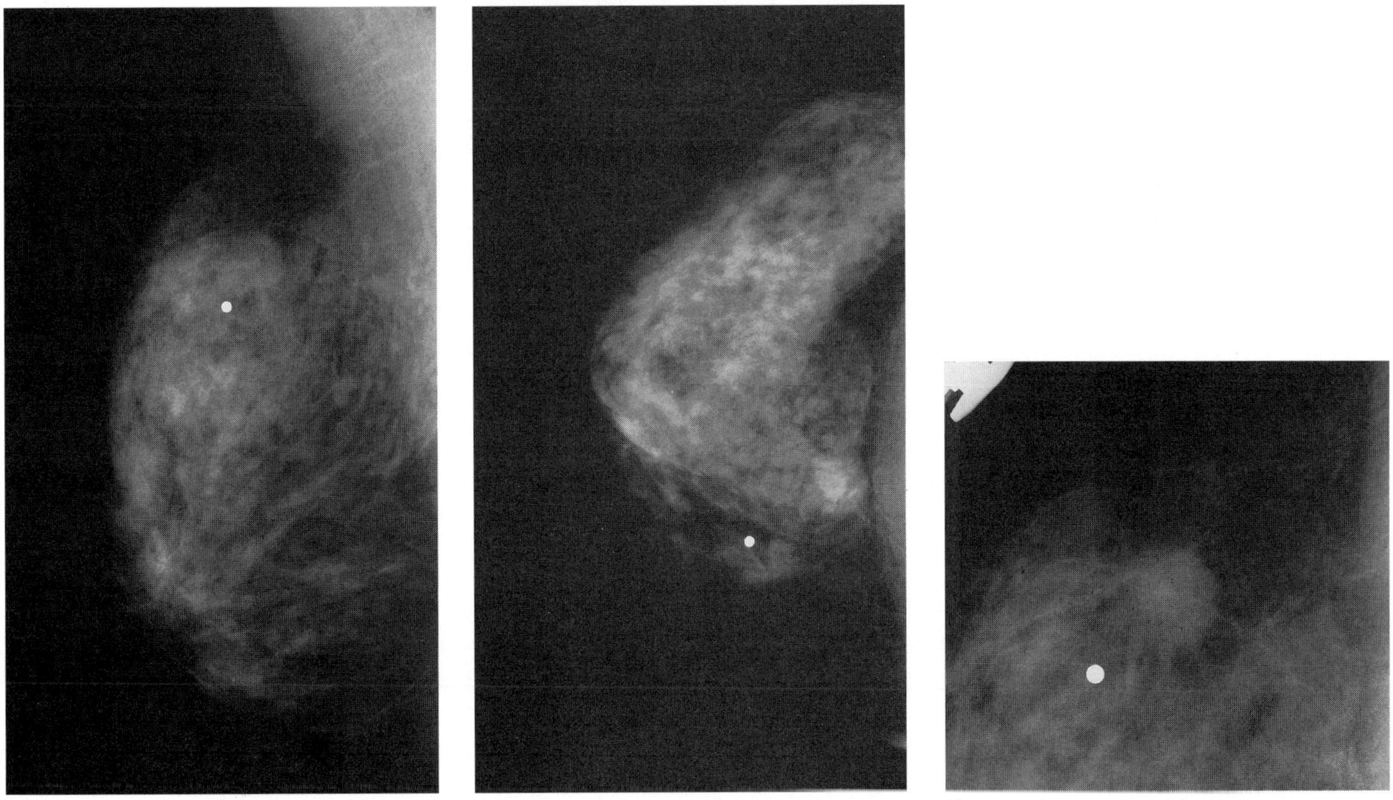

A B C

Figure 29–1. In the upper inner quadrant of the right breast, there is an oval mass that exhibits spiculated margins on the compression view. (A). Right MLO mammogram. (B). Right CC mammogram. (C). Right ML spot compression mammogram.

Ultrasound

Frequency

- 13 MHz

Mass

- margin: well defined, microlobulated
- echogenicity: hypoechoic
- retrotumoral acoustic appearance: single edge shadowing
- shape: irregular (Fig. 29–2)

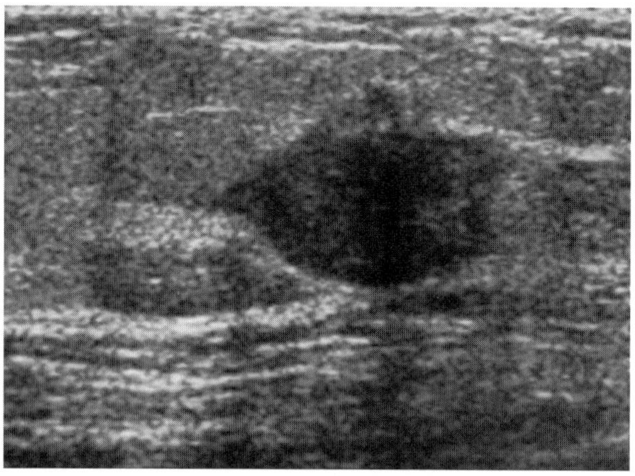

Figure 29–2. Right radial breast sonogram: The mammographic mass and the palpable lump correspond to an irregular hypoechoic solid mass.

Pathology

- infiltrating ductal carcinoma

Management

- BI-RADS Assessment Category 4, suspicious; biopsy should be considered

Pearls and Pitfalls

Only 2% of carcinomas present as well-defined masses. Furthermore, of all well-defined masses, only 5% are malignant. Infiltrating ductal is the most common histology of these circumscribed masses. Even if the malignancy initially appears circumscribed, spot compression views generally show that the mass has an ill-defined border or spiculations. Malignant circumscribed masses may also exhibit higher radiographic density compared with normal glandular tissue as in this case.

Suggested Readings

1. De Paredes ES. Well-defined masses. In: De Paredes ES. *Atlas of Film Screen Mammography.* 2nd ed. Baltimore: Williams and Wilkins; 1992:131–232.
2. Jackson VP, Dines KA, Bassett LW, et al. Diagnostic importance of radiographic density of noncalcified breast masses: analysis of 91 lesions. *AJR* 1991;157:25–28.
3. Sickles EA. Nonpalpable, circumscribed, noncalcified solid breast masses: likelihood of malignancy based on lesion size and age of patient. *Radiology* 1994;192:439–442.

Case 30

Case History

A 56-year-old woman presents with new right breast lump.

Physical Examination

- right breast: palpable lump at 2:00 position
- left breast: normal exam

Mammogram

Mass (Fig. 30–1)

- margin: spiculated
- shape: oval
- density: equal density

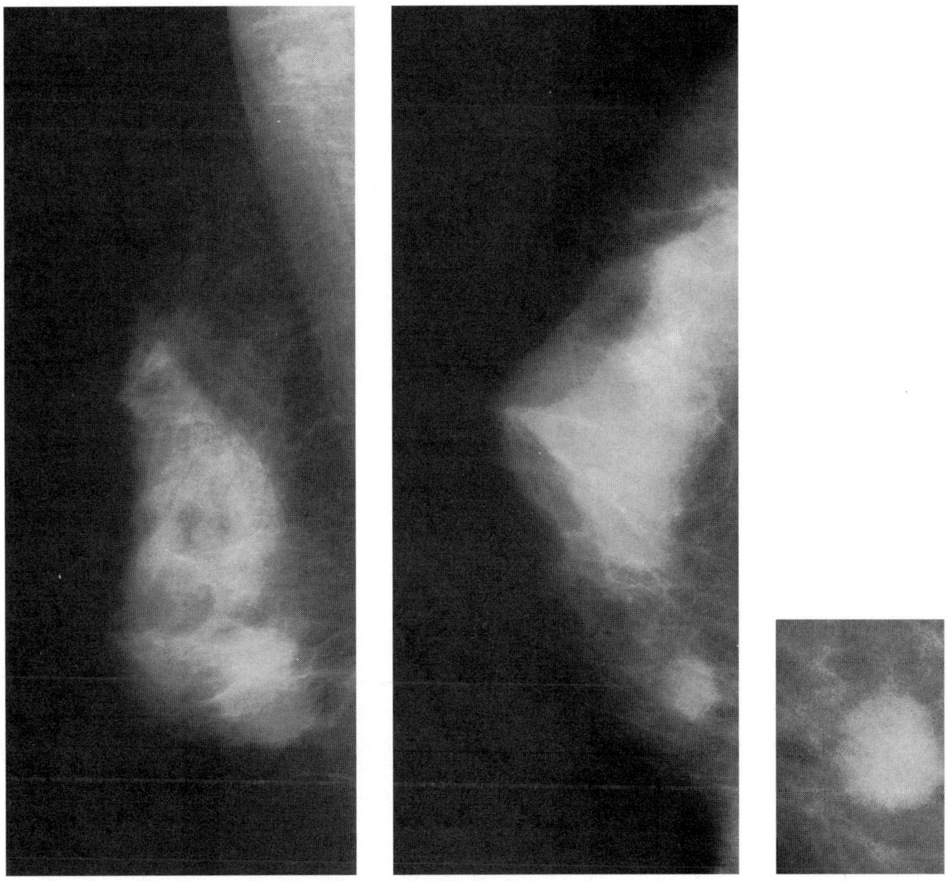

A B C

Figure 30–1. In the right upper inner breast there is an oval mass with ill-defined margins. (A). Right MLO mammogram. (B). Right CC mammogram. (C). Right CC spot compression mammogram.

Ultrasound

Low Frequency

Frequency

- 8 MHz

Mass

- margin: ill-defined
- echogenicity: hypoechoic
- retrotumoral acoustic appearance: severe shadowing, mass completely obscured
- shape: irregular (Fig. 30–2)

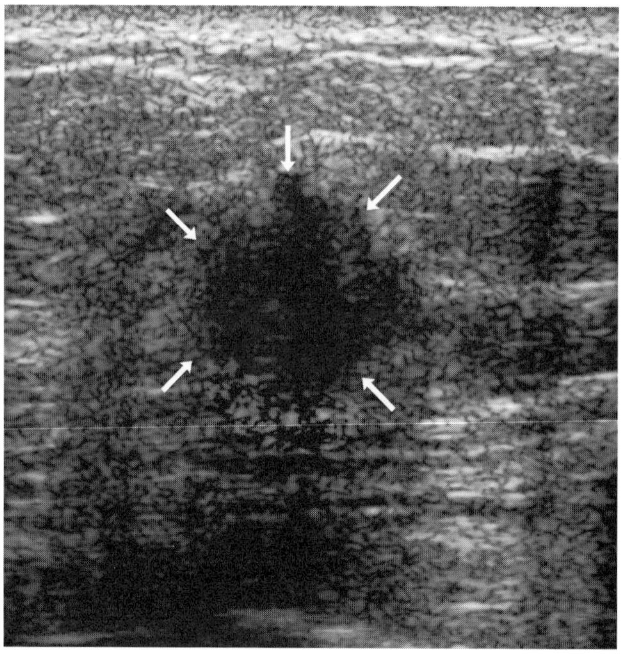

Figure 30–2. Right radial breast sonogram: Lower frequency better demonstrates the presence of an irregular mass that is causing the severe shadowing (arrows).

High Frequency

Frequency

- 13 MHz (Fig. 30–3)

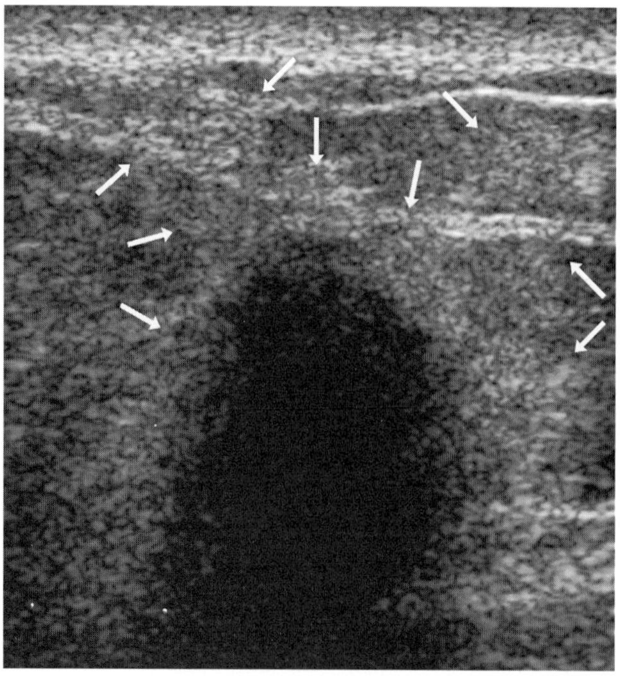

Figure 30–3. Right radial breast sonogram: with higher frequency the mass identified in Figure 30–1 corresponds to a heavily shadowing mass. Around the shadowing is hyperechoic spiculation and architectural distortion (arrows).

Pathology

- infiltrating ductal carcinoma

Management

- BI-RADS Assessment Category 4, suspicious; biopsy should be considered

Pearls and Pitfalls

Although both benign and malignant masses may produce severe shadowing, reducing the sonographic frequency improves the sonographic delineation of an associated mass. The high frequency improves detection of associated architectural distortion.

Suggested Readings

1. Leucht D, Madjar H. Analytic criteria for the interpretation of focal sonographic lesions. In: Leucht D, ed. *Teaching Atlas of Breast Ultrasound.* New York: Thieme; 1996:23–33.
2. Sohn C, Blohmer J-U, Hamper. Invasive ductal and lobular carcinoma. In: Sohn C, Blohmer J-U, Hamper UM, eds. *Breast Ultrasound.* New York: Thieme; 1999:60–66.
3. Tohno E, Cosgrove DO, Sloane JP. Invasive ductal carcinoma. In: Tohno D, Cosgrove DO, Sloane JP, eds. *Ultrasound Diagnosis of Breast Diseases.* New York: Churchill Livingston; 1994:158–171.

Case 31

Case History

A 79-year-old woman presents with enlarging left breast nodule.

Physical Examination

- normal exam

Mammogram

Mass (Fig. 31–1)

- margin: circumscribed
- shape: oval
- density: equal density

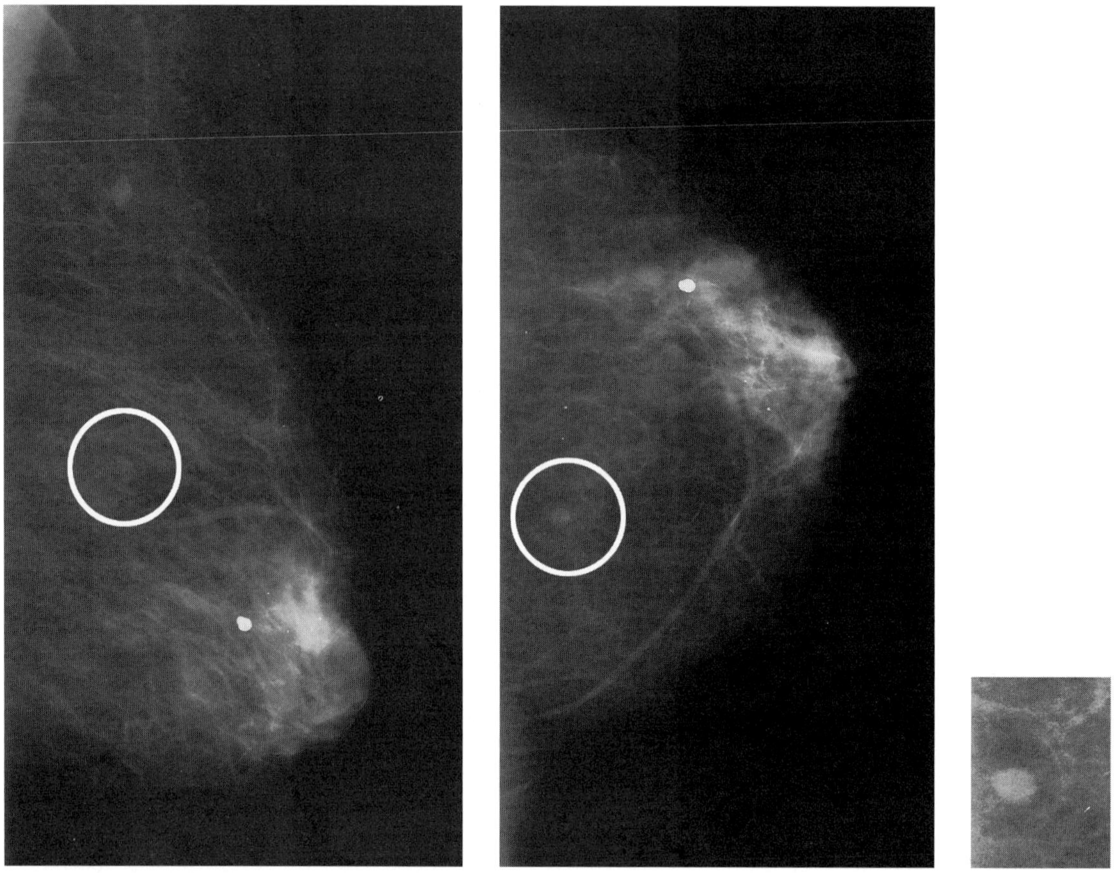

A B C

Figure 31–1. In the upper inner left breast, there is a circumscribed oval mass. This mass has increased in size since the patient's prior exam. (A). Left MLO mammogram. (B). Left CC mammogram. (C). Left MLO spot mammogram.

Ultrasound

Low Frequency

Frequency

- 7 MHz

Mass

- margin: ill defined
- echogenicity: hypoechoic
- retrotumoral acoustic appearance: posterior shadowing distal to mass
- shape: lobulated (Fig. 31–2)

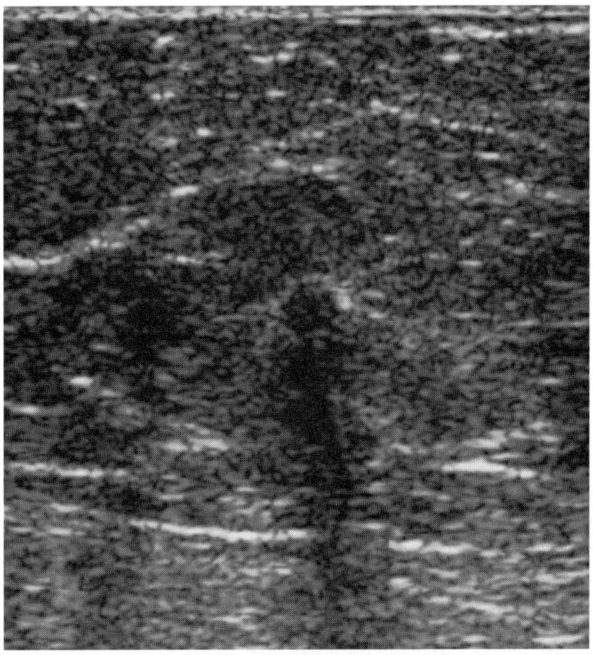

Figure 31–2. Left radial breast sonogram: The mass identified in Figure 31–1 corresponds to a round hypoechoic mass with acoustic shadowing.

High Frequency

Frequency

- 11.5 MHz

Associated Findings

The higher-frequency exam improves the definition of the mass. With the lower frequency, the mass may be mistaken as a benign round cyst or fibroadenoma with a fibrotic wall causing the shadowing. The higher frequency displays the irregular shape of the mass. (See Fig. 31–3.)

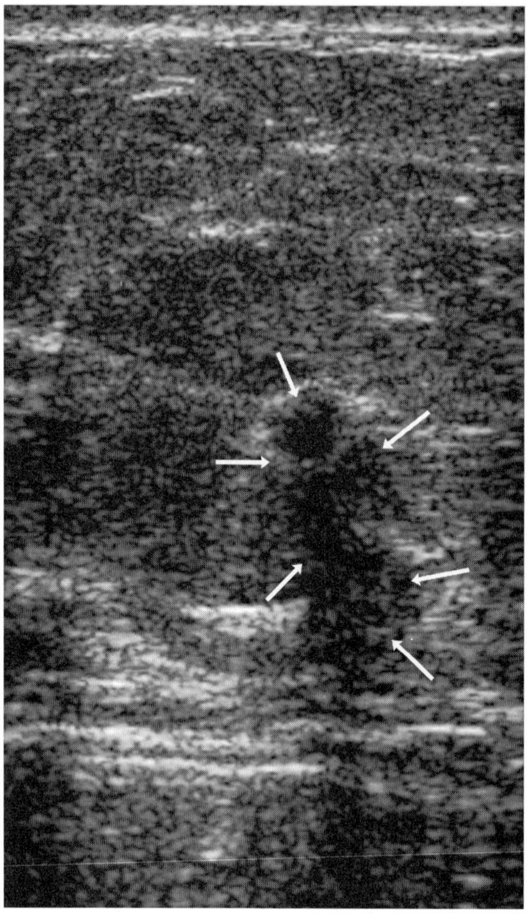

Figure 31–3. Left radial breast sonogram: The mass identified in Figure 31–2 corresponds to an irregular, ill-defined mass (arrows) with posterior acoustic shadowing.

Pathology

- infiltrating ductal carcinoma

Management

- BI-RADS Assessment Category 4, suspicious; biopsy should be considered

Pearls and Pitfalls

This case illustrates that higher-frequency sonography improves delineation of masses. If one wishes to use sonographic information to determine management assessment, one should initially use the highest ultrasound that adequately penetrates the mass.

Suggested Readings

1. Marsteller LP, Shaw de Paredes EKK. Well defined masses in the breast. *Radiographics* 1989;9:13–37.
2. Moskowitz M. The predictive value of certain mammographic signs in screening for breast cancer. *Cancer* 1983;51:1007–1011.
3. Sickles EZ. Mammographic features of 300 consecutive nonpalpable breast cancers. *AJR* 1986;146:661–663.

Case 32

Case History

A 51-year-old woman presents with a new left breast lump.

Physical Examination

- left breast: a palpable lump in the left breast at the 2:00 position
- right breast: normal exam

Mammogram

Mass (Fig. 32–1)

- margin: circumscribed
- shape: oval
- density: high

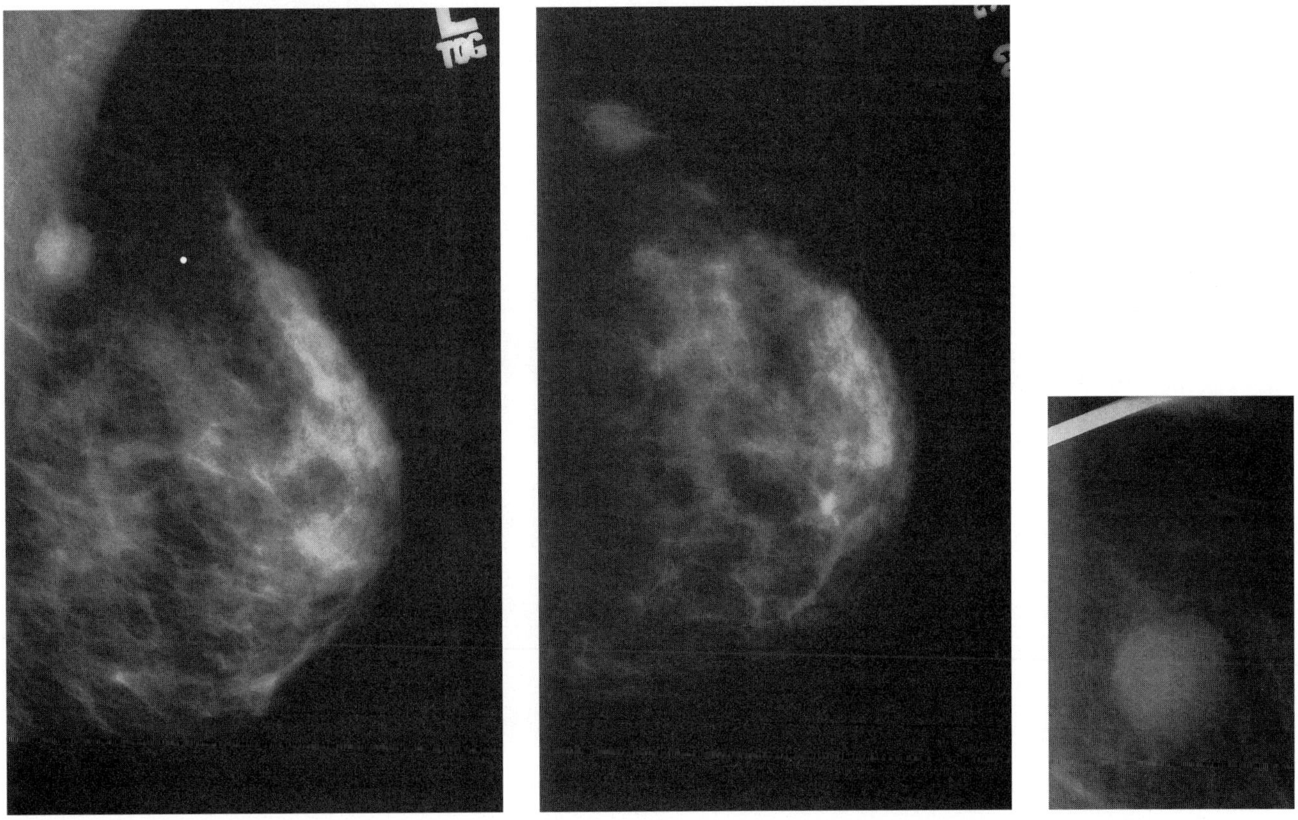

A B C

Figure 32–1. There is a well-circumscribed oval density in the left upper outer breast. This mass corresponds to a palpable lump and is new since the screening mammogram of the previous year. A small segment of the margin is indistinct even with spot compression views. (A). Left MLO mammogram. (B). Left CC mammogram. (C). Left MLO spot compression view.

Ultrasound

Frequency

- 11.5 MHz

Mass

- margin: well defined
- echogenicity: hypoechoic
- retrotumoral acoustic appearance: retrotumoral enhancement present
- shape: ellipsoid (Figs. 32–2 and 32–3)

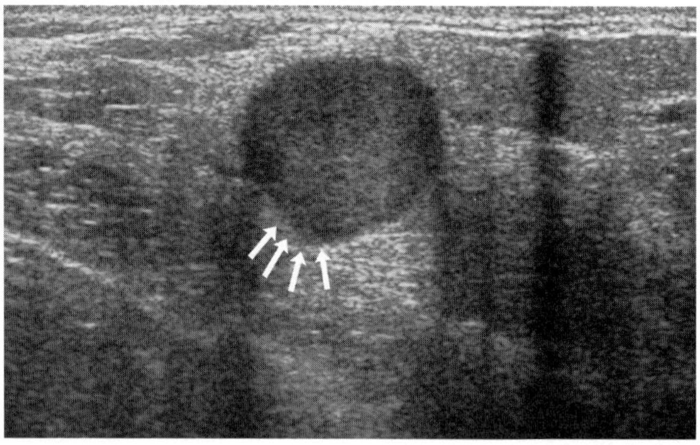

Figure 32–2. Left antiradial breast sonogram: The nodule identified in Figure 32–1 sonographically corresponds to a well-defined hypoechoic, oval mass with increased posterior acoustic enhancement. Although the margin is well defined, there is slight flattening and angularity of the deep margin of the mass (arrows). A solid or complex cystic mass may produce this appearance.

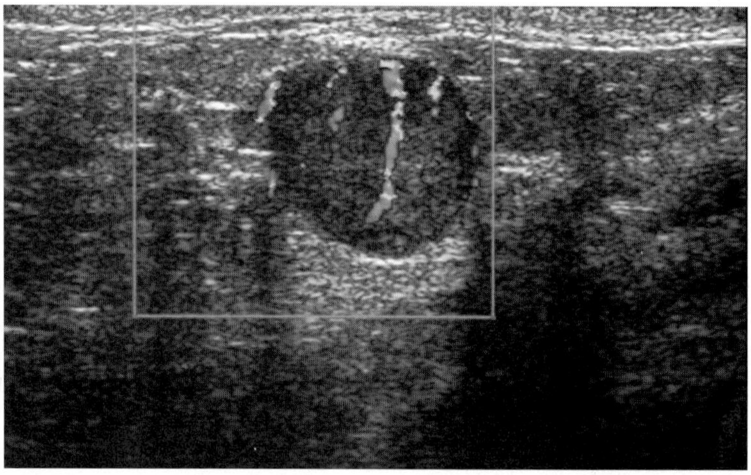

Figure 32–3. Left antiradial color Doppler breast sonogram: Color Doppler demonstrates blood flow throughout the mass indicating that this nodule is solid (see Color Plate 32–3).

Pathology

- invasive papillary carcinoma

Management

- BI-RADS Assessment Category 4, suspicious abnormality; biopsy should be considered

Pearls and Pitfalls

1. Papillary carcinoma represents about 2% of breast cancers. Most patients are between 40 and 60 years old. About 90% of central papillary carcinomas present with a palpable mass, and most patients notice bloody nipple discharge.
2. Mammographically, there are two common presentations of papillary carcinomas. One type is central in location and well circumscribed. The second type presents as nonpalpable multifocal peripheral cancers. This second type of papillary carcinoma behaves similarly to the usual ductal carcinoma in situ. Mammographically, this peripheral papillary carcinoma appears as clustered calcifications.
3. Sonographically, the first type of papillary carcinoma appears as an oval or round well-defined mass that is commonly within a cyst or duct. In this case, the shape of the mass and the ill-defined mammographic margins result in a suspicious assessment. Even if this mass displayed sonographically benign characteristics, it should be biopsied since it is increasing in size and has a mammographically suspicious appearance.

Suggested Readings

1. Deneby AS, Sanders LM, Titus JM, Kalisher L. Breast imaging case of the day. *Radiographics* 1997;17:1607–1610.
2. Merchant TE, Kievit HC, Beijerink D, van der Putte SC, de Graaf PW. MRI appearance of multiple papilloma of the breast. *Breast Cancer Res Treat* 1991;19:63–67.
3. Schneider JA. Invasive papillary breast carcinoma: mammographic and sonographic appearance. *Radiology* 1989;171:377–379.
4. Soo MS, Williford ME, Walsh R, Bentley RC, Kornguth PJ. Papillary carcinoma of the breast: imaging findings. *AJR* 1995;164:321–326.

Case 33

Case History

A 68-year-old woman presents with mammographic enlargement of a left breast nodule.

Physical Examination

- normal exam

Mammogram

Mass (Fig. 33–1)

- margin: obscured
- shape: oval
- density: equal

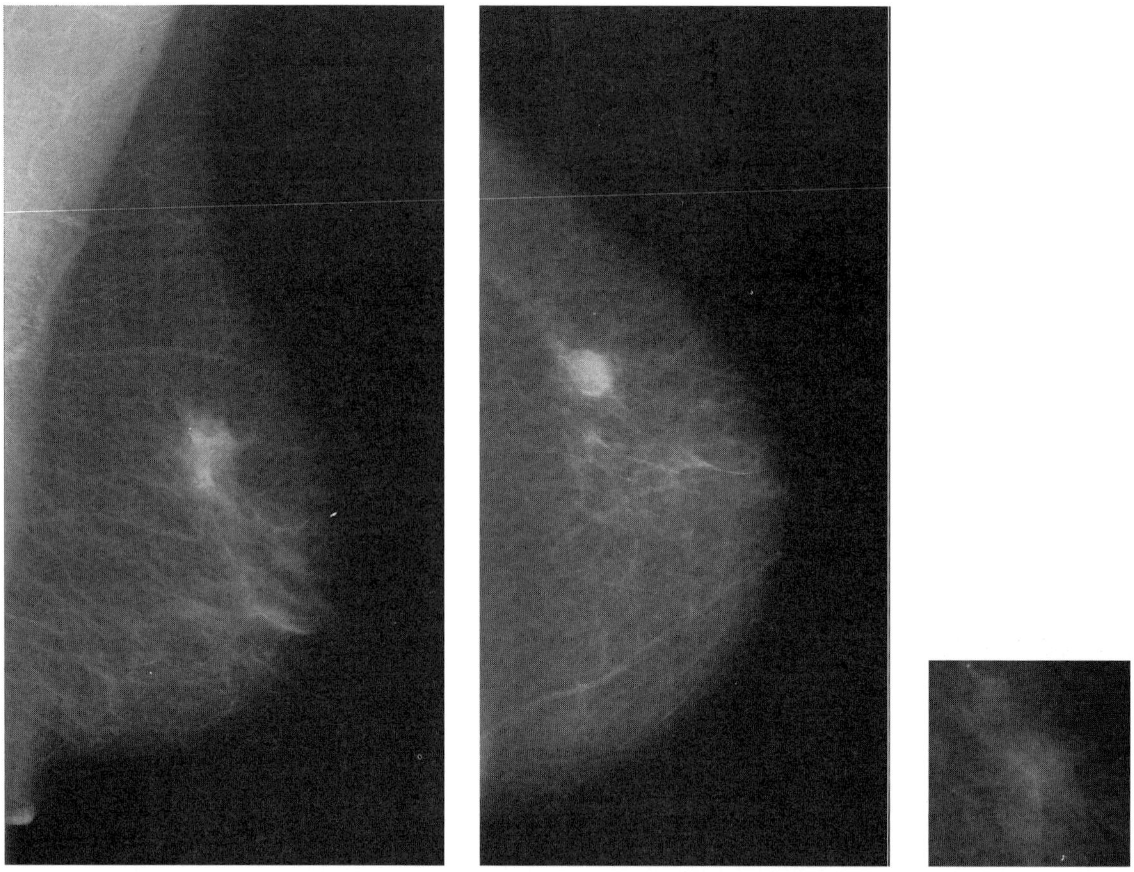

A B C

Figure 33–1. An oval circumscribed nodule with obscured margins is present in the upper outer breast. (A). Left MLO mammogram. (B). Left CC mammogram. (C). Left ML spot compression mammogram.

Ultrasound

Frequency

- 10 MHz

Mass

- margin: spiculation/architectural distortion
- echogenicity: isoechoic to fat
- retrotumoral acoustic appearance: bilateral edge shadowing
- shape: ellipsoid (Fig. 33–2)

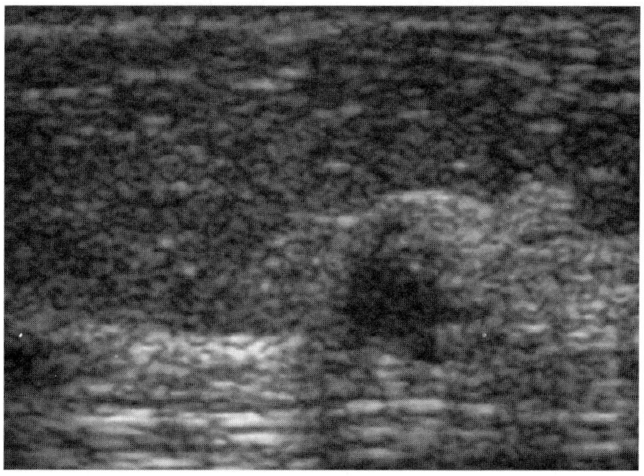

Figure 33–2. Left longitudinal breast sonogram: The mammographic nodule identified in Figure 33–1 corresponds to a mass with hypoechoic spiculations extending into the surrounding hyperechoic breast tissue.

Pathology

- invasive lobular carcinoma

Management

- BI-RADS Assessment Category 4, suspicious; biopsy should be considered

Pearls and Pitfalls

1. Mammographically 50 to 70% of lobular carcinomas appear as a spiculated or ill-defined masses. This tumor rarely (<5% of cases) appears as a circumscribed mass.
2. Sonographically, lobular carcinoma has the following appearances: a heterogeneous or hypoechoic irregular mass with ill-defined margins (60 to 85% of cases), a well-circumscribed mass (12 to 15%), or an area of severe shadowing that obscures the mass (15%).

Suggested Readings

1. Butler RS, Venta LA, Wiley EL, Ellis RL, Dempsey PJ, Rubin E. Sonographic evaluation of infiltrating lobular carcinoma. *AJR* 1999;172:325–330.
2. Cornford EJ, Wilson AR, Athanassiou E, et al. Mammographic features of invasive lobular and invasive ductal carcinoma of the breast: a comparative analysis. *Br J Radiol* 1995;68:450–453.
3. Hilleren DJ, Andersson IT, Lindholm K, Linnell FS. Invasive lobular carcinoma: mammographic findings in a 10-year experience. *Radiology* 1991;178:149–154.
4. Krecke KN, Gisvold JJ. Invasive lobular carcinoma of the breast: mammographic findings and extent of disease at diagnosis in 184 patients. *AJR* 1993;61:957–960.
5. Mendelson EB, Harris KM, Doshi N, Tobon H. Infiltrating lobular carcinoma: mammographic patterns with pathologic correlation. *AJR* 1989;153:265–271.
6. Paramagul CP, Helvie MA, Adler DD. Invasive lobular carcinoma: sonographic appearance and role of sonography in improving diagnostic sensitivity. *Radiology* 1995;195:231–234.
7. Yeh C, Titus JM, Kalisher L. Breast imaging case of the day. *Radiographics* 1997;17:1328–1332.

Case 34

Case History

A 59-year-old woman presents with palpable left axillary nodes. Biopsy of one of the nodes is consistent with breast cancer.

Physical Examination

- left breast: enlarged axillary node; no other palpable masses
- right breast: normal exam

Mammogram

Mass (Fig. 34–1)

- margin: circumscribed
- shape: lymph node
- density: high density

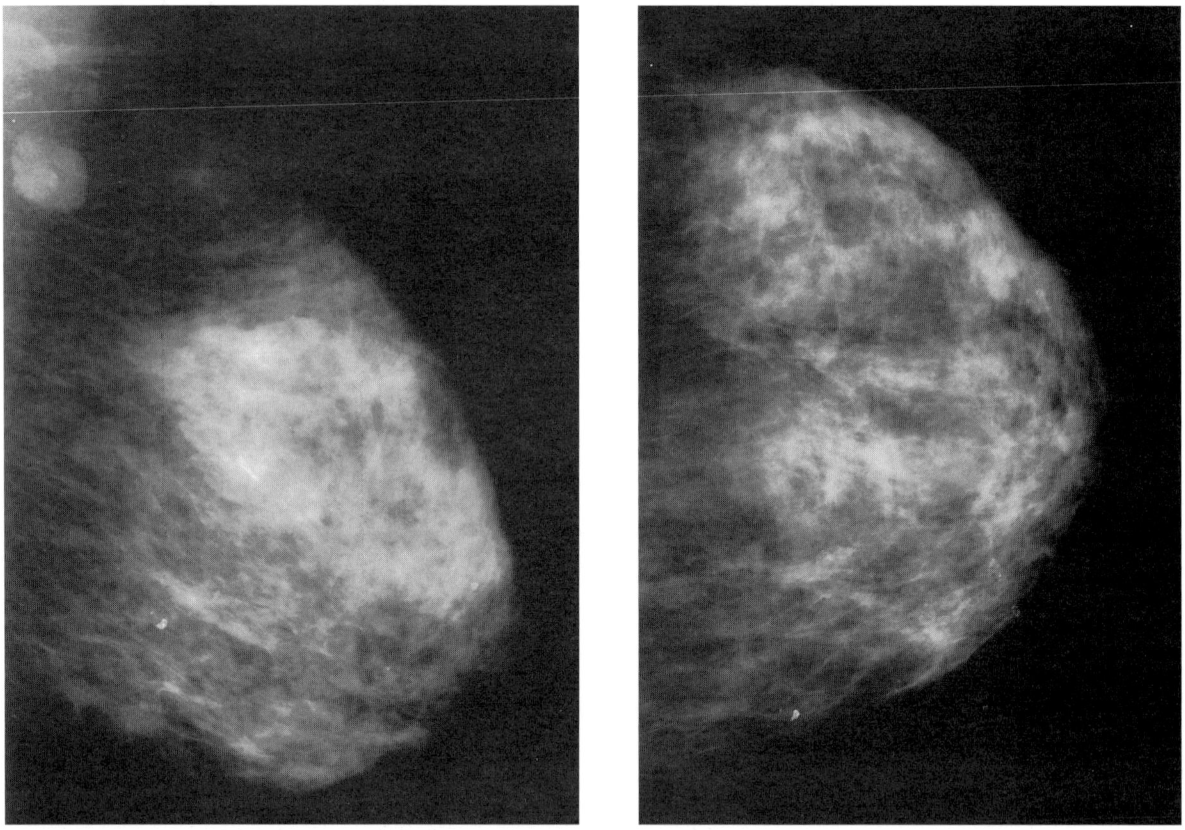

A B

Figure 34–1. In the left axilla there are multiple enlarged axillary nodes. No suspicious mammographic masses or calcifications are present. (A). Left MLO mammogram. (B). Left CC mammogram.

Ultrasound

Frequency

- 11.5 MHz

Mass

- margin: ill defined
- echogenicity: hypoechoic
- retrotumoral acoustic appearance: posterior shadowing distal to mass
- shape: irregular (Fig. 34–2)

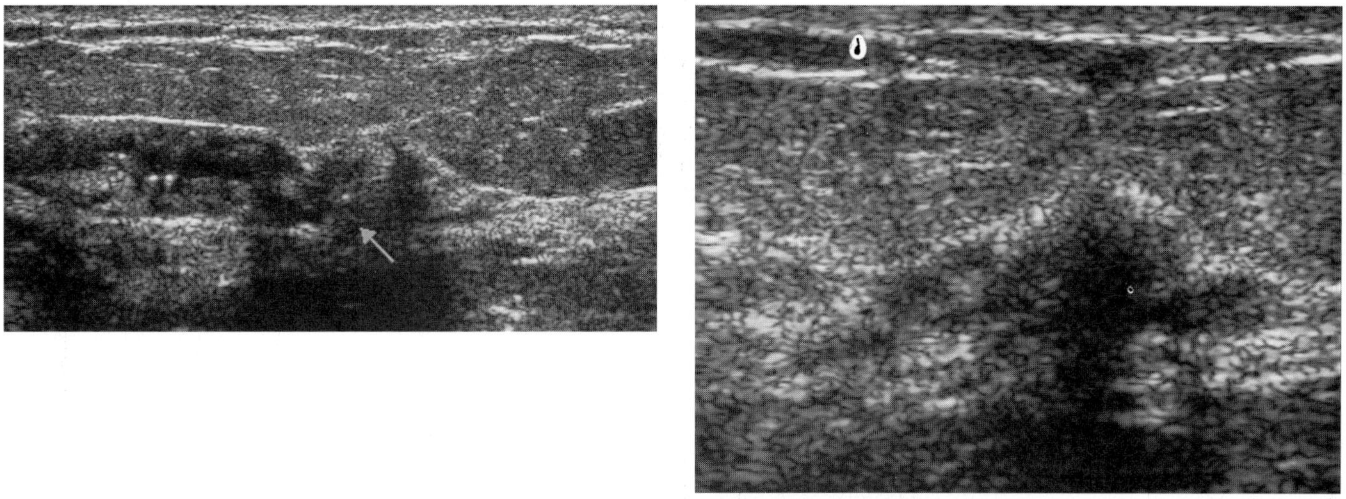

A B

Figure 34–2. At the 6:00 position of the left breast, there is a hypoechoic irregular mass. This area appears to best correlate with the area of abnormal MRI contrast enhancement (Fig. 34–3). However, percutaneous sonographic-guided biopsy of this area was benign. (A). Left radial breast sonogram. (B). Left antiradial breast sonogram.

Other Modalities (Fig. 34–3)

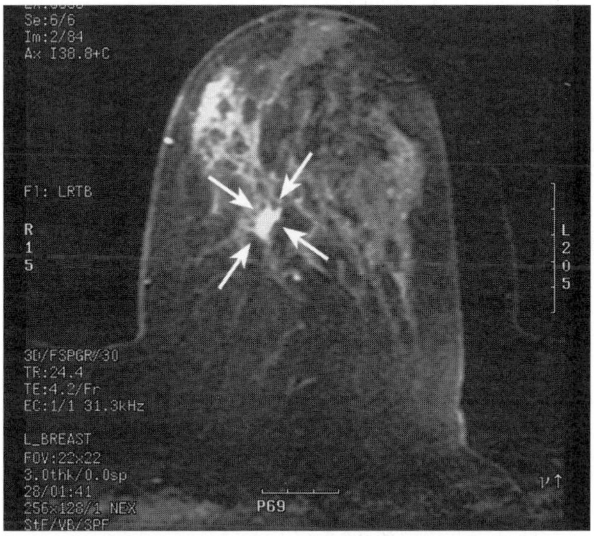

Figure 34–3. Left transverse dynamic bolus 3-D volume gradient breast MRI: In the inferior breast, there is an irregular contrast-enhancing spiculated mass (arrows).

Pathology

- invasive ductal carcinoma

Management

- BI-RADS Assessment Category 4, suspicious; biopsy should be considered

Pearls and Pitfalls

1. This case illustrates a tumor that is only detectable with MRI. Mastectomy specimen demonstrates that the MRI mass corresponds to a 1.5 cm infiltrating ductal carcinoma. No other tumors are detected within the breast. One of 12 axillary nodes are positive for metastatic disease.
2. Breast cancer presents as axillary adenopathy in 0.3 to 1% of reported series. Besides breast cancer, metastatic disease from other distant primaries may present in this manner. The most common primary is melanoma. If the adenopathy is due to breast cancer and the mammogram is normal, then the primary tumors are generally less than 2 cm. In over half of the cases, the breast tumor is in the upper outer quadrant.

Suggested Readings

1. Ashikari R, Rosen PP, Urban JA. Breast cancer presenting as an axillary mass. *Ann Surg* 1976;183:415–417.
2. Feuerman L, Attie JN, Rosenberg B. Carcinoma in axillary lymph nodes as an indicator of breast cancer. *Surg Gynecol Obstet* 1962;114:5–8.
3. Fitts WT, Steiner GC, Enterline HT. Prognosis of occult carcinoma of the breast. *Am J Surg* 1963;106:460–463.
4. Leibman AJ, Kossoff MB. Mammography I. Women with axillary lymphadenopathy and normal breasts on physical examination: value in detecting occult breast carcinoma. *AJR* 1992;159:493–495.
5. Merson M, Anderola S, Galimberti V, Bufalino R, Marchini S, Veronesi U. Breast carcinoma presenting as axillary metastases without evidence of a primary tumor. *Cancer* 1992;70:504–508.
6. Owen HW, Dockerty MB, Gray HK. Occult carcinoma of the breast. *Surg Gynecol Obstet* 1954;98:302–308.
7. Rosen PP. Axillary lymph node metastases in patients with occult noninvasive breast carcinoma. *Cancer* 1980;46:1298–1306.
8. Vilcoq JR, Calle R, Ferme R, et al. Conservative treatment of axillary adenopathy due to probable subclinical breast cancer. *Arch Surg* 1982;117:1136–1138.

Case 35

Case History

A 72-year-old woman presents with a new density on her screening mammogram.

Physical Examination

- normal exam

Mammogram

Mass (Fig. 35-1)

- margin: indistinct
- shape: oval
- density: equal density

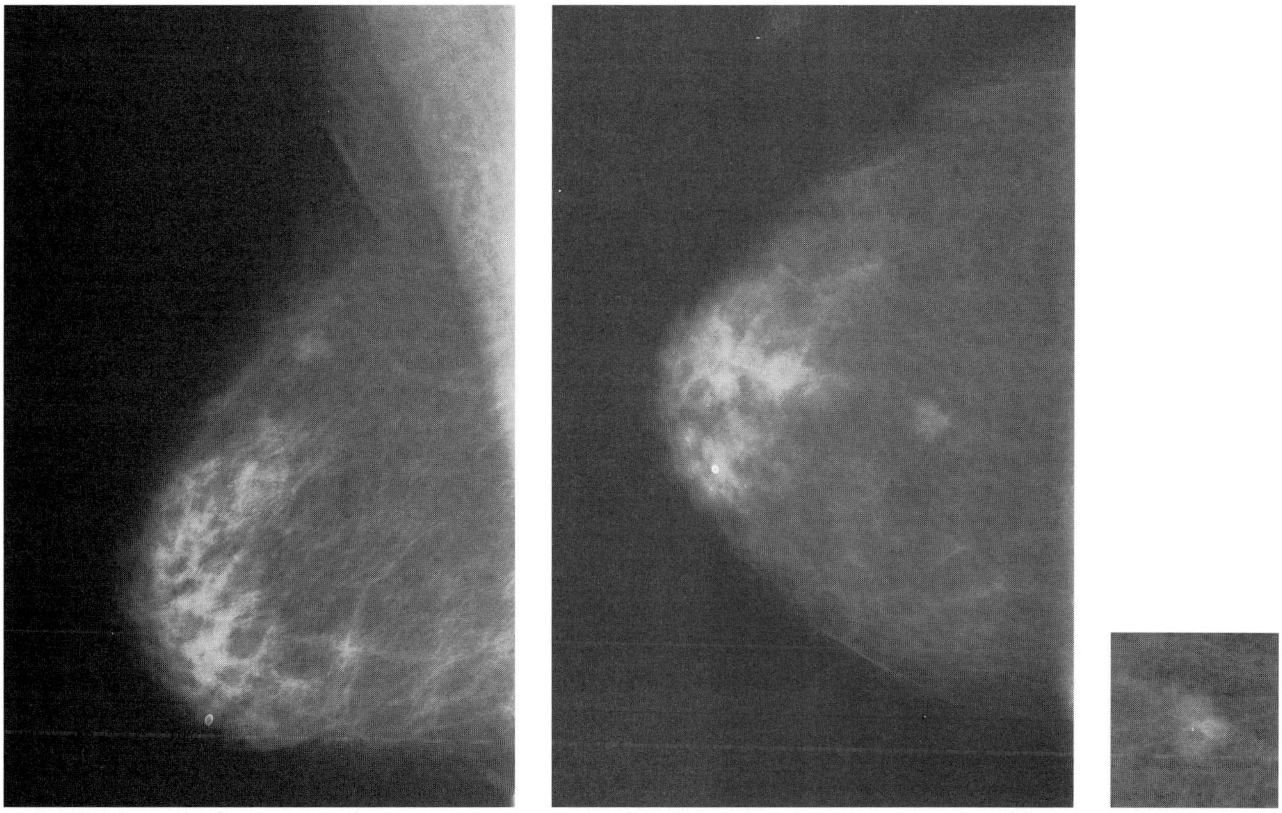

A B C

Figure 35-1. At the 12:00 position there is an oval mass. Spot compression view demonstrates that the mass is mildly lobulated and has an ill-defined margin. (A). Right MLO mammogram. (B). Right CC mammogram. (C). Right CC spot compression.

Pathology

- medullary carcinoma

Management

- BI-RADS Assessment Category 4, suspicious abnormality; biopsy should be considered

Pearls and Pitfalls

1. Medullary carcinoma represents between 5 and 7% of all breast cancers. The mean patient age is 50 years.
2. Series that describe medullary carcinoma commonly include both typical and atypical medullary carcinomas. Typical medullary carcinoma (TMC) is an uncalcified mass with either well-defined or ill-defined margins. Atypical medullary carcinoma (AMC) generally presents with ill-defined margins. Histologically, AMC is commonly mistaken for TMC.
3. Whereas TMC has a favorable prognosis (5-year survival rate of 75 %), AMC prognosis is similar to infiltrating ductal cancer (5-year survival rate of 66 %).

Suggested Readings

1. Bloom HJG, Richardson WW, Field JR. Host resistance and survival in carcinoma of breast. A study of 104 cases of medullary carcinoma in a series of 1411 cases of breast cancer followed for 20 years. *Br Med J* 1970;3:181–187.
2. Hoge A, Asal N, Owen W, Anderson P. Histologic and staging classification of breast cancer: implications for therapy. *South Med J* 1982;75:1329–1332.
3. Liberman L, LaTrenta LR, Samli B, Morris EA, Abramson AF, Dershaw DD. Overdiagnosis of medullary carcinoma: a mammographic-pathologic correlative study. *Radiology* 1996;201:443–446.
4. Lidang Jensen M, Kiaer H, Andersen J, et al. Prognostic comparison of three classifications for medullary carcinomas of the breast. *Histopathology* 1997;30:523–532.
5. Maier WP, Rosemon GP, Goldman LI, et al. A ten year study of medullary carcinoma of the breast. *Surg Obstet Gynecol* 1977;144:695–698.
6. Richardson RW. Medullary carcinoma of the breast: a distinctive tumour type with a relatively good prognosis following radical mastectomy. *Br J Cancer* 1956;10415–10423.
7. Ridolfi RE, Rosen PP, Post A, et al. Medullary carcinoma of the breast. A clinical pathological study with 10 year follow-up. *Cancer* 1977;40:1365–1385.

Case 36

Case History

A 28-year-old woman presents with a palpable right breast lump.

Physical Examination

- right breast: palpable lump at 11:00 position of right breast
- left breast: normal exam

Mammogram

Mass (Fig. 36–1)

- margin: obscured
- shape: oval
- density: equal density

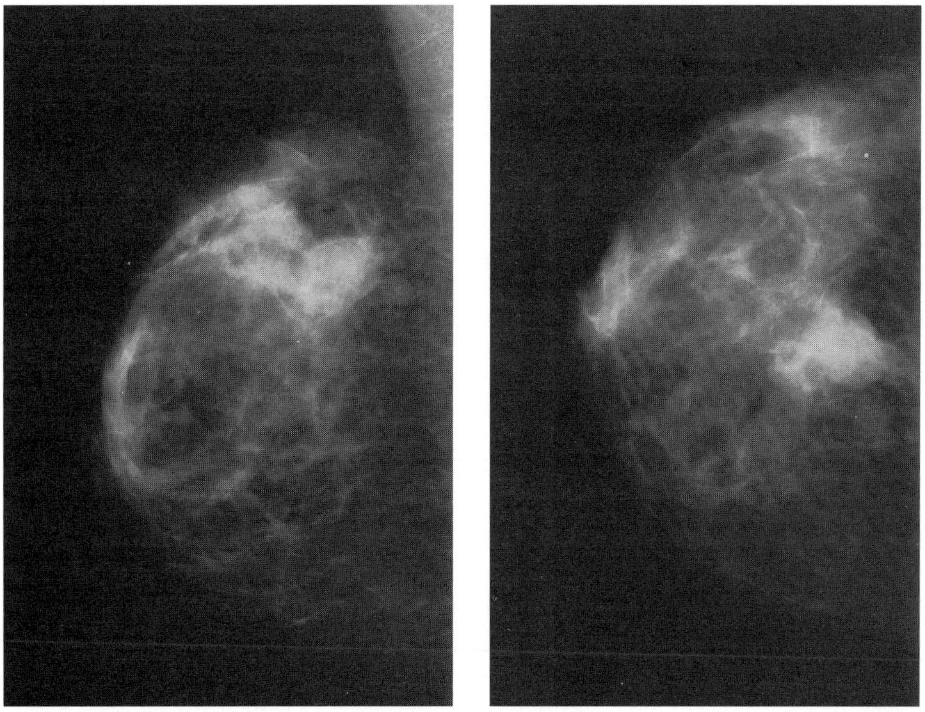

A B

Figure 36–1. At the 11:00 position of the right breast, there is an oval mass with partially obscured margins. This mass corresponds to the palpable mass. (A). Right MLO mammogram. (B). Right CC mammogram.

Ultrasound

Frequency

- 11.5 MHz

Mass

- margin: well defined
- echogenicity: hypoechoic
- retrotumoral acoustic appearance: bilateral edge shadowing
- shape: ellipsoid (Fig. 36–2)

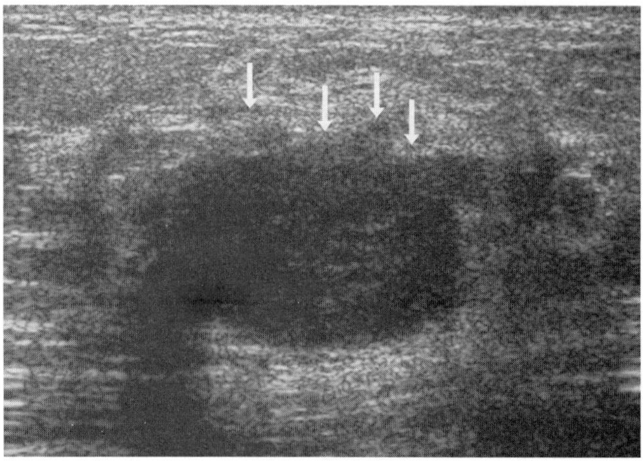

Figure 36–2. Right radial breast sonogram: The palpable lump corresponds to a hypoechoic, oval mass. Most of the margin is well defined, but mild irregularity and lobulation of the superficial margin is present (arrows).

Other Modalities (Fig. 36–3)

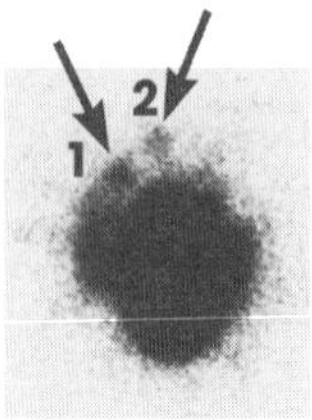

Figure 36–3. Right breast lymphoscintigraphy: Two sentinel lymph nodes (arrows) are identified after injection around the tumor illustrated in Figure 36–2. Both of these nodes were removed and no metastatic disease was identified histologically.

Pathology

- metaplastic carcinoma
- combination of high-grade infiltrating ductal carcinoma and metaplastic changes of benign osteoclastic cells, cartilage, and osteoid

Management

- BI-RADS Assessment Category 4, suspicious; biopsy should be considered

Pearls and Pitfalls

1. Metaplastic carcinoma is a combination of adenocarcinoma (such as invasive ductal) and a second epithelial (e.g., squamous, spindle) or mesenchymal (chondroid, osseous) cell type.
2. Mammographically, these tumors appear as circumscribed lobular, oval, or round masses. If there is a significant invasive ductal component, then the margins may be ill defined or spiculated.
3. Carcinomas with chondroid and osseous differentiation appear to have a better prognosis than those with infiltrating ductal carcinoma in a small series.

Suggested Readings

1. Brenner RJ, Turner GC, Valles AM, et al. Metaplastic carcinoma of the breast: report of three cases. *Cancer* 1998;82:1082–1087.
2. Chieng C, Cranor M, Lesser ME, Rosen PP. Metaplastic carcinoma of the breast with osteocartilaginous heterologous elements. *Am J Surg Pathol* 1998;22:188–194.
3. Patterson SK, Tworek JA, Roubidoux MA, et al. Metaplastic carcinoma of the breast. *Am J Roentgenol* 1997;169:709–712.
4. Tavasoli PA. Metaplastic carcinoma. In: *Pathology of the breast.* Stamford: Appleton and Lange; 1999: 481–504.

Case 37

Case History

A 50-year-old woman presents with a newly discovered lump in her left breast.

Physical Examination

- left breast: palpable 1 cm mass at 12:00
- right breast: normal exam

Mammogram

Mass (Fig. 37–1)

- margin: indistinct
- shape: oval
- density: high density

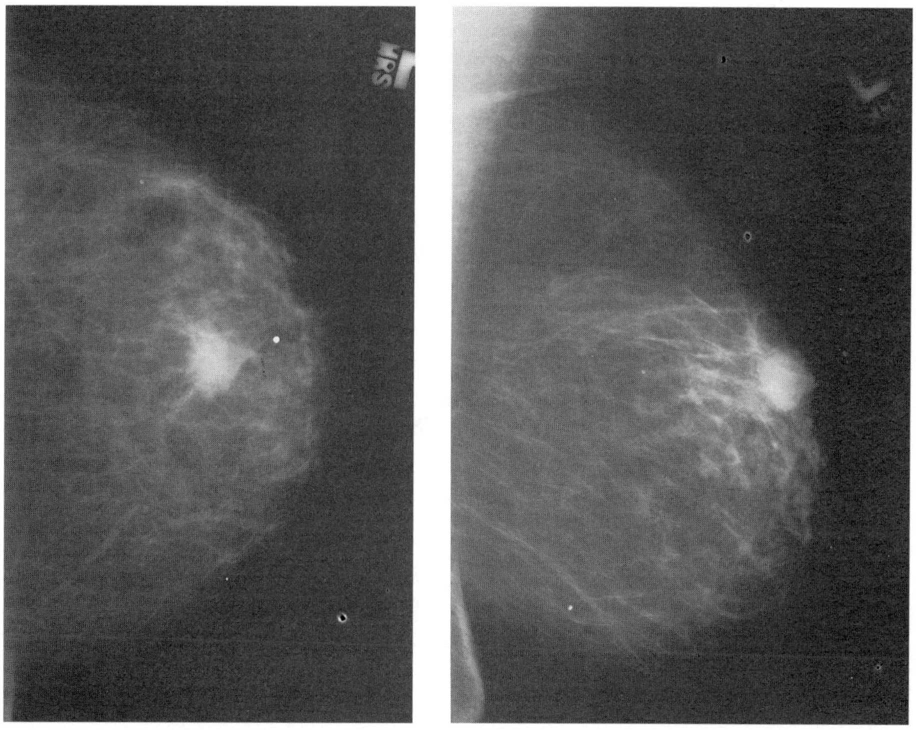

A B

Figure 37–1. At the 12:00 position of the left breast, there is an ill-defined, oval mass that corresponds to the palpable lump. (A). Left MLO mammogram. (B). Left CC mammogram.

Ultrasound

Frequency

- 10 MHz

Mass

- margin: ill defined
- echogenicity: hypoechoic
- retrotumoral acoustic appearance: increased acoustic transmission
- shape: lobulated (Fig. 37–2)

Figure 37–2. Left transverse color Doppler breast sonogram: At the 12:00 position, there is a lobulated multicystic mass. The septations within the mass have color flow and the edge of the mass consists of solid tissue that forms an ill-defined margin (arrows) (see Color Plate 37–2).

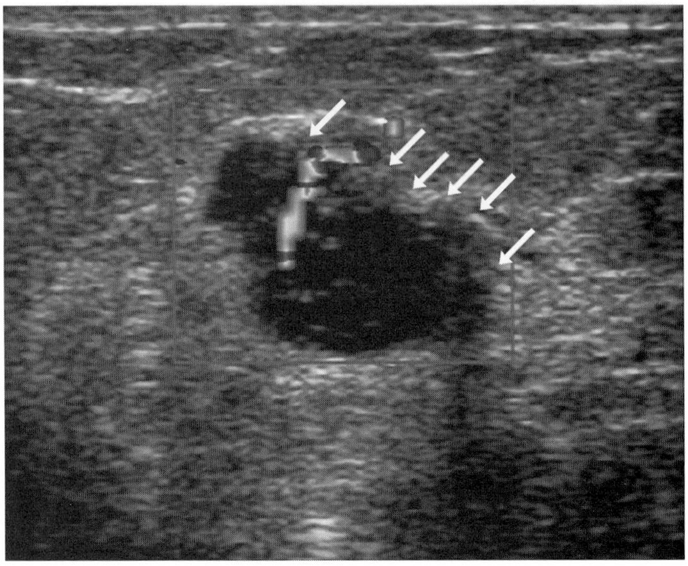

Pathology

- metastases: metastatic melanoma

Management

- BI-RADS Assessment Category 4, suspicious; biopsy should be considered

Pearls and Pitfalls

1. Extramammary metastases to the breast represent about 1% of all clinically detected breast malignancies.
2. Excluding lymphomas and leukemias, the most common extramammary types of metastases to the breast are (in decreasing order of frequency) melanoma, lung, prostate, ovary, gastrointestinal, and cervix.
3. Mammographically, metastases to the breast are noncalcified, round or oval masses with either well-defined or ill-defined margins. They are generally superficial and commonly palpable.
4. Sonographically, metastases are most commonly hypoechoic solid round, oval or lobulated masses with either well-defined or ill-defined margins. Posterior acoustic shadowing is generally not present. Melanoma has increased color flow compared to normal breast parenchyma.

Suggested Readings

1. Bohman LG. Bassett LW, Gold RH, Voet R. Breast metastases from extramammary malignancies. *Radiology* 1982;144:309–312.
2. Derchi LE, Rizzatto G, Giuseppetti GM, Dini G, Garaventa A. Metastatic tumors in the breast: sonographic findings. *J Ultrasound Med* 1985;4:69–74.
3. McCrea ES, Johnston C, Haney PJ. Metastases to the breast. *AJR* 1983;141:685–690.
4. Moncada R, Cooper RA, Garces M, Badrinath K. Calcified metastases from malignant ovarian neoplasm. *Radiology* 1974;113:31–35.
5. Paulus DD, Libshitz HI. Metastasis to the breast. *Radiol Clin North Am* 1982;20:561–568.
6. Tavassoli FA. Metastatic carcinoma. In: Tavassoli FA, Fattaneh A. *Pathology of the Breast.* 2nd ed. Stamford: Appleton and Lange; 1999:551–555.
7. Tohno E, Cosgrove DO, Sloane JP.Metastases to the Breast. In: Tohno D, Cosgrove DO, Sloane JP, eds. *Ultrasound Diagnosis of Breast Diseases.* New York: Churchill Livingston; 1994:185–186.
8. Toombs BD, Kalisher L. Mastatic disease to the breast: clinical, pathologic, and radiographic features. *Am J Roentgenol* 1977;129:673–676.

Case 38

Case History

A 39-year-old woman presents with new left breast lump.

Physical Examination

- left breast: palpable mass at the 4:00 position; a second mammographic mass is not palpable
- right breast: normal exam

Mammogram

Mass (Fig. 38–1)

- margin: circumscribed
- shape: oval
- density: high density

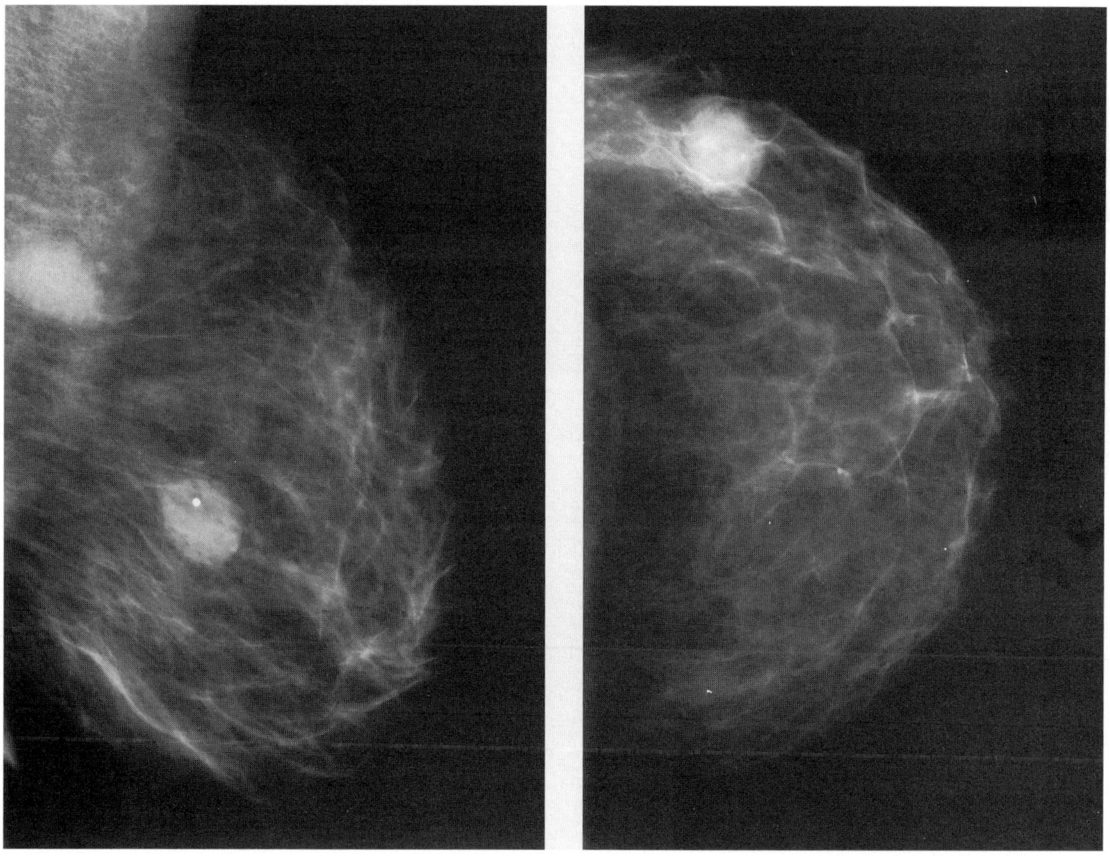

A B

Figure 38–1. Two similar circumscribed oval masses are present in the left breast. One mass is in the upper outer quadrant and the other is in the outer inferior quadrant. These masses are new since the patient's baseline mammogram 3 years ago. (A). Left MLO mammogram. (B). Left CC mammogram.

Ultrasound

Frequency

- 11.5 MHz

Mass

- margin: well defined
- echogenicity: hypoechoic
- retrotumoral acoustic appearance: bilateral edge shadowing
- shape: ellipsoid (Figs. 38–2 and 38–3)

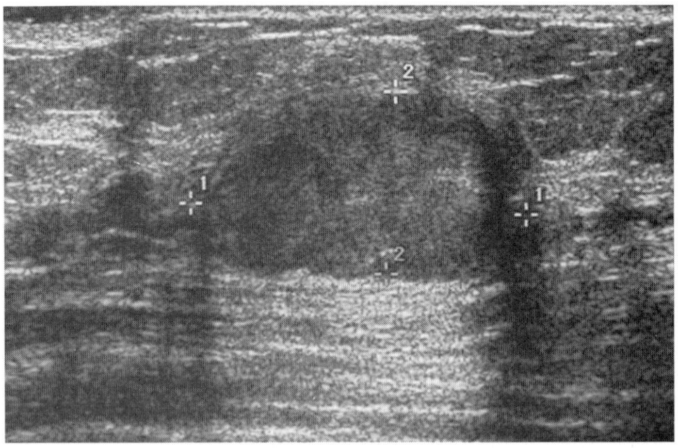

Figure 38–2. Left radial breast sonogram at 2:00: The mammographic mass in the left upper outer quadrant (Fig. 38–1) corresponds to a well-defined oval, hypoechoic mass with posterior acoustic enhancement.

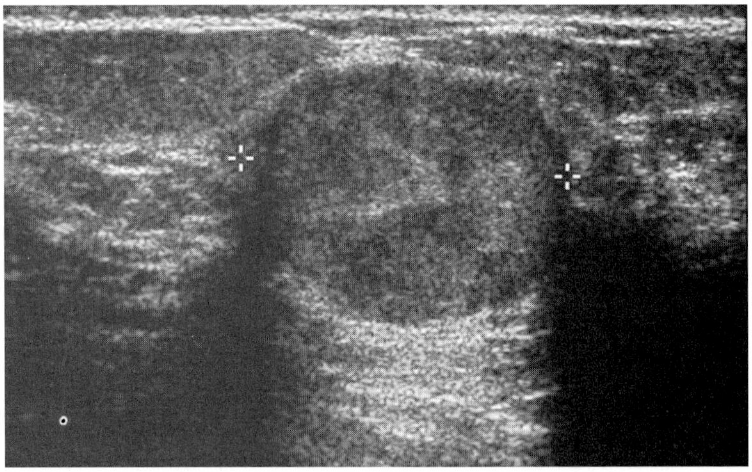

Figure 38–3. Left radial breast sonogram at 4:00: The mammographic mass in the inferior outer quadrant (Fig. 38–1) corresponds to a well-defined, oval, hypoechoic mass with increased acoustic enhancement. The appearance of this mass is similar to the 2:00 mass (Fig. 38–2).

Pathology

- mucinous carcinoma

Management

- BI-RADS Assessment Category 4, suspicious; biopsy should be considered

Pearls and Pitfalls

1. Mucinous carcinoma accounts for 1 to 7% of all breast cancers. The mean age of patients is in the seventh decade.
2. Mammographically, mucinous cancers are oval or lobulated and may have either ill-defined or well-defined margins. Low-grade, pure mucinous tumors tend to have well-defined margins.
3. Sonographically, mucinous neoplasms appear as well-defined lobulated or oval hypoechoic masses with a thin hyperechoic capsule. They may exhibit decreased, equal, or increased acoustic transmission.

Suggested Readings

1. Cardenosa G, Doudna C, Eklund GW. Mucinous (colloid) breast cancer: clinical and mammographic findings in 10 patients. *AJR* 1994;162:1077–1079.
2. Chopra S, Evans AJ, Pinder SE, et al. Pure mucinous breast cancer-mammographic and ultrasound findings. *Clin Radiol* 1996;51:421–424.
3. Conant EF, Dillon RL, Palazzo J, Ehrlish SM, Feig SA. Imaging findings in mucin-containing carcinomas of the breast: correlation with pathologic features. *AJR* 1994;163:821–824.
4. Ruggieri AM, Scola FH, Schepps B, et al. Mucinous carcinoma of the breast: mammographic findings. *Breast Dis* 1995;8:353–361.
5. Wilson TE, Helvie MA, Oberman HA, Joynt LK. Pure and mixed mucinous carcinoma of the breast: pathologic basis for differences in mammographic appearance. *AJR* 1995;165:285–289.

Case 39

Case History

A 43-year-old woman presents with a palpable lump. Lump was first detected 1 year ago and had been found to be sonographically solid.

Physical Examination

- left breast: 2 to 3 cm mass at the 1:00 position
- right breast: normal exam

Mammogram

Mass (Fig. 39–1)

- margin: circumscribed
- shape: oval
- density: equal density

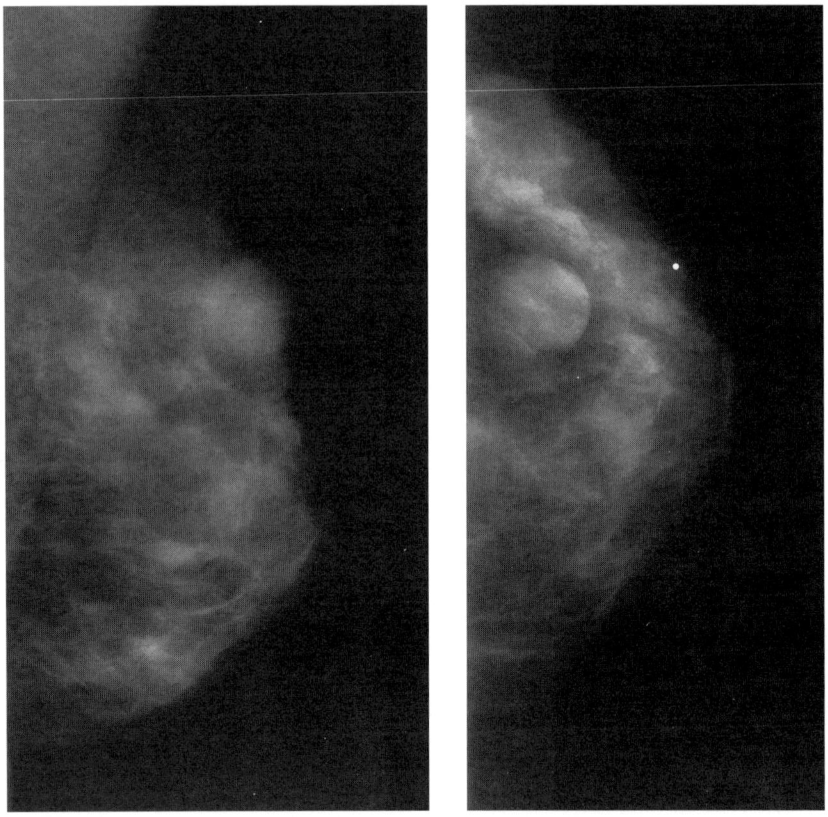

A B

Figure 39–1. At the 1:00 position of the left breast there is a predominantly circumscribed oval mass that corresponds to the patient's palpable lump. (A). Left MLO mammogram. (B). Left CC mammogram.

Ultrasound

Frequency

- 7.5 MHz

Mass

- margin: well defined
- echogenicity: heterogeneous (mixed)
- retrotumoral acoustic appearance: retrotumoral enhancement present
- shape: ellipsoid (Fig. 39–2)

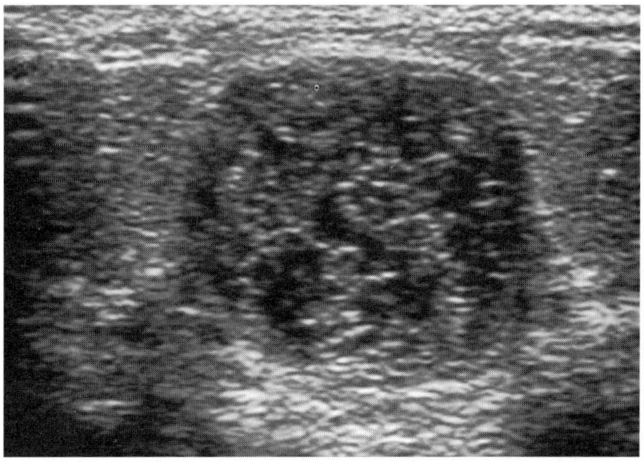

Figure 39–2. Left longitudinal breast sonogram: The palpable mass corresponds to a well-defined, oval, solid mass with heterogenous echogenicity and increased acoustic transmission. Irregular cystic spaces are present thoughout the mass. Since the previous sonogram (1 year prior) the mass has doubled in size.

Pathology

- phyllodes tumor (cystosarcoma phyllodes)

Management

- BI-RADS Assessment Category 4, suspicious abnormality; biopsy should be considered

Pearls and Pitfalls

1. Phyllodes tumors constitute 0.3% of all breast tumors. Women with this tumor are generally older than women with fibroadenomas. The average age is 45. About 30% of phyllodes tumors recur and 10% metastasize. This tumor most frequently metastasizes to lungs (66%), skeleton (28%), and lymph nodes (15%).
2. Mammographically, phyllodes tumors are generally well defined, uncalcified, and are lobulated, round, or oval. They are similar to fibroadenomas, but should be considered if the mass is greater than 6 to 8 cm or is rapidly growing.
3. Sonographically, these masses are hypoechoic or heterogeneous echogenicity with posterior acoustic enhancement. Unlike fibroadenomas, phyllodes tumors commonly have thin, irregular cystic spaces within them.

Suggested Readings

1. Buchberger W, Strasser K, Heim D, Muller E, Schrocksnadel H. Phylloides tumor: findings on mammography, sonography, and aspiration cytology in 10 cases. *AJR* 1991;157:715–719.
2. Czum JM, Sanders LM, Titus JM, Kalisher L. Breast imaging case of the day. *Radiographics* 1997;17:548–551.
3. Liberman L, Bonaccio E, Hamele-Bena D, Abramson AF, Cohen MA, Dershaw DD. Benign and malignant phyllodes tumors: mammographic and sonographic findings. *Radiology* 1996;198:121–124.
4. Tavassoli FA, Fattaneh A. *Pathology of the Breast.* 2nd ed. Stamford: Appleton and Lange; 1999:598–631.

Case 40

Case History

A 45-year-old woman presents for screening mammogram.

Physical Examination

- normal exam

Mammogram

Mass (Fig. 40–1)

- margin: indistinct
- shape: oval
- density: high density

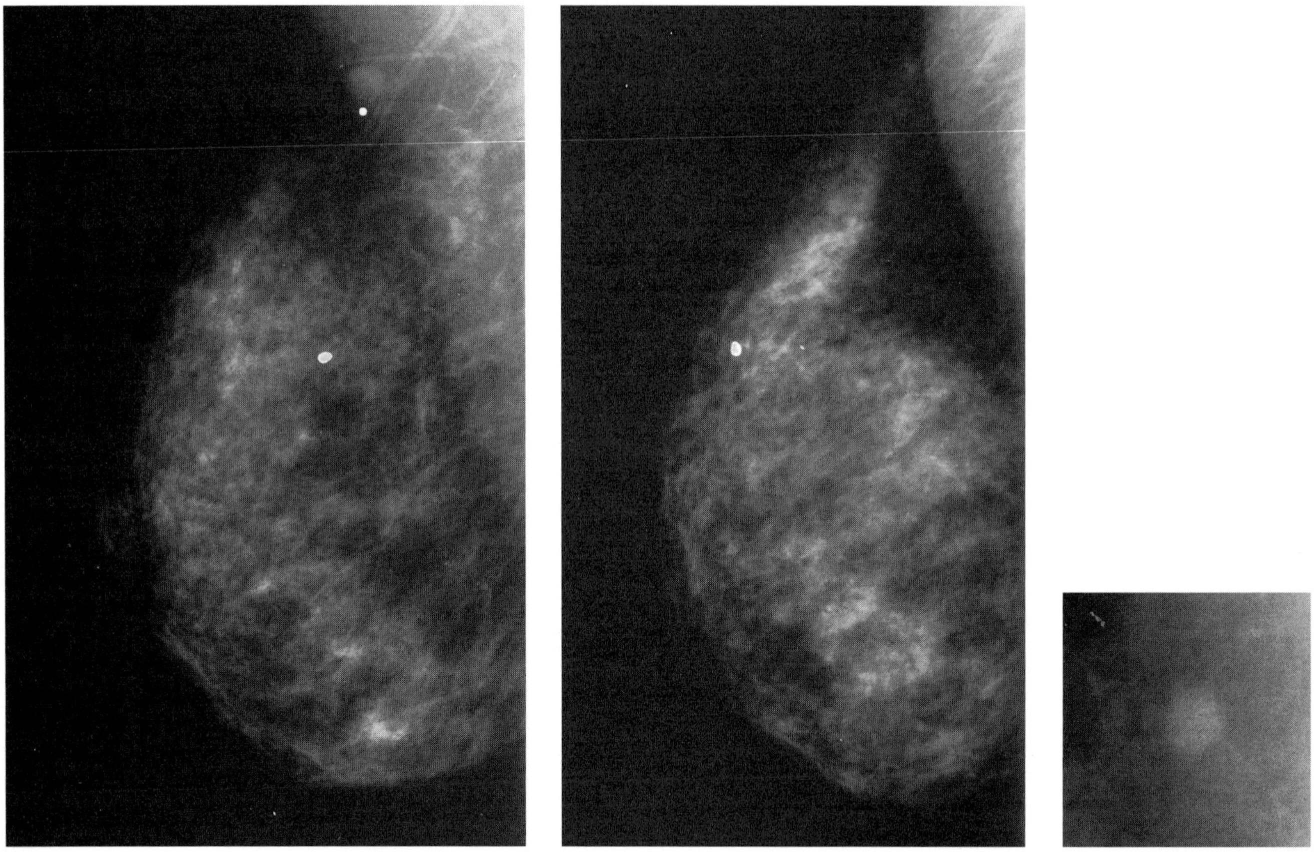

A B C

Figure 40–1. In the right upper outer quadrant, there is an ill-defined oval mass. (A). Right MLO mammogram. (B). Right exaggerated CC mammogram. (C). Right MLO spot compression mammogram.

Ultrasound

Frequency

- 13 MHz

Mass

- margin: ill defined
- echogenicity: hypoechoic
- retrotumoral acoustic appearance: bilateral edge shadowing
- shape: ellipsoid (Figs. 40-2 and 40-3)

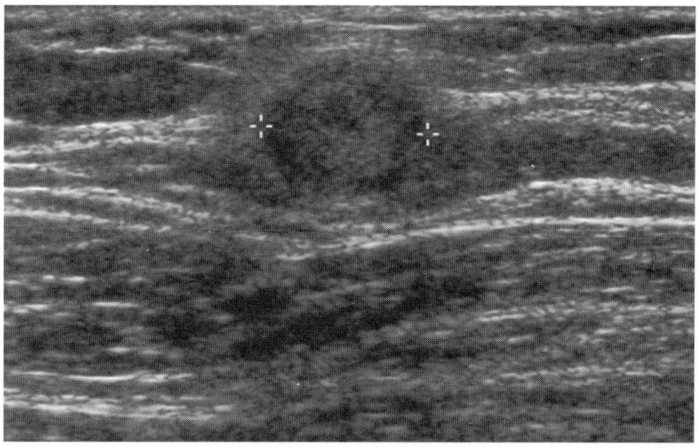

Figure 40-2. Right radial breast sonogram: The mammographic mass corresponds to an oval hypoechoic solid mass. In this view, the mass has a subtle hyperechoic irregular halo.

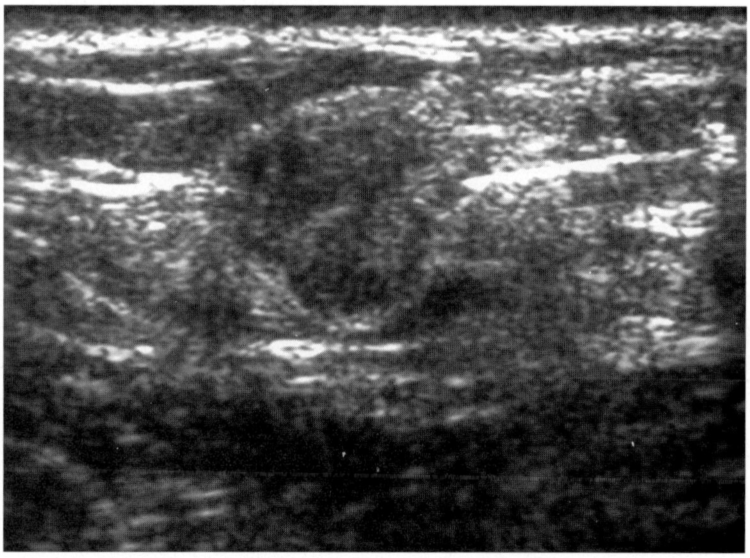

Figure 40-3. Right antiradial breast sonogram: The irregular margin of the mass is better demonstrated in this view.

Pathology

- granular cell tumor

Management

- BI-RADS Assessment Category 4, suspicious; biopsy should be considered

Pearls and Pitfalls

1. Granular cell tumors represent $<0.1\%$ of breast lesions. Although the tumor has been reported in a wide age range (17 to 75 years), it tends to present in younger women (average age in the 30s).
2. Mammographically and sonographically, this tumor presents as an oval or round mass with ill-defined or spiculated margins.
3. Although this mass may simulate carcinoma, it rarely metastasizes. It may be infiltrative so local excision is required.

Suggested Readings

1. Bassett LW, Cove HC. Myoblastoma of the breast. *AJR* 1979;132:122–123.
2. Baum JK, Robins JR, Schnitt S, Houlihan MJ. The ultrasound appearance of granular cell tumor of the breast: a case report. *Breast Dis* 1994;7:281–285.
3. Ilkhanipour ZS, Harris KM, Kanbour AI. Granular cell tumor of the breast: two case reports mimicking carcinoma. *Breast Dis* 1993;6:221–225.
4. Tavassoli FA, Fattaneh A. *Pathology of the Breast.* 2nd ed. Stamford: Appleton and Lange; 1999:697.

Section IV

Irregular Masses

This is an outline of the approach to mammographic irregular masses. For further discussion, see Chapter 1.

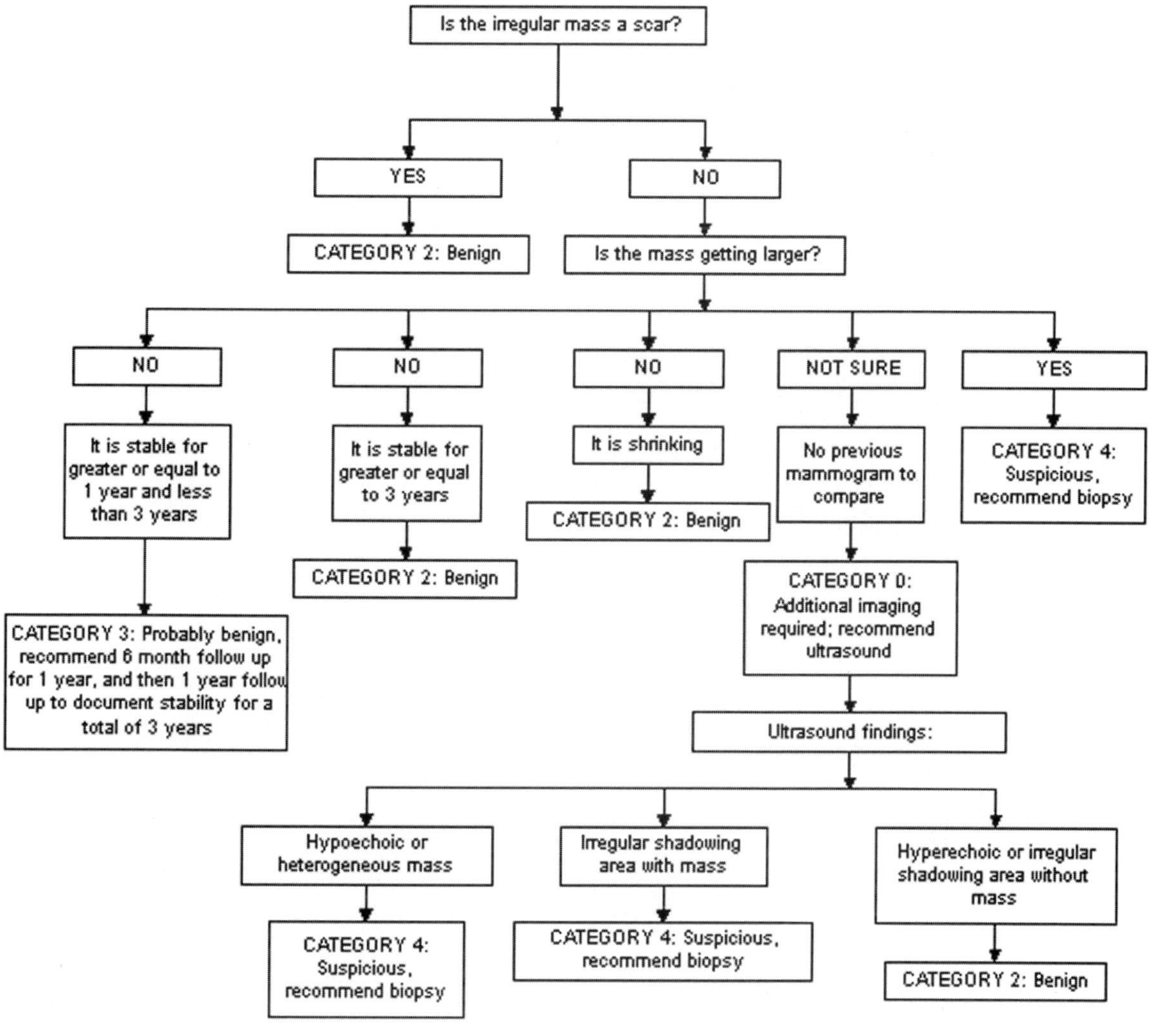

Case 41

Case History

An 86-year-old woman presents with a new left breast palpable lump.

Physical Examination

- left breast: palpable lump in upper outer quadrant
- right breast: normal exam

Mammogram

Mass (Fig. 41-1)

- margin: indistinct
- shape: irregular
- density: equal density

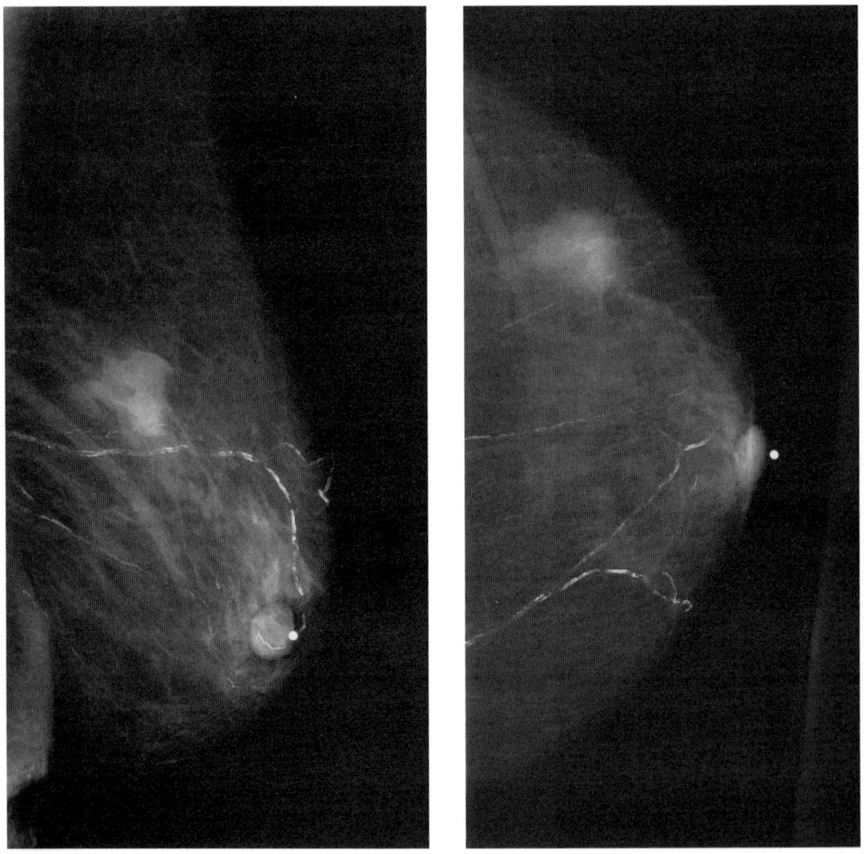

A B

Figure 41-1. In the left upper outer quadrant, there is an irregular mass that corresponds to the palpable lump. (A). Left MLO mammogram. (B). Left CC mammogram.

Ultrasound

Frequency (Fig. 41–2)

- 8 MHz
- margin: ill-defined
- echogenicity: hyperechoic
- retrotumoral acoustic appearance: posterior shadowing distal to mass
- shape: ellipsoid

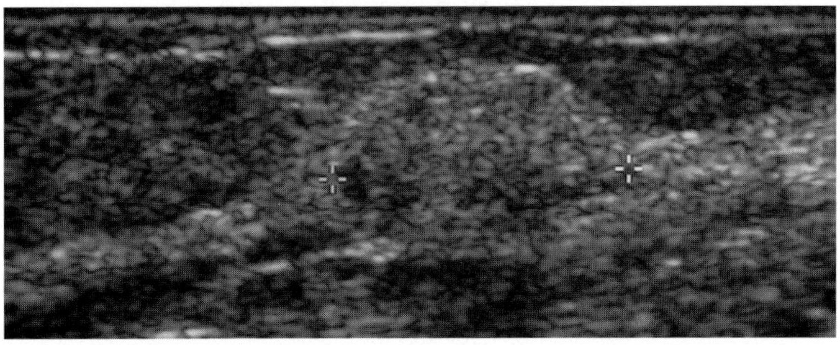

Figure 41–2. Left radial breast sonogram: The palpable mammographic mass corresponds to a hyperechoic oval mass, which has a partially ill-defined margin.

Pathology

- microglandular adenosis

Management

- BI-RADS Assessment Category 4, suspicious; biopsy should be considered

Pearls and Pitfalls

1. Microglandular adenosis is a rare type of adenosis. Most patients present with a palpable lump.
2. There are no specific radiographic or sonographic patterns for this disease due to its rarity.
3. Microglandular adenosis has been associated with infiltrating carcinoma so lesions that increase in size should be critically reevaluated.

Suggested Readings

1. James BA, Cranor ML, Rosen PP. Carcinoma of the breast arising in microglandular adenosis. *Am J Clin Pathol* 1993;100:507–513.
2. Rosen PP. Microglandular adenosis: a benign lesion simulating invasive mammary carcinoma. *Am J Surg Pathol* 1983;7:137–144.
3. Rosenblum MK, Purazella R, Rosen PP. Is microglandular adenosis a precancerous disease? A study of carcinoma arising therein. *Am J Surg Pathol* 1986;10:237–245.
4. Tavassoli FA. Benign lesions. In: Tavasolli FA, Fattaneh A, eds. *Pathology of the Breast.* 2nd ed. Stamford: Appleton and Lange; 1999:115–204.

Case 42

Case History

A 60-year-old woman presents with a new right breast lump. She has no previous trauma, breast surgery, or biopsy.

Physical Examination

- right breast: palpable lump at 11:00
- left breast: normal exam

Mammogram

Mass (Fig. 42–1)

- margin: indistinct
- shape: irregular
- density: equal density

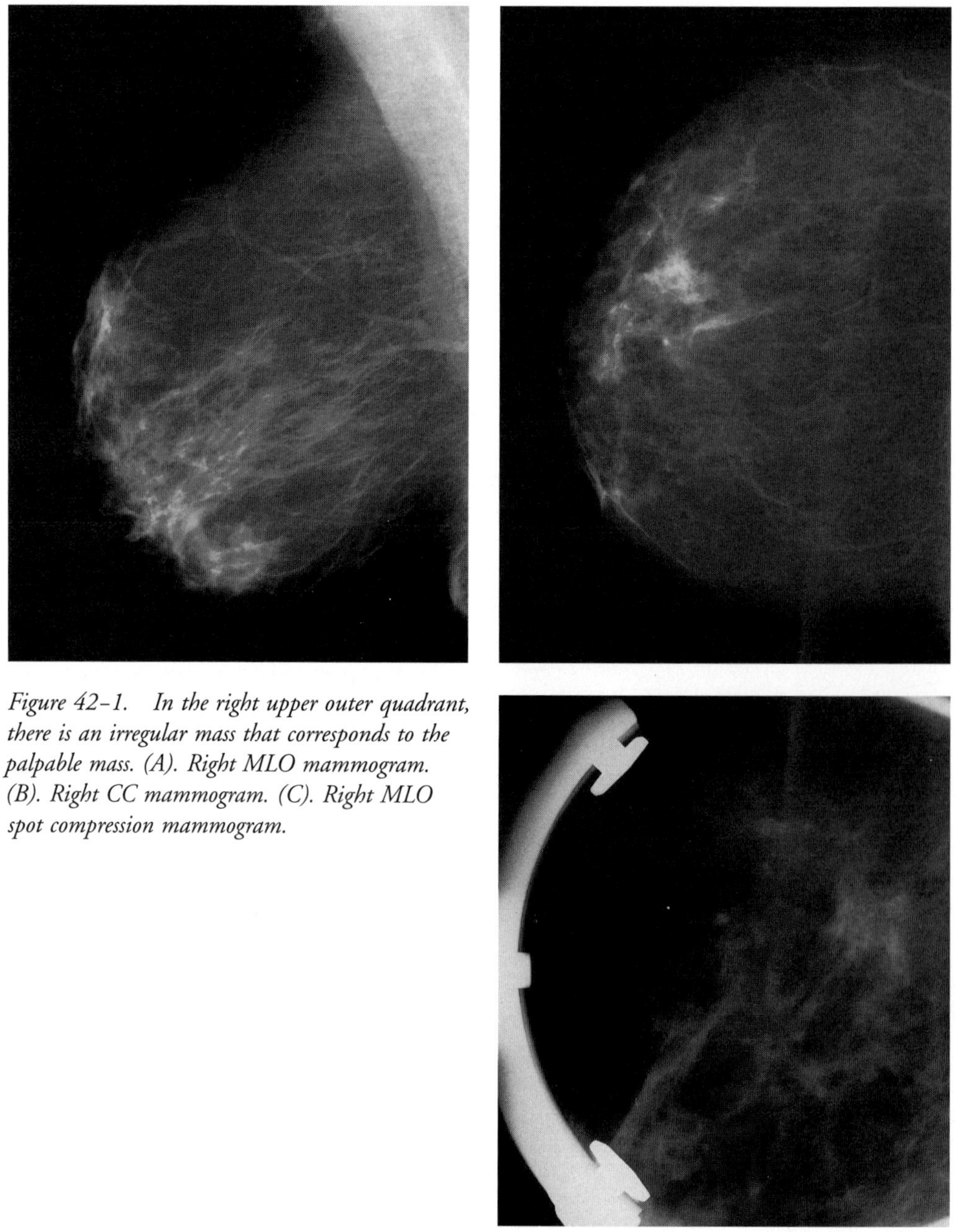

Figure 42–1. In the right upper outer quadrant, there is an irregular mass that corresponds to the palpable mass. (A). Right MLO mammogram. (B). Right CC mammogram. (C). Right MLO spot compression mammogram.

Ultrasound

Frequency

- 11.5 MHz

Mass

- margin: ill defined
- echogenicity: heterogeneous
- retrotumoral acoustic appearance: posterior shadowing distal to mass
- shape: irregular (Fig. 42–2)

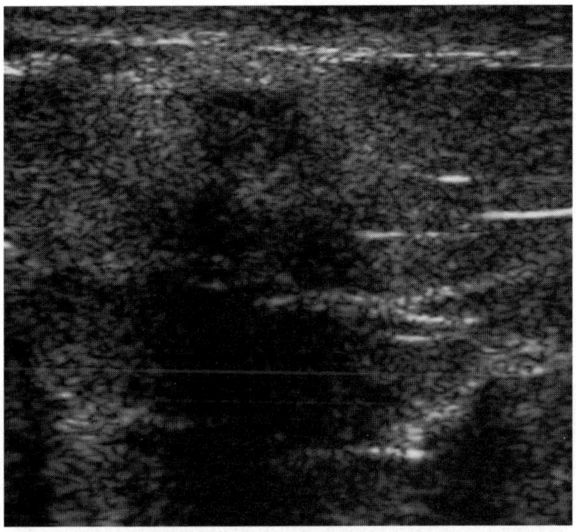

Figure 42–2. Right radial breast sonogram: The palpable mammographic mass corresponds to an ill-defined irregular mass with a hyperechoic rim and hypoechoic center. The mass exhibits severe acoustic shadowing.

Pathology

- fat necrosis

Management

- BI-RADS Assessment Category 4, suspicious; biopsy should be considered

Pearls and Pitfalls

Although only 40% of patients with fat necrosis have a history of previous breast injury, this lesion has a traumatic origin. Fat necrosis has two different appearances. In some patients, the fat necrosis causes a fibrotic response that results in an irregular solid mass (illustrated in this case), which may be associated with skin thickening and nipple retraction. This form cannot be distinguished mammographically or sonographically from carcinoma. The other form results in a lipid collection without an inflammatory response. This form results in a round or oval nodule (oil cyst) that is either calcium or fat density mammographically.

Suggested Readings

1. Bassett LW, Gold RH, Cove HC. Mammographic spectrum of traumatic fat necrosis: the fallibility of "pathognomonic" signs of carcinoma. *AJR* 1978;130:119–122.
2. Evers K, Troupin RH. Lipid cyst: classic and atypical appearances. *AJR* 1991;157:271–273.
3. Orson LW, Cigtay OS. Fat necrosis of the breast: characteristic xeromammographic appearance. *Radiology* 1983;146:35–38.

Case 43

Case History

A 72-year-old woman status post–right lumpectomy and radiation therapy has developed a new mammographic finding near the surgical site.

Physical Examination

- right breast: subareolar scar
- left breast: normal exam

Mammogram

Mass (Fig. 43–1)

- margin: spiculated
- shape: irregular
- density: equal density

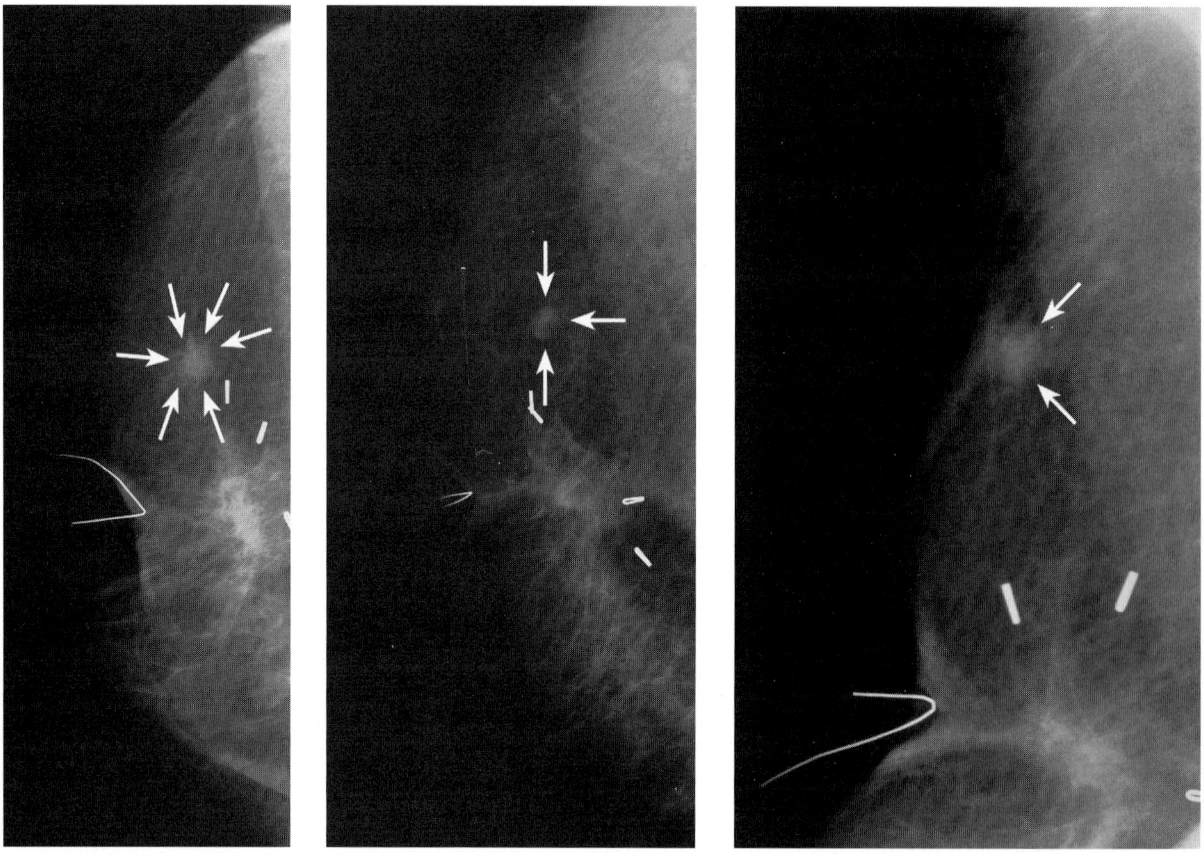

A B C

Figure 43–1. There is a spiculated density deep to the right nipple. This density corresponds to the scar from the patient's lumpectomy. In the upper outer breast, there is a spiculated mass (arrows), which is separate from the main scar. This spiculated mass is new since the patient's previous exam. (A). Right LM mammogram. (B). Right CC mammogram. (C). Right mammogram tangential to spiculated mass (arrows).

Ultrasound

Frequency

- 10 MHz

Mass

- margin: ill defined
- echogenicity: hypoechoic
- retrotumoral acoustic appearance: severe shadowing
- shape: irregular (Figs. 43–2 and 43–3)

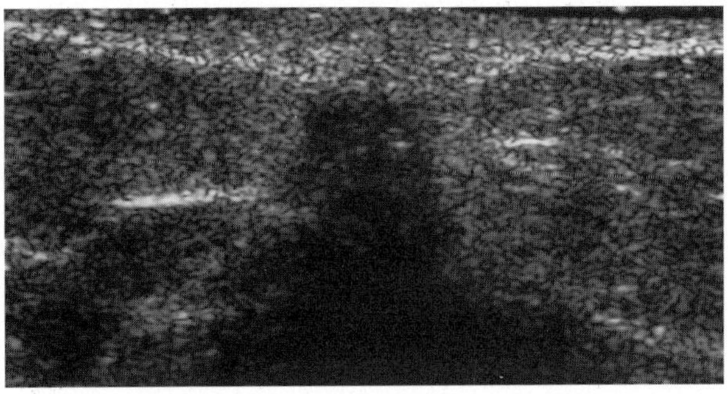

Figure 43–2. Right radial breast sonogram: In the upper outer quadrant, the new small spiculated mammographic mass corresponds to an ill-defined hypoechoic shadowing mass. The hyperechoic halo around the mass corresponds to the mammographic spiculations.

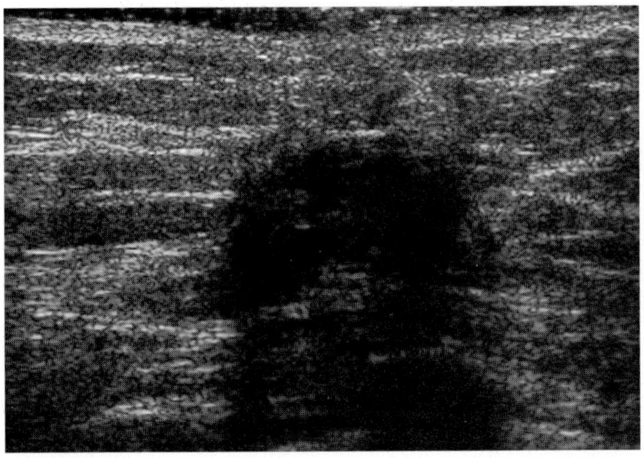

A

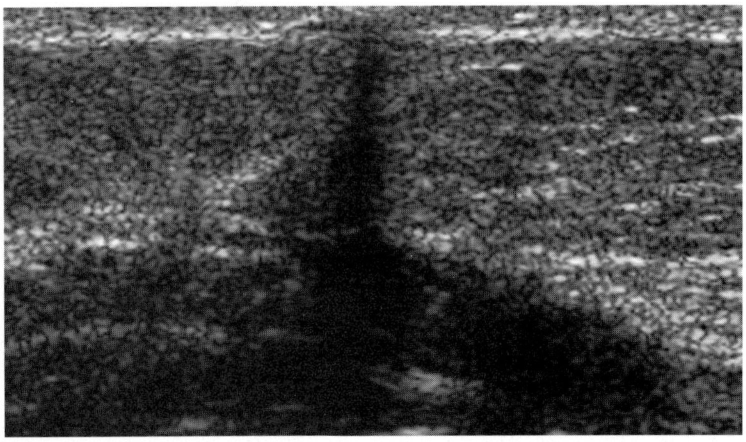

B

Figure 43–3. The lumpectomy scar is distinguished from the adjacent spiculated mass by both its location and appearance. Although the scar is wide in the antiradial view (A), it is extremely narrow in the radial view (B). The adjacent spiculated mass depicted in Figure 43–2 is the same width in both views. (A). Right antiradial breast sonogram. (B). Right radial breast sonogram.

Pathology

- fat necrosis: the new spiculated mass in the right upper outer quadrant corresponded to fat necrosis.
- scar: the lumpectomy scar showed no evidence of recurrence and was not rebiopsied.

Management

- BI-RADS Assessment Category 4, suspicious; biopsy should be considered

Pearls and Pitfalls

1. When fat necrosis causes new irregular masses in the area of a lumpectomy site, this abnormality cannot be distinguished from malignancy mammographically or sonographically.
2. Sonographically, scars are irregular spiculated masses. They can be distinguished from malignancy when the scar produces architectural distortion without a mass. This case illustrates the appearance of a benign scar. Although one view exhibits hypoechoic architectural distortion, the other view demonstrates no mass, only a thin line of tissue irregularity. However, if a scar develops a hypoechoic mass from fibrosis or fat necrosis, then malignancy cannot be excluded.

Suggested Readings

1. Sohn C, Blohmer J-U, Hamper UM. Sonography in the follow-up of breast cancer. In: Sohn C, Blohmer J-U, Hamper UM, eds. *Breast Ultrasound.* New York: Thieme; 1999:98–102.
2. Tohno E, Cosgrove DO, Sloane JP. Postoperative scarring. In: Tohno D, Cosgrove DO, Sloane JP, eds. *Ultrasound Diagnosis of Breast Diseases.* New York: Churchill Livingston; 1994:146–147.

Case 44

Case History

A 49-year-old woman presents with a new density on her right screening mammogram.

Physical Examination

- normal exam

Mammogram

Mass (Fig. 44-1)

- margin: indistinct
- shape: irregular
- density: equal

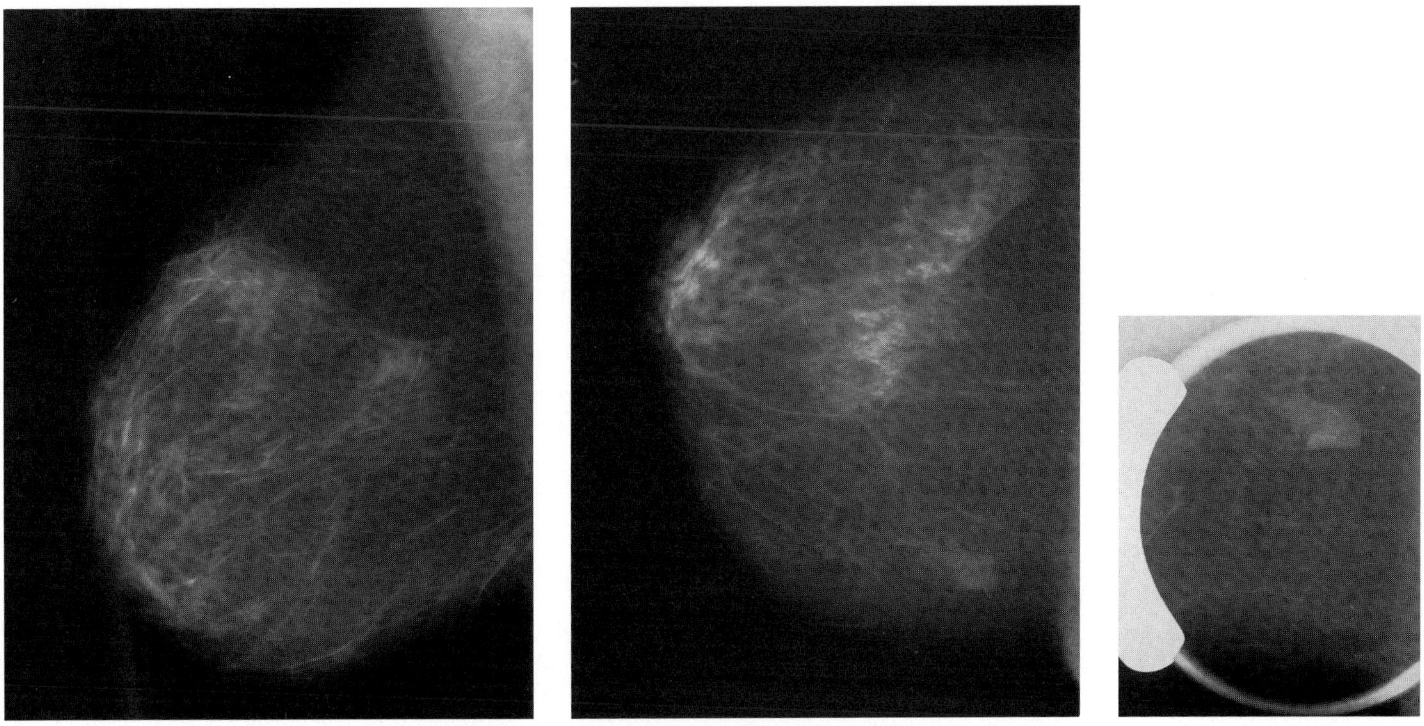

A B C

Figure 44-1. In the right upper medial breast there is an irregular mass that is partially obscured by the dense overlapping breast tissue. (A). Right MLO mammogram. (B). Right CC mammogram. (C). Right CC spot compression mammogram.

Ultrasound

Frequency

- 7.5 MHz

Mass

- margin: ill defined
- echogenicity: hyperechoic
- retrotumoral acoustic appearance: posterior shadowing distal to mass
- shape: irregular (Fig. 44-2)

Figure 44–2. Right breast sonogram: The irregular density identified in Figure 44–1 corresponds to a homogeneously hyperechoic irregular mass. (A). Right radial breast sonogram. (B). Right aradial breast sonogram.

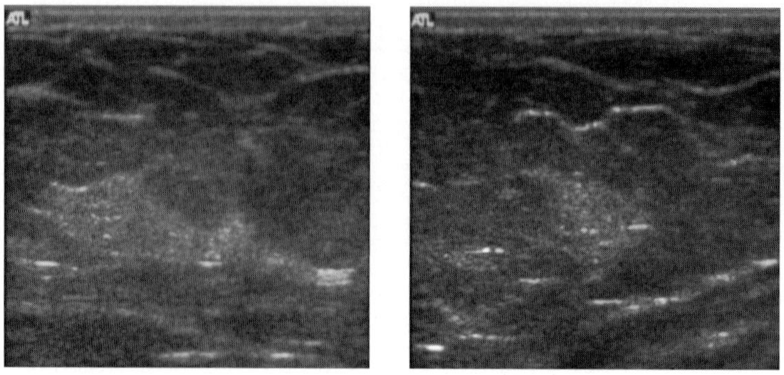
A B

Pathology

- fibroadenoma

Management

- BI-RADS Assessment Category 4, suspicious; biopsy should be considered

Pearls and Pitfalls

1. Fibroadenomas are the most common mass in women younger than 40 years. Researchers have reported that these masses are present in 9 to 25% of autopsy cases. The highest incidence of fibroadenomas is in women younger than 25 years.
2. Mammographically, fibroadenomas are most commonly oval, round, or lobular circumscribed masses. Sometimes, they appear irregular as in this case. Fibroadenomas may have large popcorn calcifications. Rarely, their calcifications similate malignant microcalcifications.
3. Sonographically, these masses are generally oval, round, or lobular, well-defined solid masses. Less than one third of fibroadenomas have irregular margins. Echogenicity of fibroadenomas are generally hypoechoic (92%). Less commonly, they are hyperechoic (4%), heterogeneous (2%), or anechoic (1%).

Suggested Readings

1. Cole-Beuglet C, Skoriano RZ, Kurtz AB, Goldberg BB. Fibroadenoma of the breast: sonogrammography correlated with pathology in 122 patients. *AJR* 1983;140:369–375.
2. Fornage BD, Lorigan JB, Andry E. Fibroadenoma of the breast: sonographic appearance. *Radiology* 1989;172:671–675.
3. Frantz VK, Pickren JW, Melcher GE, et al. Incidence of chronic cystic disease in so called “normal breasts.” A study based on 225 postmortem examinations. *Cancer* 1951;4:762–783.
4. Jackson VP, Rothschild PA, Kreipke DL, et al. The spectrum of sonographic findings of fibroadenoma of the breast. *Invest Radiol* 1986;21:34–40.
5. Meyer JE, Frenna TH, Polger M, Sonnenfeld MR, Shaffer K. Enlarging occult fibroadenomas. *Radiology* 1992;183:639–641.

Case 45

Case History

An 84-year-old woman presents for screening mammogram.

Physical Examination

- normal exam

Mammogram

Mass (Fig. 45-1)

- margin: indistinct
- shape: irregular
- density: equal density

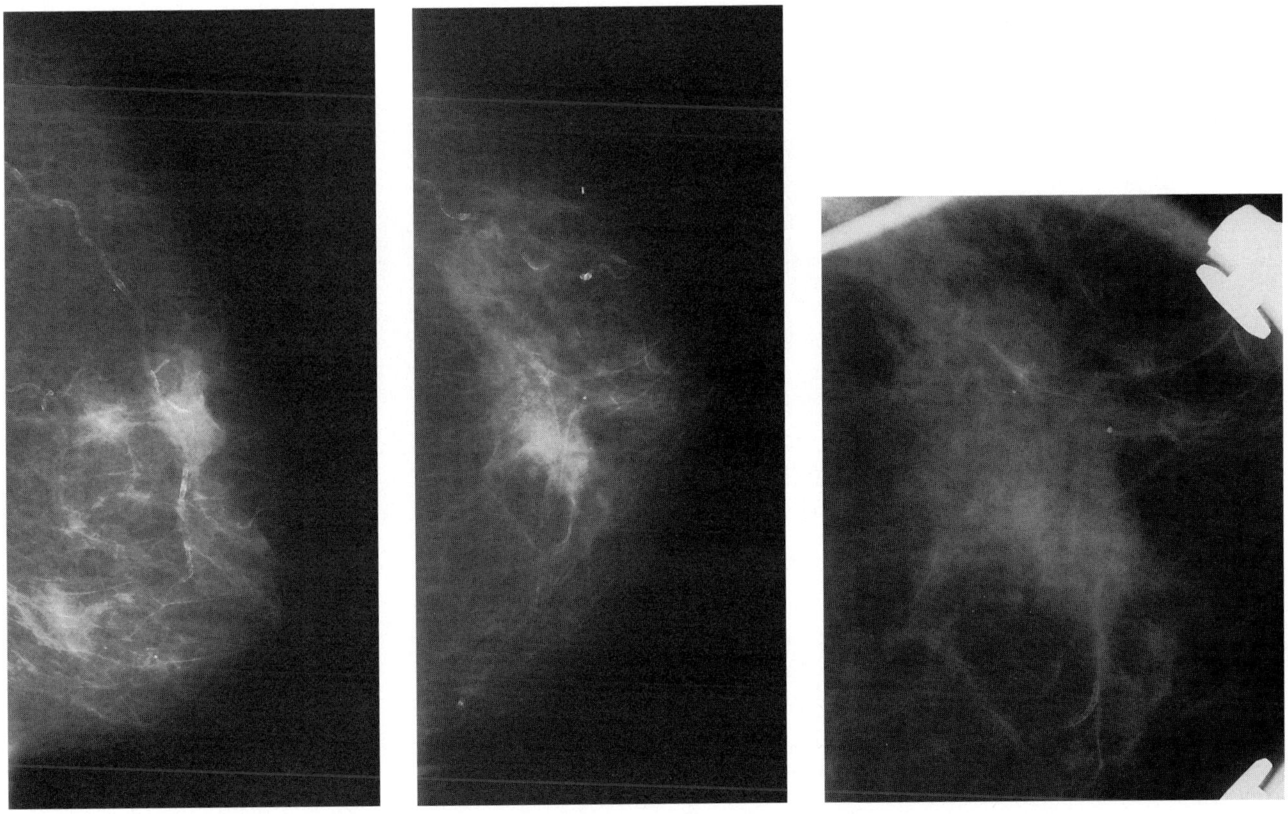

A B C

Figure 45-1. In the left upper inner breast, there is an ill-defined mass. (A). Left ML mammogram. (B). Left CC mammogram. (C). Left CC spot compression mammogram.

Ultrasound

Frequency

- 10 MHz

Mass

- margin: ill defined
- echogenicity: hypoechoic
- retrotumoral acoustic appearance: posterior shadowing distal to mass
- shape: irregular (Fig. 45-2)

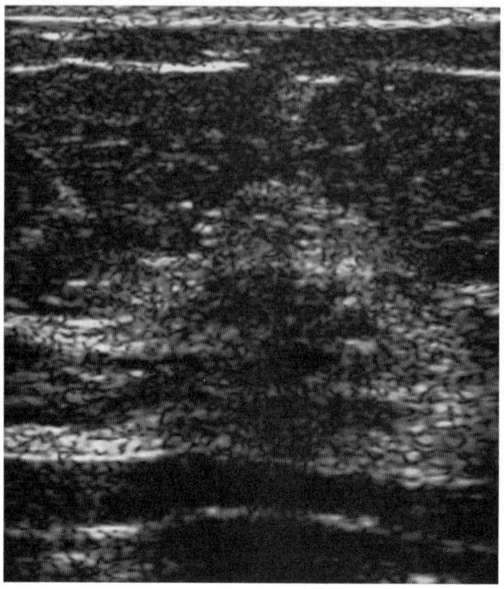

Figure 45–2. Left radial breast sonogram: The mammographic mass in Figure 45–1 corresponds to a solid hypoechoic irregular mass with posterior acoustic shadowing.

Other Modalities (Fig. 45–3)

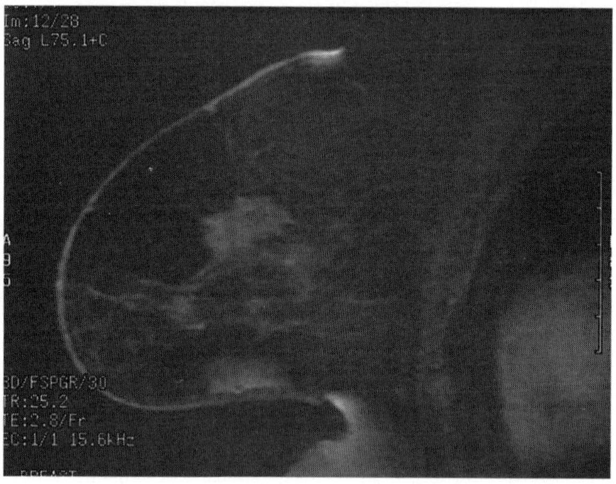

Figure 45–3. Left sagital dynamic bolus three-dimensional (3-D) volume gradient series breast magnetic resonance imaging (MRI): The mass does not exhibit early contrast enhancement and cannot be separated from the surrounding breast parenchyma.

Pathology

- fibroadenoma

Management

- BI-RADS Assessment Category 4, suspicious; biopsy should be considered

Pearls and Pitfalls

In this case, the MRI was the most helpful test in predicting the benign nature of the mass. Although the mass has an irregular shape, the fibroadenoma did not exhibit early gadolinium contrast enhancement, which is characteristic of malignancies.

Suggested Readings

1. Hochman MG, Orel SG, Powell CM, Schnall MD, Reynolds CA, White LN. Fibroadenomas: MR imaging appearances with radiologic-histopathologic correlation. *Radiology* 1997;204:123–129.
2. Kvistad KA, Rydland J, Vainio J, et al. Breast lesions: evaluation with dynamic contrast-enhanced T1-weighted MR imaging and with T2*-weighted first-pass perfusion MR imaging. *Radiology* 2000;216:545–553.
3. Stelling CBKK, Powell DE, Mattingly SS. Fibroadenomas: histopathologic and MR imaging features. *Radiology* 1987;167:399–407.

Case 46

Case History

A 42-year-old woman has a bruised right breast from a recent seat belt injury.

Physical Examination

- right breast: large ecchymosis, covering the upper outer quadrant, that is associated with a 3 cm palpable mass
- left breast: normal exam

Mammogram

Mass

- margin: indistinct
- shape: irregular
- density: high density

Associated Findings (Fig. 46–1)

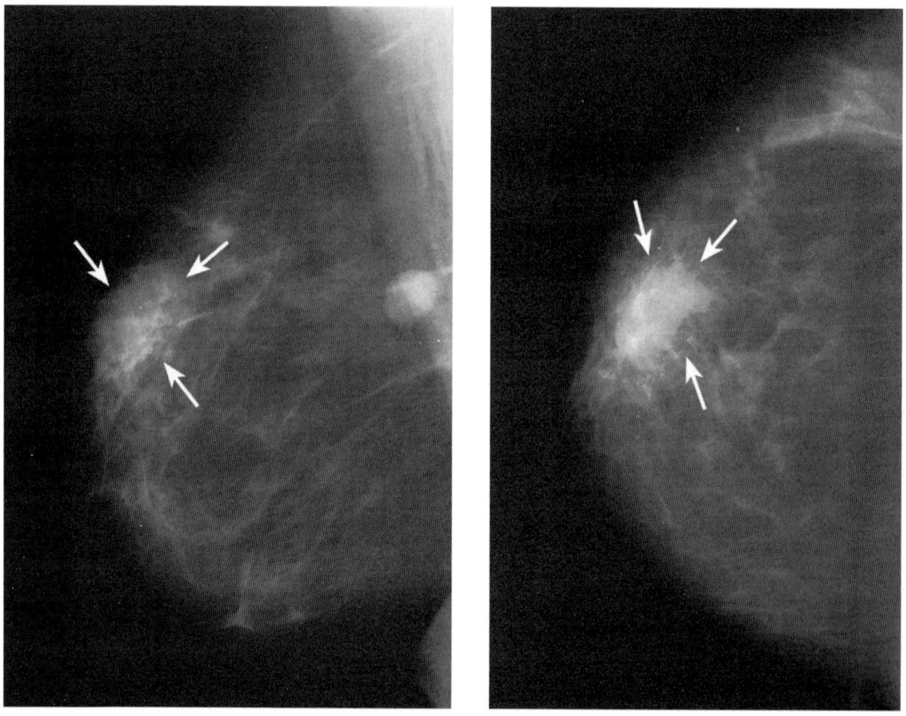

Figure 46–1. In the anterior upper outer quadrant of the right breast, there is an ill-defined mass (arrows), which is in the same position as the ecchymosis and palpable lump. The well-defined oval mass in the posterior upper outer quadrant is a benign fibroadenoma. (A). Right MLO mammogram. (B). Right CC mammogram.

A B

Ultrasound

Frequency

- 7 MHz

Mass

- margin: well defined
- echogenicity: hypoechoic
- retrotumoral acoustic appearance: increased acoustic transmission
- shape: ellipsoid (Figs. 46–2 and 46–3)

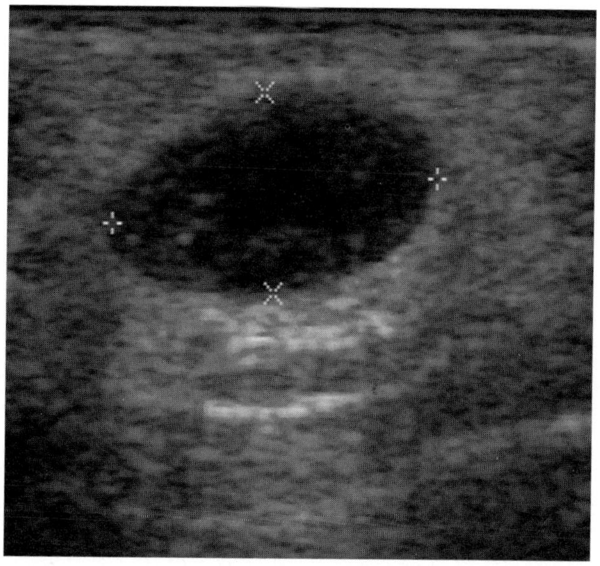

Figure 46–2. Right longitudinal breast sonogram: The palpable lump associated with the ecchymosis is a well-defined hypoechoic complex fluid collection.

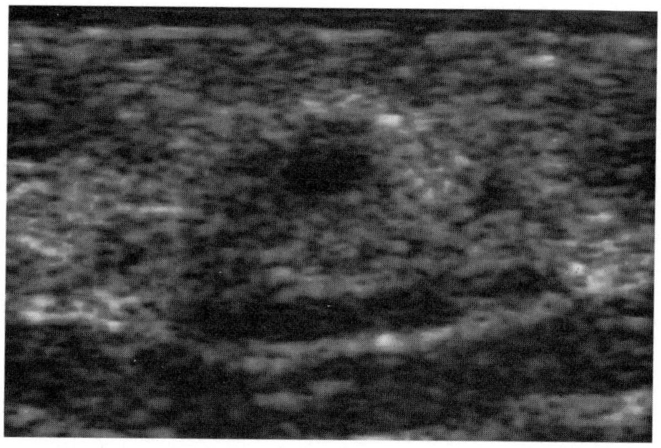

Figure 46–3. Right longitudinal breast sonogram: Two months after the first sonogram (Fig. 46–2), the palpable lump is smaller and corresponds to a heterogeneous solid mass. This change in appearance is consistent with a hematoma.

Pathology

- hematoma

Management

- BI-RADS Assessment Category 3, probably benign; short-interval follow-up

Pearls and Pitfalls

1. Mammographically, acute hematomas present as either ill-defined or circumscribed masses.
2. Sonographically, hematomas are usually anechoic or hypoechoic. Rarely, a hematoma will be uniformly hyperechoic or have echogenic debris, which either layers or adheres to one wall. Inflamed tissues around the hematoma may produce a hyperechoic halo. The differential diagnosis of a hematoma is abscess. If adherent debris is present, then intracystic neoplasm should be considered.

Suggested Readings

1. Jackson VP, Jahan R, Fu YS. Benign breast lesions. In: Bassett LW, Jackson VP, Jahan R, Fu YS, Gold RH, eds. *Diagnosis of Diseases of the Breast.* Philadelphia: WB Saunders Company; 1997:357–443.
2. Kopans DB. Ultrasound and breast evaluation. In: Kopans DB. *Breast Imaging.* 2nd ed. Philadelphia: Lippincott-Raven; 1998:409–443.
3. Tohno E, Cosgrove DO, Sloane JP. Haematoma. In: Tohno D, Cosgrove DO, Sloane JP, eds. *Ultrasound Diagnosis of Breast Diseases.* New York: Churchill Livingston; 1994:144–145.

Case 47

Case History

A 46-year-old woman presents for screening mammogram. After mammogram is done, patient's physician detects a palpable lump in the same area as the mammographic abnormality.

Physical Examination

- left breast: palpable lump in the upper outer quadrant
- right breast: normal exam

Mammogram

Mass

- margin: indistinct
- shape: irregular
- density: equal density

Associated Findings (Fig. 47–1)

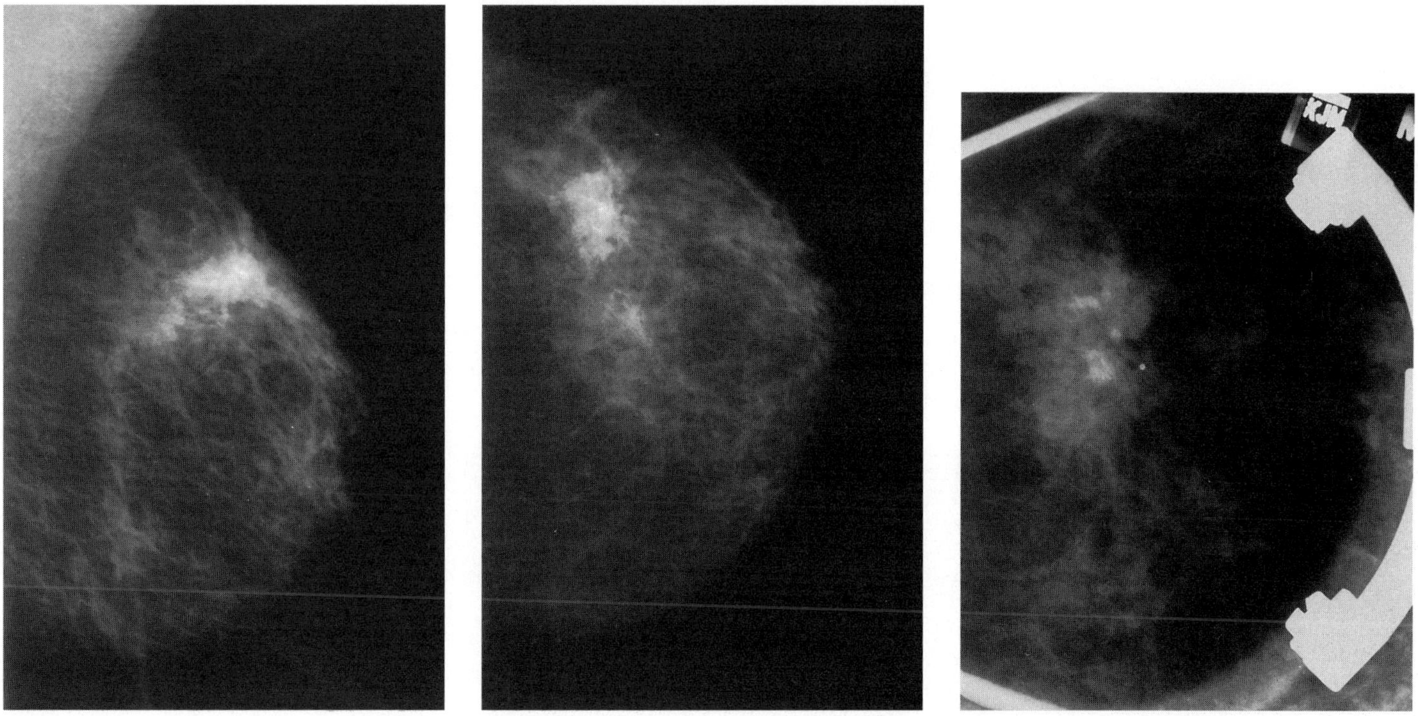

A B C

Figure 47–1. In the upper outer quadrant of the left breast, there is an irregular mass with architectural distortion. (A). Left MLO mammogram. (B). Left CC mammogram. (C). Left CC spot mammogram.

Ultrasound

Low Frequency

Frequency

- 6 MHz

Mass

- margin: ill defined
- echogenicity: hypoechoic
- retrotumoral acoustic appearance: severe shadowing, mass completely obscured
- shape: irregular (Fig. 47–2)

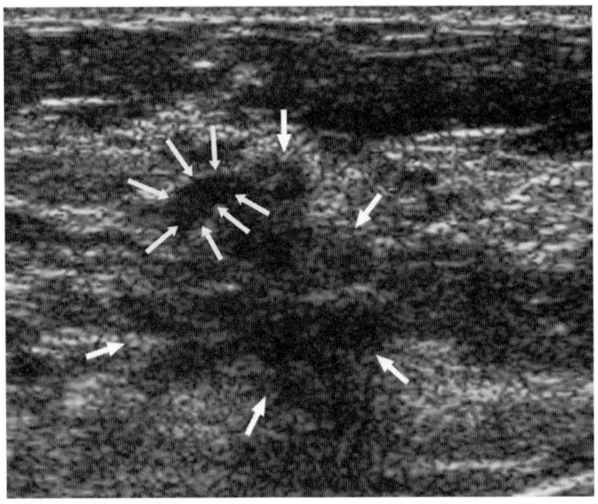

Figure 47–2. Left radial breast sonogram: Lower frequency examination demonstrates that the lesion identified in Figure 47–3 corresponds to a mass (large arrows) that consists of a collection of multiple short tubular structures. Small arrows outline one tubular structure.

High Frequency

Frequency

- 10 MHz

Associated Findings

In this case, the higher frequency is less useful because the fibrotic tissue around the thick walled ducts produces severe shadowing so the internal structures cannot be identified (Fig. 47–3).

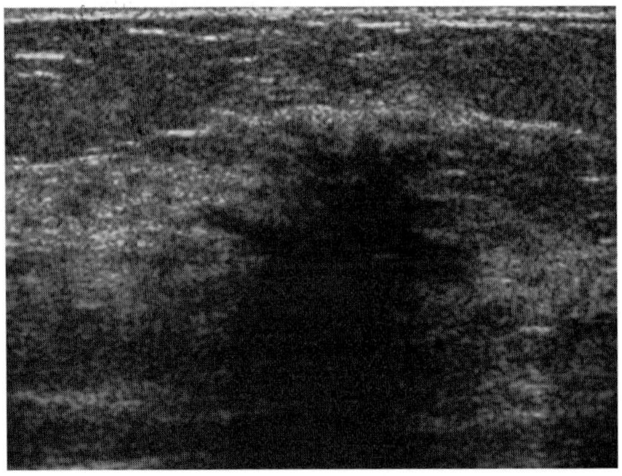

Figure 47–3. Left radial breast sonogram: The palpable lump corresponding to the mammographic mass is hypoechoic with severe shadowing.

Pathology

- papilloma (multiple fibrous walled ducts surrounding sclerosing papillomas)

Management

- BI-RADS Assessment Category 4, suspicious; biopsy should be considered

Pearls and Pitfalls

1. Papillomas may develop sclerosis. Microscopically, these sclerosing papillomas generally do not appear as intracystic masses. The sclerotic papillomas are surrounded by thickened duct walls.
2. Sclerosing papillomas produce a palpable lump. These lesions are rarely associated with nipple discharge or pain.
3. Mammographically, sclerosing papillomas present as a circumscribed mass or as an ill-defined mass with spiculation and architectural distortion.
4. Sonographically, this lesion presents as an ill-defined hypoechoic shadowing mass. This lesion consists of several sclerotic papillomas that appear as short tubular structures.

Suggested Readings

1. Fenoglio C, Lattes R. Sclerosing papillary proliferations in the female breast. *Cancer* 1974;33:691-700.
2. Tavasoli FA. Papillary lesions. In: Tavassoli FA, Fattaneh A. *Pathology of the Breast.* 2nd ed. Stamford: Appleton and Lange; 1999:325-371.

Case 48

Case History

A 63-year-old woman presents for a screening mammogram.

Physical Examination

- normal exam

Mammogram

Mass (Fig. 48–1)

- margin: spiculated
- shape: irregular
- density: equal density

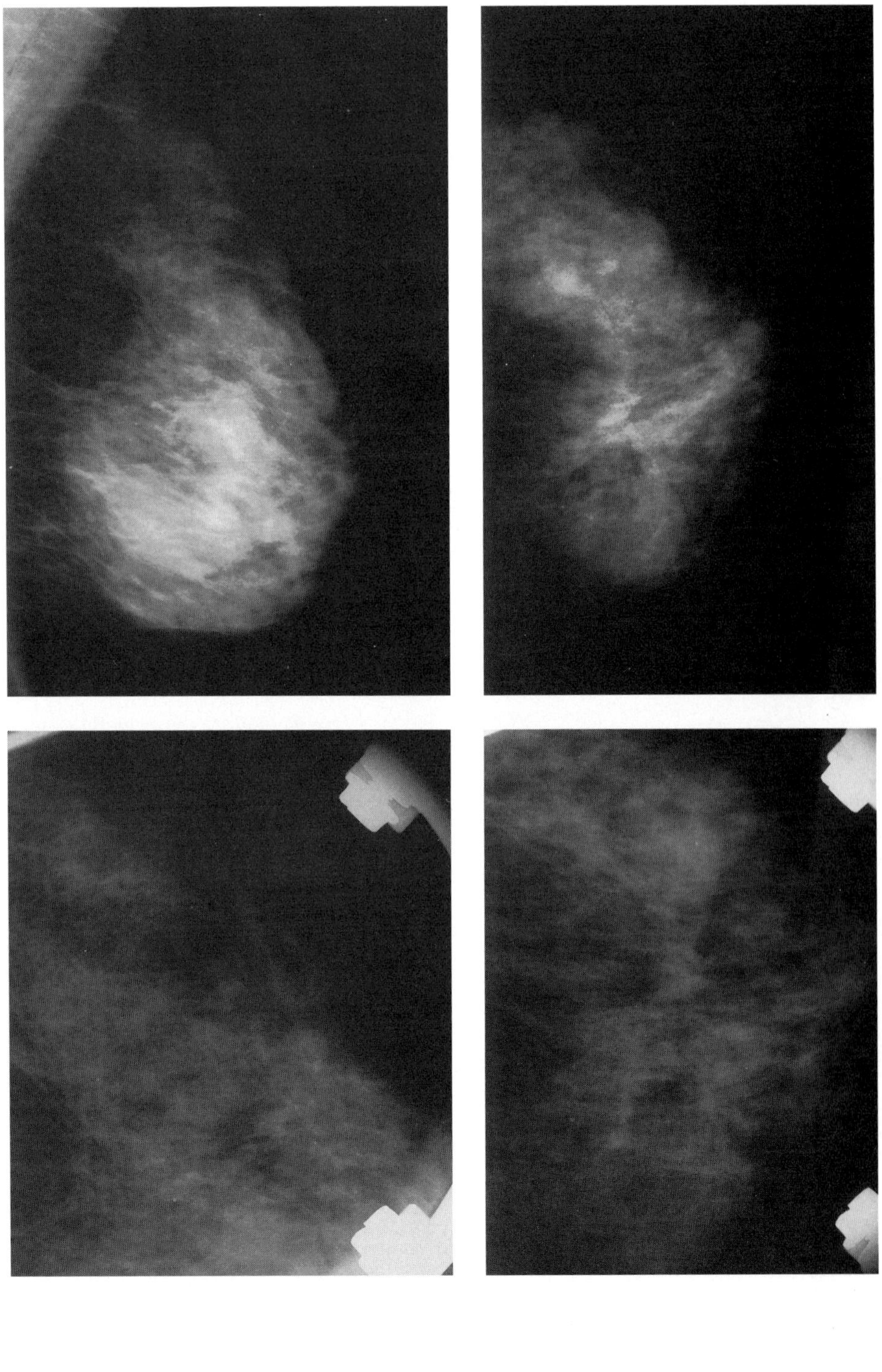

A B C D

Figure 48–1. In the left upper medial breast, there is a spiculated mass that is more prominent on the CC view compared with the MLO or ML views. (A). Left MLO mammogram. (B). Left CC mammogram. (C). Left ML spot compression mammogram. (D). Left CC spot compression mammogram.

Ultrasound

Frequency

- 11.5 MHz

Mass (Fig. 48-2)

- margin: ill defined
- echogenicity: hypoechoic
- retrotumoral acoustic appearance: severe shadowing, mass completely obscured
- shape: irregular (Fig. 48-2)

A

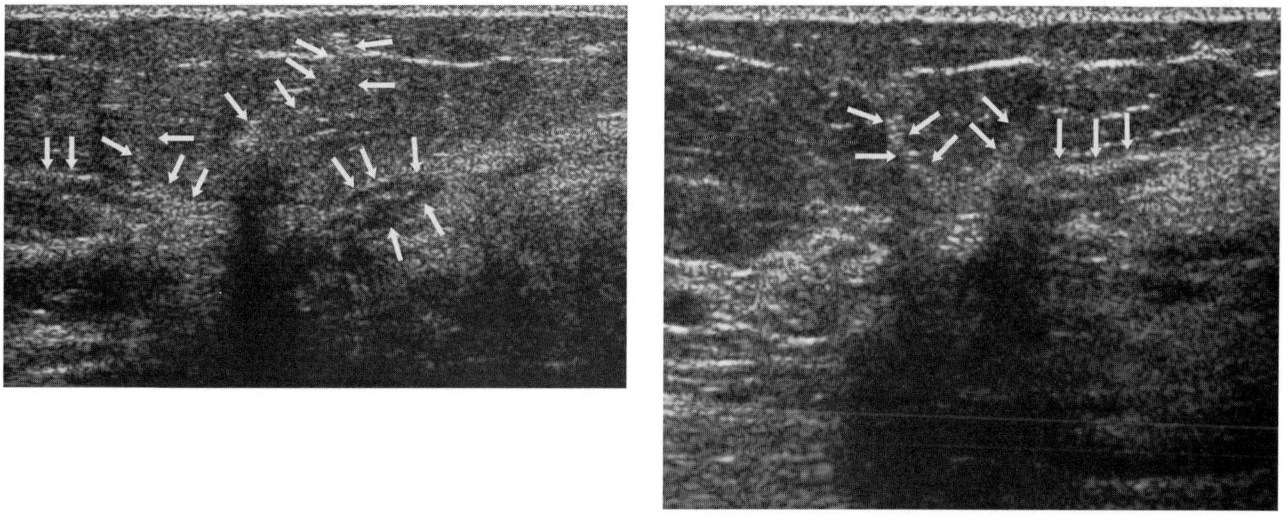

B

Figure 48-2. Sonographically the mammographic mass corresponds to an irregular hypoechoic shadowing mass with prominent spiculations (arrows). The mass is much narrower in the radial compared with the antiradial orientation. This asymmetric configuration may explain the difference in conspicuity between the mammographic images. (A). Left radial breast sonogram. (B). Left antiradial breast sonogram.

Other Modalities (Fig. 48-3)

Pathology

- radial sclerosing lesion (radial scar)

Management

- BI-RADS Assessment Category 4, suspicious; biopsy should be considered

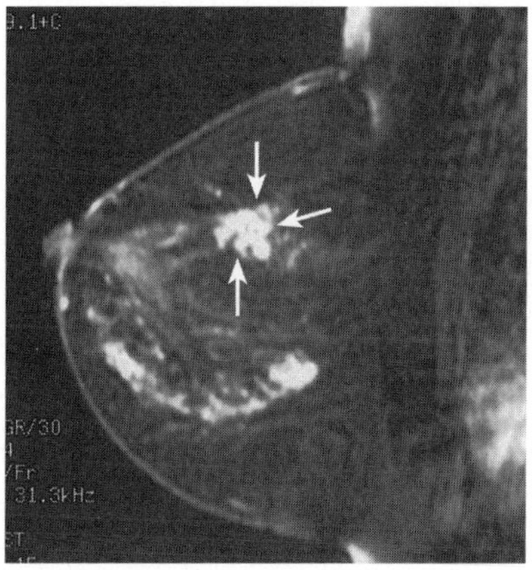

Figure 48-3. Left sagittal dynamic bolus 3-D volume gradient series breast MRI: In the upper medial breast, there is an irregular enhancing mass (arrows) that corresponds to the mammographic and sonographic masses.

Pearls and Pitfalls

1. Radial scars are common lesions. They have been identified in 28% of autopsied women. Women with radial scars have about twice the risk of malignancy compared with those without this lesion. Therefore, radial scars should be completely excised for thorough pathologic examination.
2. Mammographically, radial scars exhibit spiculations and architectural distortion. The center is less dense than the usual carcinoma. Spot compression reveals multiple oval and linear lucencies within the central area. Commonly, this lesion is either only visible or much better identified on one view.
3. Sonographically, the radial scar is an irregular hypoechoic mass associated with architectural distortion and severe shadowing with high frequencies. With low frequencies (<7 MHz), the radial scar may be an irregular, hyperechoic area with little or no shadowing. Sonographically, this lesion cannot be differentiated from either a surgical scar or malignant mass.
4. On MRI, radial scars may enhance in a pattern similar to malignancies.

Suggested Readings

1. Cohen MA, Sferlazza SJ. Role of sonography in evaluation of radial scars of the breast. *AJR* 2000;174:1075–1078.
2. Jacobs TW, Byrne C, Colditz G, Connolly JL, Schnitt SJ. Radial scars in benign breast-biopsy specimens and the risk of breast cancer. *N Engl J Med* 1999;340:430–436.
3. Tabar L, Dean PB. Stellate/spiculated lesions. In: Tabar L, Dean PB. *Teaching Atlas of Mammography.* 3rd ed. New York: Thieme; 2001:93–147.
4. Weissman BN, Wong M, Smith DN. Image interpretation session: 1996. *Radiographics* 1997;17:243–267.

Case 49

Case History

A 72-year-old woman status post–right lumpectomy and radiation therapy has developed a new mammographic finding near the surgical site.

Physical Examination

- right breast: subareolar scar
- left breast: normal exam

Mammogram

Mass (Fig. 49–1)

- margin: spiculated
- shape: irregular
- density: equal density

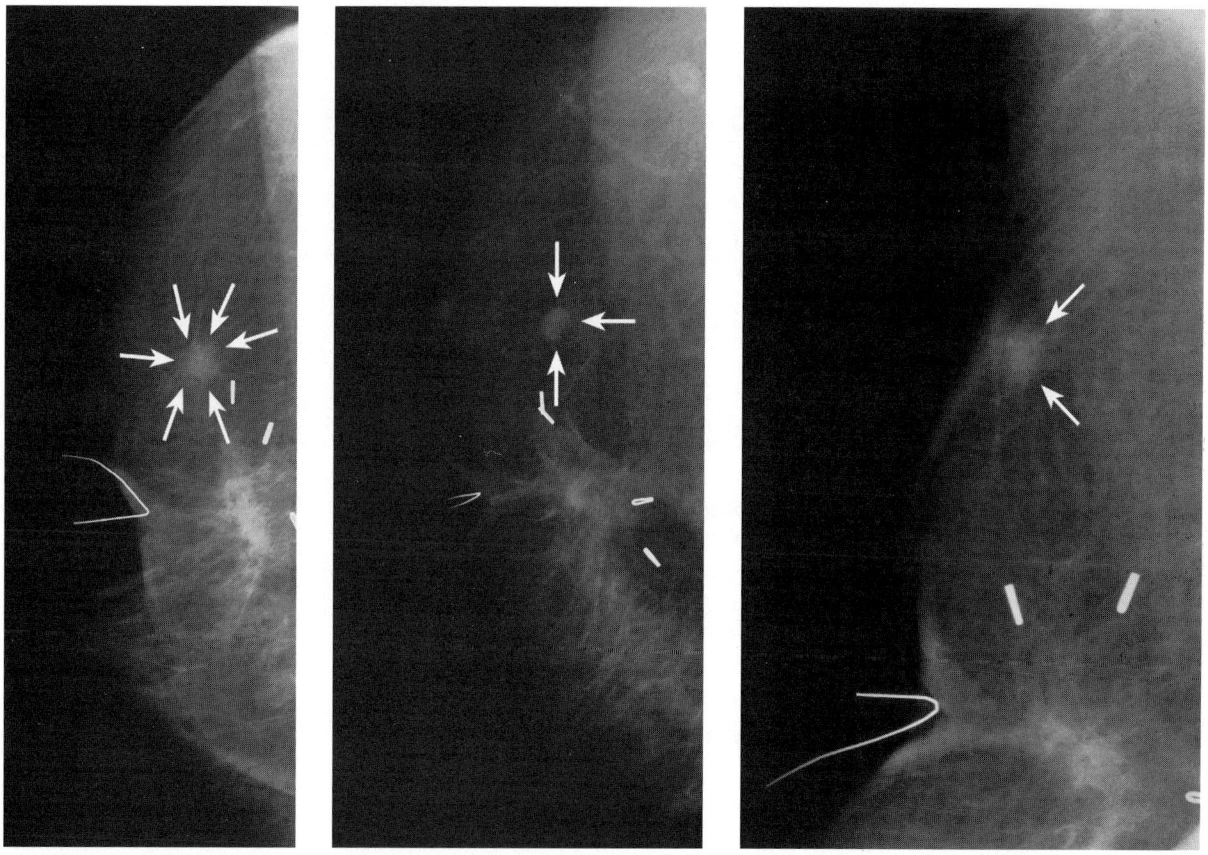

A B C

Figure 49–1. There is a spiculated density deep to the right nipple. This density corresponds to the scar from the patient's lumpectomy. In the upper outer breast, there is a spiculated mass (arrows) that is separate from the main scar. This spiculated mass is new since the patient's previous exam. (A). Right LM mammogram. (B). Right CC mammogram. (C). Right mammogram tangential to spiculated mass (arrows).

Ultrasound

Frequency

- 10 MHz

Mass

- margin: ill defined
- echogenicity: hypoechoic
- retrotumoral acoustic appearance: severe shadowing
- shape: irregular (Figs. 49–2 and 49–3)

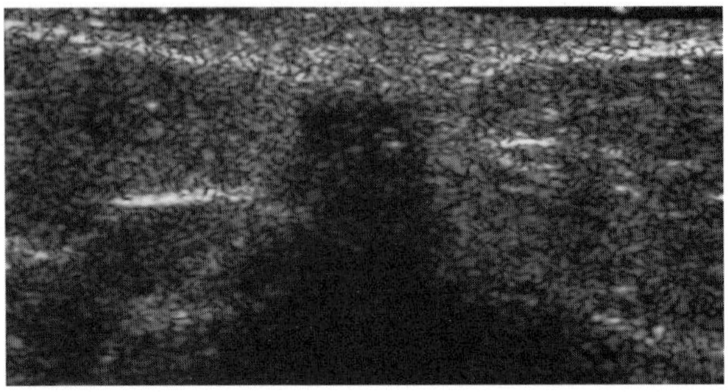

Figure 49–2. Right radial breast sonogram: In the upper outer quadrant, the new small spiculated mammographic mass corresponds to an ill-defined hypoechoic shadowing mass. The hyperechoic halo around the mass corresponds to the mammographic spiculations.

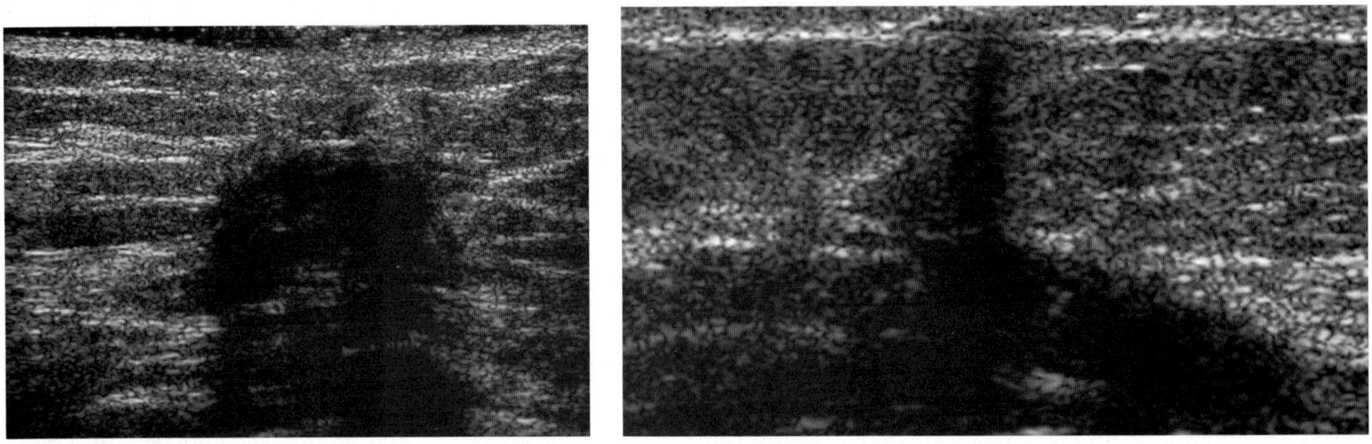

A B

Figure 49–3. The lumpectomy scar is distinguished from the adjacent spiculated mass by both its location and appearance. Although the scar is wide in the antiradial view (A), it is extremely narrow in the radial view (B). The adjacent spiculated mass depicted in Figure 49–2 is the same width in both views. (A). Right antiradial breast sonogram. (B). Right radial breast sonogram.

Pathology

- fat necrosis (the new spiculated mass in the right upper outer quadrant)
- scar (showed no evidence of recurrence and was not rebiopsied)

Management

- BI-RADS Assessment Category 4, suspicious; biopsy should be considered

Pearls and Pitfalls

1. When fat necrosis causes new irregular masses in the area of a lumpectomy site, this abnormality cannot be distinguished from malignancy mammographically or sonographically.

2. Sonographically, scars are irregular spiculated masses. They can be distinguished from malignancy when the scar produces architectural distortion without a mass. This case illustrates the appearance of a benign scar. Although one view exhibits hypoechoic architectural distortion, the other view demonstrates no mass, only a thin line of tissue irregularity. However, if a scar develops a hypoechoic mass from fibrosis or fat necrosis, then malignancy cannot be excluded.

Suggested Readings

1. Sohn C, Blohmer J-U, Hamper UM. Sonography in the follow-up of breast cancer. In: Sohn C, Blohmer J-U, Hamper UM, eds. *Breast Ultrasound.* New York: Thieme; 1999:98–102.
2. Tohno E, Cosgrove DO, Sloane JP. Postoperative scarring. In: Tohno D, Cosgrove DO, Sloane JP, eds. *Ultrasound Diagnosis of Breast Diseases.* New York: Churchill Livingston; 1994:146–147.

Case 50

Case History

A 50-year-old woman presents with erythema and a new mass in the upper outer quadrant of the left breast. Physical exam and mammogram 6 months earlier were negative.

Physical Examination

- left breast: palpable mass at 3:00
- right breast: normal exam

Mammogram

Mass (Fig. 50–1)

- margin: spiculated
- shape: irregular
- density: high

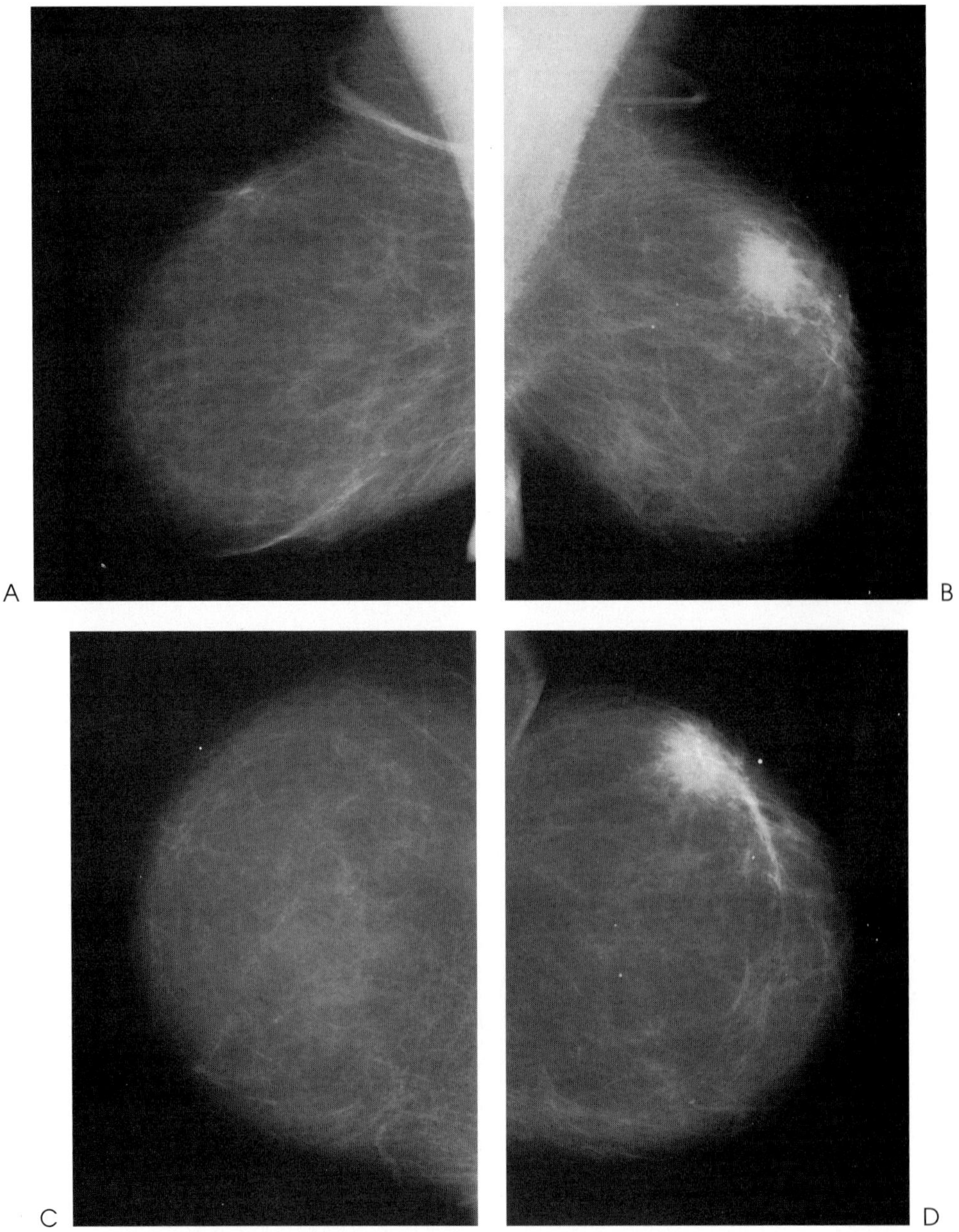

Figure 50–1. There is an ill-defined mass with irregular margins in the upper outer left breast. (A). Right MLO mammogram. (B). Left MLO mammogram. (C). Right CC mammogram. (D). Left CC mammogram.

Ultrasound

Frequency

- 8 MHz

Mass

- margin: ill defined
- echogenicity: hypoechoic
- retrotumoral acoustic appearance: bilateral edge shadowing
- shape: irregular (Fig. 50–2)

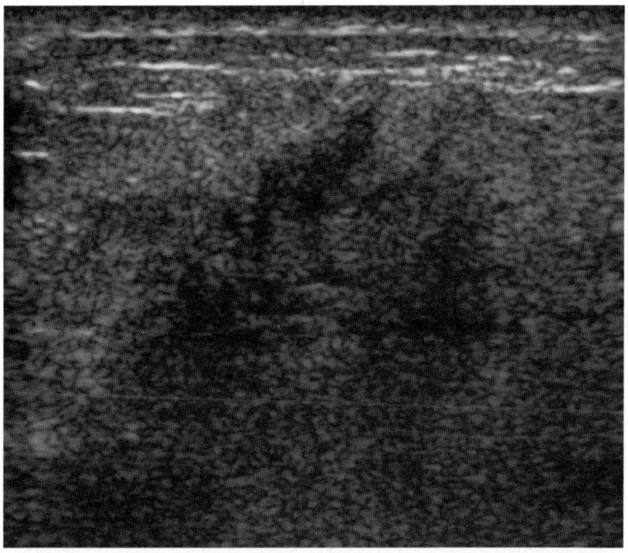

Figure 50–2. Left radial breast sonogram: The mammographic mass (Fig. 50–1) corresponds to a palpable ill-defined hypoechoic mass.

Pathology

- myofibroblastoma

Management

- BI-RADS Assessment Category 4, suspicious; biopsy should be considered

Pearls and Pitfalls

1. Myofibroblastoma is a benign tumor composed of breast stromal fibroblasts and/or myofibroblasts. This lesion most commonly presents as a palpable mass in patients 50 to 70 years old. Men are affected more often than women.
2. Mammographically, these lesions are most commonly noncalcified, oval, or lobulated masses with either well-defined or ill-defined margins.
3. Sonographically, myofibroblastomas are generally oval or lobular well-defined hypoechoic masses with variable decreased acoustic transmission. This case has an unusual mammographic and sonographic appearance.

Suggested Readings

1. Greenberg JS, Kaplan SS, Grady C. Myofibroblastoma of the breast in women: imaging appearances. *AJR* 1998;171:71–72.
2. Pina L, Apesteguia L, Cojo R, et al. Myofibroblastoma of male breast: report of three cases and review of the literature. *Eur Radiol* 1997;7:931–934.

Case 51

Case History

A 64-year-old woman presents with back pain, abnormal bone scan, and a right breast lump.

Physical Examination

- right breast: palpable lump in the outer breast
- left breast: normal exam

Mammogram

Mass (Fig. 51-1)

- margin: spiculated
- shape: irregular
- density: high density

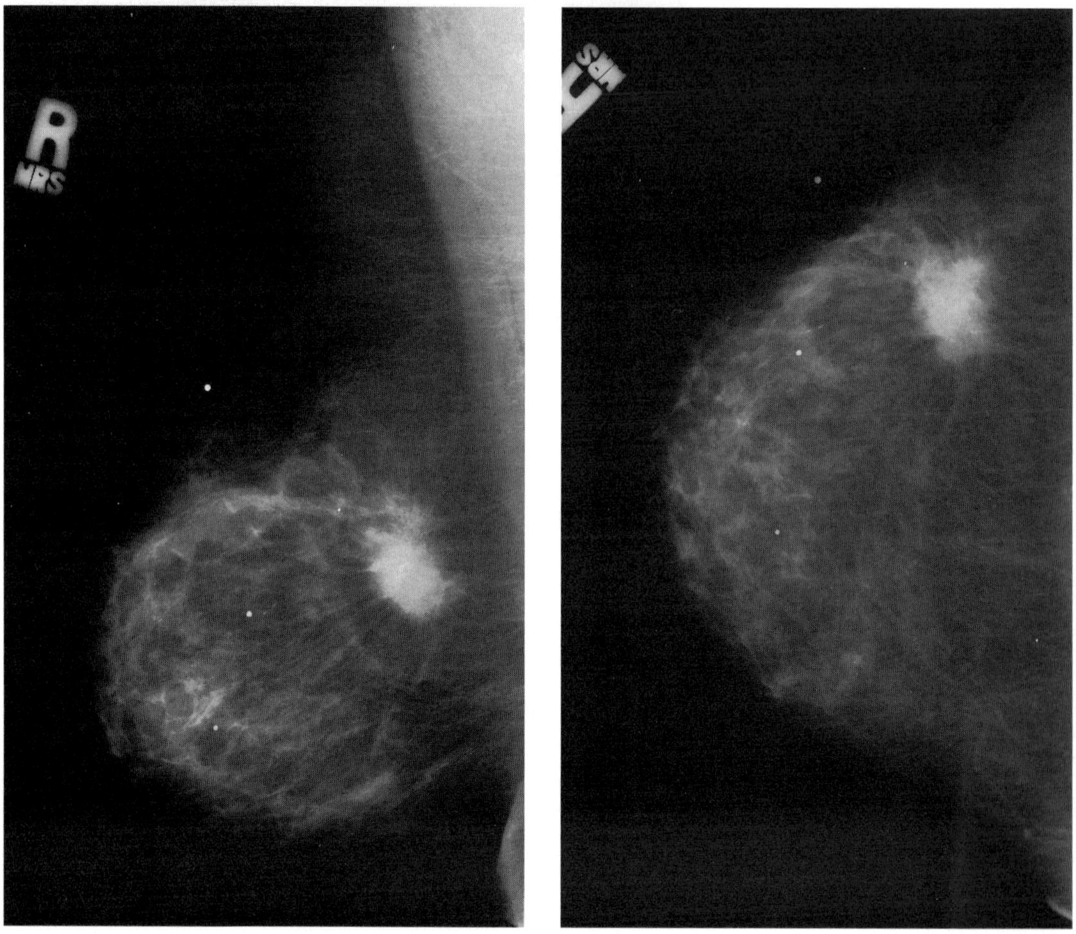

A B

Figure 51-1. In the upper outer quadrant, there is a spiculated mass that corresponds to the patient's palpable mass. (A). Right MLO mammogram. (B). Right CC mammogram.

Other Modalities

Findings

The bone scan demonstrates that the patient's back pain is due to metastatic disease. Biopsies confirmed that these bone metastases originated from her breast cancer (Fig. 51–2).

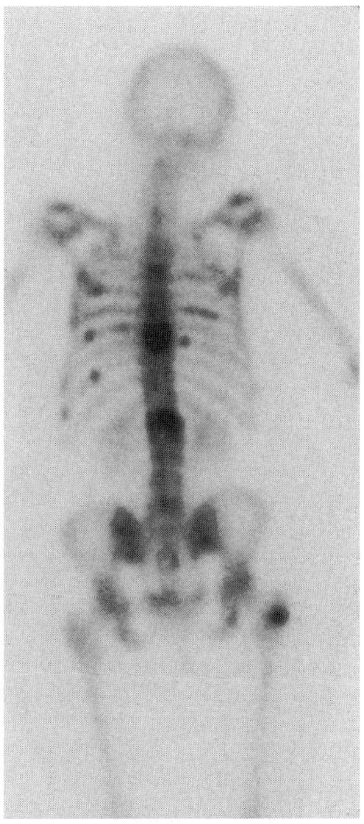

Figure 51–2. Tc-99m whole-body bone scan, posterior view: There are multiple areas of abnormal uptake in the ribs, spine, and right hip consistent with metastatic bony disease.

Pathology

- infiltrating ductal carcinoma

Management

- BI-RADS Assessment Category 5, highly suggestive of malignancy

Pearls and Pitfalls

1. Infiltrating ductal carcinoma is the most common breast cancer histology. This cell type represents between 47 and 79% of all invasive breast cancers. The lower percentage has been reported in Japan and the higher percentages in the United States and Scandinavia.
2. Two thirds of invasive ductal carcinomas appear as irregular mammographic masses. The spiculations consist of a combination of fibrosis and infiltrating tumor. This case illustrates this classic presentation.
3. Because this mass is highly suggestive of malignancy, no other imaging of the breast is necessary. However, if the surgeon wishes to obtain a biopsy prior to excision, then one may perform sonographically guided biopsy as these lesions are generally easily identified with this method.

Suggested Readings

1. Tabar L, Dean PB. Stellate/spiculated lesions. In: Tabar L, Dean PB. *Teaching Atlas of Mammography.* 3rd ed. New York: Thieme; 2001:93–147.
2. Tavassoli FA. Infiltrating carcinoma: common and familiar special types. In: Tavassoli FA, Fattaneh A. *Pathology of the Breast.* 2nd ed. Stamford: Appleton and Lange; 1999:401–480.

Case 52

Case History

An 80-year-old woman presents with left nipple retraction.

Physical Examination

- left breast: retracted nipple, associated with skin thickening; no definite mass identified
- right breast: normal exam

Mammogram

Mass

- margin: spiculated
- shape: irregular
- density: high

Calcifications

- type: dystrophic
- distribution: grouped/clustered

Associated Findings

- architectural distortion, skin retraction, skin thickening, trabecular thickening, nipple retraction (Fig. 52–1)

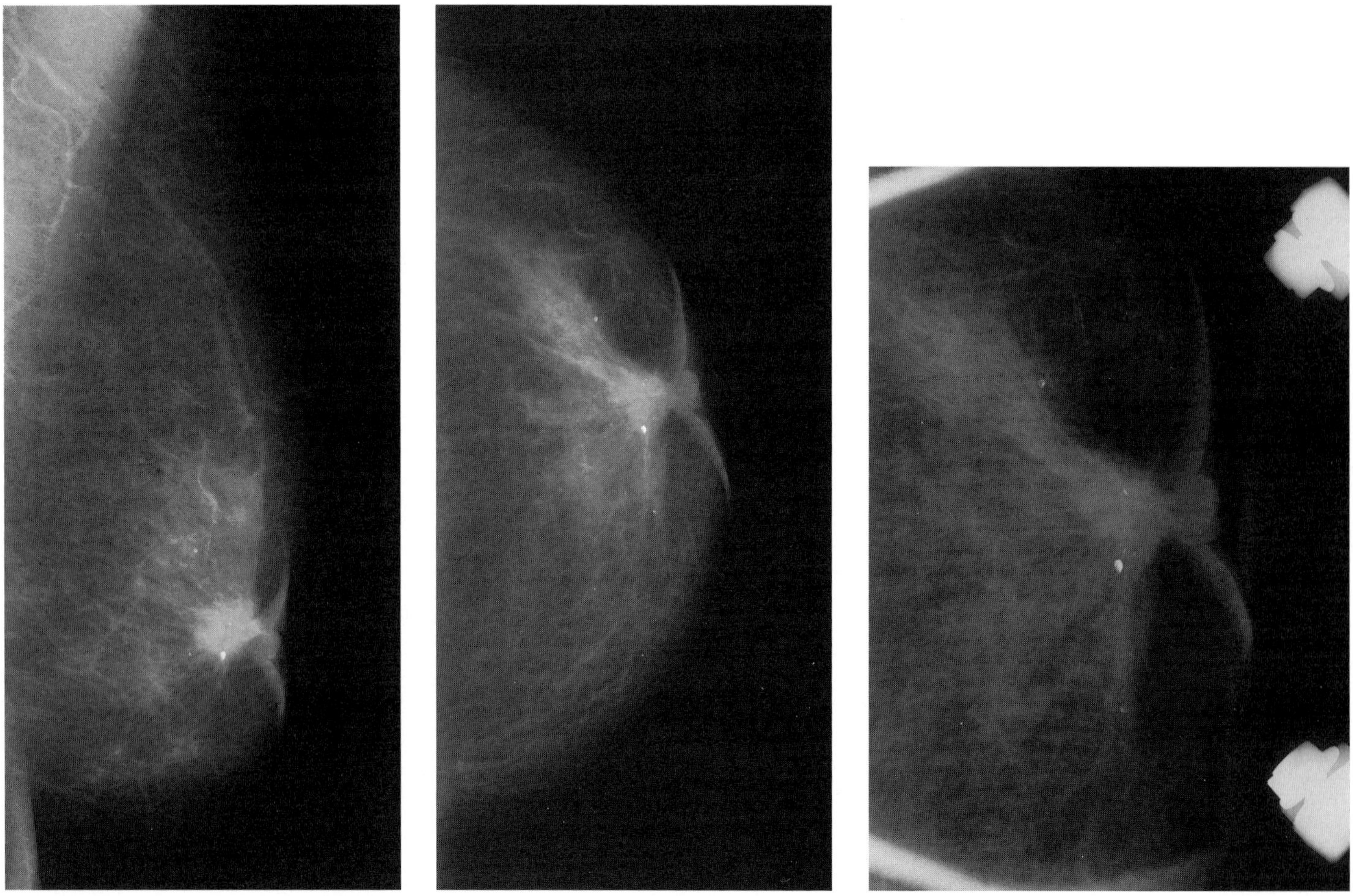

A B C

Figure 52–1. There is a spiculated subareolar mass associated with calcifications, skin thickening, and nipple retraction. (A). Left MLO mammogram. (B). Left CC mammogram. (C). Left CC spot magnification mammogram.

Ultrasound

Frequency

- 8 MHz

Mass

- margin: spiculation/architectural distortion
- echogenicity: hypoechoic
- retrotumoral acoustic appearance: bilateral edge shadowing
- shape: irregular (Fig. 52–2)

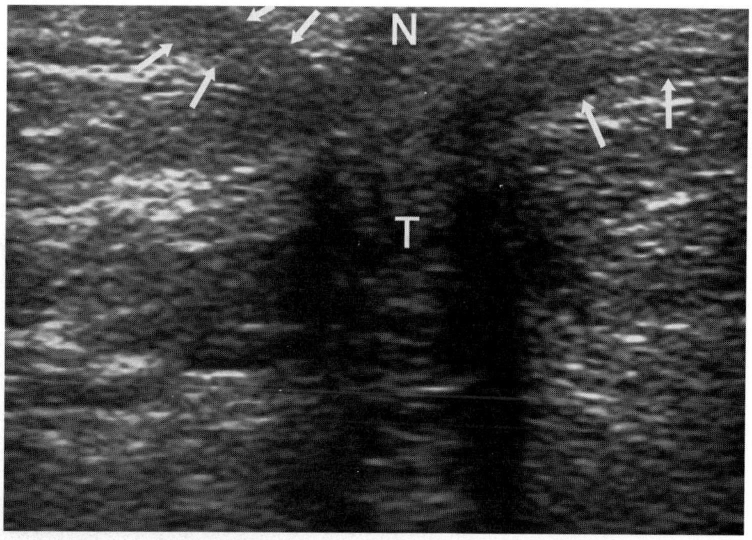

Figure 52–2. Left transverse breast sonogram: The sonogram is centered over the nipple (N). Superficially, skin thickening is present (arrows). Deep to the nipple is a solid, irregular, ill-defined, hypoechoic tumor (T).

Pathology

- invasive ductal carcinoma

Management

- BI-RADS Assessment Category 5, highly suggestive of malignancy

Pearls and Pitfalls

1. Nipple inversion is due to many etiologies. Benign causes include congenital position, duct ectasia, subareolar abscess, granulomatous mastitis, and postoperative scarring. If the inversion is relatively recent, then carcinoma should be considered.
2. The mass in this case is highly suggestive of malignancy so sonography is not needed for characterization of the mass. Sonography was performed for biopsy guidance.

Suggested Readings

1. Evans AJ, Wilson ARM, Blamey RW, Robertson JFR, Ellis IO, Elston CW. *Atlas of Breast Disease Management.* Philadelphia: WB Saunders; 1998:32–34.
2. Tavassoli FA, Fattaneh A. *Pathology of the Breast.* 2nd ed. Stamford: Appleton and Lange; 1999:792–793.

Case 53

Case History

A 54-year-old woman presents for screening mammogram.

Physical Examination

- normal exam

Mammogram

Mass (Fig. 53-1)

- margin: spiculated
- shape: irregular
- density: equal

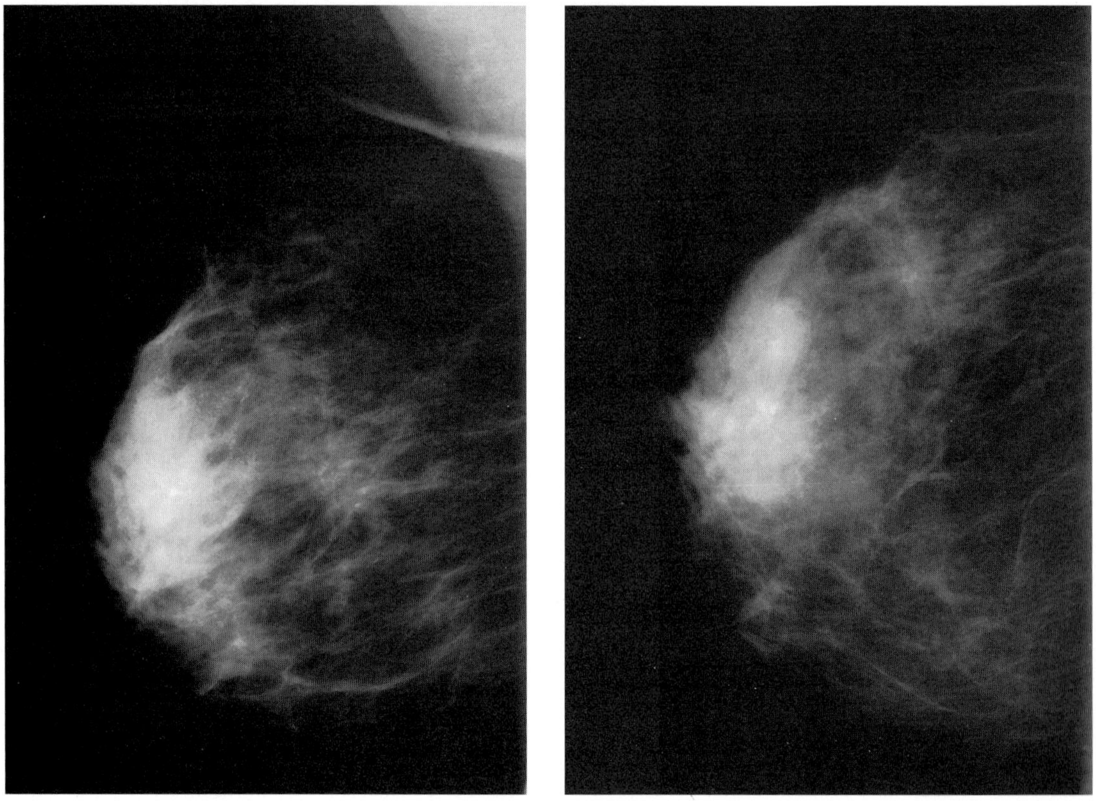

A B

Figure 53-1. A spiculated mass is in the right upper outer quadrant. (A). Right MLO mammogram. (B). Right CC mammogram.

Ultrasound

Frequency

- 11.5 MHz

Mass (Figs. 53-2 and 53-3)

- margin: ill defined
- echogenicity: hypoechoic
- retrotumoral acoustic appearance: severe shadowing, mass completely obscured
- shape: irregular

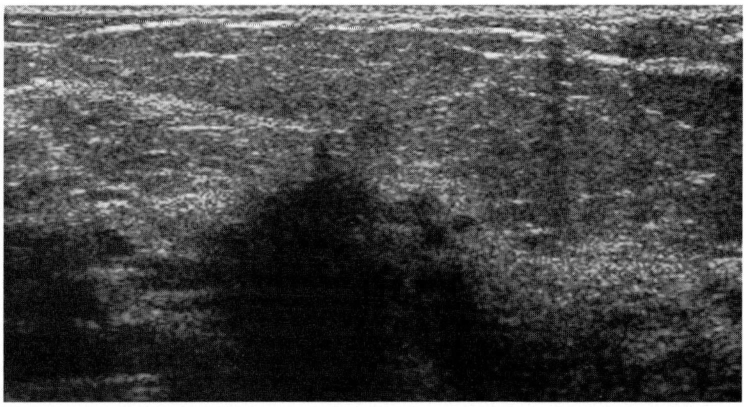

Figure 53–2. Right radial breast sonogram: The spiculated mass identified in Figure 53–1 corresponds to an irregular hypoechoic mass with severe acoustic shadowing.

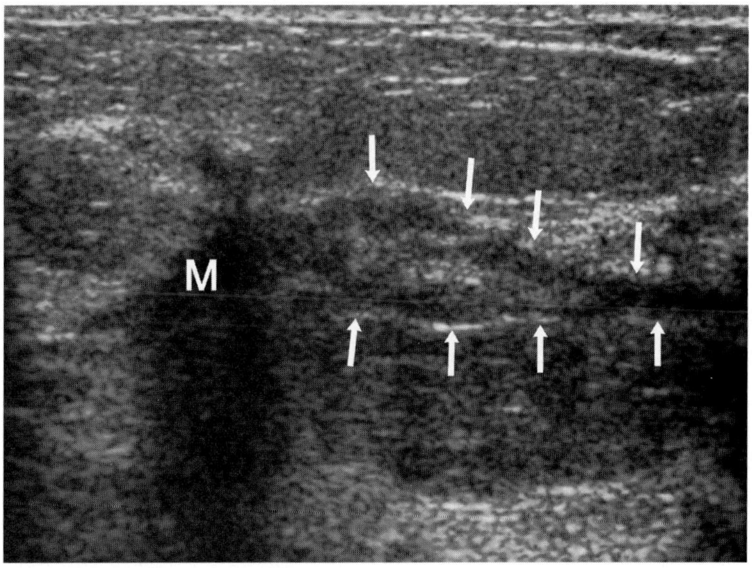

Figure 53–3. Right radial breast sonogram: A few dilated ducts (arrows) extend from the main mass (M) (shown in Fig. 53–2) toward the nipple. The size of the main sonographic mass matches the mammographic size (about 2.5 cm). However, if one adds the length of the abnormal ducts, the total length of the abnormality is 5 cm. Only a small portion of the main mass is displayed in this image.

Pathology

Infiltrating ductal carcinoma. The main mass consisted of well-differentiated infiltrating ductal carcinoma. The sonographically dilated ducts histologically corresponded to dilated ducts with infiltrating carcinoma within the walls. (See Fig. 53–4.)

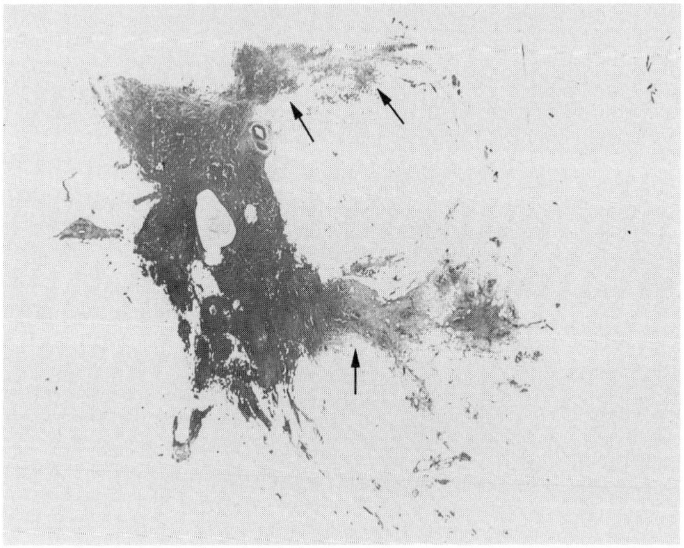

Figure 53–4. Low-power microscopic image of the malignancy demonstrates direct infiltration of tumor cells creating spiculation (arrows) (see Color Plate 53–4).

Management

- BI-RADS Assessment Category 5, highly suggestive of malignancy

Pearls and Pitfalls

1. The breast sonogram suggests that the malignancy is larger than the mammographic density. To confirm this information, sonographically guided biopsies of both the mass and the abnormal ducts were performed. Both the biopsies and the excisional specimen confirmed that the tumor size matched the sonographic size.
2. Sonographically dilated ducts that extend from a tumor mass should be viewed as suspicious for additional carcinoma.

Suggested Readings

1. Tohno D, Cosgrove DO, Sloane JP, eds. *Ultrasound Diagnosis of Breast Diseases.* New York: Churchill Livingston; 1994:165–166.

Case 54

Case History

A 65-year-old woman has right breast microcalcifications that have been stereotactically mammographically biopsied and are malignant. She now presents for needle localization of these microcalcifications before lumpectomy.

Physical Examination

- normal exam

Mammogram

Mass (Fig. 54–1)

- margin: indistinct
- shape: irregular
- density: equal density

Calcifications

- type: fine linear/branching
- distribution: grouped/clustered

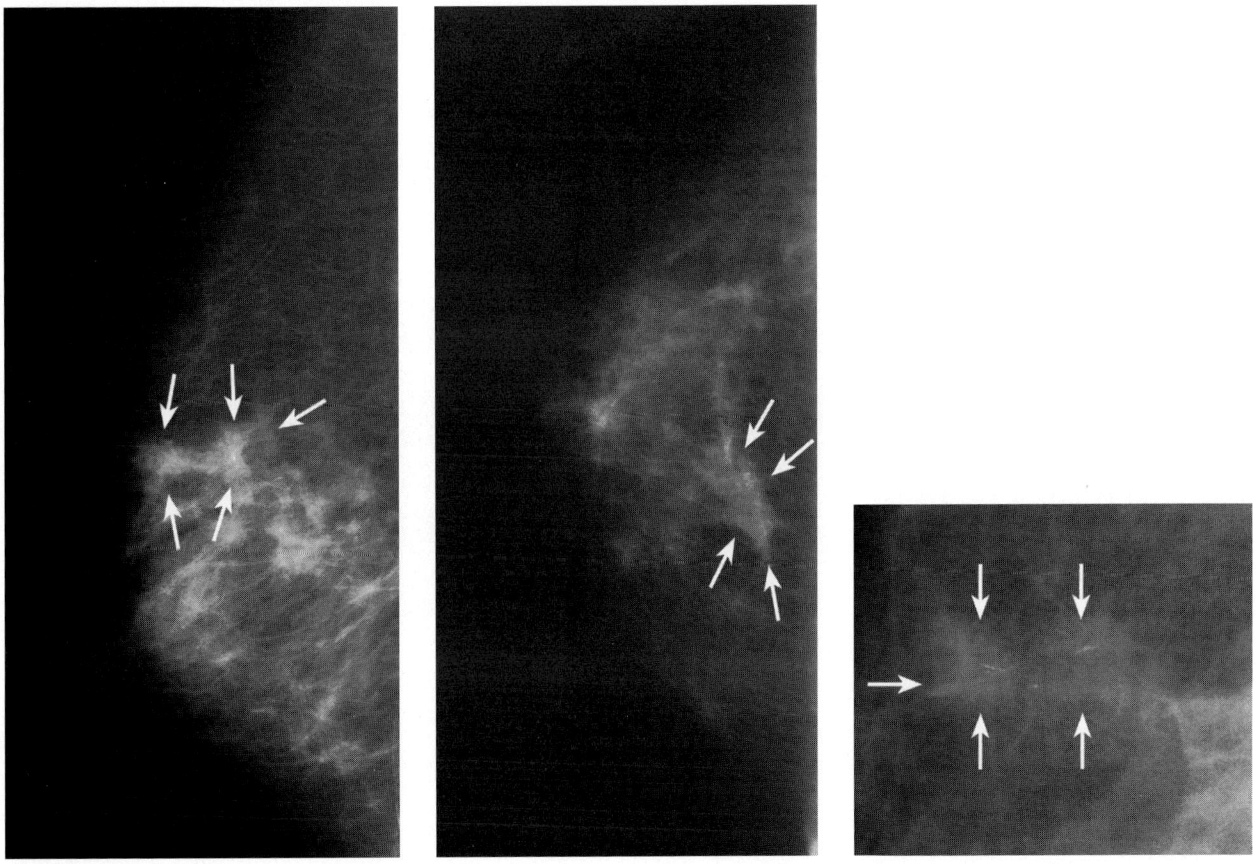

A B C

Figure 54–1. In the upper inner quadrant, there is a cluster of fine linear calcifications. These calcifications are associated with a dumbbell-shaped ill-defined mass (arrows). The shape of this mass and the subtle multinodular pattern of the surrounding parenchyma suggest that the tumor may be multifocal. (A). Right ML mammogram. (B). Right CC mammogram. (C). Right MLO magnification mammogram.

Ultrasound

Frequency

- 10 MHz

Mass

- margin: ill defined
- echogenicity: hypoechoic
- retrotumoral acoustic appearance: posterior shadowing distal to mass
- shape: irregular (Figs. 54–2, 54–3, and 54–4)

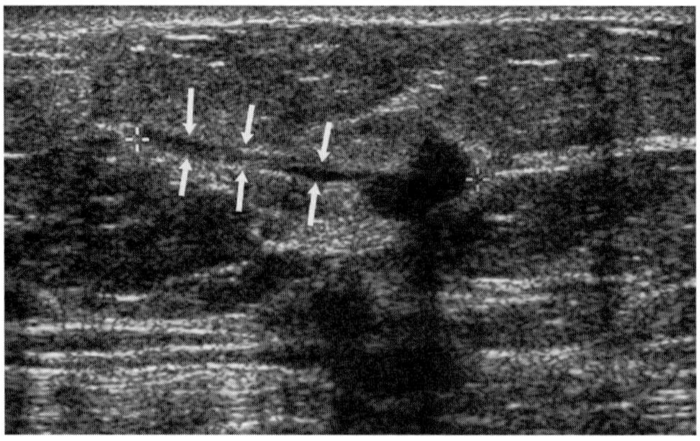

Figure 54–2. Right radial breast sonogram: At 2:00, a spiculated mass is associated with the stereotactic biopsy track (arrows). This mass corresponds to the mammographic mass containing the microcalcifications (Fig. 54–1).

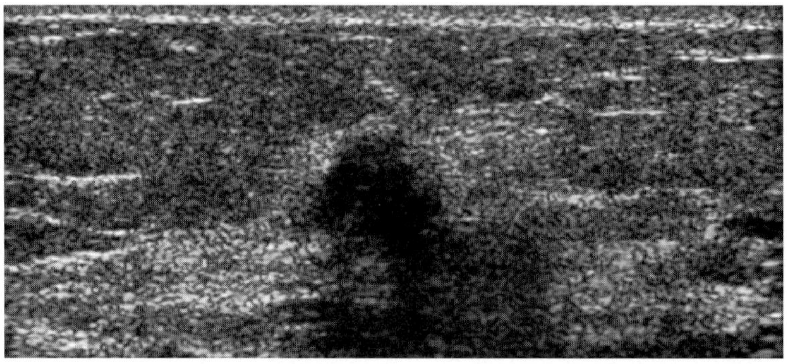

Figure 54–3. Right radial breast sonogram: At 12:00, a second spiculated solid mass is present. This mass may be part of the dumbbell structure identified mammographically (Fig. 54–1).

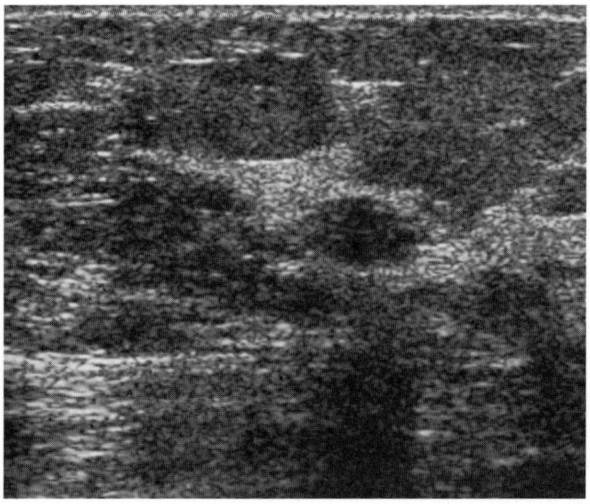

Figure 54-4. Right radial breast sonogram: At the 9:00 position there is an oval, ill-defined, solid shadowing mass. This mass is not mammographically identifiable. Sonographically guided biopsies of the masses in Figures 54-3 and 54-4 confirmed that they were both malignant.

Pathology

Infiltrating ductal carcinoma. Mastectomy specimen: Grossly the tumor was 4 cm but random sections outside this mass demonstrated small foci of infiltrating and in situ ductal carcinoma so the overall size of the malignancy could not be defined. The tumor appeared to be an extensive multifocal malignancy.

Management

- BI-RADS Assessment Category 4, suspicious; biopsy should be considered

Pearls and Pitfalls

1. Although the terms *multifocal* and *multicentric* appear to be synonymous, they refer to two distinct meanings when applied to malignancy. Multifocality refers to one tumor appearing with multiple closely spaced foci. Multicentricity refers to the simultaneous development of multiple different malignancies. Usually, a tumor is considered multifocal if the foci are either within the same quadrant of the breast or within 5 cm of each other.
2. Mammographically, it is important to consider multifocality if there is a suggestion of multiple ill-defined masses closely related to a highly suspicious mass. Sometimes, with multiple oblique magnification views, one can identify spiculations extending from one mass to another. Sonography is a useful method to clarify multifocality and guide for biopsy.

Suggested Readings

1. Berg WA, Gilbreath PL. Multicentric and multifocal cancer: whole breast use in preoperative evaluation. *Radiology* 2000;214:59–66.
2. Johnson JE, Dutt PL, Page DL. Extent and multicentricity of in situ and invasive carcinoma. In: Bland KI, Copeland EM, eds. *The Breast.* Philadelphia: WB Saunders; 1998:296–306.
3. Lagios MD. Multicentricity of breast carcinoma demonstrated by routine correlated serial subgross and radiographic examination. *Cancer* 1997;40:1726–1734.

Case 55

Case History

A 57-year-old woman with an new right breast dimpling. Mammographically, two suspicious abnormalities are identified: lesion A in the medial inferior breast (which corresponds to the skin dimpling) and mass B at 12:00. Unfortunately, only the 12:00 mass (B) is adequately localized for biopsy. The medial inferior abnormality (A) is not confidently identified during an attempt to perform mammographic stereotactic biopsy and is not localized on the initial breast sonogram. Lesion A is only identified sonographically after breast MRI demonstrates the mass.

Physical Examination

- right breast: subtle skin dimpling in medial breast associated with vague firmness
- left breast: normal exam

Mammogram

Mass (Fig. 55-1)

- margin: indistinct
- shape: irregular
- density: equal density

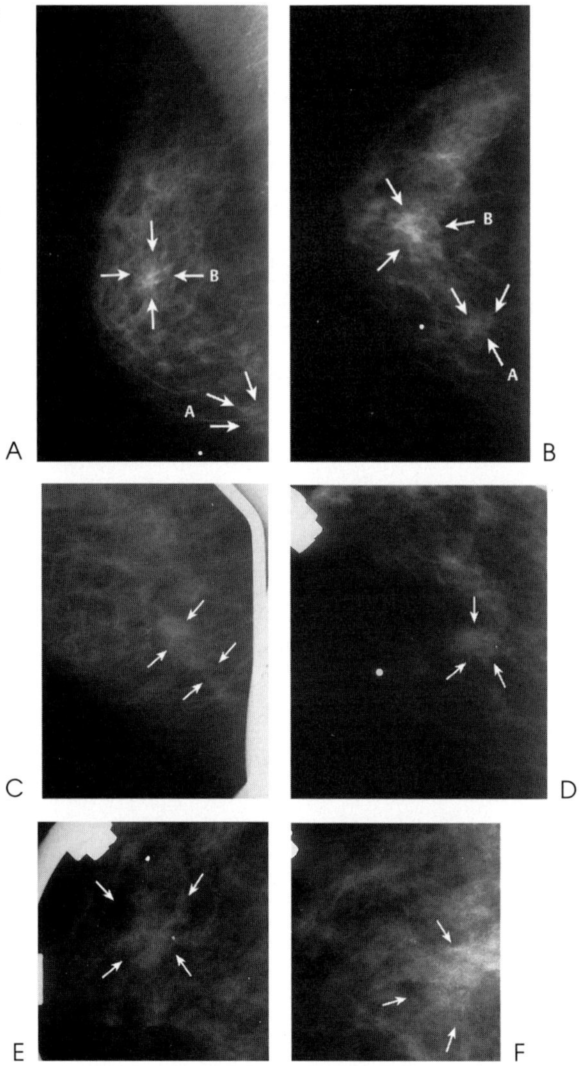

Figure 55-1. The skin dimpling in the medial inferior quadrant (marked by a radiopaque dot) is associated with an ill-defined mass (A), which is better identified on the CC spot compression (D). Lesion A appears as a subtle density associated with architectural distortion in Figure 55-1C, MLO spot compression (arrows). A second ill-defined mass (B) is demonstrated at the 12:00 position. (A). Right MLO mammogram. (B). Right CC mammogram. (C). Right MLO spot compression of medial inferior area of skin dimpling (lesion A; arrows). (D). Right CC spot compression of medial inferior area of skin dimpling (lesion A; arrows). (E). Right MLO spot compression of 12:00 mass (lesion B; arrows). (F). Right CC spot compression of 12:00 mass (lesion B; arrows).

Ultrasound

Frequency

- 11.5 MHz

Mass (Figs. 55–2 and 55–3)

- margin: ill-defined
- echogenicity: hypoechoic
- retrotumoral acoustic appearance: posterior shadowing distal to mass
- shape: irregular

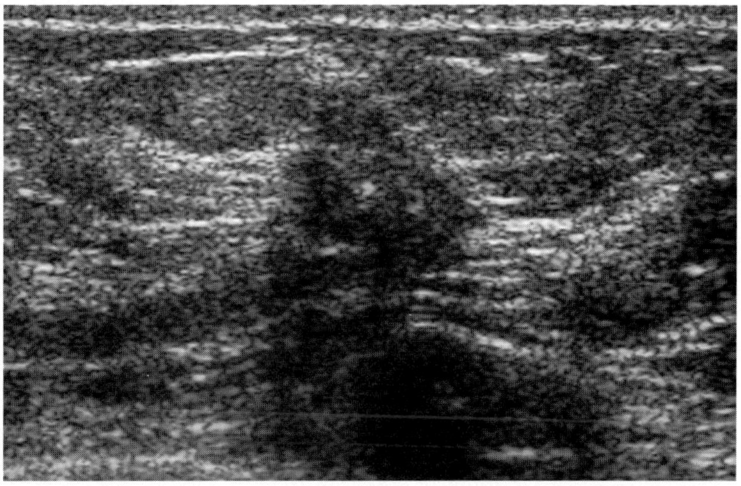

Figure 55–2. Right radial breast sonogram: This ill-defined hypoechoic mass (lesion A) was initially missed sonographically. After the right breast MRI (Fig. 55–4) demonstrated the mass, the patient was reexamined sonographically and this mass was identified.

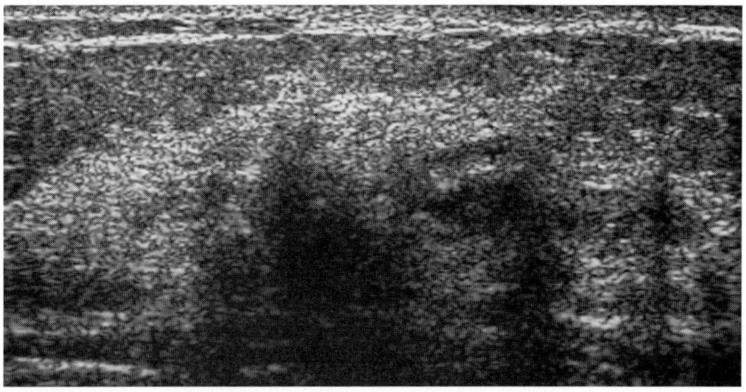

Figure 55–3. Right radial breast sonogram: This irregular hypoechoic mass corresponds to the mammographic mass at 12:00 (lesion B).

Other Modalities (Figs. 55–4 and 55–5)

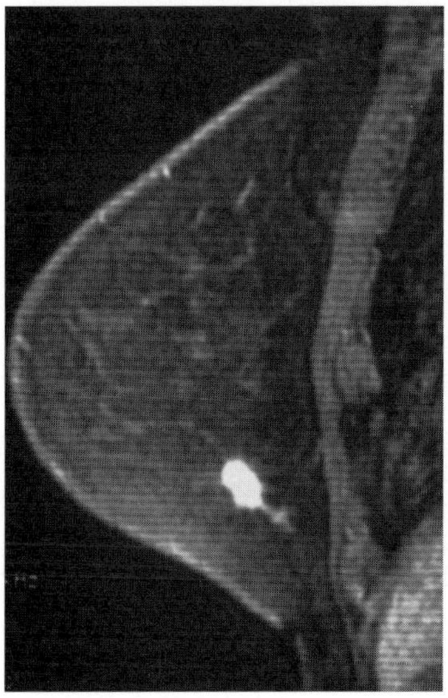

Figure 55–4. Right sagittal dynamic bolus 3-D volume gradient series breast MRI: In the inferior medial breast, a mass exhibits abnormal early enhancement. This mass corresponds to the area of skin dimpling (lesion A).

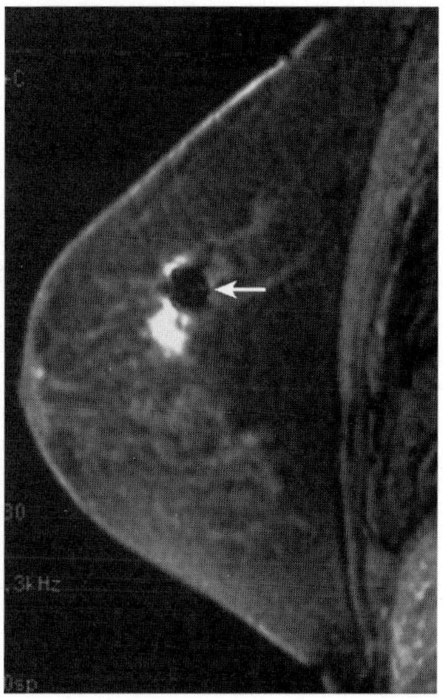

Figure 55–5. Right sagittal dynamic bolus 3-D volume gradient series breast MRI: Lesion B is in the upper breast at 12:00. Lesion B exhibits low-intensity clip artifact from previous mammographic stereotactic core biopsy.

Pathology

- infiltrating ductal carcinoma
- Mastectomy specimen showed 3 separate tumor masses. Two of the masses matched the MRI tumors. The third malignancy was identified pathologically in the inferior breast and could not be identified retrospectively by MRI.

Management

- BI-RADS Assessment Category 4, suspicious; biopsy should be considered

Pearls and Pitfalls

This case illustrates multicentric malignancies. Due to differences in pathologic examination and definition of multicentricity, studies have reported the prevalence of multicentricity between 9 and 75%. The probable true prevalence is between 25 and 50% for all histologies. Invasive ductal carcinoma has a lower rate of multicentricity (19%) compared with other histologies.

Suggested Readings

1. Gump FE, Habif DV, Logergo P, et al. The extent and distribution of cancer in breasts with palpable primary tumors. *Ann Surg* 1986;204:384–388.
2. Johnson JE, Dutt PL, Page DL. Extent and multicentricity of in situ and invasive carcinoma. In: Bland KI, Copeland EM, eds. *The Breast*. Philadelphia: WB Saunders; 1998:296–306.
3. Tavassoli FA, Fattaneh A. *Pathology of the Breast*. 2nd ed. Stamford: Appleton and Lange; 1999:56–74.

Case 56

Case History

A 73-year-old woman presents with a palpable left breast mass.

Physical Examination

- left breast: palpable mass at the 5:00 position
- right breast: normal exam

Mammogram

Mass (Fig. 56–1)

- margin: indistinct
- shape: irregular
- density: equal

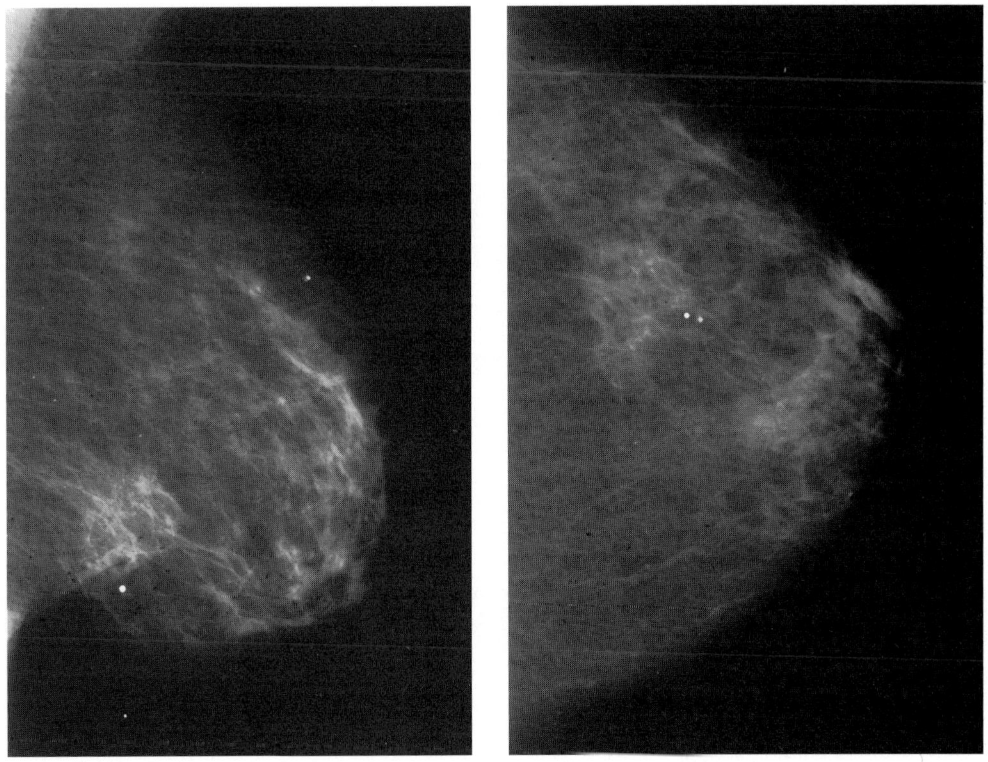

A B

Figure 56–1. *An ill-defined mass is in the lower outer quadrant. This mass is associated with skin retraction. This mass corresponds to the palpable lump. (A). Left MLO mammogram. (B). Left CC mammogram.*

Ultrasound

Frequency

- 7 MHz

Mass

- margin: spiculation/architectural distortion
- echogenicity: heterogeneous (mixed)
- retrotumoral acoustic appearance: severe shadowing, mass partially obscured
- shape: irregular (Fig. 56–2)

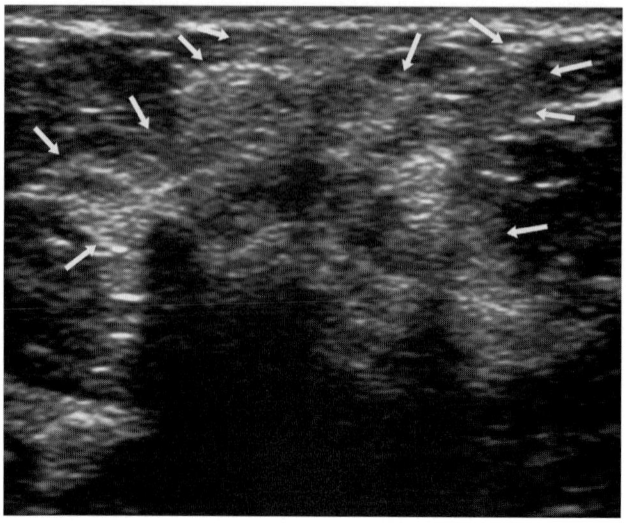

Figure 56–2. Left radial breast sonogram: The palpable mass corresponds to an irregular mass (arrows) of heterogeneous echogenicity. Posterior acoustic shadowing partially obscures the mass.

Pathology

- invasive lobular carcinoma (Fig. 56–3)

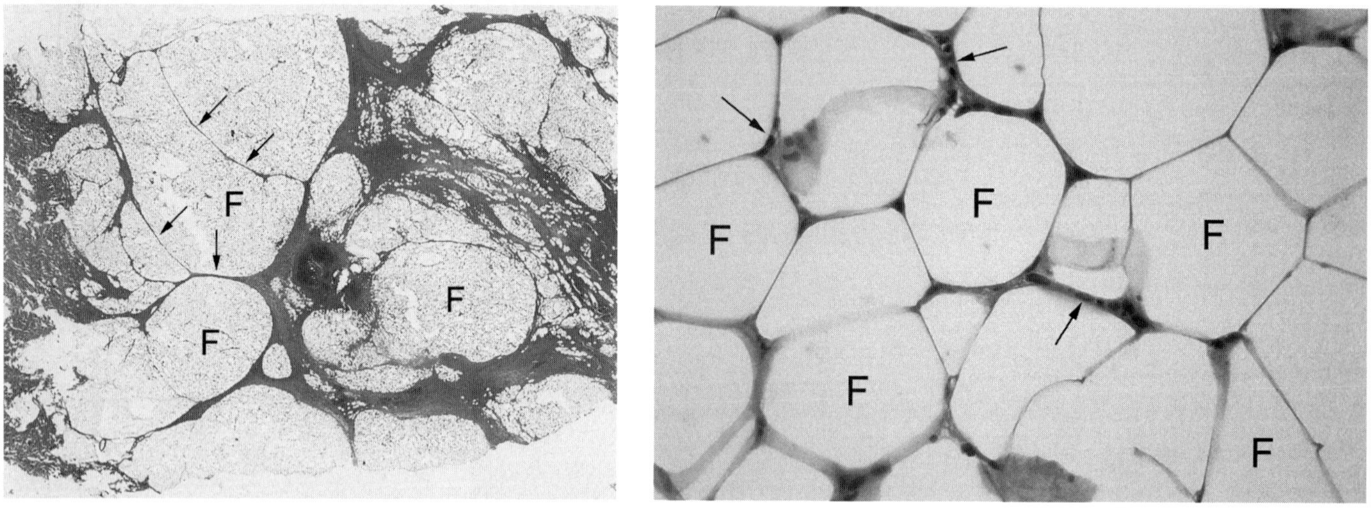

A B

Figure 56–3. Surgical specimen demonstrates that the malignant cells infiltrate the normal breast tissues without distorting the structure of the tissues. Normal fat cells (F) are distributed between thin collumns (arrows) of malignant cells and produce the low-density mammographic mass. (A). Low-power microscopic view. (B). High-power microscopic view (see Color Plate 56–3A and B).

Management

- BI-RADS Assessment Category 4, suspicious abnormality; biopsy should be considered

Pearls and Pitfalls

1. Studies report that lobular carcinoma accounts for 1 to 15% of all breast malignancies. The median age of patients is between 45 and 57 years.
2. Mammographically, this tumor may exhibit relatively low density because the malignancy extends into the breast stroma via small cords of cells or as isolated single cells. If the malignant cells are surrounded by fat (as in this case), the radiographic density is relatively low for a large mass.
3. Sonographically, lobular carcinoma may be missed since it may present (particularly at lower frequencies) as a predominantly hyperechoic mass with shadowing. The mass may blend into the surrounding hyperechoic parenchyma. The main clue that helps one differentiate this mass from the surrounding parenchyma is focal shadowing from the mass.

Suggested Readings

1. Butler RS, Venta LA, Wiley EL, Ellis RL, Dempsey PJ, Rubin E. Sonographic evaluation of infiltrating lobular carcinoma. *AJR* 1999;172:325–330.
2. Rissanen T, Tikkakoski T, Autio AL, Apaja-Sarkkinen M. Ultrasonography of invasive lobular breast carcinoma. *Acta Radiologica* 1998;39:285–291.
3. Tavassoli FA. Infiltrating carcinoma: common and familiar special types. In: Tavassoli FA, Fattaneh A. *Pathology of the Breast.* 2nd ed. Stamford: Appleton and Lange; 1999:401–480.

Case 57

Case History

A 59-year-old woman presents with a new density identified by screening mammography.

Physical Examination

- normal exam

Mammogram

Mass (Fig. 57–1)

- margin: indistinct
- shape: irregular
- density: equal

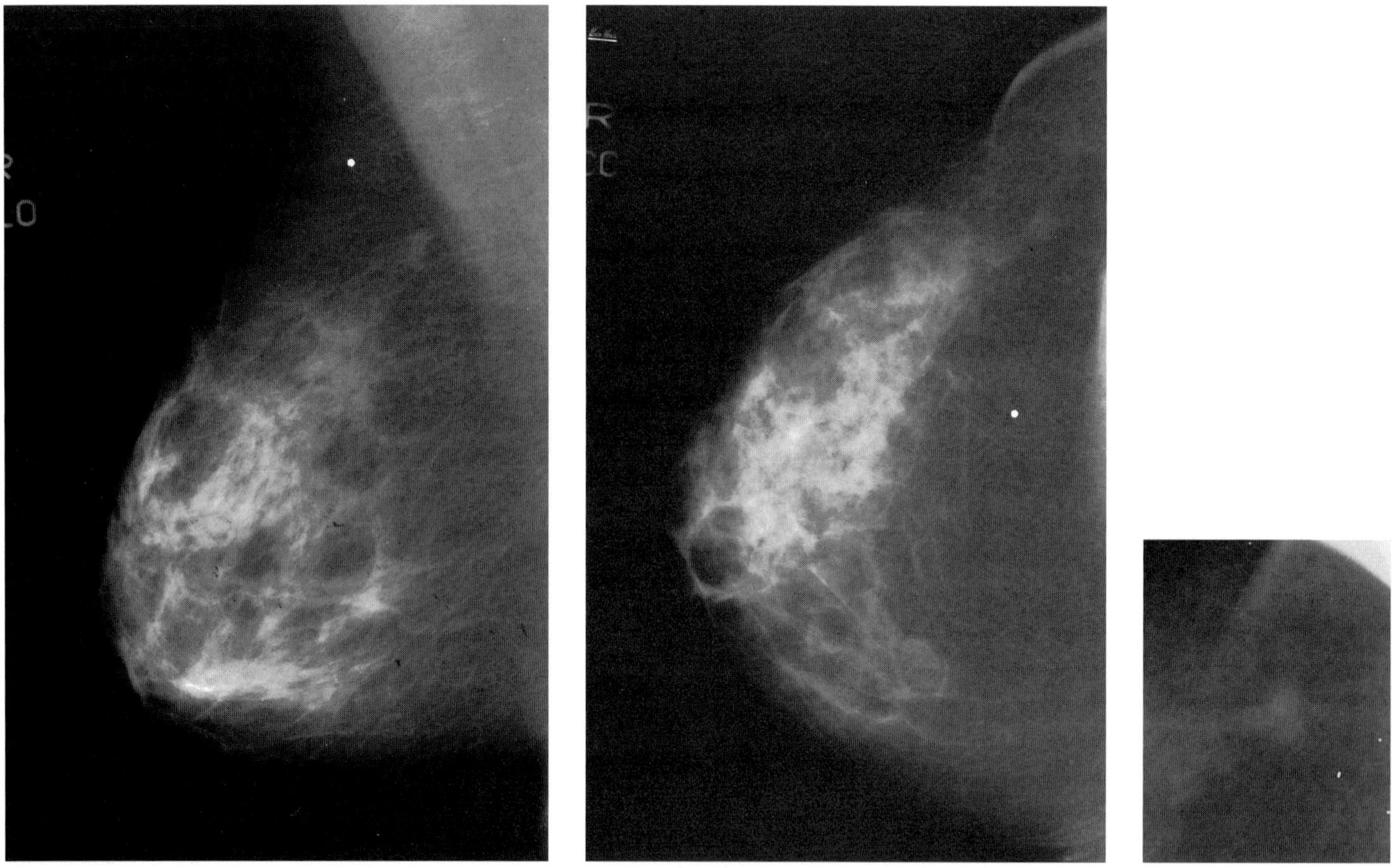

A B C

Figure 57–1. There is a small irregular mass in the right upper outer breast. Radiopaque marker (dot) labels a skin mole. (A). Right MLO mammogram. (B). Right CC mammogram. (C). Right CC spot compression mammogram.

Ultrasound

Low Frequency

Frequency

- 7 MHz

Mass

- margin: ill defined
- echogenicity: heterogeneous (mixed)
- retrotumoral acoustic appearance: posterior shadowing distal to mass
- shape: irregular (Fig. 57–2)

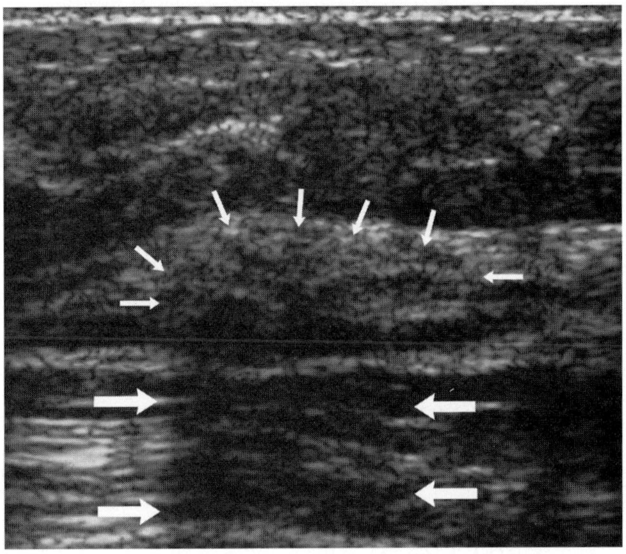

Figure 57–2. Right radial breast sonogram: The mass identified in Figure 57–1 corresponds to minimal sonographic architectural distortion (small arrows) and posterior acoustic shadowing (large arrows).

High Frequency

Frequency

- 10 MHz

Associated Findings

The mass is much easier to identify on the higher-frequency examination (Fig. 57–3) compared with the lower-frequency exam (Fig. 57–2) because the heterogeneous echogenicity of the mass is subtle on the lower-frequency study. (See Fig. 57–3.)

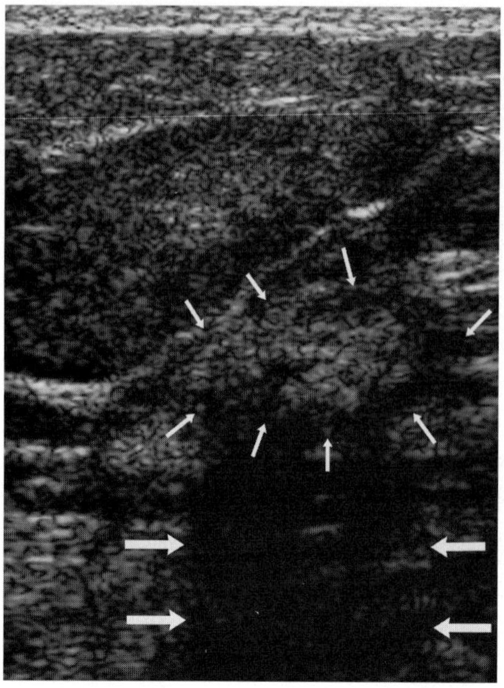

Figure 57–3. Right radial breast sonogram: Higher-frequency sonographic examination of same mass as Figures 57–1 and 57–2 demonstrates a mass with heterogeneous echogenicity (small arrows) and acoustic shadowing (large arrows).

Pathology

- invasive lobular carcinoma

Management

- BI-RADS Assessment Category 4, suspicious abnormality; biopsy should be considered

Pearls and Pitfalls

This case illustrates that higher-frequency sonographic technique greatly improves the detectability of breast masses.

Suggested Readings

1. Evans N, Lyons K. The use of ultrasound in the diagnosis of invasive lobular carcinoma of the breast less than 10 mm in size. *Clin Radiol* 2000;55:261–263.
2. Skaane P, Skjorten F. Ultrasonographic evaluation of invasive lobular carcinoma. *Acta Radiologica* 1999;40:369–375.

Case 58

Case History

A 70-year-old woman presents with non-Hodgkin's lymphoma and a new right breast mammographic mass.

Physical Examination

- breasts: no palpable masses
- bilateral palpable cervical, axillary, and inguinal adenopathy

Mammogram

Mass (Fig. 58–1)

- margin: indistinct
- shape: irregular
- density: equal density

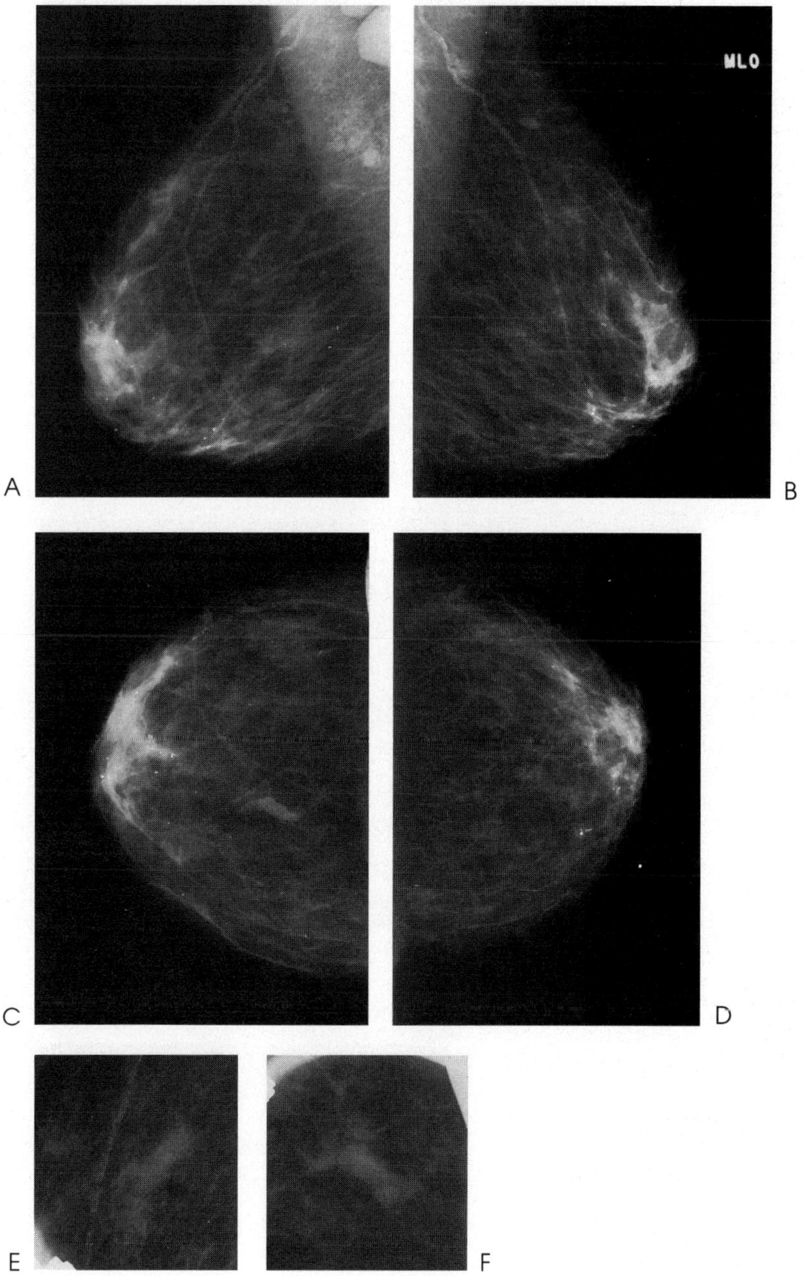

Figure 58–1. In the 12:00 position of the right breast, there is an irregular, ill-defined mass. Large right axillary lymph nodes are also evident. (A). Right MLO mammogram. (B). Left MLO mammogram. (C). Right CC mammogram. (D). Left CC mammogram. (E). Right MLO spot compression mammogram. (F). Right CC spot compression mammogram.

Ultrasound

Frequency

- 13 MHz

Mass

- margin: ill defined
- echogenicity: hypoechoic
- retrotumoral acoustic appearance: no shadowing
- shape: irregular (Figs. 58–2 and 58–3)

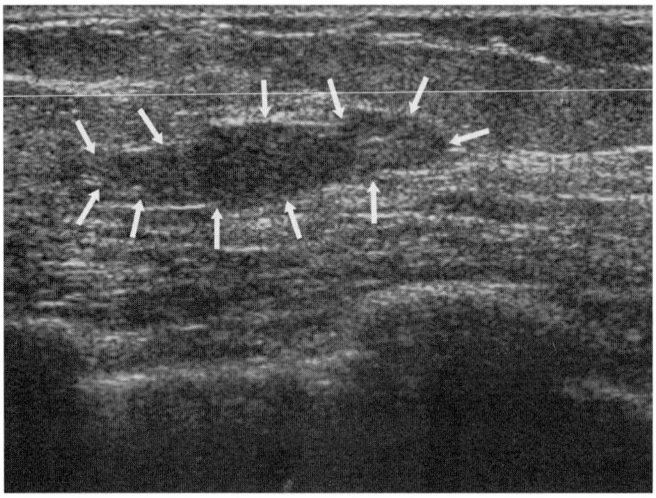

Figure 58–2. Right radial breast sonogram: The mammographic mass (Fig. 58–1) corresponds to an ill-defined hypoechoic mass (arrows).

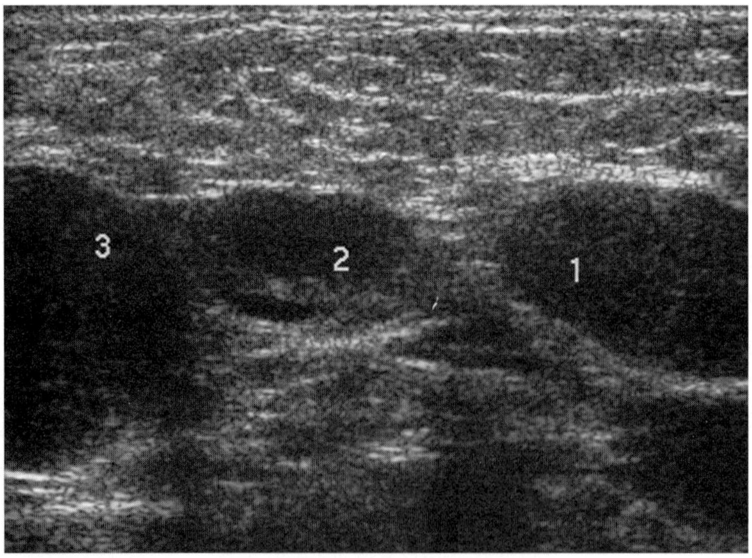

Figure 58–3. Right radial breast sonogram: In the axilla, there are numerous enlarged lymph nodes (labeled 1, 2, 3).

Pathology

- lymphoma
- non-Hodgkin's lymphoma, which matches the cell type of the patient's systemic lymphoma

Management

- BI-RADS Assessment Category 4, suspicious; biopsy should be considered

Pearls and Pitfalls

1. Lymphoma is one of the most common metastatic malignancies of the breast. Non-Hodgkin's is more common than Hodgkin's lymphoma. Generally, the patients present with unilateral breast involvement.
2. Mammographically, lymphoma presents as a circumscribed, irregular mass or as an ill-defined density associated with skin thickening.
3. Sonographically, lymphoma generally is a circumscribed or irregular hypoechoic mass. Sometimes the mass simulates a cyst by appearing anechoic with increased acoustic transmission.

Suggested Readings

1. Kiziltepe TT, Erden GA, Dingil G, Ince A. Breast metastasis from non-Hodgkin's lymphoma: evaluation with color Doppler sonography. *AJR* 1996;167:1595–1596.
2. Liberman L, Giess CS, Dershaw DD, Louie DC, Deutch BM. Non-Hodgkin lymphoma of the breast: imaging characteristics and correlation with histopathologic findings. *Radiology* 1994;192:157–160.
3. McCrea ES, Johnston C, Haney PJ. Metastases to the breast. *AJR* 1983;141:685–690.
4. Meyer JE, Kopans DB, Long JC. Mammographic appearance of malignant lymphoma of the breast. *Radiology* 1980;135:623–626.

Case 59

Case History

A 75-year-old woman presents for a screening mammogram.

Physical Examination

- normal exam

Mammogram

Mass (Fig. 59–1)

- margin: indistinct
- shape: irregular
- density: equal density

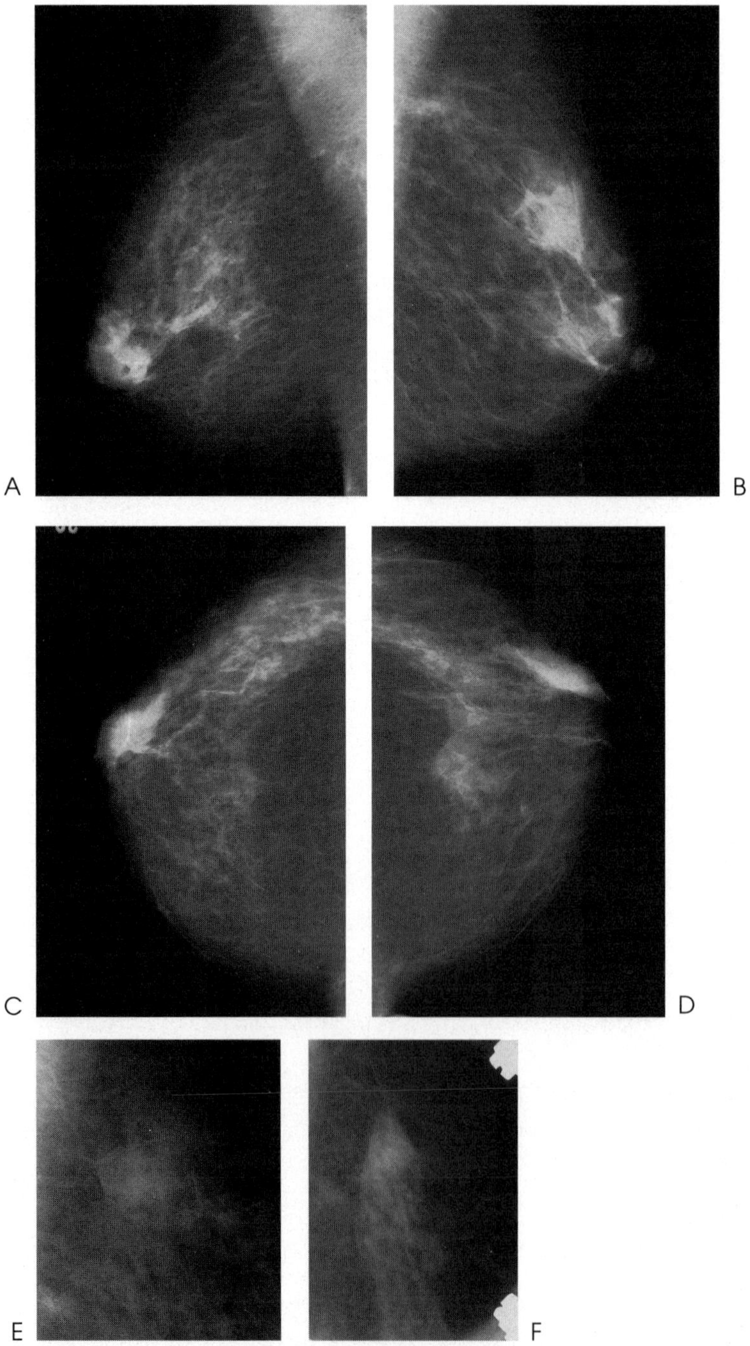

Figure 59–1. In the left upper outer quadrant, there is an ill-defined mass. The mass is not visible on the routine CC view (D) but is identified on the exaggerated CC (F) view. (A). Right MLO mammogram. (B). Left MLO mammogram. (C). Right CC mammogram. (D). Left CC mammogram. (E). Left MLO spot compression mammogram. (F). Left exaggerated CC spot compression mammogram.

Ultrasound

Frequency

- 7 MHz

Mass

- margin: ill defined
- echogenicity: hypoechoic
- retrotumoral acoustic appearance: bilateral edge shadowing
- shape: irregular (Fig. 59–2)

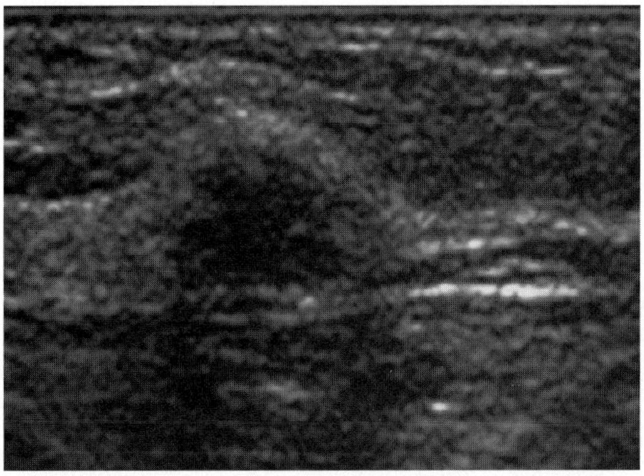

Figure 59–2. Left radial breast sonogram: The mammographic mass corresponds to an irregular, hypoechoic mass.

Pathology

- tubular carcinoma

Management

- BI-RADS Assessment Category 4, suspicious; biopsy should be considered

Pearls and Pitfalls

1. Tubular carcinoma comprises 1 to 10% of all breast malignancies.
2. Mammographically, tubular carcinomas are generally noncalcified, irregular masses with spiculated margins. They are commonly high density and less than 1 cm in size.
3. Sonographic findings of tubular carcinoma are similar to irregular masses produced by infiltrating ductal carcinoma. The mass is irregular, hypoechoic with posterior acoustic shadowing. High-frequency sonography may be necessary to detect very small masses. In this case, sonography was used to localize for percutaneous biopsy.

Suggested Readings

1. Elson BC, Helvie MA, Frank TS, Wilson TE, Adler DD. Tubular carcinoma of the breast: mode of presentation, mammographic appearance, and frequency of nodal metastases. *AJR* 1993;161:1173–1176.
2. Feig SA, Shaber GS, Patchefsky AS, Schwartz GF, Edeiken J, Nerlinger R. Tubular carcinoma of the breast. *Radiology* 1978;129:311–314.
3. Leibman AJ, Lewis M, Druse B. Tubular carcinoma of the breast: mammographic appearance. *AJR* 1993;160:263–265.

Case 60

Case History

A 55-year-old woman presents for screening mammogram.

Physical Examination

- normal exam

Mammogram

Mass (Fig. 60–1)

- margin: spiculated
- shape: irregular
- density: equal density

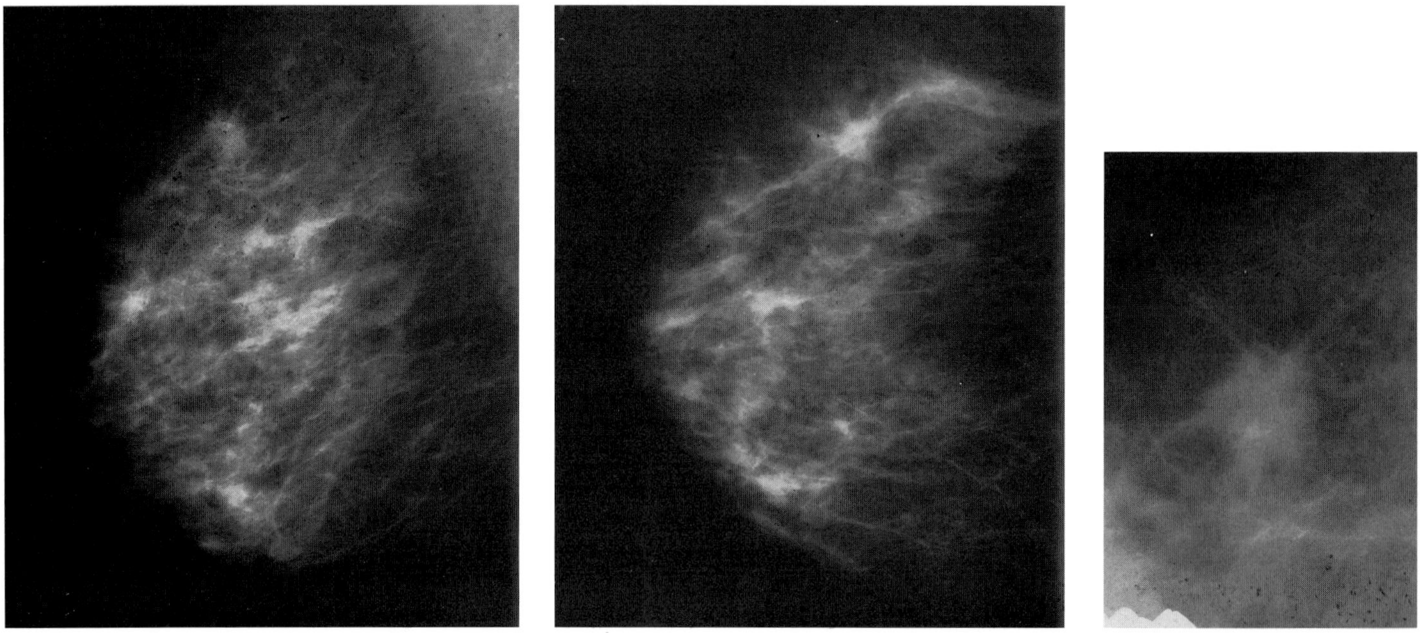

A B C

Figure 60–1. There is a spiculated mass in the right upper outer quadrant. (A). Right MLO mammogram. (B). Right CC mammogram. (C). Right MLO spot magnification mammogram.

Ultrasound

Frequency

- 11.5 MHz

Mass

- margin: ill defined
- echogenicity: hypoechoic
- retrotumoral acoustic appearance: severe shadowing, mass completely obscured
- shape: irregular (Fig. 60–2)

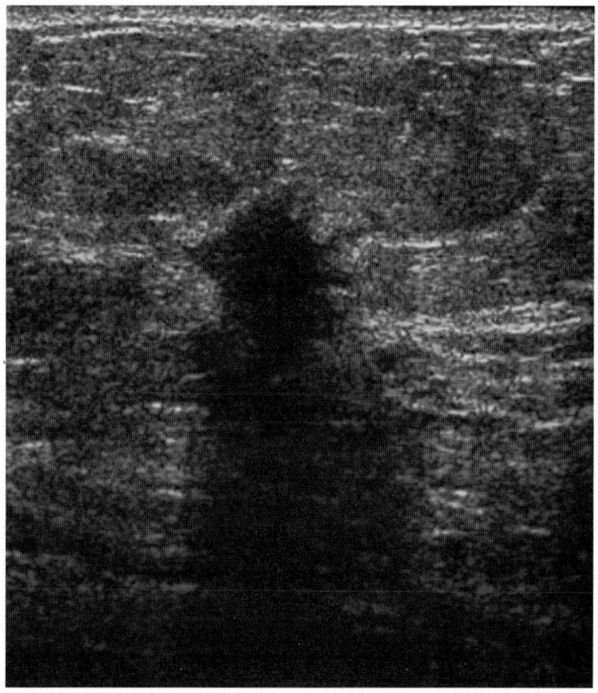

Figure 60–2. Right radial breast sonogram: Sonographic examination of the mammographic spiculated mass (Fig. 60–1) demonstrates an irregular, hypoechoic mass with severe shadowing.

Pathology

- tubular carcinoma (Fig. 60–3)

Management

- BI-RADS Assessment Category 4, suspicious; biopsy should be considered

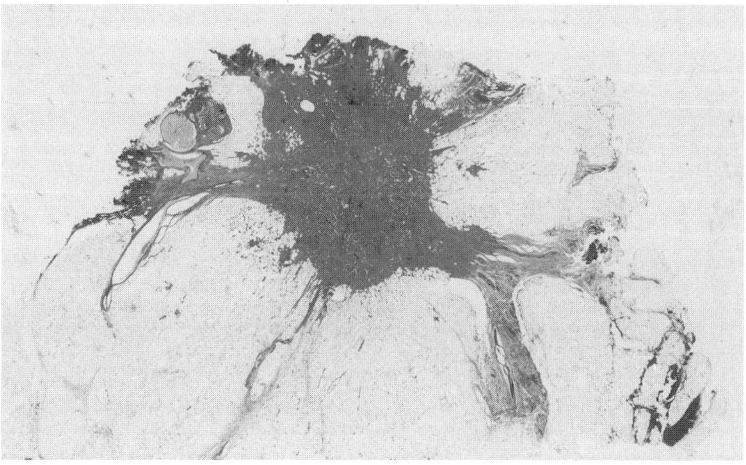

Figure 60–3. Low-power microscopic image: The irregular shape of the pathologic specimen corresponds to the mammographic spiculated mass (see Color Plate 60–3).

Pearls and Pitfalls

1. Sonography detects between 88 and 100% of cases of tubular carcinomas. Sonography is useful when the tumor is mamographically occult or for guiding biopsy.
2. Tubular carcinoma has been reported to be multicentric in 15 to 60% of patients and has been associated with another malignancy in the contralateral breast in 10 to 40% of patients. This patient also had abnormal calcifications in the left breast due to ductal carcinoma in situ.

Suggested Readings

1. Mitnick JS, Gianutsos R, Pollack AH, et al. Tubular carcinoma of the breast: sensitivity of diagnostic techniques and correlation with histopathology. *AJR* 1999;172:319–323.
2. Sheppard DG, Whitman GJ, Huynh PT, Sahin AA, Fornage BD, Stelling CB. Tubular carcinoma of the breast: mammographic and sonographic features. *AJR* 2000;174:253–257.

Case 61

Case History

A 57-year-old woman presents with a new left breast lump.

Physical Examination

- left breast: two palpable lumps at the 1:00 position; skin is thickened, red, and erythematous
- right breast: normal exam

Mammogram

Mass (Fig. 61–1)

- margin: indistinct
- shape: irregular
- density: high density

Figure 61–1. In the left upper outer breast there is an area of increased density associated with a dominant ill-defined irregular mass. (A). Right MLO mammogram. (B). Left MLO mammogram. (C). Right CC mammogram. (D). Left CC mammogram. (E). Left CC spot compression mammogram.

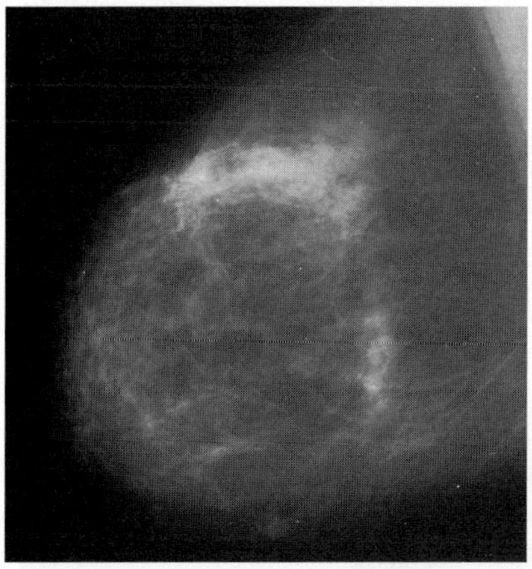
A

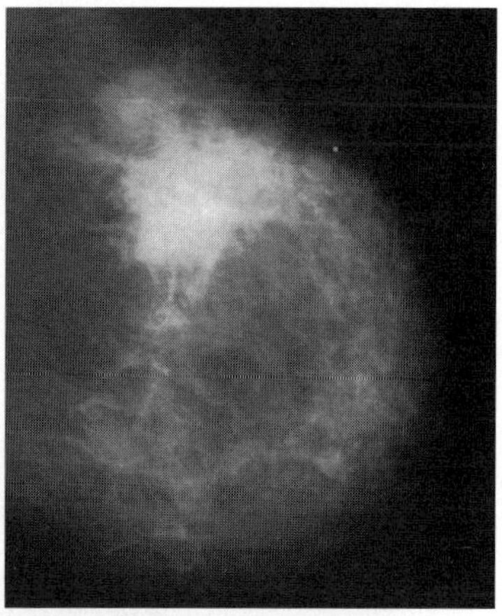
B

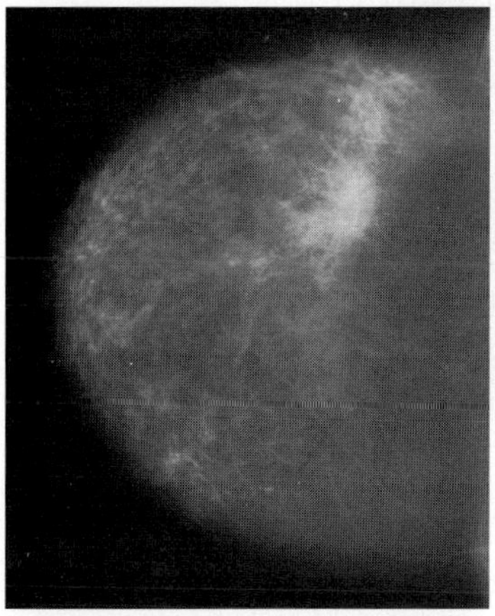
C

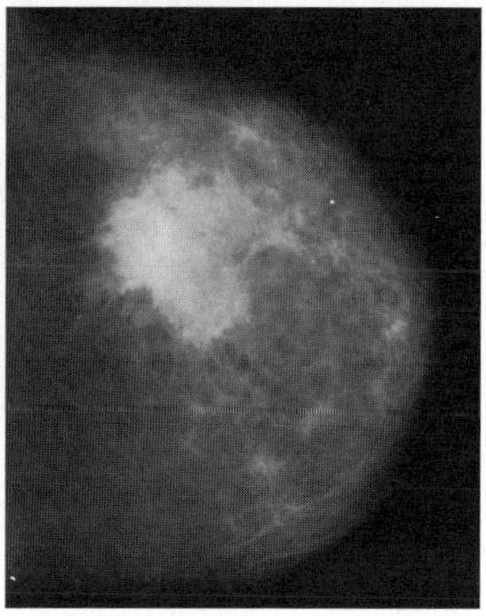
D

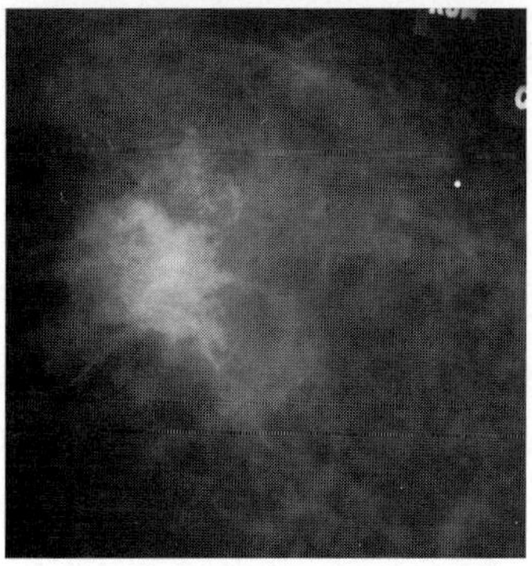
E

Ultrasound

Frequency

- 10 MHz

Mass

- margin: ill defined
- echogenicity: hypoechoic
- retrotumoral acoustic appearance: posterior shadowing distal to mass
- shape: irregular (Figs. 61–2 and 61–3)

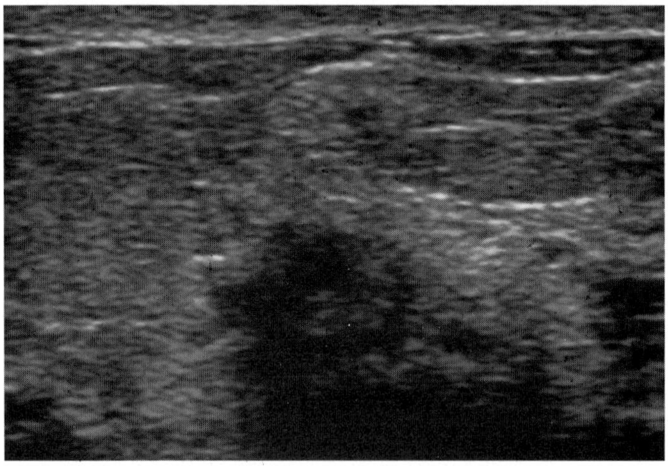

Figure 61–2. Left radial breast sonogram: In the left upper outer quadrant, there are two palpable masses. The mass in this image corresponds to the dominant mammographically identified mass (Fig. 61–1).

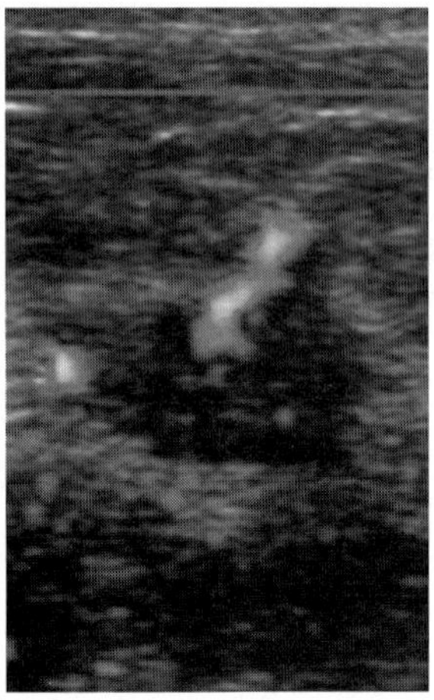

Figure 61–3. Left radial color Doppler breast sonogram: A second palpable lump corresponds to this smaller, irregular, spiculated mass, which is a satellite lesion of the dominant mass in Figure 61–2 (see Color Plate 61–3).

Pathology

Inflammatory carcinoma. Mastectomy specimen demonstrated a 5 cm lobular carcinoma associated with lymphatic invasion of the deep dermis; 12 of 12 lymph nodes were positive for metastatic disease.

Management

- BI-RADS Assessment Category 5, highly suggestive of malignancy

Pearls and Pitfalls

1. Clinically, inflammatory carcinoma presents with diffuse erythema, edema over two thirds of the breast, peau d'orange, tenderness, induration, warmth, enlargement, and a diffusely palpable mass. Pathologically, this entity is defined by invasion of the dermal lymphatics.
2. Mammographically, the findings of inflammatory carcinoma include: skin thickening, nipple inversion, diffuse increased breast density, trabecular thickening, axillary adenopathy, architectural distortion or focal asymmetric density, malignant calcifications and mass.
3. Sonographically, the neoplasm will appear as an irregular, hypoechoic, ill-defined mass. Associated findings include skin thickening, increased echogenicity of the subcutaneous fat, and dilated tubular structures under the skin due to dilated veins or lymphatics. The tissues will exhibit strong color Doppler due to inflammatory hyperemia.

Suggested Readings

1. Dershaw DD, Moore MP, Liberman L, Deutch BM. Inflammatory breast carcinoma: mammographic findings. *Radiology* 1994;190:831–834.
2. Kushwaha AC, Whitman GJ, Stelling CB, Cristofanilli M, Buzdar AU. Primary inflammatory carcinoma of the breast: retrospective review of mammographic findings. *AJR* 2000;174:535–538.
3. Tardivon AA, Viala J, Rudelli AC, Guinebretiere J-M, Vanel D. Mammographic patterns of inflammatory breast carcinoma: a retrospective study of 92 cases. *Eur J Radiol* 1997;24:124–130.
4. Tohno E, Cosgrove DO, Sloane JP. Inflammatory carcinoma. In: Tohno D, Cosgrove DO, Sloane JP, eds. *Ultrasound Diagnosis of Breast Diseases.* New York: Churchill Livingston; 1994:176–177.

Section V

Calcifications

When one evaluates calcifications, one should first exclude benign calcifications. They are Category 2, benign, if they have the following characteristics:

1. large size (smallest thickness or diameter >1 mm)
2. scattered distribution
3. special type of calcification (e.g., milk of calcium, dermal calcification)

If the calcifications do not have the above characteristics or if they are small and clustered, then analyze the *shape* of the calcifications.

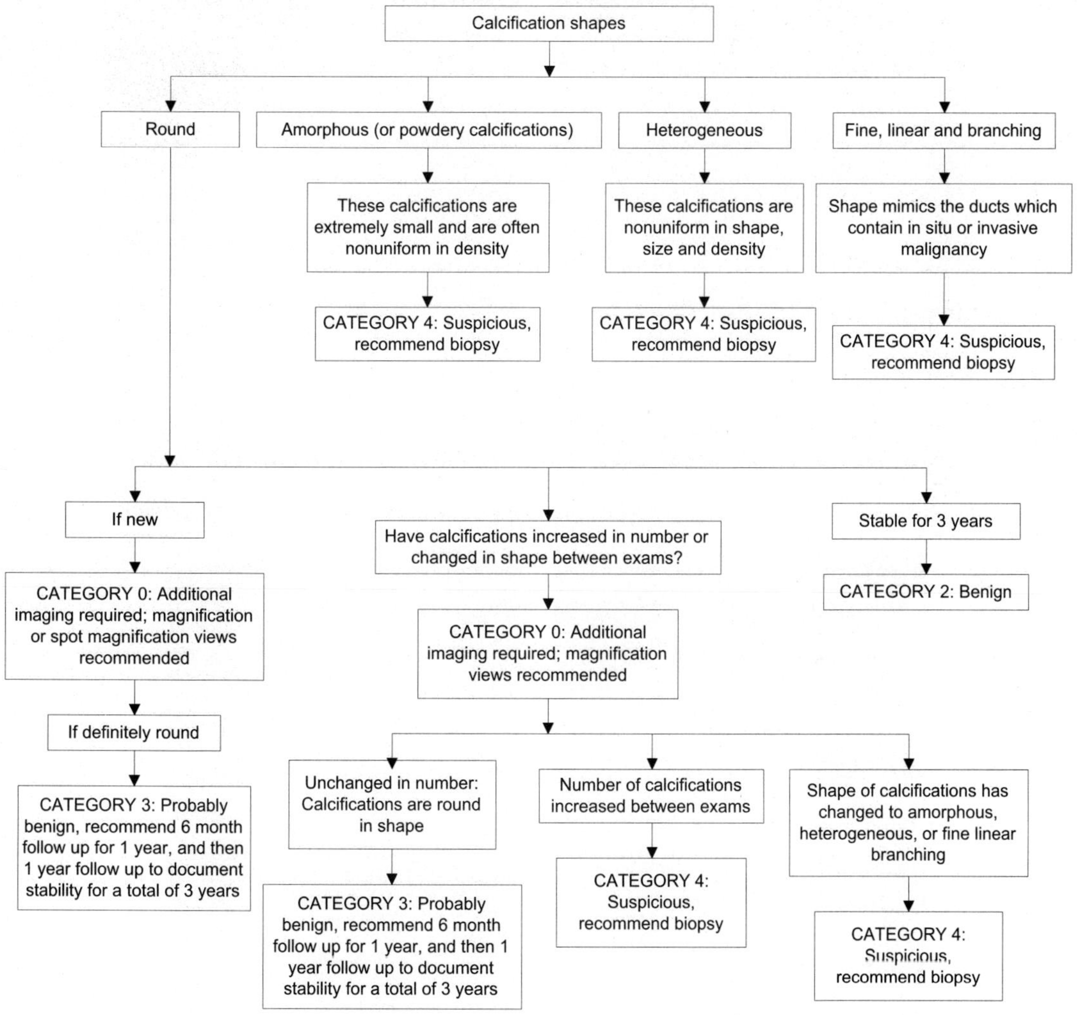

Case 62

Case History

A 61-year-old woman presents for a screening mammogram.

Physical Examination

- normal exam

Mammogram

Calcifications (Fig. 62–1)

- type: vascular
- distribution: diffuse/scattered

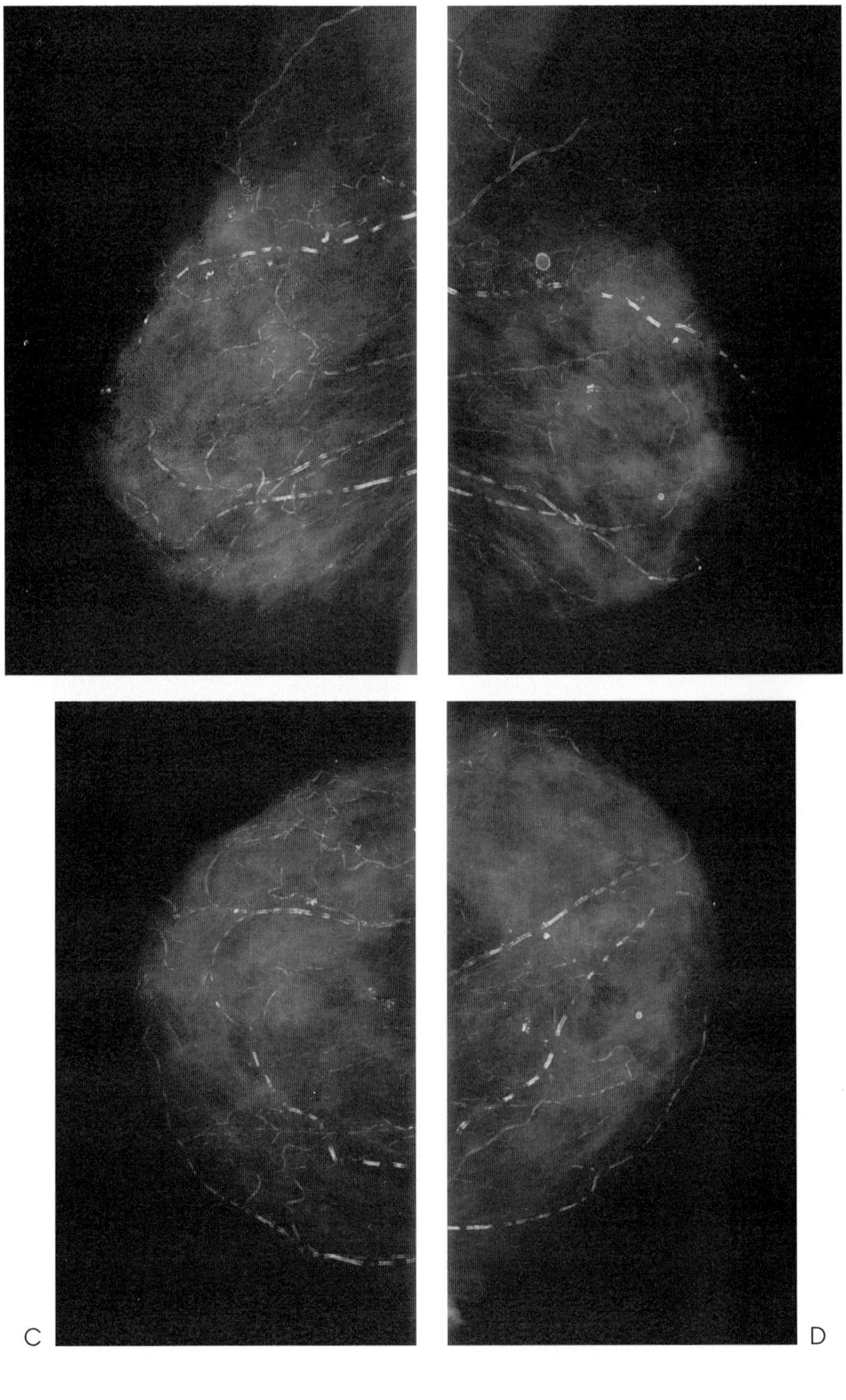

A B C D

Figure 62–1. Both breasts exhibit numerous linear vascular calcifications. (A). Right MLO mammogram. (B). Left MLO mammogram. (C). Right CC mammogram. (D). Left CC mammogram.

Pathology

- atherosclerosis

Management

- BI-RADS Assessment Category 1, negative

Pearls and Pitfalls

Atherosclerosis is the most common cause of vascular calcifications in the breast. These calcifications are linear and generally are easy to differentiate from malignant calcifications. Vascular calcifications may be increased in patients with renal failure. Occasionally, vessels that are poorly calcified may appear worrisome but, generally, magnification views clarify the etiology of the calcification.

Suggested Readings

1. Cooper RA, Berman S. Extensive breast calcification in renal failure. *J Thorac Imaging* 1988;3:81–82.
2. Kemmeren JM, Beijerinck D, van Noord PA, et al. Breast arterial calcifications: association with diabetes mellitus and cardiovascular mortality. *Radiology* 1996;201:75–78.
3. Kragel PJ, Aquino MO, Fiorella R, et al. Clinical radiographic and pathologic features of medical calcific sclerosis in the breast. *South Med J* 1997;90:518–521.
4. Meybehm M, Pfeifer U. Vascular calcifications mimicking grouped microcalcifications on mammography. *Breast Dis* 1990;3:81–86.
5. Sommer G, Kopsa H, Zazgornik J, et al. Breast calcifications in renal hyperparathyroidism. *AJR* 1987; 48:855–857.

Case 63

Case History

A 76-year-old woman presents for routine mammogram.

Physical Examination

- normal exam

Mammogram

Calcifications (Fig. 63–1)

- type: large rodlike
- distribution: diffuse/scattered

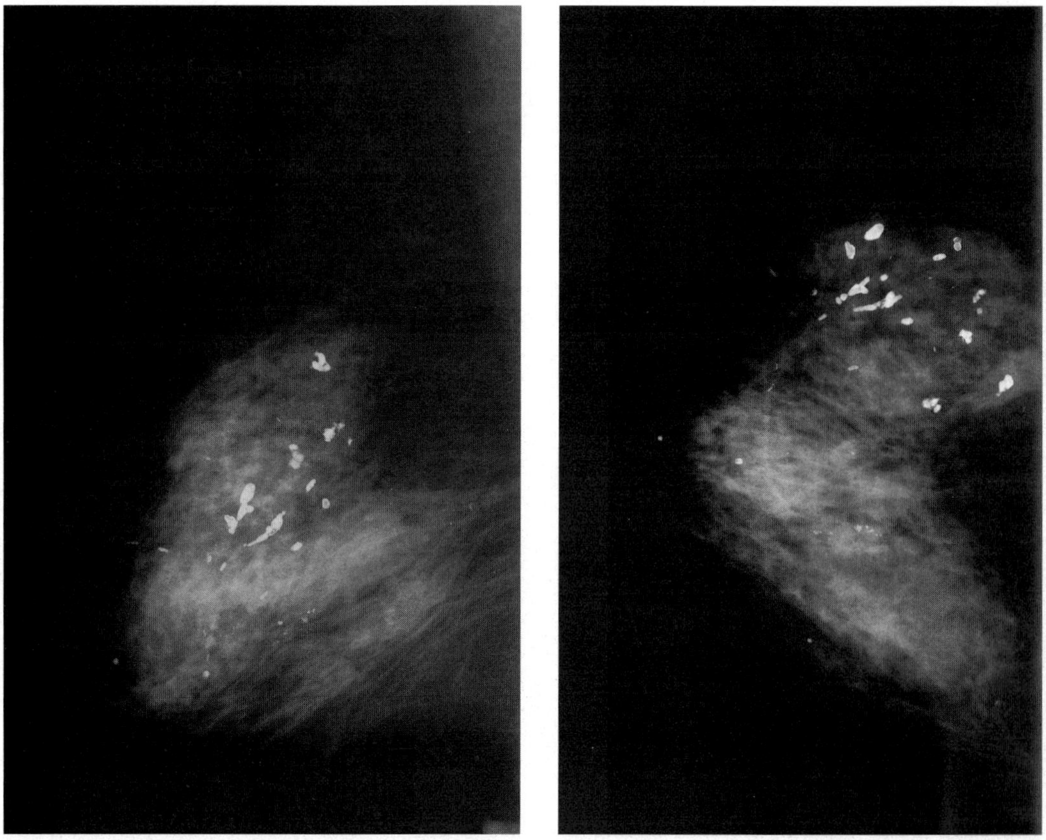
A B

Figure 63–1. There are diffuse, scattered, thick, linear, large oval and round calcifications in the upper half of the breast oriented toward the nipple. These calcifications are smooth bordered and some have central lucencies. Most of the linear calcifications do not branch. (A). Right MLO mammogram. (B). Right CC mammogram.

Pathology

- plasma cell mastitis

Management

- BI-RADS Assessment Category 2, benign finding

Pearls and Pitfalls

1. Secretory calcifications result from ductal inflammation and are benign. This process is commonly bilateral. The large size, scattered distribution, and smooth borders distinguish these calcifications from malignant calcifications.
2. Secretory calcifications may present in one of two forms. They may be primarily linear, either with or without central lucency, or they may be spherical or globular in configuration with lucent centers. In this latter form, they are sometimes difficult to differentiate from multiple oil cysts. This case illustrates the spherical form.

Suggested Readings

1. De Paredes ES. *Atlas of Film-Screen Mammography*, 2nd ed. Baltimore: Urban & Schwarzenberg 1988:191–276.
2. Gershon-Cohen J, Ingleby H, Hermel MB. Calcifications in secretory disease of the breast. *AJR* 1956;76:132–135.

Case 64

Case History

A 79-year-old woman presents for a screening mammogram.

Physical Examination

- normal exam

Mammogram

Calcifications (Fig. 64-1)

- type: large rodlike
- distribution: diffuse/scattered

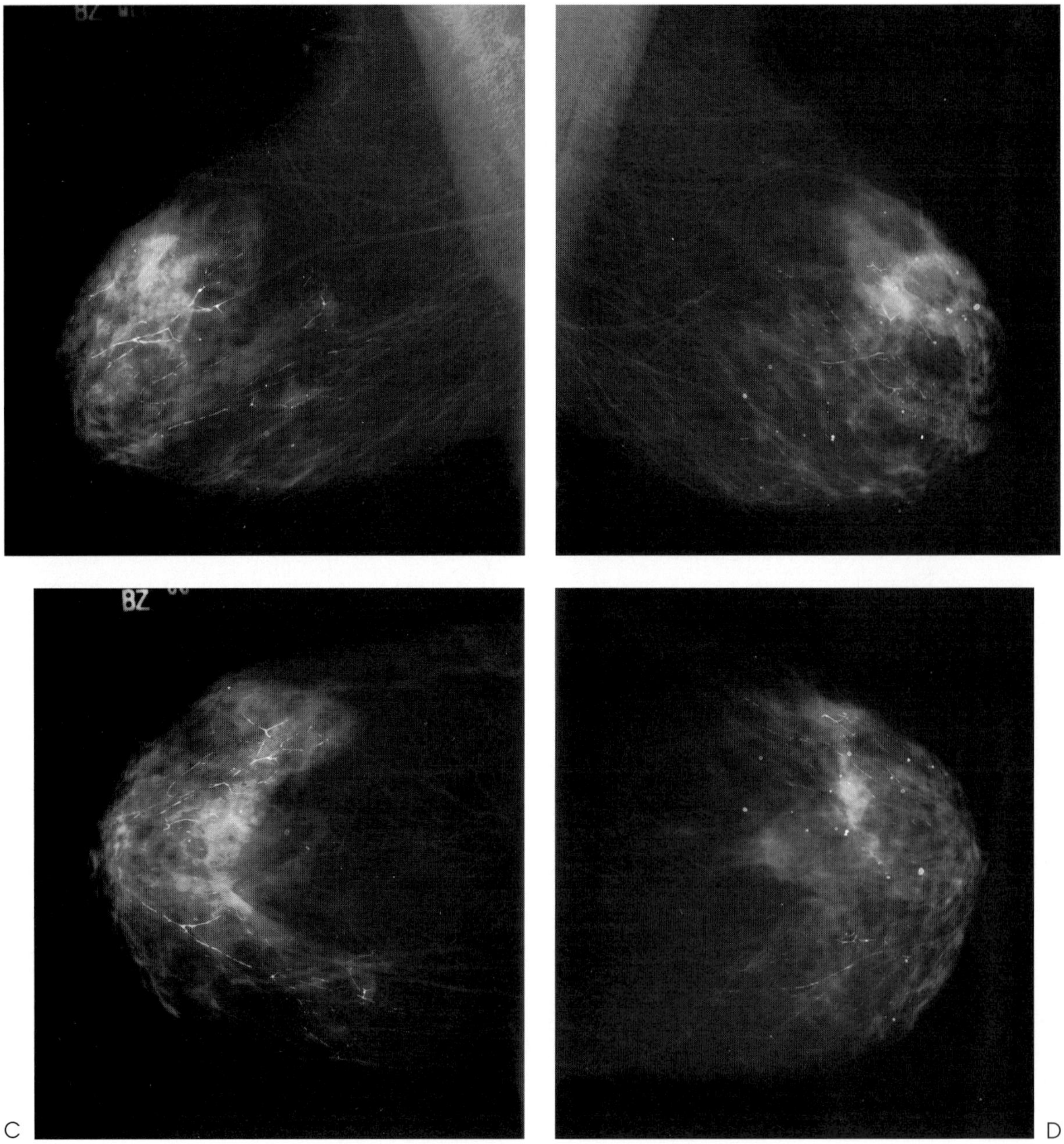

A B C D

Figure 64-1. *There are numerous, large, smooth-bordered, solid, linear calcifications in both breasts. The calcifications are oriented toward the nipple and some of the calcifications exhibit a branching pattern. (A). Right MLO mammogram. (B). Left MLO mammogram. (C). Right CC mammogram. (D). Left CC mammogram.*

Pathology

- plasma cell mastitis

Management

- BI-RADS Assessment Category 2, benign finding

Pearls and Pitfalls

Secretory calcifications result from plasma cell mastitis, which is a periductal inflammatory condition. Since the calcifications may be within the ducts, in the walls of the ducts, or adjacent to the walls, the calcification pattern parallels the ductal pattern. These large calcifications are oriented toward the nipple and may branch. This case illustrates the predominantly linear form of this condition.

Suggested Readings

1. Asch T, Fry C. Radiographic appearance of mammary duct ectasia with calcification. *N Engl J Med* 1962;266:86–87.
2. Kopans DB. Pathologic, mammographic, and sonographic correlation. In: Kopans DB. *Breast Imaging.* 2nd ed. Philadelphia: Lippincott-Raven; 1998:511–516.
3. Levitan LH, Witten DM, Harrison EG. Calcification in breast disease: mammographic-pathologic correlation. *Am J Roentgenol Radium Ther Nucl Med* 1964;92:29–39.

Case 65

Case History

A 50-year-old woman presents with right breast calcifications on her baseline mammogram.

Physical Examination

- normal exam

Mammogram

Calcifications (Fig. 65–1)

- type: milk of calcium
- distribution: grouped/clustered

A

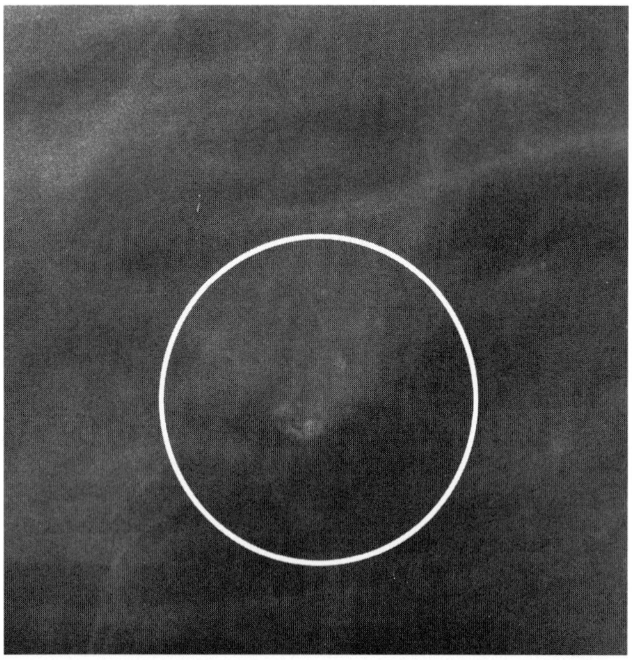

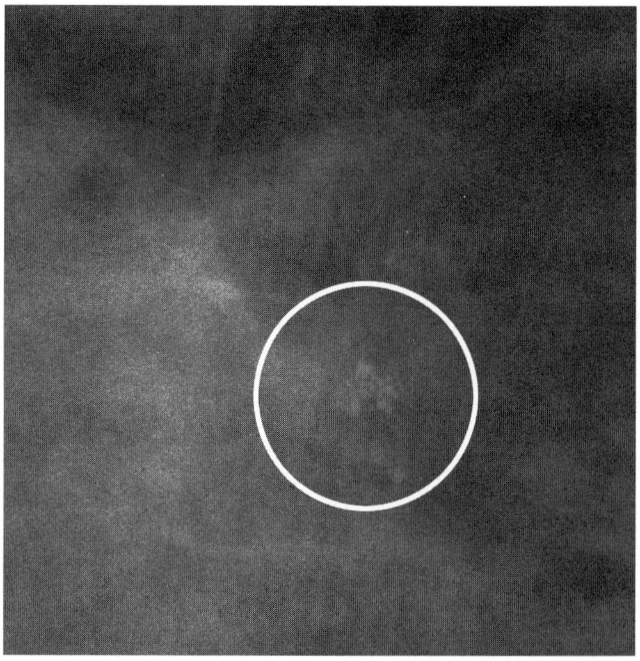

B

C

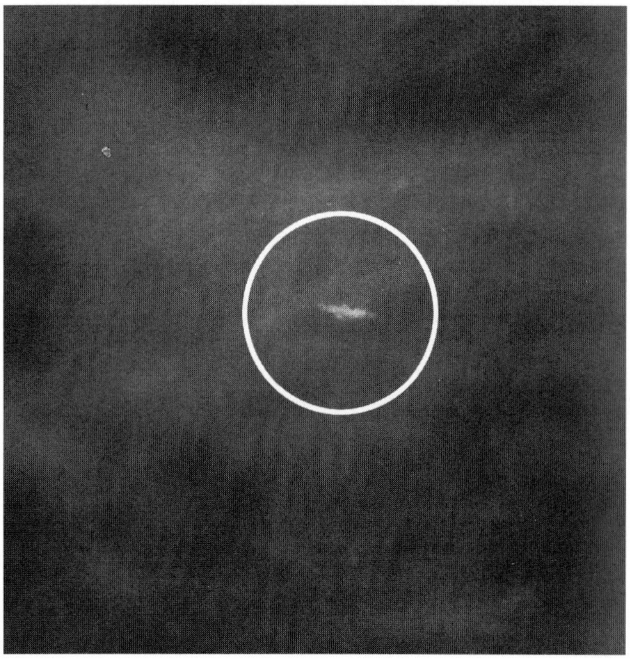

Figure 65–1. A cluster of calcifications is present in the right inner inferior quadrant (circled). On both the right MLO magnification view (A) and the right CC magnification view (B), the calcifications are predominantly round or oval. In the right ML magnification view (C), the calcifications produce a linear layer consistent with milk of calcium. (A). Right MLO magnification mammogram. (B). Right CC magnification mammogram. (C). Right ML magnification mammogram.

Ultrasound

Frequency

- 10 MHz (Fig. 65–2)

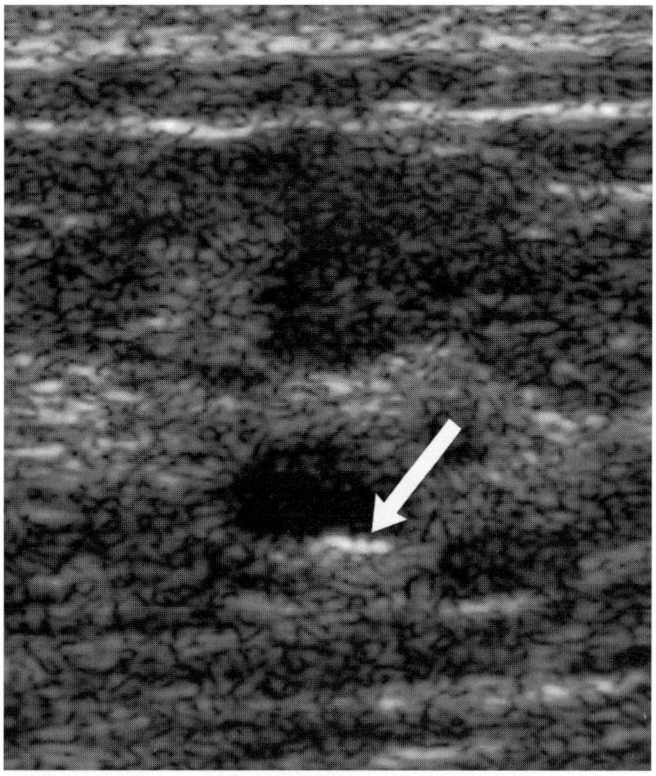

Figure 65–2. Right radial breast sonogram: The sonographic image of milk of calcium mirrors the mammographic image. In the area of the mammographic calcifications identified in Figure 65–1, sonographically, there is a cyst with hyperechoic material layering on the bottom of the cyst (arrow).

Pathology

- milk of calcium in microcysts

Management

- BI-RADS Assessment Category 2, benign finding

Pearls and Pitfalls

Milk of calcium calcifications are the result of microcysts with calcium suspended in liquid. The microcysts produce tiny, ill defined round calcifications on the craniocaudal view and linear or saucer-shaped layers of calcifications on the upright mediolateral view.

Suggested Readings

1. Homer MJ, Cooper AG, Spellman ER. Milk of calcium in breast microcysts: manifestation as a solitary focal disease. *AJR* 1988;150:789–790.
2. Pennes DR, Rebner M. Layering granular calcifications in macroscopic breast cysts. *Breast Dis* 1988;1:109–112.

Case 66

Case History

A 36-year-old woman presents for baseline mammogram.

Physical Examination

- bilateral numerous palpable lumps, sonographically shown to be cysts

Mammogram

Calcifications (Fig. 66–1)

- type: milk of calcium
- distribution: diffuse/scattered

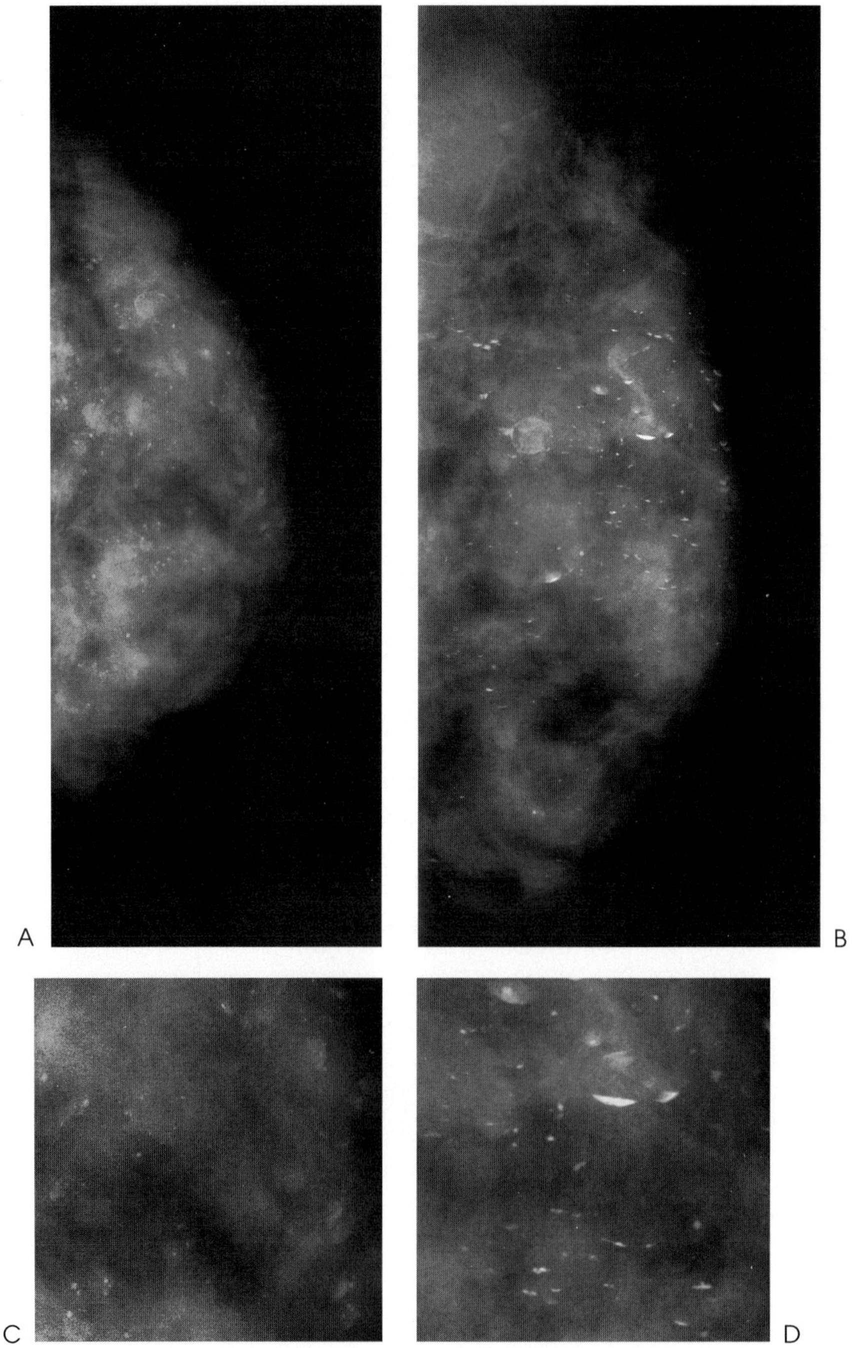

Figure 66–1. There are diffuse calcifications throughout the left breast. On the CC view (A), the calcifications are predominantly ill defined and round. However, in the ML view (B), the calcifications are linear or saucer-shaped. (A). Left CC mammogram. (B). Left ML mammogram. (C). Enlargement of left CC mammogram. (D). Enlargement of left MLO mammogram.

Ultrasound

Frequency

- 10 MHz (Fig. 66–2)

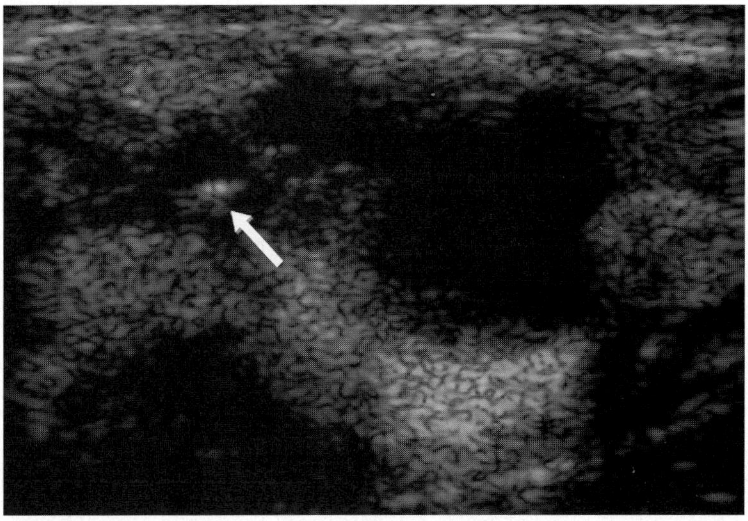

Figure 66–2. Left longitudinal left breast sonogram: Sonographically, this breast has numerous cysts. In some of these cysts, hyperechoic layering material is present (arrow). This hyperechoic material corresponds to the mammographic milk of calcium calcifications.

Pathology

- microcysts with milk of calcium

Management

- BI-RADS Assessment Category 2, benign finding

Pearls and Pitfalls

In this case, macrocysts have sonographic evidence of milk of calcium. Sonographically, milk of calcium may appear as a hyperechoic material that layers in the dependent portion of the cyst. Milk of calcium may also appear as punctate high-intensity foci, which are "piled up" within a cyst.

Suggested Readings

1. Sickles EA, Abele JS. Milk of calcium within tiny benign breast cysts. *Radiology* 1981;141:655–658.

Case 67

Case History

A 72-year-old woman presents for screening mammogram.

Physical Examination

- normal exam

Mammogram

Calcifications (Fig. 67–1)

- type: round
- distribution: diffuse/scattered

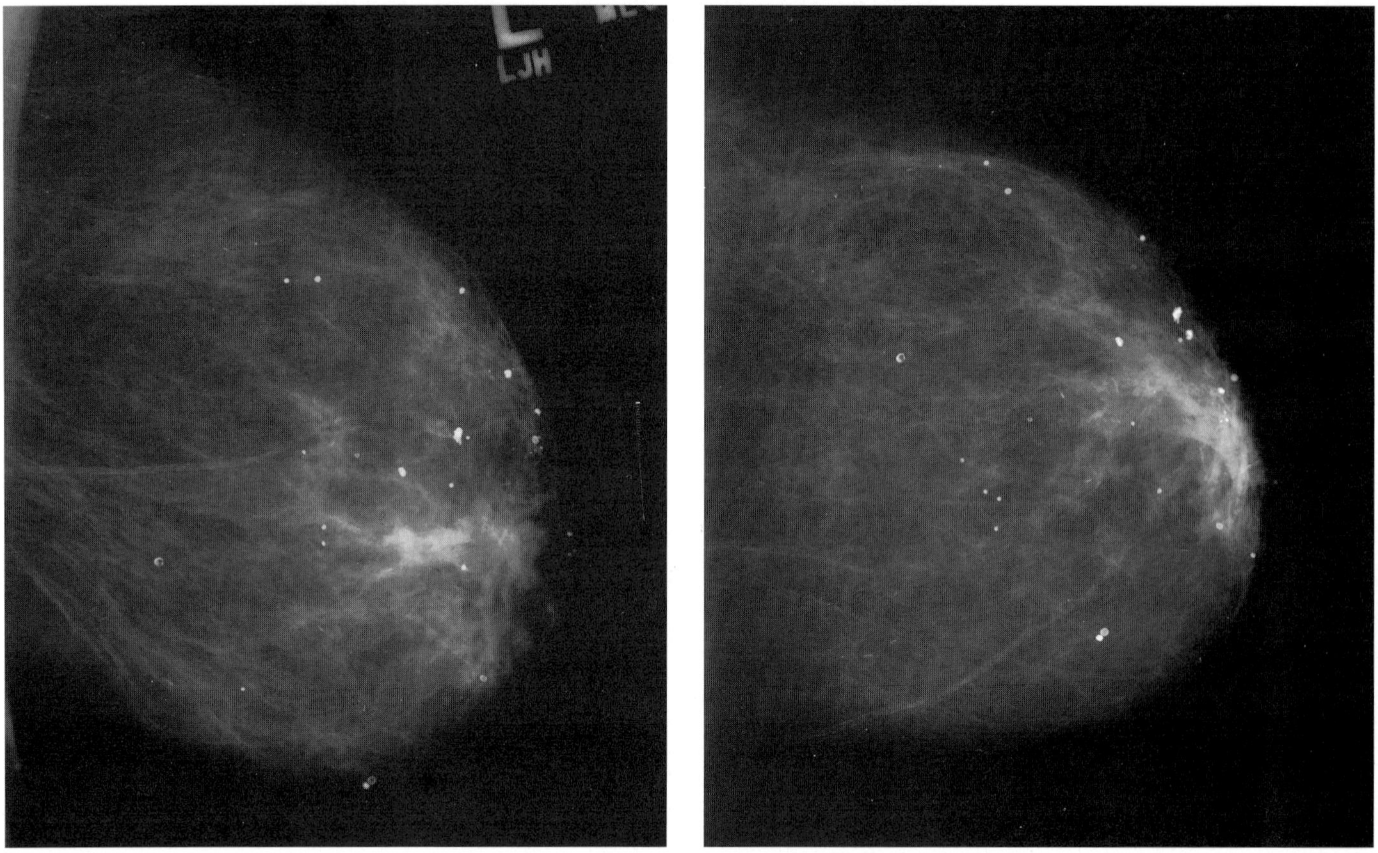

A B

Figure 67–1. In the left breast there are scattered round, oval calcifications. Some are solid and others have lucent centers. (A). Left MLO mammogram. (B). Left CC mammogram.

Pathology

- oil cyst

Management

- BI-RADS Assessment Category 2, benign finding

Pearls and Pitfalls

When the walls of an oil cyst calcifies, the calcification is round or oval and may either have a solid white or lucent center. Sometimes, only part of the wall is calcified so only a curvilinear calcification is evident.

Suggested Readings

1. Monsees BS. Evaluation of breast microcalcifications. *Radiol Clin North Am* 1995;33:1109–1121.

Case 68

Case History

A 30-year-old woman presents with a small lump near her nipple.

Physical Examination

- right breast: 5 mm palpable lump next to nipple
- left breast: normal exam

Mammogram

Calcifications (Fig. 68–1)

- type: lucent center
- distribution: diffuse/scattered

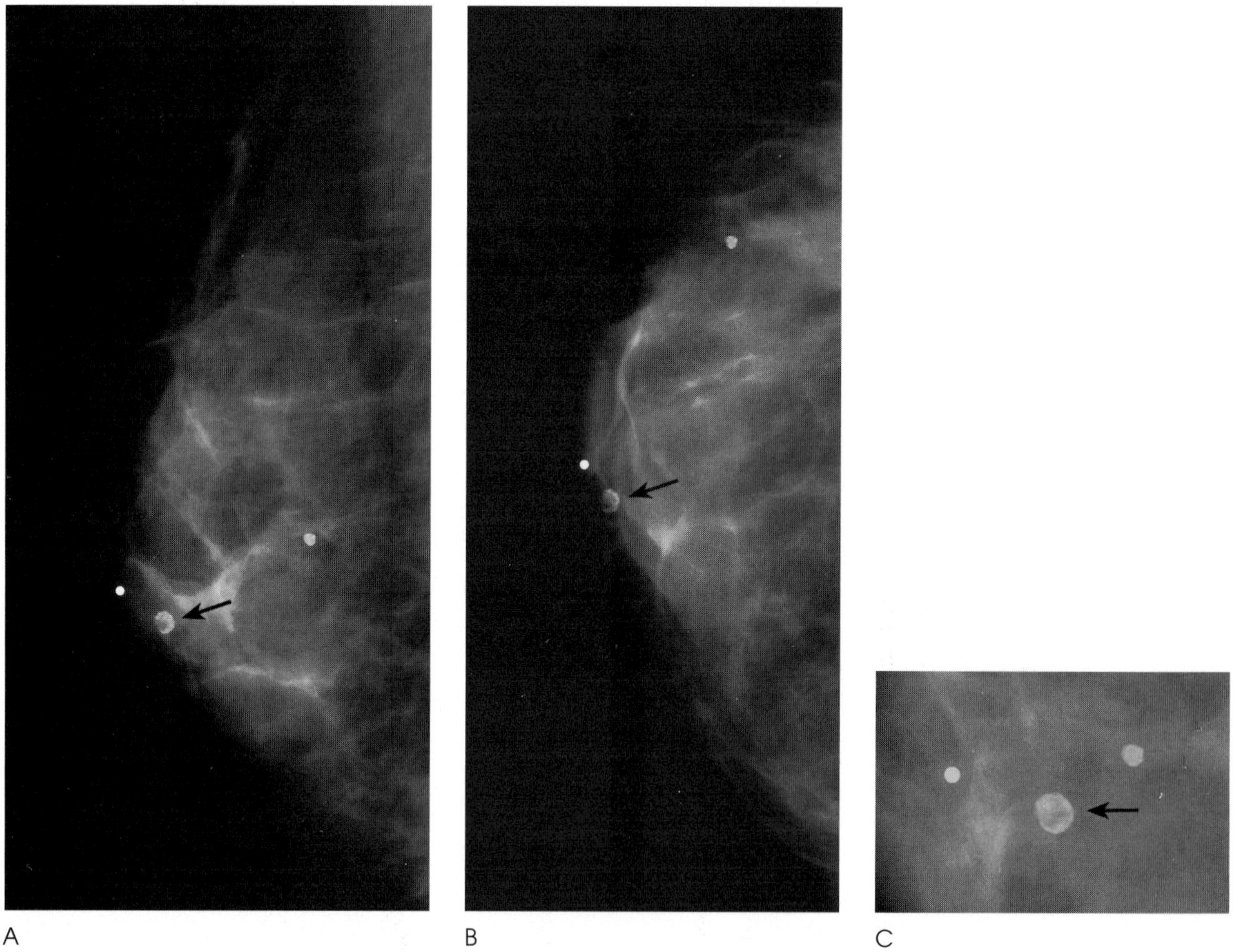

A B C

Figure 68–1. There are two large, round calcifications. A radiopaque marker is adjacent to the larger calcification (arrow) near the nipple. The marker indicates a palpable mass is present. (A). Right MLO mammogram. (B). Right CC mammogram. (C). Right MLO spot compression mammogram.

Ultrasound

Frequency

- 13 MHz (Fig. 68–2)

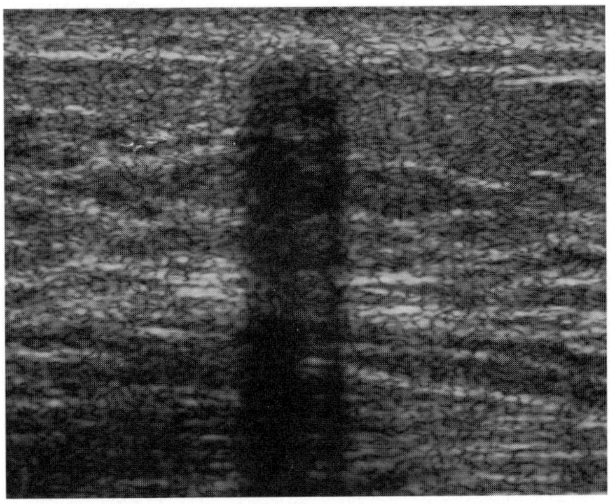

Figure 68–2. Right antiradial breast sonogram: The palpable lump near the nipple corresponds to a well-defined hypoechoic nodule with posterior acoustic shadowing. This sonographic nodule corresponds to the mammographic oil cyst.

Pathology

- oil cyst

Management

- BI-RADS Assessment Category 2, benign finding

Pearls and Pitfalls

1. The sonographic appearances of oil cysts include a well-defined heavily shadowing oval or round mass (as in this case) or a nonshadowing hypoechoic well-defined cystic mass.
2. The differential diagnosis of the sonographic mass in this case is either oil cyst or a simple cyst surrounded by a fibrotic capsule.

Suggested Readings

1. Carlisle LM, Trought WS, Peete W. Xeromammographic and ultrasonic diagnosis of a traumatic oil cyst. *AJR* 1978;130:1189–1190.

Case 69

Case History

A 45-year-old woman presents for screening mammogram. She had a benign breast biopsy several years ago.

Physical Examination

- right breast: faint scar at the 5:00 position near the areola
- left breast: normal exam

Mammogram

Calcifications (Fig. 69-1)

- type: lucent center
- distribution: regional

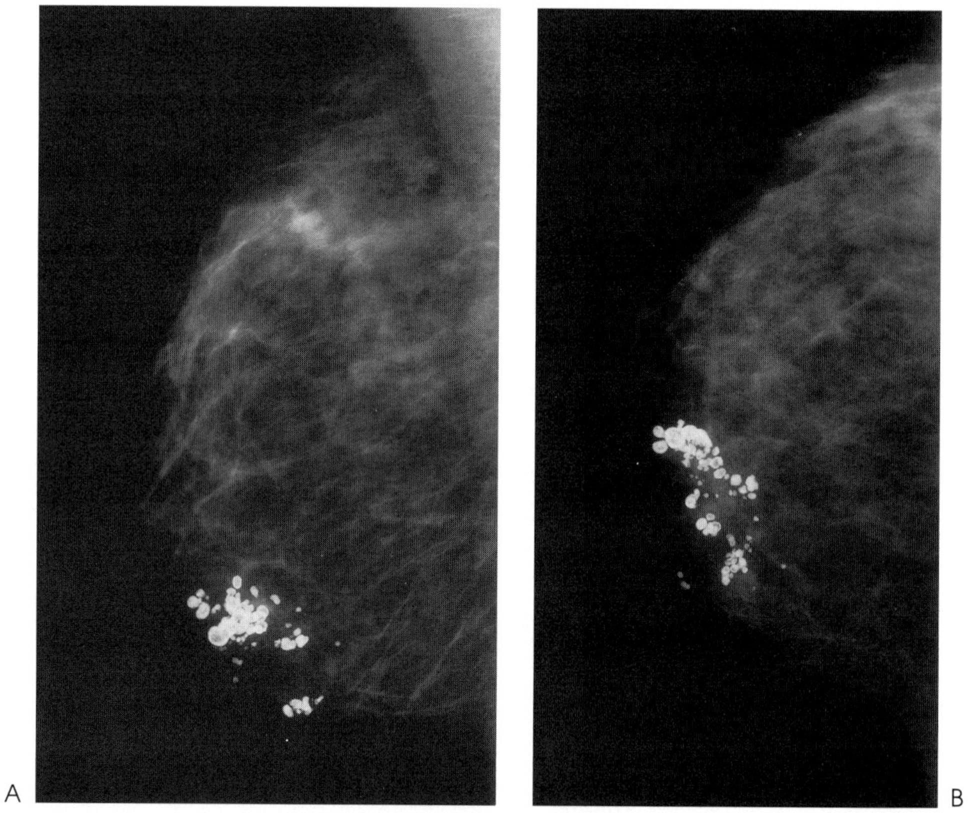

Figure 69-1. In the inferior medial right breast there are numerous round calcifications with lucent centers. (A). Right MLO mammogram. (B). Right CC mammogram.

Pathology

- oil cyst

Management

- BI-RADS Assessment Category 2, benign finding

Pearls and Pitfalls

1. Oil cysts result from fat necrosis. In this case, the fat necrosis was the consequence of a previous biopsy.
2. Oil cysts may be solitary, scattered, or regional as in this case. They may appear as solid round, eggshell, lucent centered, or partial rim calcifications. The lucent center form is the most common presentation.

Suggested Readings

1. Bassett LW, Gold RH, Cove HC. Mammographic spectrum of traumatic fat necrosis: the fallibility of "pathognomonic" signs of carcinoma. *AJR* 1978;130:119–122.
2. Jackson VP, Jahan R, Fu YS. Benign breast lesions. In: Bassett LW, Jackson VP, Jahan R, Fu YS, Gold RH, eds. *Diagnosis of Diseases of the Breast*. Philadelphia: WB Saunders Company; 1997:357–443.

Case 70

Case History

A 58-year-old woman arrives for screening mammogram.

Physical Examination

- normal exam

Mammogram

Calcifications (Fig. 70–1)

- type: eggshell/rim
- distribution: single

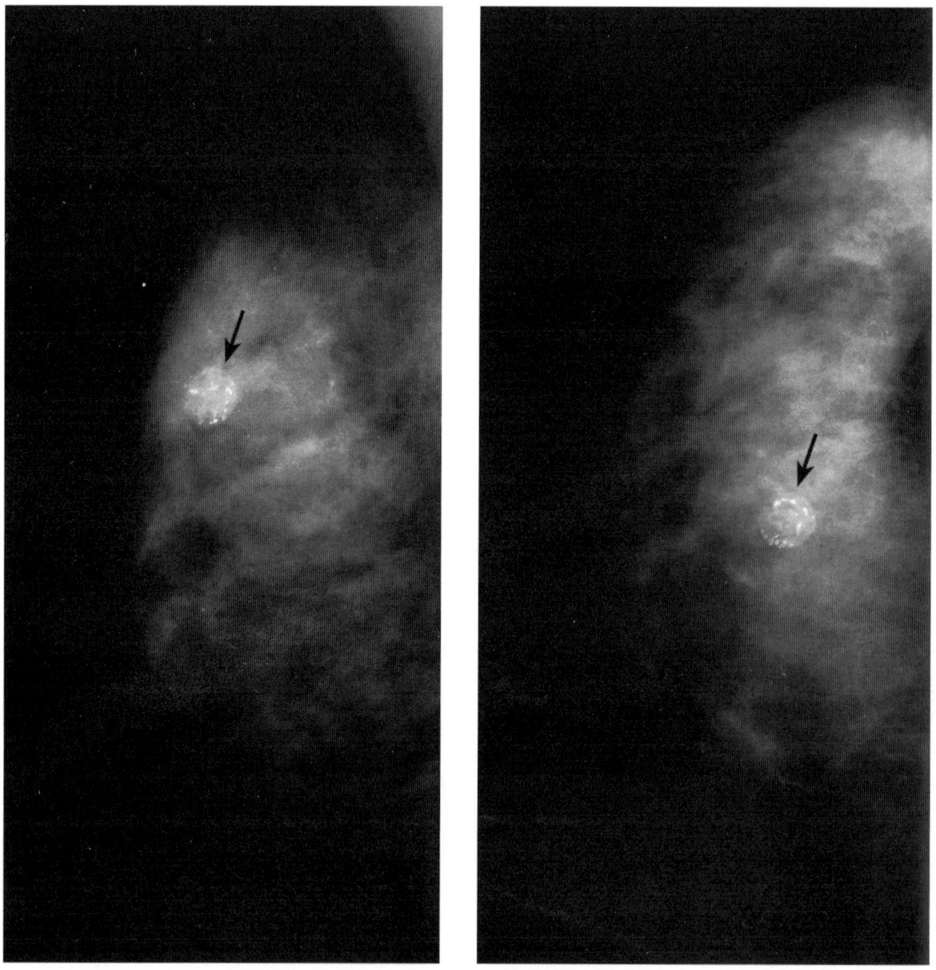

A B

Figure 70–1. *In the 12:00 position of the right breast (arrow) there is a spherical calcification characteristic of a calcified cyst. (A). Right MLO mammogram. (B). Right CC mammogram.*

Pathology

- cyst

Management

- BI-RADS Assessment Category 2, benign finding

Pearls and Pitfalls

Calcification of cyst walls appears as spherical or as a dense rim with a more lucent center (eggshell).

Suggested Readings

1. De Paredes ES. *Atlas of Film Screen Mammography.* 2nd ed. Baltimore: Williams & Wilkins; 1992:299–416.
2. Jackson VP, Jahan R, Fu YS. Benign breast lesions. In: Bassett LW, Jackson VP, Jahan R, Fu YS, Gold RH, eds. *Diagnosis of Diseases of the Breast.* Philadelphia: WB Saunders Company; 1997:357–443.

Case 71

Case History

An 84-year-old woman presents, status post-left lumptectomy and radiation therapy 3 years ago.

Physical Examination

- left breast: lumpectomy scar in the left upper outer quadrant
- right breast: normal exam

Mammogram

Calcifications (Fig. 71–1)

- type: eggshell/rim
- distribution: single

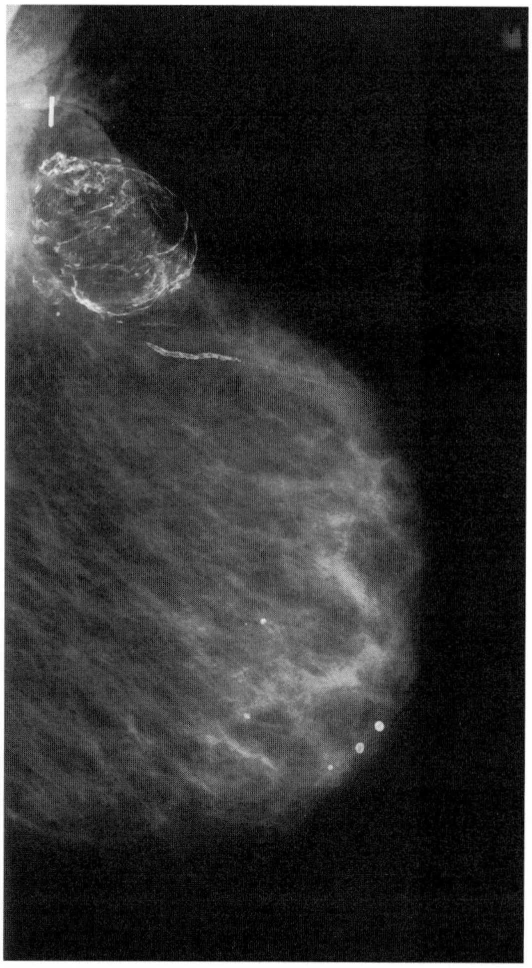
A

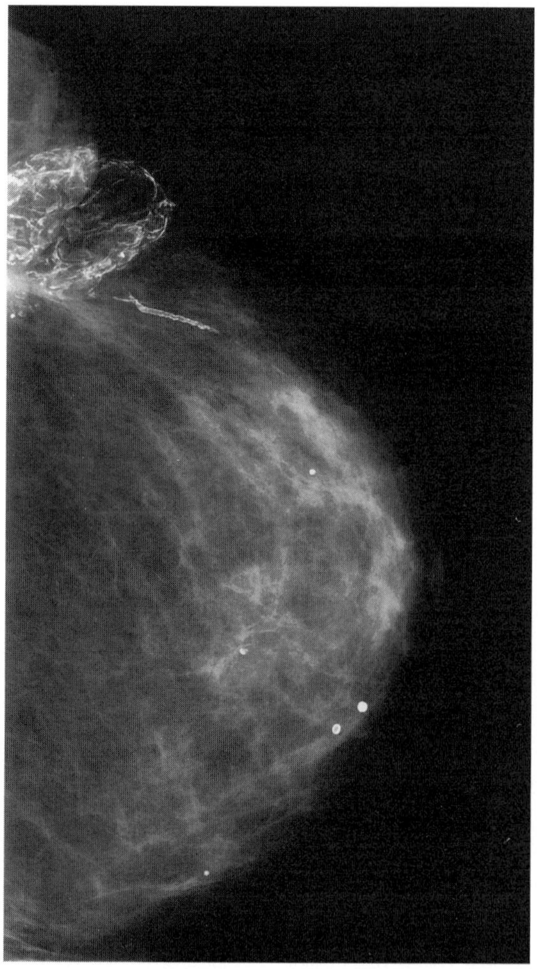
B

Figure 71–1. In the left upper outer quadrant there is a spherical rim calcification in the area of the patient's lumpectomy site. (A). Left MLO mammogram. (B). Left exaggerated CC mammogram.

Pathology

- fat necrosis

Management

- BI-RADS Assessment Category 2, benign finding

Pearls and Pitfalls

Calcifications from fat necrosis may appear as round lucent center, coarse irregular dystrophic, thin rim, or eggshell calcifications.

Suggested Readings

1. Bassett LW, Gold RH, Cove HC. Mammographic spectrum of traumatic fat necrosis: the fallibility of "pathognomonic" signs of carcinoma. *AJR* 1978;130:119–122.
2. Bassett LW, Gold RH, Mirra JM. Noneoplastic breast calcifications in lipid cysts: development after excision and primary irradiation. *AJR* 1982;138:335–338.

Case 72

Case History

A 69-year-old woman presents for screening mammogram.

Physical Examination

- normal exam

Mammogram

Calcifications (Figs. 72-1 and 72-2)

- type: coarse/popcorn
- distribution: single

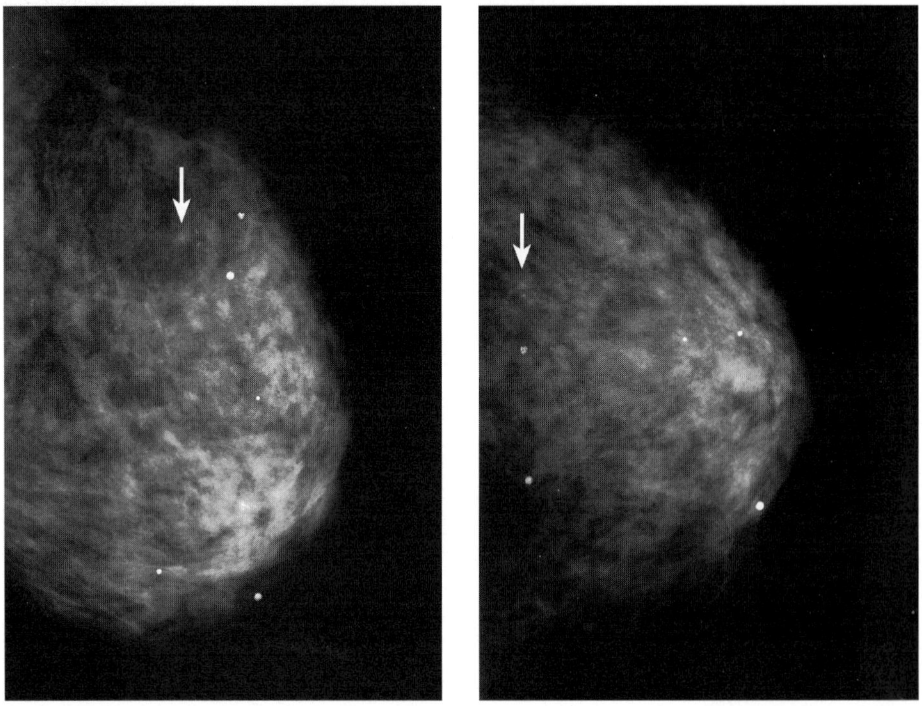

Figure 72-1. Faint coarse calcifications are present in the upper outer breast (arrow). (A). Left MLO mammogram. (B). Left CC mammogram.

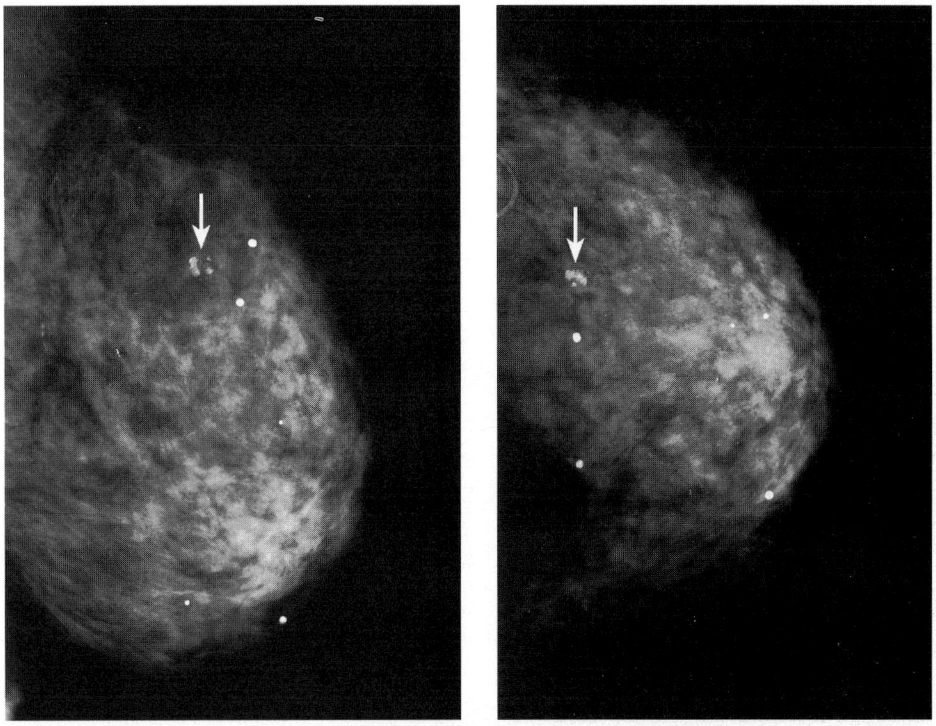

A B

Figure 72–2. Exam performed 3 years after Figure 72–1. The calcifications (arrow) have enlarged and are now characteristic of an involuting fibroadenoma. (A). Left MLO mammogram. (B). Left CC mammogram.

Pathology

- fibroadenoma

Management

- BI-RADS Assessment Category 2, benign finding

Pearls and Pitfalls

Differential diagnosis of large coarse calcifications includes fibroadenoma, fat necrosis, and calcium deposition from hypercalcemia (i.e., hyperparathyroidism, renal failure).

Suggested Readings

1. Gershon-Cohen J, Ingleby H. Roentgenography of fibroadenoma of the breast. *Radiology* 1952;59:77 86.
2. Han SY, Witten DM. Diffuse calcification of the breast in chronic renal failure. *AJR* 1977;129:341–342.

Case 73

Case History

A 43-year-old woman presents, status 2 years post–right lumpectomy for breast cancer, now with left breast lump.

Physical Examination

- right breast: surgical scar in the inferior right breast
- left breast: 1 cm lump near the left nipple

Mammogram

Calcifications (Fig. 73–1)

- type: coarse/popcorn
- distribution: single

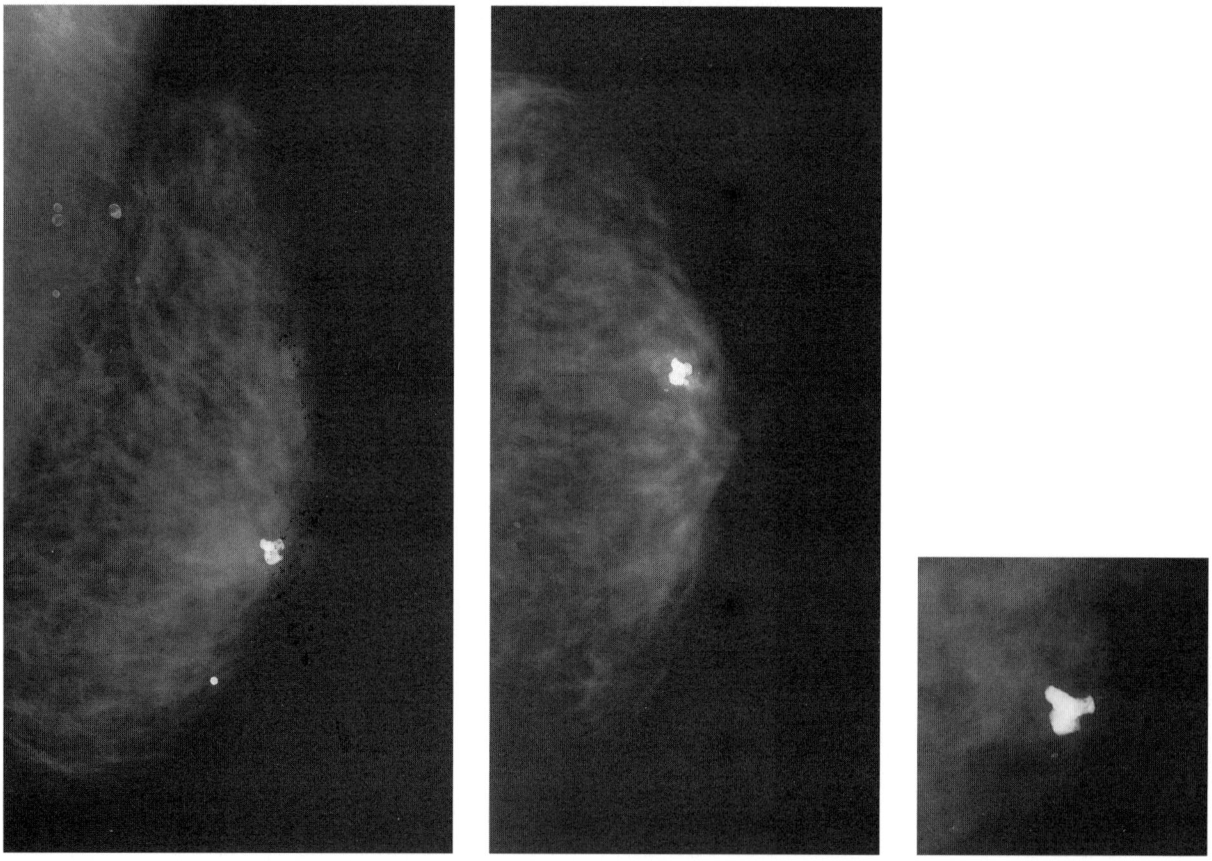

A B C

Figure 73–1. *In the subareolar region of the left breast there is a large, coarse, lobulated calcification characteristic of a fibroadenoma. (A). Left MLO mammogram. (B). Left CC mammogram. (C). Left MLO spot magnification mammogram.*

Ultrasound

Frequency

- 13 MHz

Mass

- margin: ill defined
- echogenicity: hypoechoic
- retrotumoral acoustic appearance: posterior shadowing distal to mass
- shape: ellipsoid (Fig. 73–2)

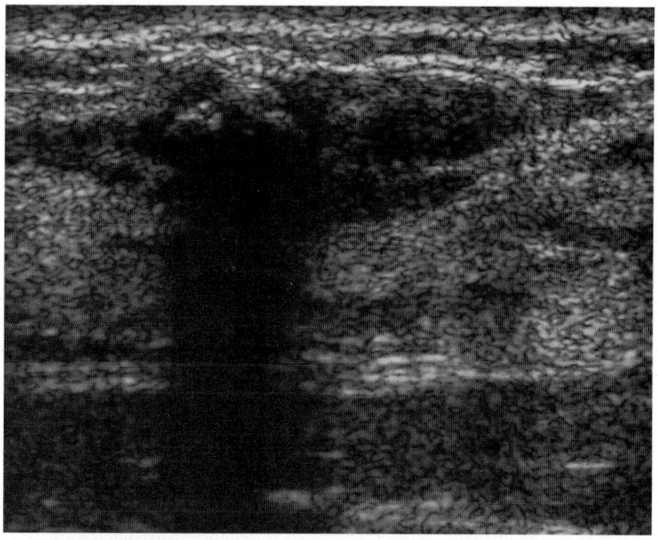

Figure 73–2. Antiradial left breast sonogram: Sonographic appearance of the palpable lump in the subareolar region demonstrates an ill-defined hypoechoic solid mass with a large calcification. The calcification is associated with shadowing. This calcification corresponds to the calcification mammographically identified in Figure 73–1.

Other Modalities

Findings

Although the magnetic resonance imaging (MRI) mass has ill-defined borders, this subareolar mass exhibits relatively slow enhancement that supports the mammographic evidence that the mass is a fibroadenoma. A low-intensity punctate mass within the enhancing mass focus corresponds to the mammographic calcification (Figs. 73-3 and 73-4).

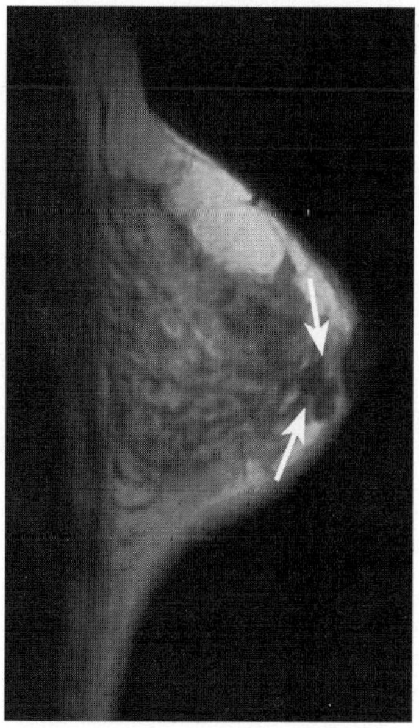

Figure 73–3. Left longitudinal T2-weighted breast MRI: With this technique the mass presents as a low-intensity lobulated mass (arrows).

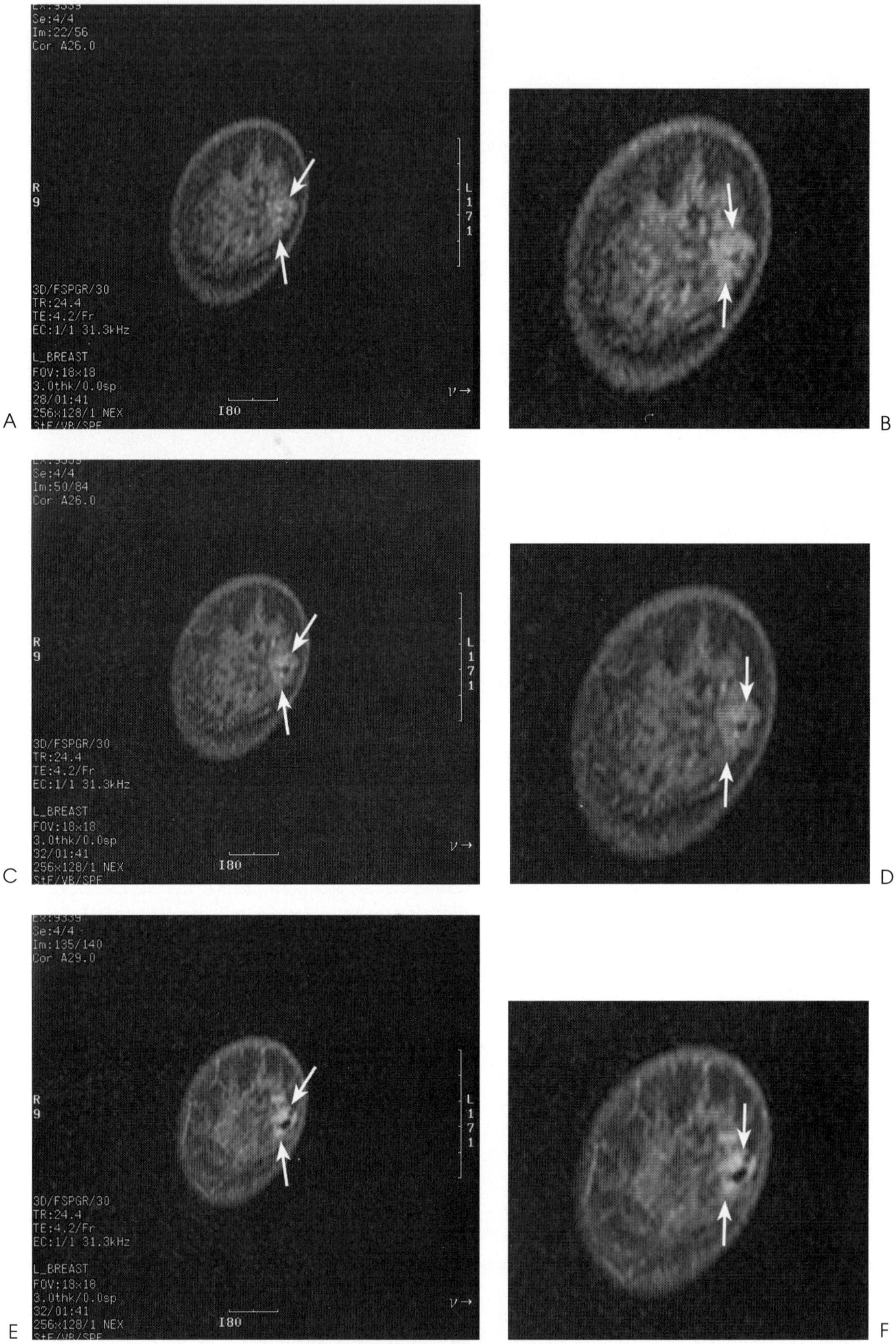

Figure 73–4. These coronal images before (A) and after (B) gadolinium injection demonstrate that the mass (arrows) identified in the sonogram (Fig. 73–2) shows no enhancement 1 minute (B) after injection. The mass (arrows) does not enhance until 6 minutes after injection (C). (A). Left coronal three-dimensional (3-D) volume gradient breast MRI before gadolinium injection. (B). Left coronal dynamic bolus 3-D volume gradient breast MRI, 1 minute after gadolinium injection. (C). Left coronal dynamic bolus 3-D volume gradient breast MRI, 6 minutes after gadolinium injection.

Pathology

- fibroadenoma

Management

- BI-RADS Assessment Category 2, benign finding

Pearls and Pitfalls

The classic mammographic appearance of fibroadenoma calcification is the key evidence for management. Once the palpable mass could be linked to the mammographic calcification, one may be comfortable that the mass is benign. Furthermore, the MRI contrast enhancement pattern supports this benign conclusion. Sonographically, fibroadenomas have a wide variety of appearances. Therefore, an indeterminate appearance sonographically should not deter one from making the diagnosis of fibroadenoma when there is excellent mammographic evidence.

Suggested Readings

1. Bassett LW. Mammographic analysis of calcifications. *Radiol Clin North Am* 1992;30:93–105.
2. De Paredes ES. *Atlas of Film Screen Mammography*. 2nd ed. Baltimore: Williams & Wilkins; 1992:299–416.
3. Gershon-Cohen J, Ingleby H. Roentgenography of fibroadenoma of the breast. *Radiology* 1952;59:77–87.

Case 74

Case History

An 84-year-old woman presents for screening mammogram.

Physical Examination

- scars in both breasts from previous reduction mammoplasties

Mammogram

Calcifications (Fig. 74–1)

- type: dystrophic
- distribution: diffuse/scattered

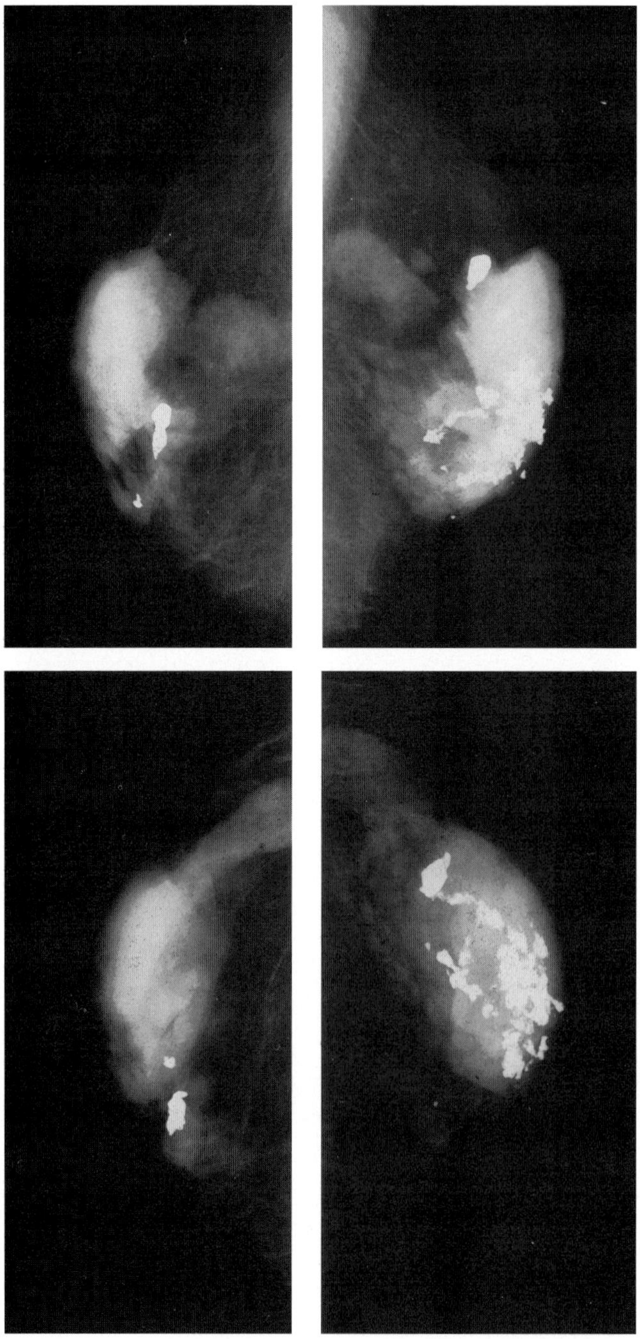

A B C D

Figure 74–1. In both breasts there are large, coarse, dystrophic calcifications that have resulted from this patient's bilateral reduction mammoplasties. (A). Right MLO mammogram. (B). Left MLO mammogram. (C). Right CC mammogram. (D). Left CC mammogram.

Pathology

- fat necrosis

Management

- BI-RADS Assessment Category 2, benign finding

Pearls and Pitfalls

Fat necrosis may be associated with either round (oil cyst), eggshell/rim, or large irregular calcifications. This case is an example of the last type of calcification.

Suggested Readings

1. Sickles EA. Breast calcifications: mammographic evaluation. *Radiology* 1986;160:289–293.

Case 75

Case History

A 79-year-old woman presents with right breast calcifications.

Physical Examination

- normal exam

Mammogram

Calcifications (Figs. 75-1 and 75-2)

- type: dystrophic
- distribution: grouped/clustered

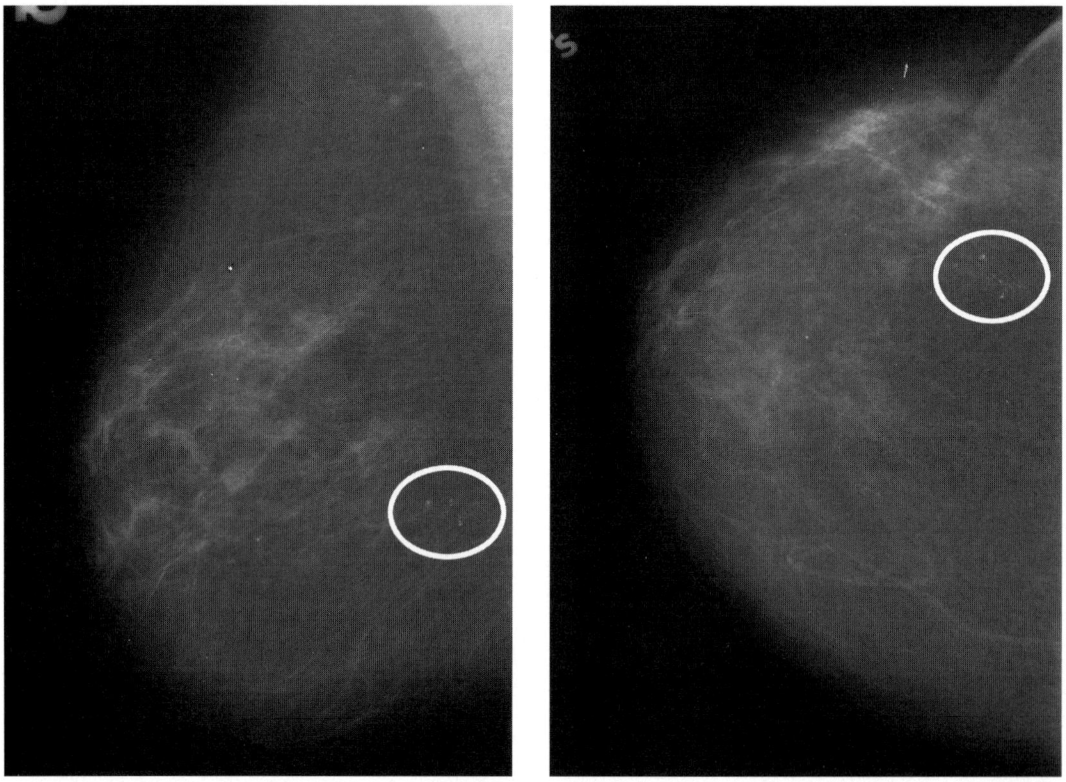
A B

Figure 75-1. In the right outer breast there is a cluster of calcifications (circled) that was biopsied after this examination. (A). Right MLO mammogram. (B). Right CC mammogram.

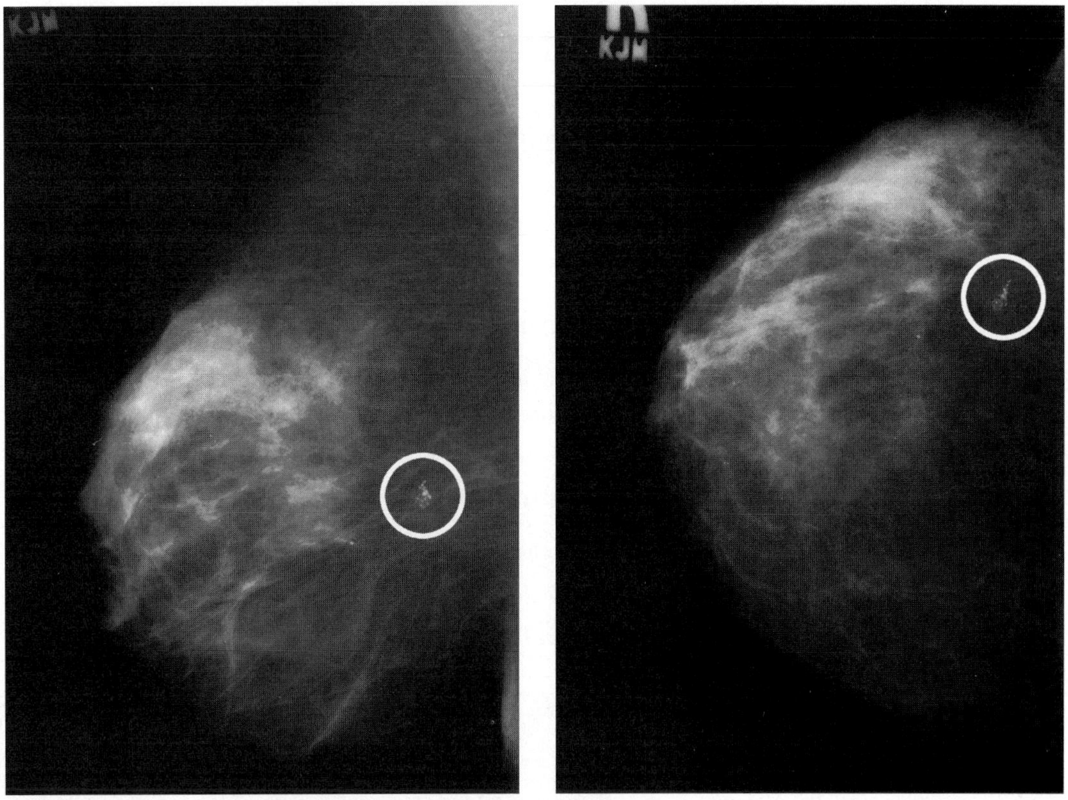

A B

Figure 75–2. Five years after the mammographic examination shown in Figure 75–1, the calcifications (circled) have become large and coarse. (A). Right MLO mammogram. (B). Right CC mammogram.

Pathology

- scar

Management

- BI-RADS Assessment Category 2, benign finding

Pearls and Pitfalls

Early dystrophic scar calcifications may be difficult to differentiate from ductal carcinoma in situ (DCIS) or invasive malignancy. However, when the calcifications are large and coarse, one can confidently consider them benign.

Suggested Readings

1. Bassett LW. Mammographic analysis of calcifications. *Radiol Clin North Am* 1992;30:93–105.
2. De Paredes ES. *Atlas of Film Screen Mammography*. 2nd ed. Baltimore: Williams & Wilkins; 1992:299–416.

Case 76

Case History

A 70-year old-woman, who is 9 years status post–right lumpectomy and radiation therapy, presents with increasing calcifications in the lumpectomy site.

Physical Examination

- right breast: well-healed right upper breast scar; no new masses
- left breast: normal exam

Mammogram

Calcifications (Fig. 76–1)

- type: dystrophic
- distribution: grouped/clustered

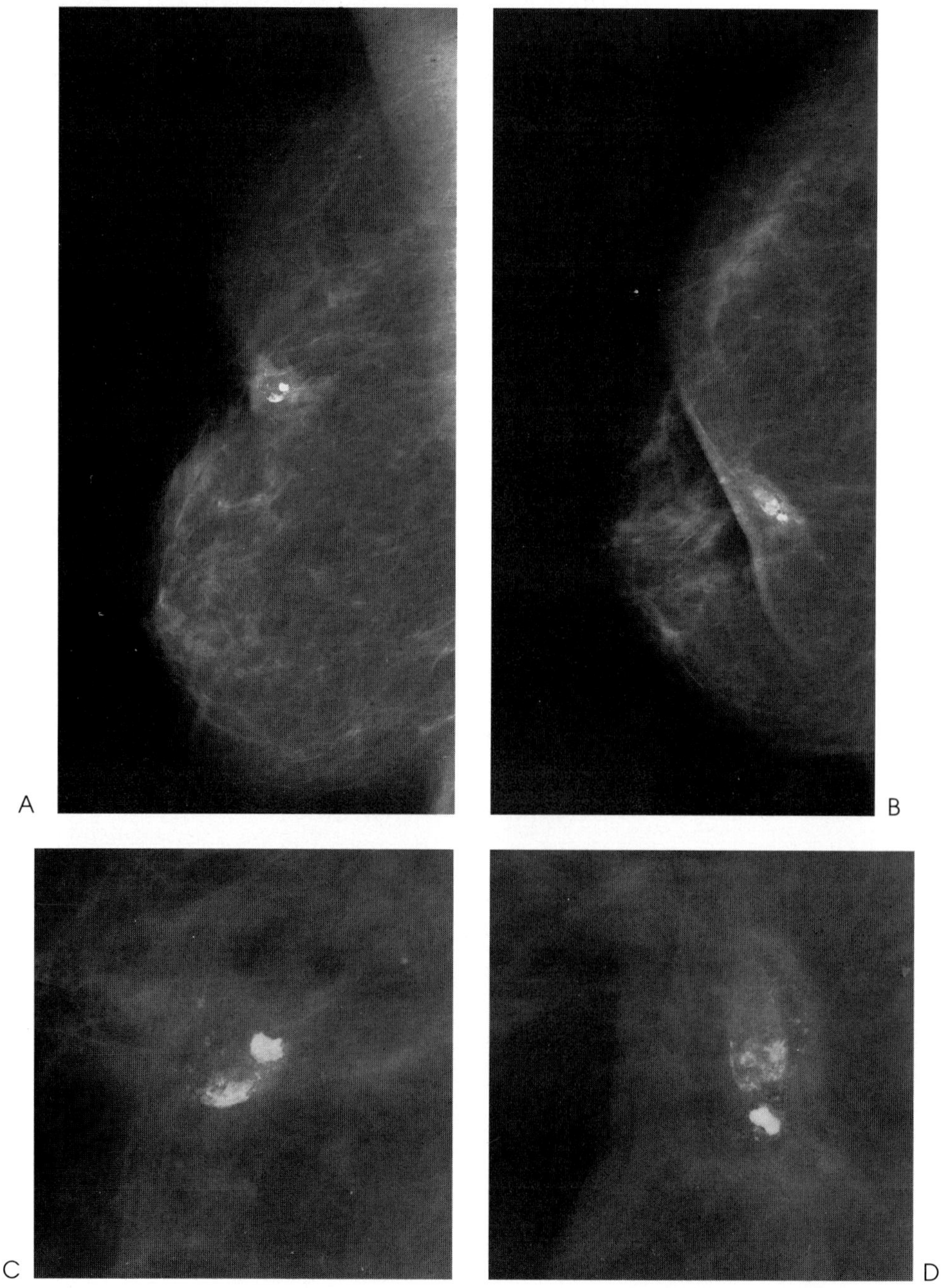

Figure 76–1. In the 12:00 position of the right breast there is a scar associated with calcifications from the patient's previous lumpectomy. There has been an increase in the number of calcifications since the previous year. (A). Right MLO mammogram. (B). Right CC mammogram. (C). Right MLO magnification mammogram. (D). Right CC magnification mammogram.

Ultrasound

Frequency

- 10 MHz

Mass

- margin: ill defined
- echogenicity: hypoechoic
- retrotumoral acoustic appearance: severe shadowing, mass completely obscured
- shape: irregular (Fig. 76–2)

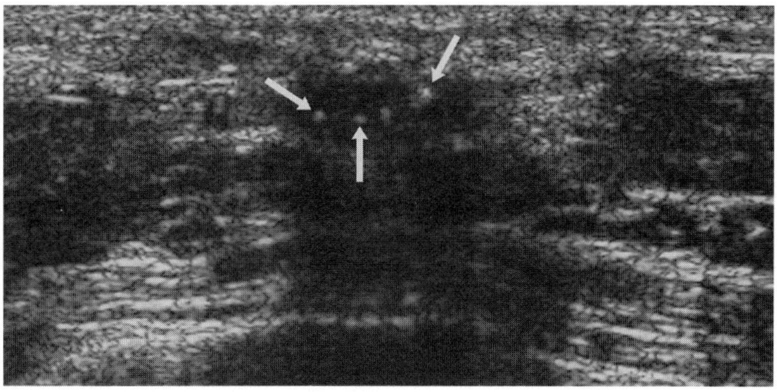

Figure 76–2. Right antiradial breast sonogram: In area of the lumpectomy scar, the sonographic findings include architectural distortion of the superficial tissue lines, calcifications (arrows), and an irregular hypoechoic mass with posterior acoustic shadowing (see Color Plate 76–2).

Pathology

- scar

Management

- BI-RADS Assessment Category 2, benign finding

Pearls and Pitfalls

In this case the sonographic findings confuse the management. Because there is a faint density associated with the scar on the mammogram, one should anticipate that the sonogram will demonstrate a mass and that it would be difficult to differentiate fibrosis from recurrent neoplasm. Therefore, if one is concerned about the increasing calcifications, then the management should be determined with the mammographic appearance of the calcifications.

Suggested Readings

1. Dershaw DD. Evaluation of the breast undergoing lumpectomy and radiation therapy. *Radiol Clin North Am* 1995;33:1147–1160.
2. Dershaw DD, Shank B, Reisinger S. Mammographic findings after breast cancer treatment with local excision and definitive irradiation. *Radiology* 1987;164:455–461.

Case 77

Case History

A 43-year-old woman, status postchemotherapy for aplastic anemia, presents for screening mammogram.

Physical Examination

- normal exam

Mammogram

Mass

- margin: circumscribed
- shape: square
- density: high

Calcifications (Fig. 77–1)

- type: dystrophic
- distribution: single

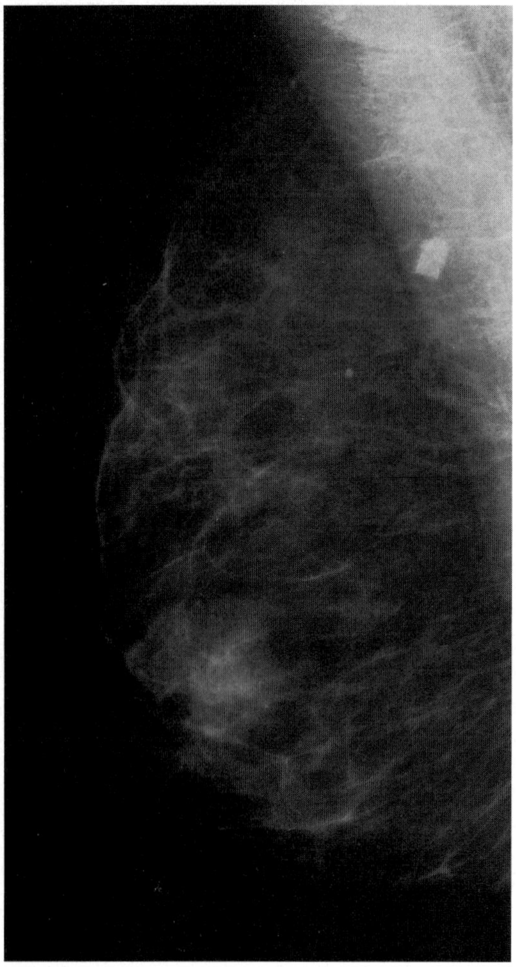

A

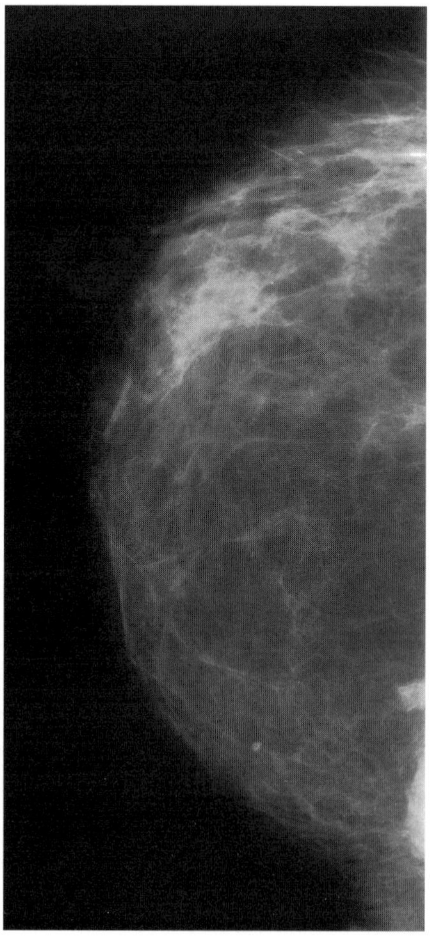

B

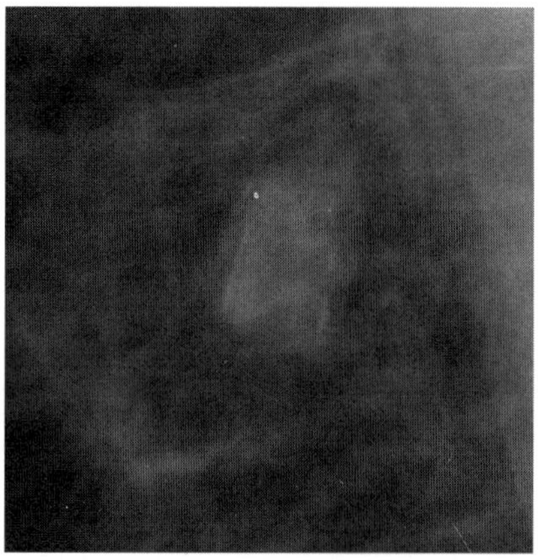

C

Figure 77–1. In the upper medial breast there is a well-defined square density with associated coarse dystrophic calcifications. (A). Right MLO mammogram. (B). Right exaggerated medial CC mammogram. (C). Right MLO magnification mammogram.

Pathology

- foreign body reaction

Management

- BI-RADS Assessment Category 2, benign finding

Pearls and Pitfalls

This is an example of a foreign body causing breast calcification.The density identified in Figure 77–1 is a Hickman catheter hub. The patient had been treated with IV chemotherapy through a Hickman catheter for aplastic anemia. The hub was inadvertently retained in the chest after the Hickman catheter was removed. Other foreign bodies such as sutures will produce irregular breast calcifications.

Suggested Readings

1. Beyer GA, Thorsen MK, Shaffer KA, et al. Mammographic appearance of the retained Dacron cuff of a Hickman catheter. *AJR* 1990;155:1203–1204.
2. Davis SP, Stomper PC, Weidner N, et al. Suture calcification mimicking recurrence in the irradiated breast: a potential pitfall in mammographic evaluation. *Radiology* 1989;172:247–248.
3. Jackson VP, Jahan R, Fu YS. Benign breast lesions. In: Bassett LW, Jackson VP, Jahan R, Fu YS, Gold RH, eds. *Diagnosis of Diseases of the Breast.* Philadelphia: WB Saunders Company; 1997:357–443.

Case 78

Case History

A 41-year-old woman presents for baseline screening mammogram.

Physical Examination

- normal exam

Mammogram

Calcifications (Fig. 78–1)

- type: skin calcifications
- distribution: scattered, difuse

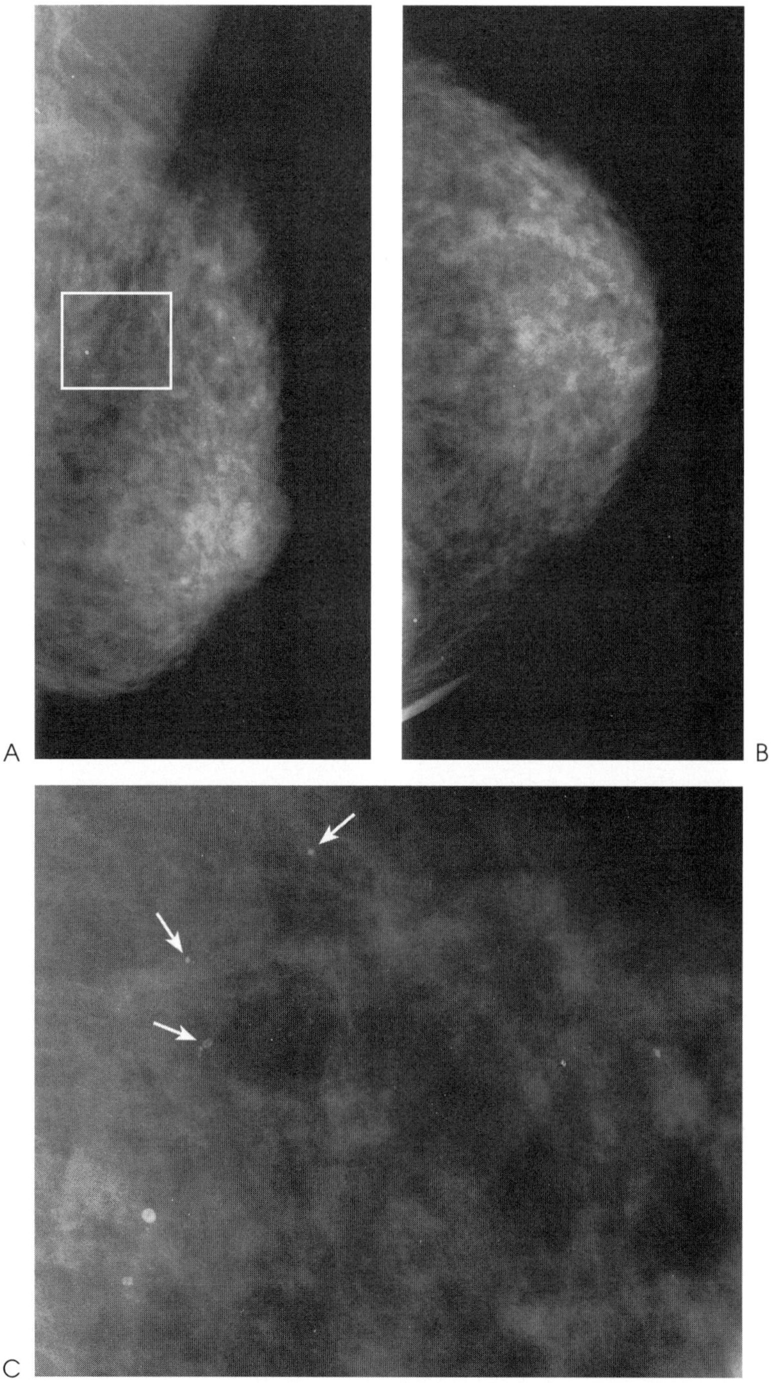

Figure 78–1. In the upper medial breast there are multiple scattered round calcifications. Some calcifications have lucent centers. (A). Left MLO mammogram. (B). Left CC mammogram. (C). Left MLO magnification mammogram.

Pathology

- skin calcifications

Management

- BI-RADS Assessment Category 2, benign finding

Pearls and Pitfalls

1. Skin calcifications are commonly in the medial side of the breast. They are well-defined, round or polygonal in shape, with lucent centers. If they are superimposed upon the breast parenchyma, they may be mistaken for intraparenchymal calcifications. Tangential views will distinguish skin calcifications from intraparenchymal ones.
2. These calcifications are within the sebaceous glands and may be the result of chronic folliculitis.

Suggested Readings

1. Kopans DB, Meyer JE, Homer MJ, et al. Dermal deposits mistaken for breast calcifications. *Radiology* 1983;149:592–594.

Case 79

Case History

A 49-year-old woman presents with new left subareolar calcifications on her screening mammogram.

Physical Examination

- normal exam

Mammogram

Calcifications (Figs. 79–1 and 79–2)

- type: punctate
- distribution: regional

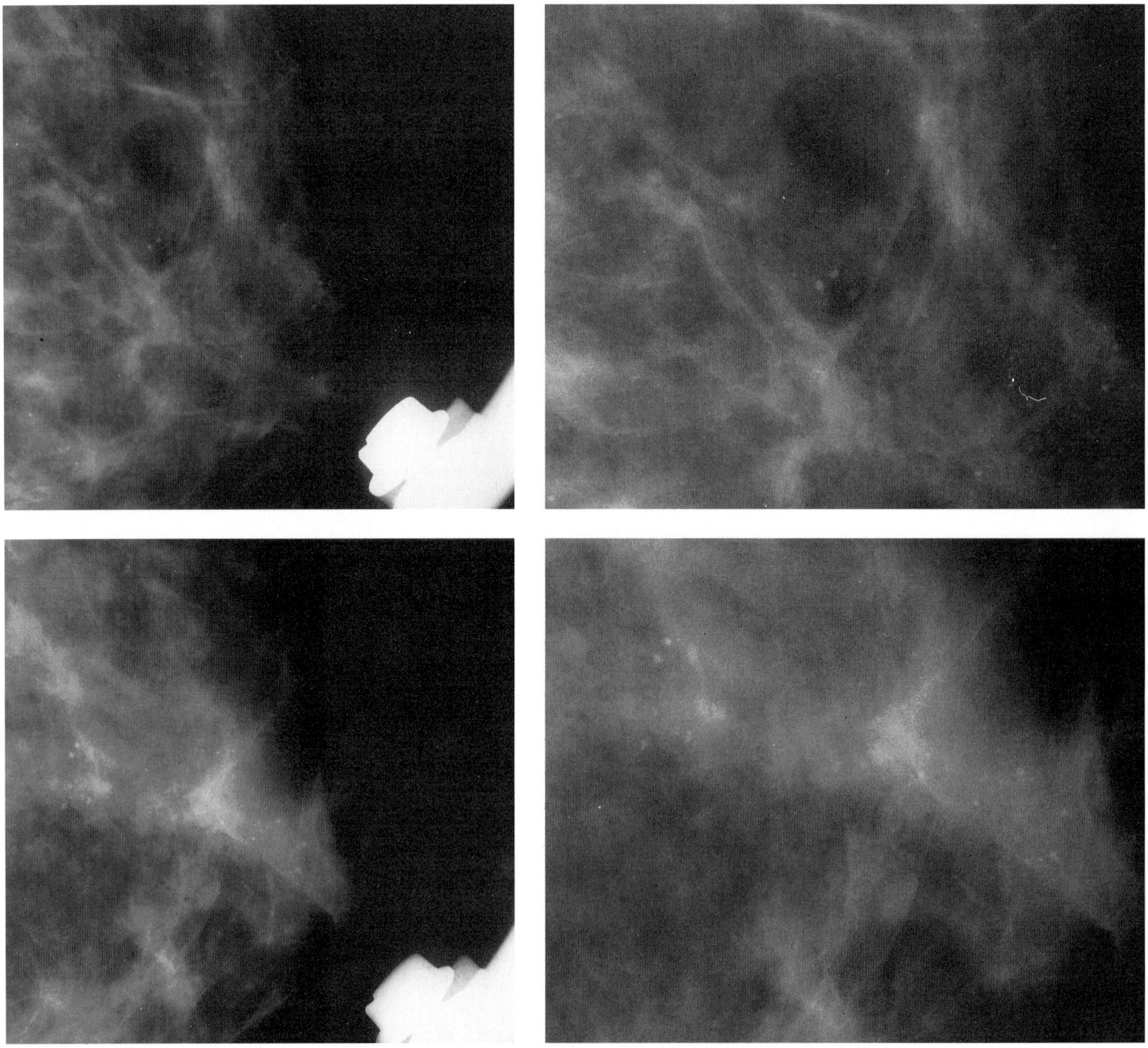

A

B

Figure 79–1. *Numerous round punctate calcifications are present in the subareolar region. (A). Left MLO magnification mammogram. (B). Left CC magnification mammogram.*

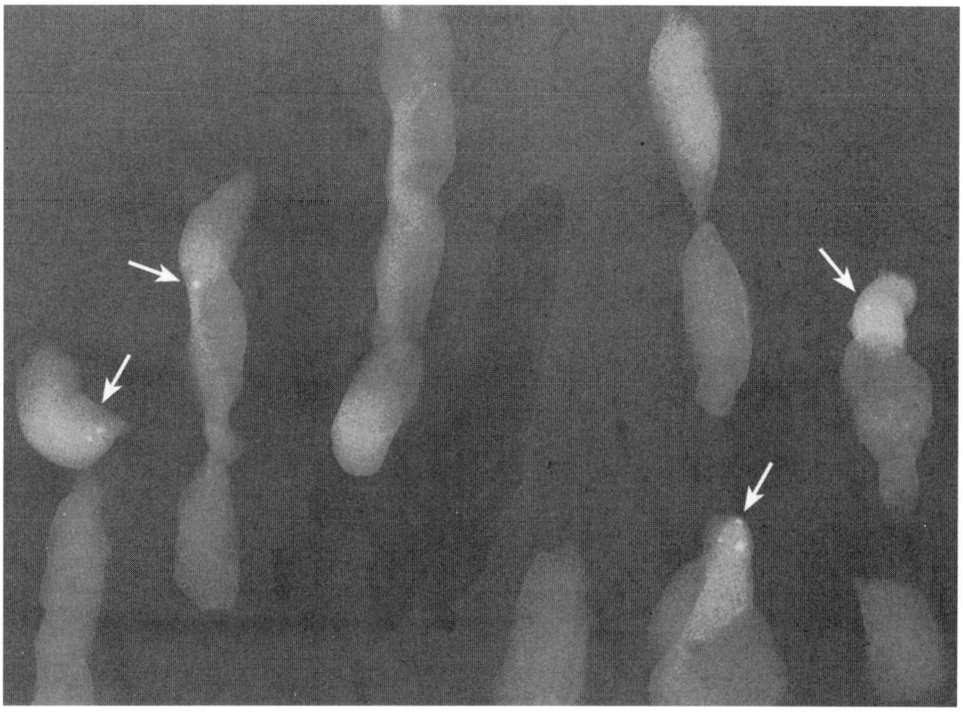

Figure 79–2. Specimen needle core biopsy radiograph: The punctate, round calcifications (arrows) are easily identified within this biopsy specimen.

Ultrasound

Frequency

- 10 to 13 MHz (Figs. 79–3 and 79–4)

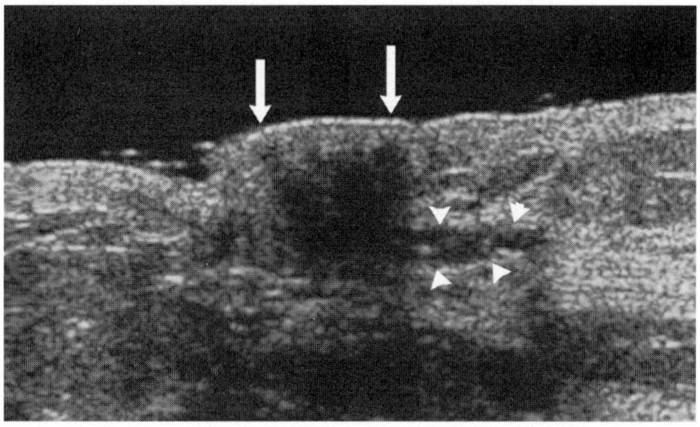

Figure 79–3. Left radial breast sonogram: Under the nipple (large arrows) there were several main ducts (arrowheads).

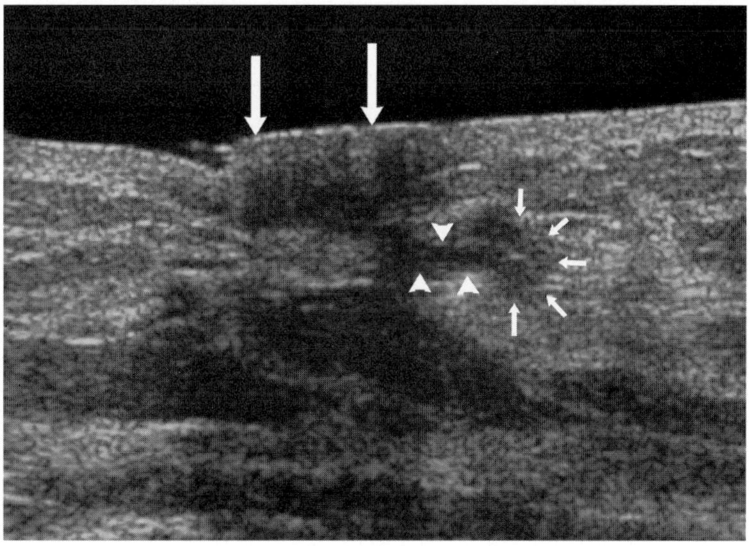

Figure 79–4. Left radial breast sonogram: The main ducts (arrowheads) led to lobulated structures (small arrows) consistent with lobular hyperplasia. Nipple (large arrows).

Pathology

Cysts. Besides calcifications within microcysts, atypical lobular hyperplasia was present.

Management

- BI-RADS Assessment Category 3, probably benign; short-interval follow-up

Pearls and Pitfalls

1. The calcifications in this case are round because they are within microcysts. This atypical lobular hyperplasia was inadvertently adjacent to these microcysts.
2. High-frequency sonography is able to delineate ductal and lobular details that were not visible with lower-resolution equipment.

Suggested Readings

1. Gershon-Cohen DS, Berger SM, Curcio BM. Breast cancer with microcalcifications: diagnostic difficulties. *Radiology* 1966;87:613–622.
2. Teboul M, Halliwell M. *Atlas of Ultrasound and Ductal Echography of the Breast.* 2nd ed. Cambridge: Blackwell Science; 1996:154–201.

Case 80

Case History

A 45-year-old woman presents with right breast calcifications that have increased in number since her prior screening mammogram performed 2 years ago.

Physical Examination

- normal exam

Mammogram

Calcifications (Figs. 80–1 and 80–2)

- type: punctate
- distribution: diffuse/scattered

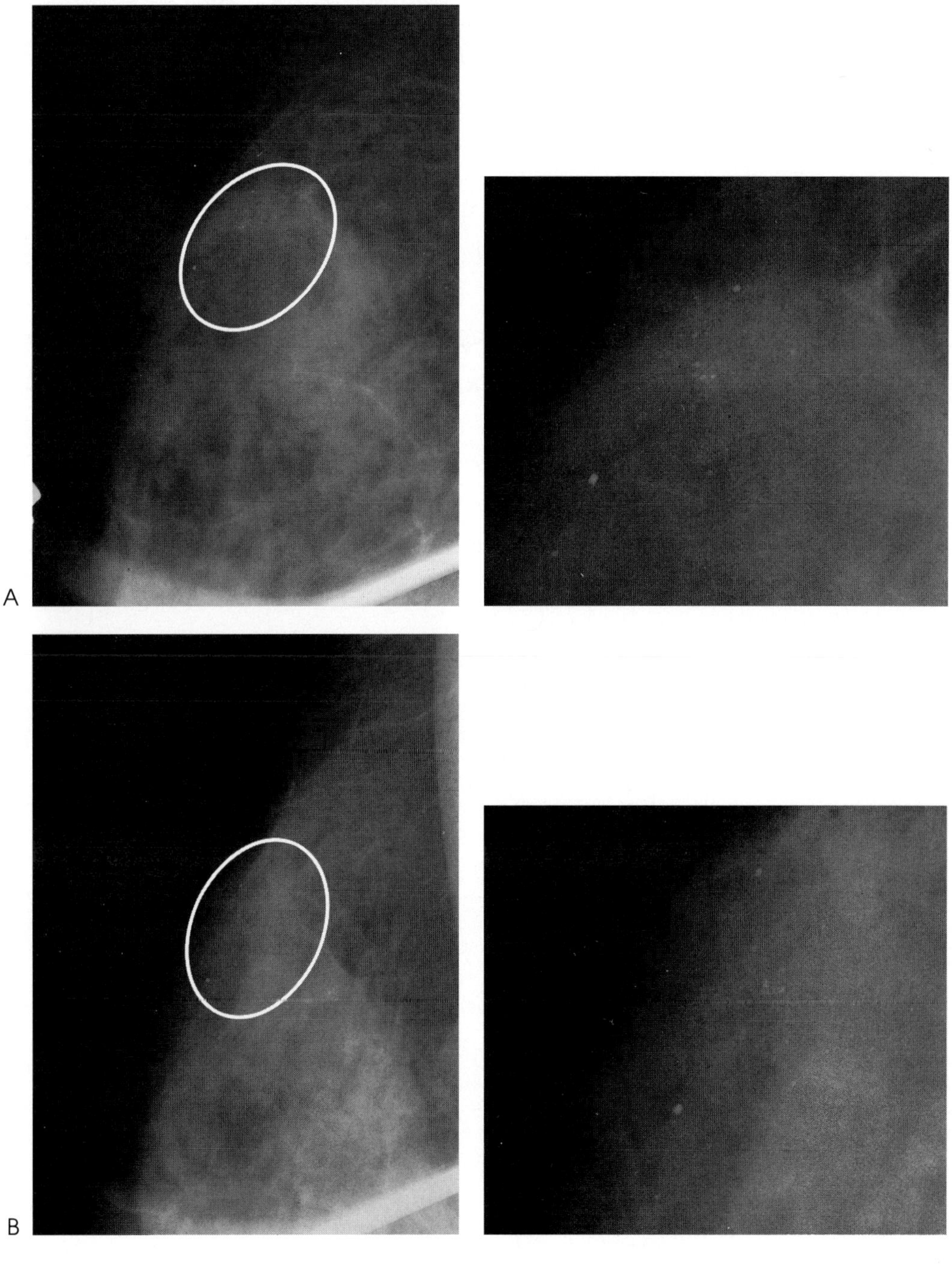

Figure 80–1. In the upper outer quadrant there are scattered round, punctate calcifications (circled). (A). Right MLO magnification view. (B). Right accentuated CC magnification view.

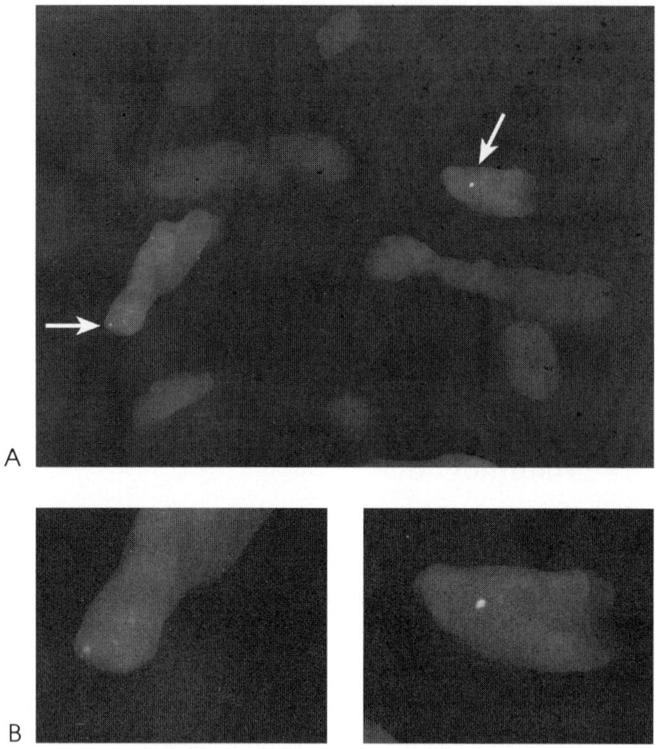

Figure 80–2. Specimen radiograph of breast tissue cores from percutaneous biopsy: The punctate calcifications in the the specimen (arrows) mirror the appearance of the punctate calcifications in Figure 80–1.

Pathology

- cysts; benign fibrous and cystic changes with calcifications in cysts

Management

- BI-RADS Assessment Category 2, benign finding

Pearls and Pitfalls

Scattered punctate or round microcalcifications are produced by a variety of benign conditions including cystic hyperplasia, papillomatosis, sclerosing adenosis, adenosis, and atypical lobular hyperplasia.

Suggested Readings

1. Gershon-Cohen DS, Berger SM, Curcio BM. Breast cancer with microcalcifications: diagnostic difficulties. *Radiology* 1966;87:613–622.

Case 81

Case History

A 57-year-old woman presents with new right breast calcifications.

Physical Examination

- normal exam

Mammogram

Calcifications (Fig. 81–1)

- type: punctate
- distribution: grouped/clustered

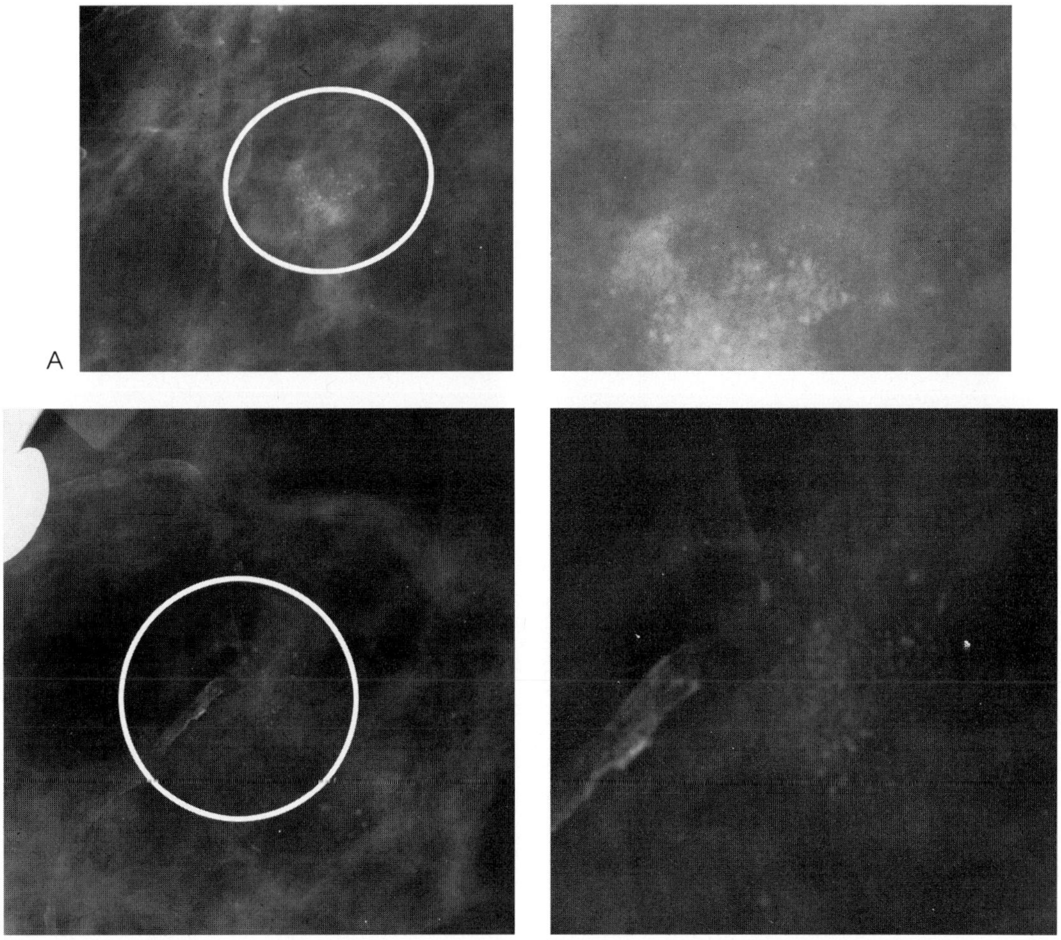

A

B

Figure 81–1. In the upper outer quadrant of the right breast, there is a cluster of punctate calcifications (circled). (A). Right MLO magnification mammogram. (B). Right CC magnification mammogram.

Pathology

- fibrocystic changes
- calcifications in adenosis

Management

- BI-RADS Assessment Category 4, suspicious abnormality; biopsy should be considered

Pearls and Pitfalls

1. One of the common problems faced by mammographers is to assign assessment categories to small round, punctate, and amorphous clusters of calcifications. If the calcifications are uniform in density and size and are clearly round in shape with smooth borders, then the cluster may be assigned a Category 3 (or Category 2 if they have been stable for 2 to 3 years). However, if the calcifications are too small (punctate) or ill defined (amorphous) to identify the shape or borders then a Category 4 is appropriate.
2. Punctate calcifications are produced by fibrocystic changes, lobular hyperplasia, atypical lobular hyperplasia, or ductal carcinoma in situ.

Suggested Readings

1. MacErlean DP, Nathan BE. Calcification in sclerosing adenosis simulating malignant breast calcification. *Br J Radiol* 1972;45:944–945.

Case 82

Case History

A 54-year-old woman presents with new calcifications on her screening mammogram.

Physical Examination

- normal exam

Mammogram

Calcifications (Fig. 82–1)

- type: punctate
- distribution: linear

A
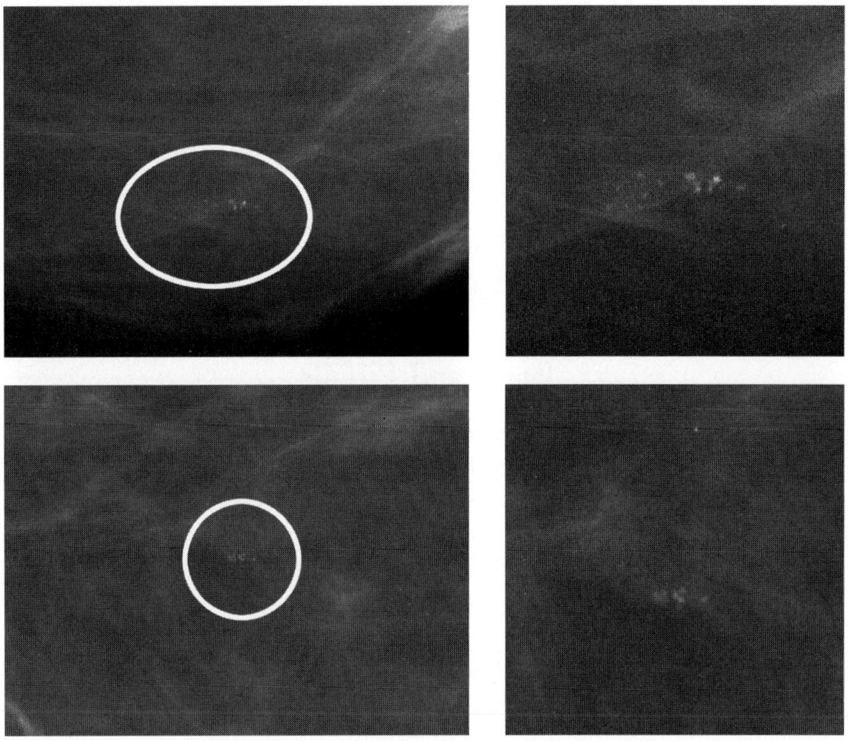
B

Figure 82–1. *A linear cluster of punctate round calcifications is present in the inner inferior quadrant of the left breast (circled). (A). Left LM magnification mammogram. (B). Left CC magnification mammogram.*

Ultrasound

Frequency

- 7 MHz (Fig. 82–2)

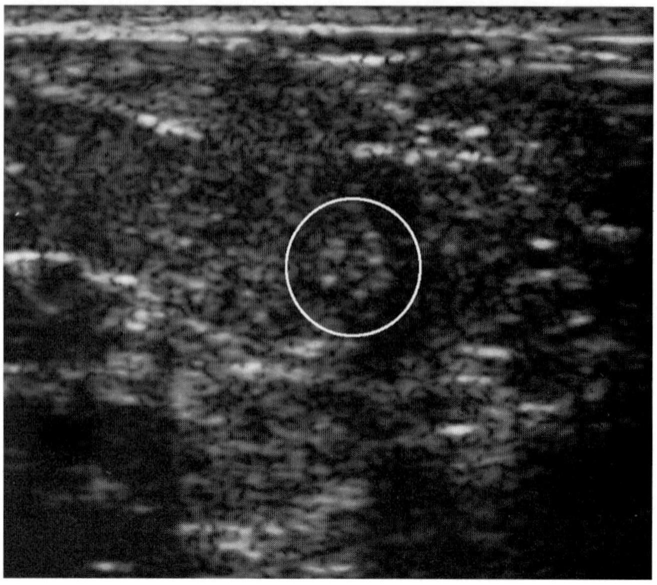

Figure 82–2. Left antiradial breast sonogram: The mammographic calcifications identified in Figures 82–1A and 1B correspond to a group of high acoustic intensity foci (circled). Sonographically, this group of calcifications were grouped in a cylindrical pattern that matched the linear pattern of the mammogram. No associated abnormal ducts or masses were present (see Color Plate 82–2).

Pathology

- fibroadenoma (not otherwise specified)

Management

- BI-RADS Assessment Category 4, suspicious abnormality; biopsy should be considered

Pearls and Pitfalls

Punctate shape of the calcifications tends to suggest a benign etiology. However, the linear arrangement may be produced by DCIS. The calcifications in this case are separate from the adjacent calcified vessel, so vascular calcifications are unlikely. As there is no sonographic abnormality other than the calcifications, the sonographic findings are nonspecific, so the management is based upon the mammographic features of the calcifications.

Suggested Readings

1. Bassett LW. Mammographic analysis of calcifications. *Radiol Clin North Am* 1992;30:93–105.
2. De Paredes E. Calcifications. In: De Paredes E, ed. *Atlas of Film-Screen Mammography.* Baltimore: Williams and Wilkins; 1992:299–416.
3. Gershon-Cohen J, Ingleby H. Roentgenography of fibroadenoma of the breast. *Radiology* 1952;59:77–86.

Case 84

Case History

A 72-year-old woman developed a cluster of calcifications that increased in number when followed at 6-month intervals for 1 year.

Physical Examination

- normal exam

Mammogram

Calcifications (Figs. 84–1 and 84–2)

- type: punctate
- distribution: grouped/clustered

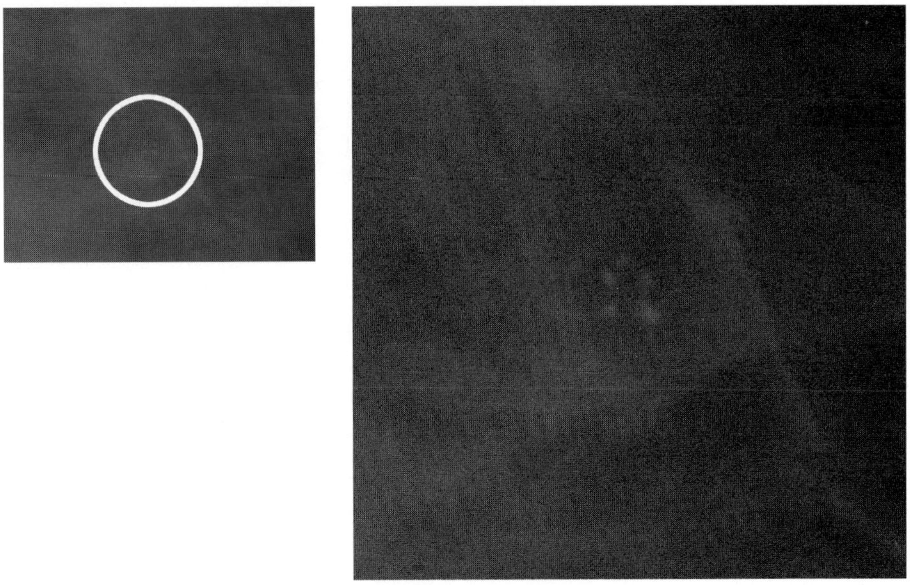

Figure 84–1. Left MLO magnification mammogram: A cluster of fairly uniform punctate calcifications is present inferior to the nipple (circle). No associated mass is appreciated on the mammogram.

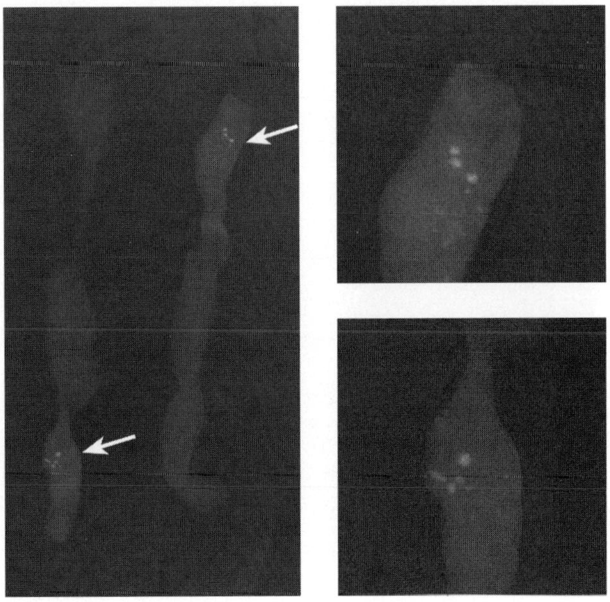

Figure 84–2. Specimen radiograph of 11 gauge core biopsy samples of the calcifications identified in Figure 84–1: In addition to the smooth, fairly round calcifications, there are numerous, smaller, fainter, punctate microcalcifications (arrows). These small calcifications cannot be appreciated on the prebiopsy magnification view (Fig. 84–1).

Ultrasound

Low Frequency

Frequency

- 7 MHz

Mass

- margin: ill defined
- echogenicity: hypoechoic
- retrotumoral acoustic appearance: single edge shadowing
- shape: oval (Fig. 84–3)

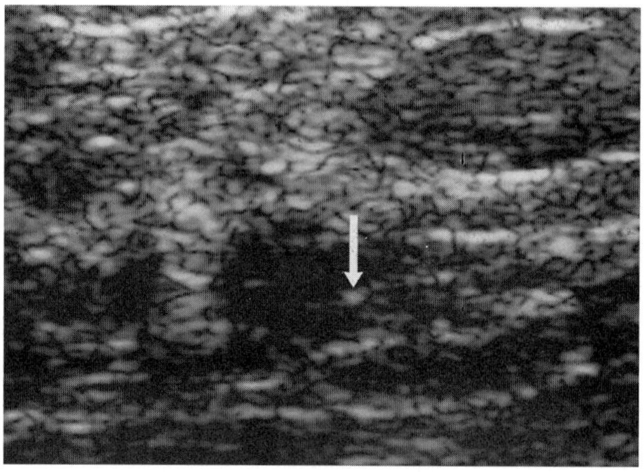

Figure 84–3. Left breast radial sonogram: The calcifications (arrow) shown in Figure 84–1 were located within a 5 mm, oval, ill-defined hypoechoic solid mass. The mass is not well characterized sonographically because this sonographic frequency exhibits inadequate resolution due to the small size of this mass.

High Frequency

Frequency

- 13 MHz

Associated Findings

The high-frequency sonographic study demonstrates an irregular ill-defined hypoechoic mass associated with the mammographic calcifications. The sonographic malignant features of the mass are better characterized by the high-frequency examination compared with the lower-frequency study. Although the calcifications are also more conspicuous with higher-frequency sonography, their sonographic appearance is still nonspecific (Fig. 84–4).

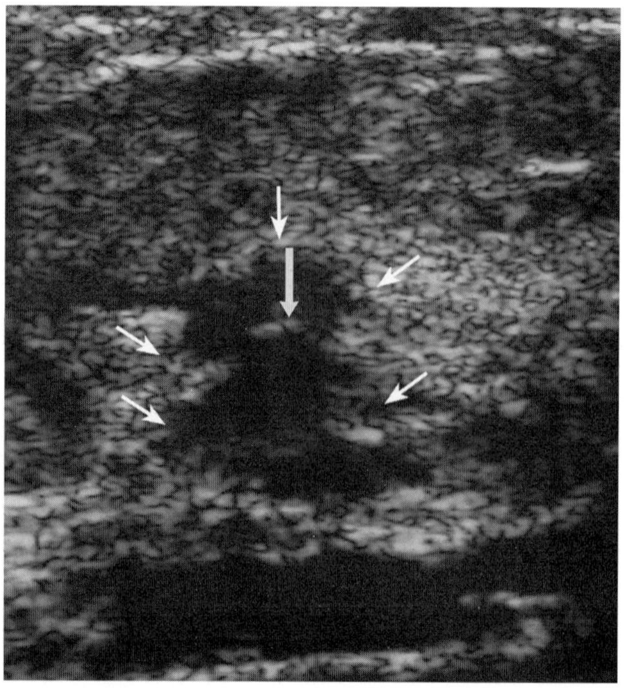

Figure 84–4. Right breast radial sonogram of same mass as Figure 84–3: The borders of the mass are irregular and associated with spiculations. The calcifications (large arrow) are easily identified.

Pathology

Invasive ductal carcinoma with a predominant intraductal component. At excision a 3 mm area of invasive and intraductal carcinoma was evident.

Management

- BI-RADS Assessment Category 4, suspicious abnormality; biopsy should be considered

Pearls and Pitfalls

Although sonographic examination would not normally be performed, this case illustrates that high-frequency sonography may identify masses in association with calcifications, even when a mass is not apparent mammographically. With high-frequency sonography, 50 to 60% of mammographic malignant calcifications without density or mass are associated with a sonographic mass.

Suggested Readings

1. Cox BA, Kelly KM, Ko P, et al. Ultrasound characteristics of breast carcinoma. *Am Surg* 1998;64:934–938.
2. Huang CS, Wu CY, Chu JS, et al. Microcalcifications of non-palpable breast lesions detected by ultrasonography: correlation with mammography and histopathology. *Ultrasound Obstetrical Gynecology* 1999;13:431–436.

Case 85

Case History

A 53-year-old woman presents with new calcifications on her screening mammogram.

Physical Examination

- normal exam

Mammogram

Calcifications (Fig. 85–1)

- type: punctate
- distribution: grouped/clustered

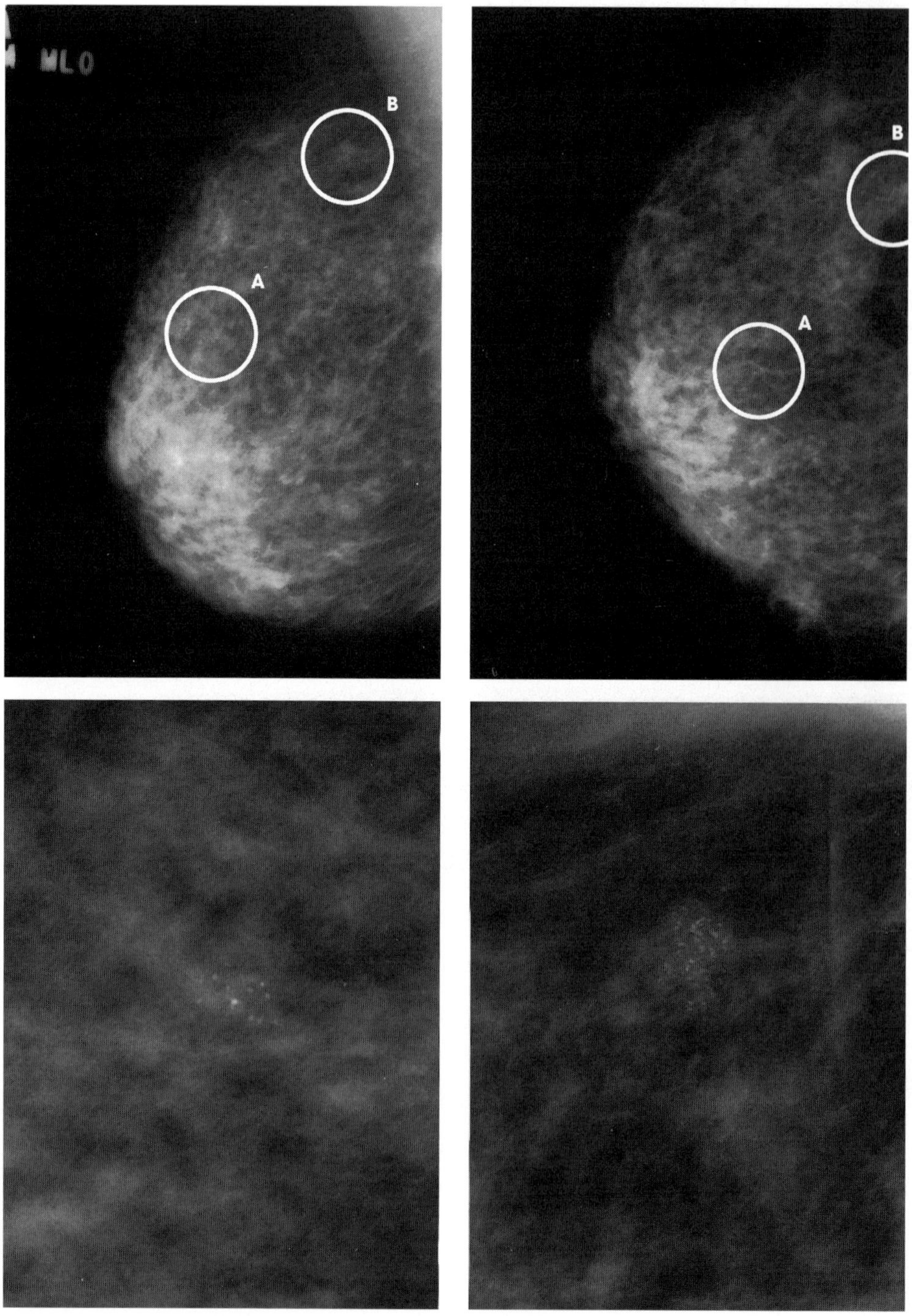

A B C D

Figure 85–1. *Two clusters of calcifications are present in the right breast. Cluster A (circled) is a cluster of punctate calcifications at the 12:00 position. Cluster B (circled) is a cluster of heterogeneous calcifications in the upper outer breast. (A). Right MLO mammogram. (B). Right XCCL mammogram. (C). Right MLO magnification mammogram. (D). Right CC magnification mammogram.*

Pathology

- ductal carcinoma in situ
- cluster A: ductal carcinoma in situ, low nuclear grade
- cluster B: invasive and in situ ductal carcinoma

Management

- BI-RADS Assessment Category 4, suspicious; biopsy should be considered

Pearls and Pitfalls

The cluster of punctate calcifications are commonly due to benign etiologies. However, because the patient has a second highly suspicious area of heterogeneous calcifications, the punctate cluster should also be biopsied. DCIS is multifocal in about one third of women. The risk of multifocal DCIS increases with increasing tumor size. Only 12 to 17% of patients with lesions 25 mm have multifocal disease compared with 47% with tumors larger than 25 mm.

Suggested Readings

1. Anastassiades O, Iakovou E, Stavridou N, et al. Multicentricity in breast cancer: a study of 366 cases. *Am J Clin Pathol* 1993;99:238–243.
2. Dershaw DD, Abramson A, Kinne DW. Ductal carcinoma in situ: mammographic findings and clinical implications. *Radiology* 1989;170:411–415.
3. Lagios MD. Multicentricity of breast carcinoma demonstrated by routine correlated serial subgross and radiographic examination. *Cancer* 1997;40:1726–1734.
4. Lagios MD, Westdahl PR, Margolin FR, et al. Duct carcinoma in situ: relationship of extent of noninvasive disease to the frequency of occult invasion, multicentricity, lymph node metastases, and short-term treatment failures. *Cancer* 1982;50:1309–1314.
5. Swain SW. Ductal carcinoma in situ. *Cancer Invest* 1992;10:443–454.
6. Zavotsky J, Gardner B. Postexcisional recurrence of carcinoma of the breast. *J Am Coll Surg* 1996;182:71–77.

Case 86

Case History

A 56-year-old woman presents with increasing right breast calcifications.

Physical Examination

- normal exam

Mammogram

Calcifications (Fig. 86–1)

- type: punctate
- distribution: linear

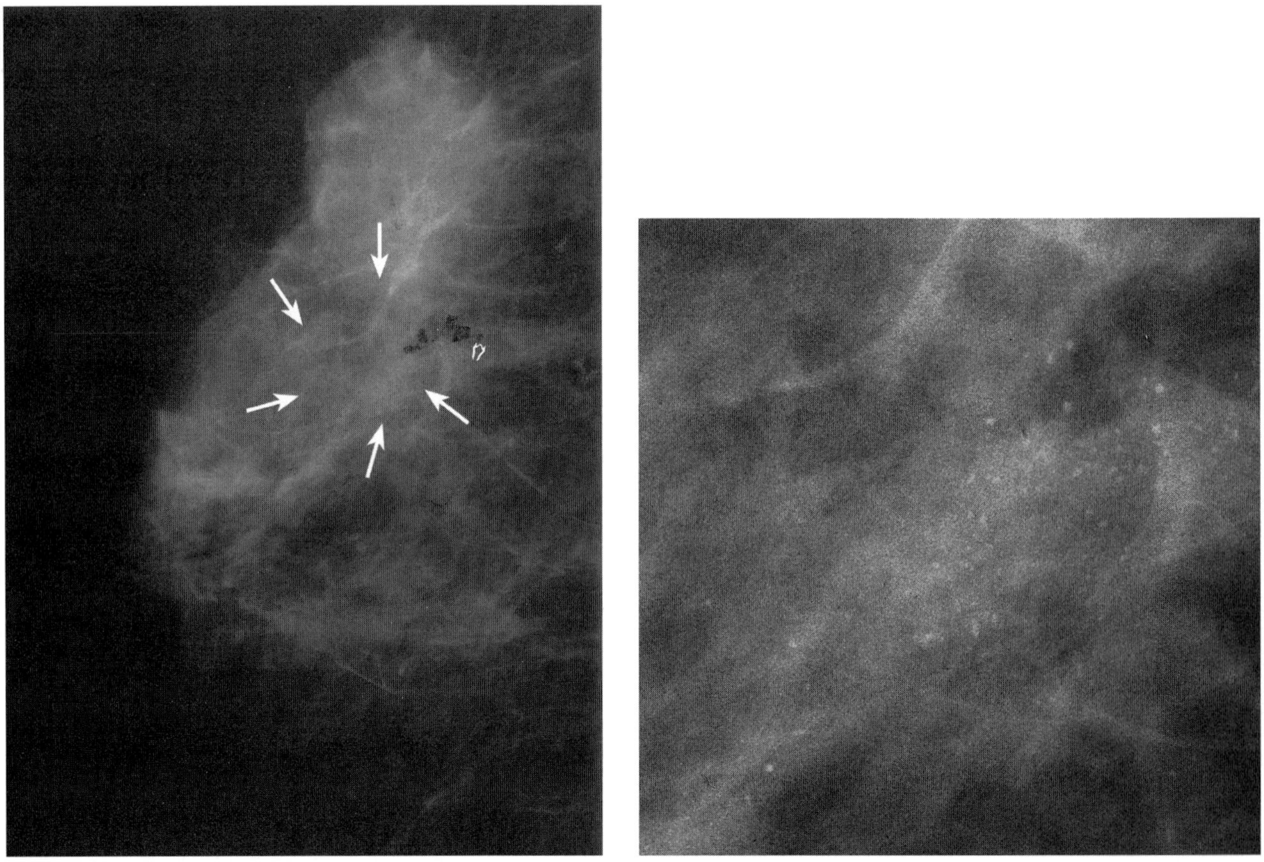

Figure 86–1. Right LM magnification mammogram: Numerous punctate calcifications are segmentally localized in the upper breast (arrows). Clip was placed after her percutaneous biopsy.

Pathology

- invasive ductal carcinoma with a predominant intraductal component
- greater than 20 mm area of DCIS with a 3 mm area of invasive ductal carcinoma
- extensive involvement of lobules with DCIS

Management

- BI-RADS Assessment Category 4, suspicious abnormality; biopsy should be considered

Pearls and Pitfalls

Punctate calcifications are a less common presentation of malignancy. They sometimes result from extension of the neoplasm into the lobules.

Suggested Readings

1. Homer MJ, Safaii H. Cancerization of the lobule: implication regarding analysis of microcalcification shape. *Breast Dis* 1990;3:131–133.
2. Lagios MD, Page DL. In situ carcinomas of the breast: ductal carcinoma in situ, Paget's disease, lobular carcinoma in situ. In: Bland KI, ed. *The Breast: Comprehensive Management of Benign and Malignant Diseases.* Philadelphia: WB Saunders; 1998:261–283.

Case 87

Case History

A 48-year-old woman presents with new densities on her right mammogram.

Physical Examination

- normal exam

Mammogram

Calcifications (Figs. 87–1 and 87–2)

- type: amorphous/indistinct
- distribution: grouped/clustered

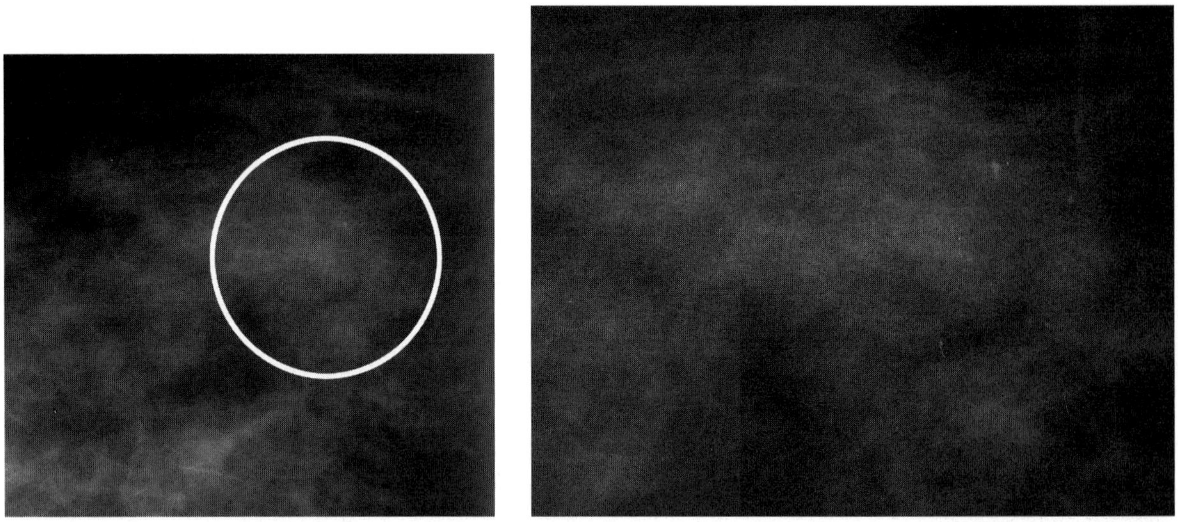

Figure 87–1. Right CC mammogram: In the outer breast, multiple amorphous densities were present (circled). These densities could only be identified on this view.

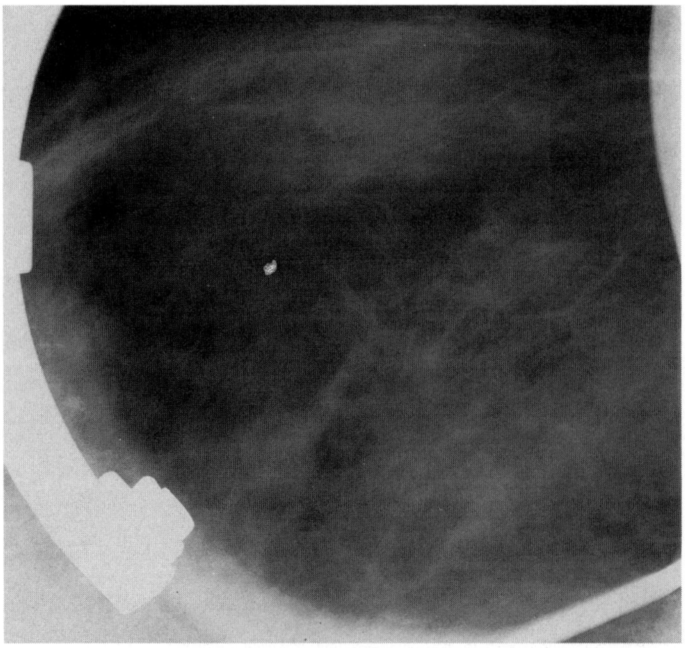

Figure 87–2. Right CC spot magnification mammogram: Patient returned 5 days later and the densities are no longer present.

Pathology

- deodorant material on skin

Management

- BI-RADS Assessment Category 2, benign finding

Pearls and Pitfalls

This case is an example of the appearance of skin powder. Various creams, powders, tattoos, and aluminum deodorants can produce densities that may appear to represent intraparenchymal calcifications. When the densities are extremely small and only visible on one view, this etiology should be considered.

Suggested Readings

1. Bartton III JW, Kornguth PJ. Mammographic deodorant and powder artifact: is there confusion with malignant microcalcifications? *Breast Dis* 1990;3:121–126.
2. Pamilo M, Soiva M, Suramo I. New artifacts simulating malignant microcalcifications in mammography. *Breast Dis* 1989;1:321–327.

Case 88

Case History

A 64-year-old woman with new calcifications on her screening mammogram.

Physical Examination

- normal exam

Mammogram

Calcifications (Fig. 88–1)

- type: amorphous/indistinct
- distribution: grouped/clustered

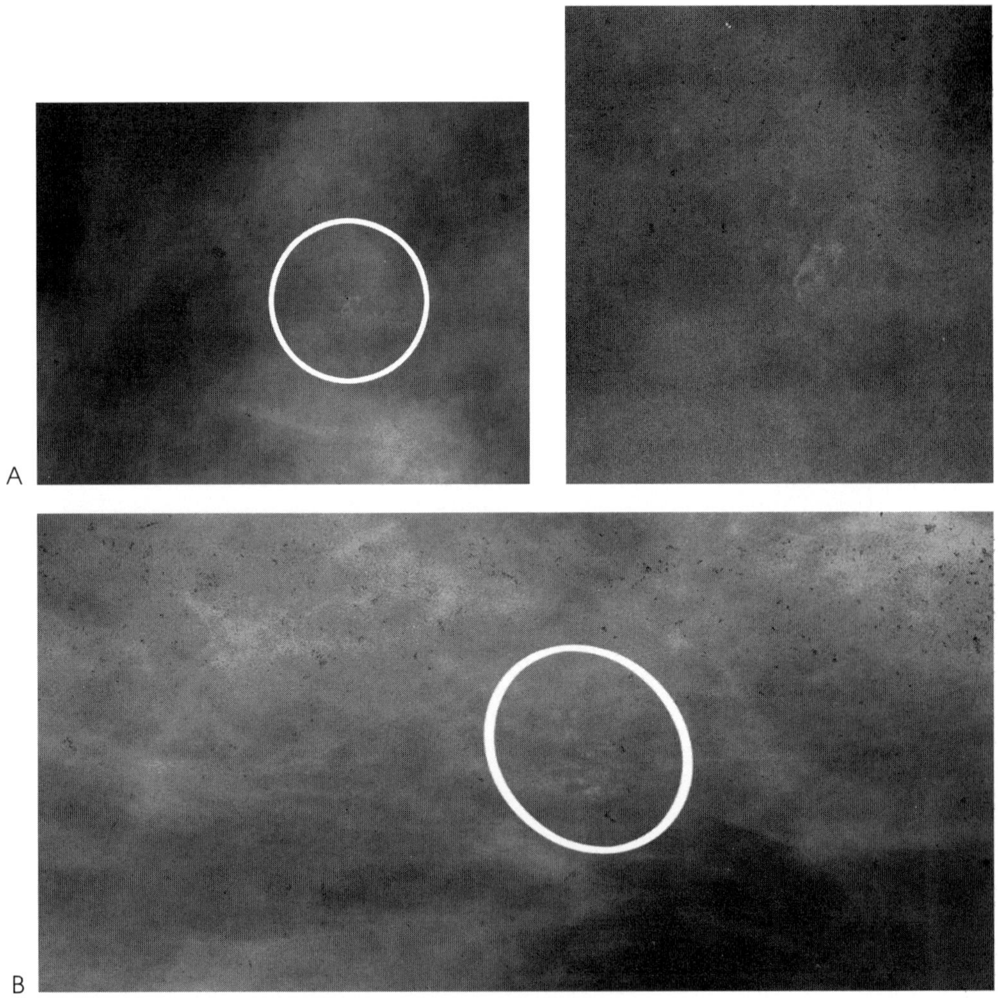

Figure 88–1. In the upper outer quadrant of the right breast, there is a cluster of indistinct amorphous calcifications (circled). (A). Right MLO magnification mammogram. (B). Right CC magnification mammogram.

Ultrasound

Low Frequency

Frequency

- 7 MHz (Fig. 88–2)

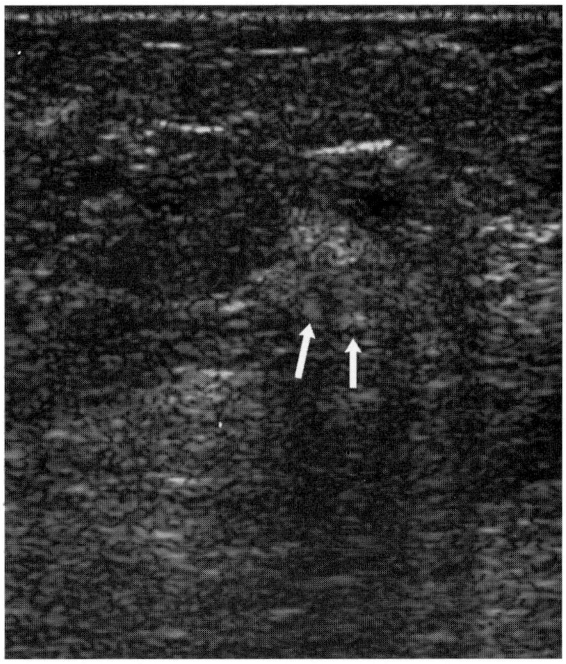

Figure 88–2. Right radial breast sonogram: The calcifications (arrows) identified in Figure 88–1 were localized sonographically. Lower-frequency sonography is generally more helpful when the breast tissue is extremely attenuating. In this case of fibroadenomatous hyperplasia, the lower frequency demonstrates that there is no mass in the area of the calcifications. Only benign-appearing hyperechoic tissue is present (see Color Plate 88–2).

High Frequency

- 10 MHz (Fig. 88–3)

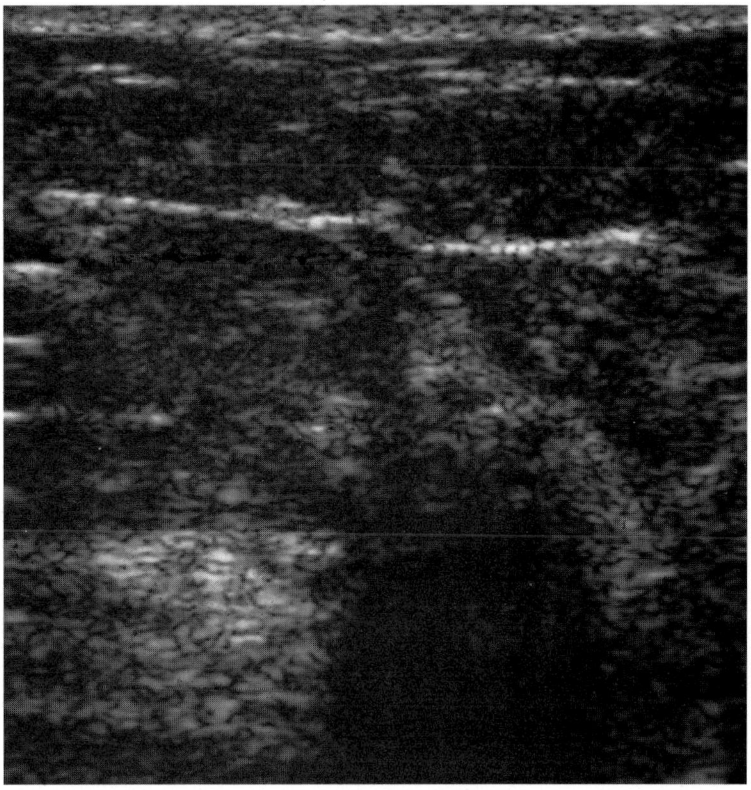

Figure 88–3. Right radial breast sonogram: When using the higher frequency, the area of calcification heavily shadows due to the highly attenuating fibrous tissue. The shadowing prevents one from differentiating attenuating benign tissue from malignant tissue.

Pathology

- fibroadenomatoid hyperplasia

Management

- BI-RADS Assessment Category 4, suspicious abnormality; biopsy should be considered

Pearls and Pitfalls

1. These amorphous calcifications are moderately suspicous. Conditions that may produce these calcifications include fibrocystic changes, fibroadenomas, fat necrosis, or intraductal carcinoma.
2. Fibrosis highly attenuates sound and commonly produces focal shadowing. To differentiate diffuse fibrosis from a focal malignant mass, one should utilize a lower frequency. A lower frequency may penetrate the tissue and demonstrate either the presence of a mass or the presence of benign tissue.

Suggested Readings

1. Kamal M, Evans AJ, Denley H, et al. Fibroadenomatoid hyperplasia: a cause of suspicious microcalcification on mammographic screening. *AJR* 1998;171:1331–1334.

Case 89

Case History

A 49-year-old woman presents with left breast calcifications that are new since her previous screening mammogram 4 years ago.

Physical Examination

- normal exam

Mammogram

Calcifications (Figs. 89–1 and 89–2)

- type: amorphous/indistinct
- distribution: segmental

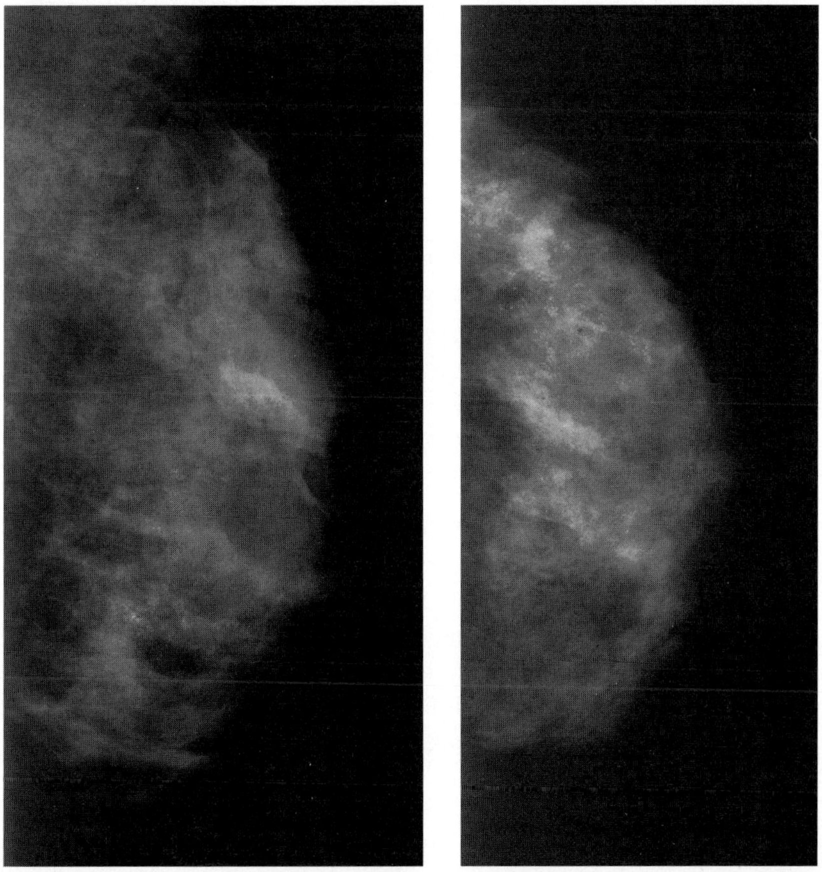

A B

Figure 89–1. Amorphous calcifications are present throughout the entire left upper outer quadrant. (A). Left MLO mammogram. (B). Left CC mammogram. (C). Left LM magnification mammogram.

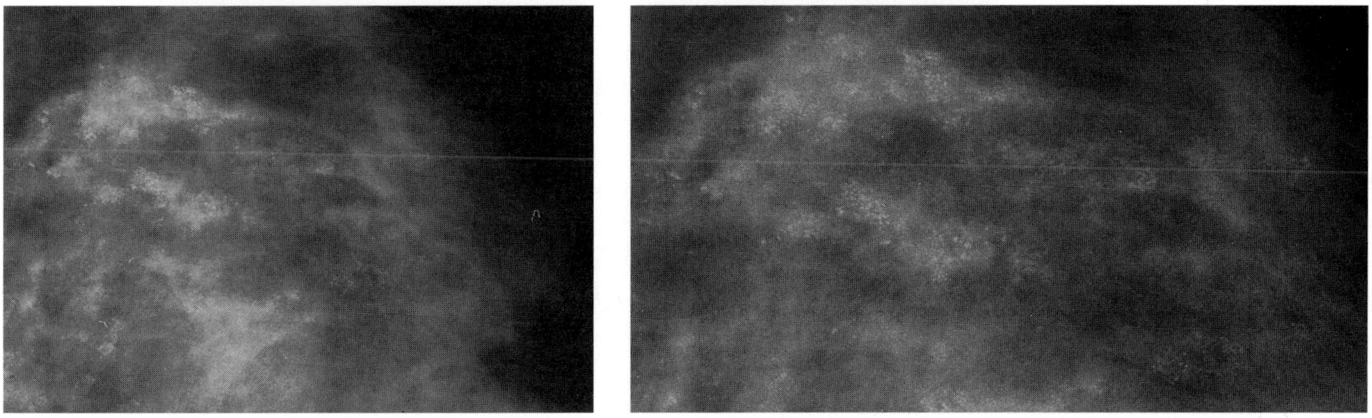

C

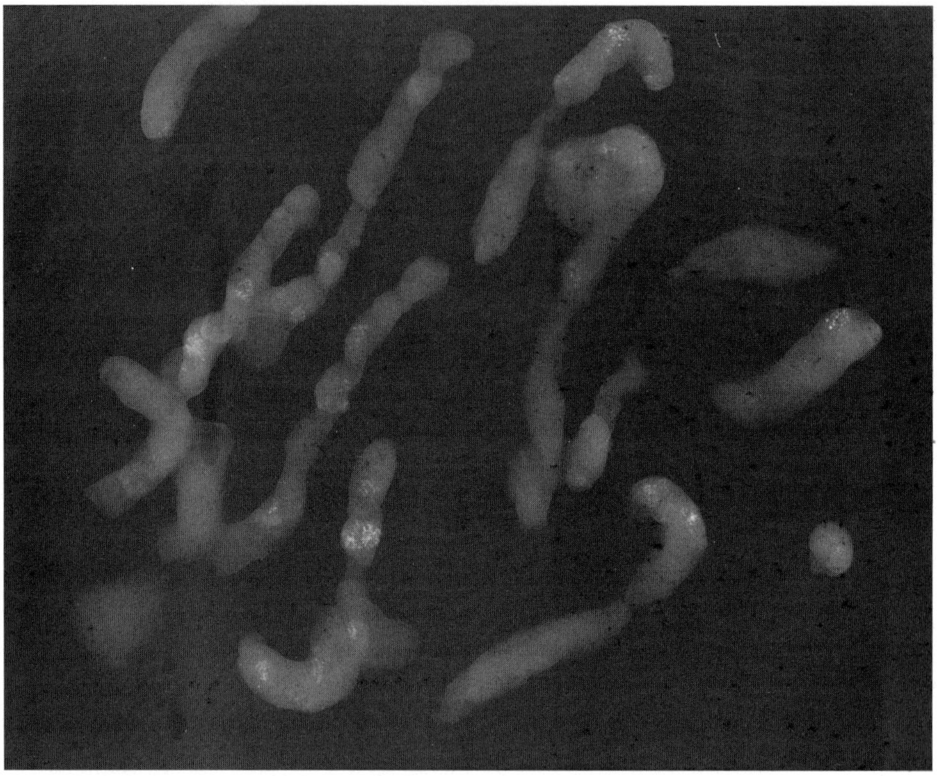

Figure 89–2. Specimen radiograph from percutaneous mammographically guided stereotactic core biopsy: Most of the cores exhibit amorphous calcifications.

Pathology

Atypical ductal hyperplasia. Both the percutaneous core biopsy and the partial mastectomy specimens demonstrated atypical duct epithelial hyperplasia without evidence of in situ or invasive carcinoma.

Management

- BI-RADS Assessment Category 4, suspicious; biopsy should be considered

Pearls and Pitfalls

Atypical ductal hyperplasia (ADH) is commonly associated with biopsied calcifications. If the sampled tissue only demonstrates ADH, reexcision of the tissue is recommended. About 50% of percutaneous biopsies showing only ADH are associated with malignancy after subsequent surgical excision. Larger tissue core sampling devices appear to reduce the chance of inadequate sampling to 10 to 20%.

Suggested Readings

1. Brem RF, Behrndt VS, Sanow L, et al. Atypical ductal hyperplasia: histologic underestimation of carcinoma in tissue harvested from impalpable breast lesions using 11-gauge stereotactically guided directional vacuum-assisted biopsy. *AJR* 1999;172:1405–1407.
2. Burbank F. Stereotactic breast biopsy of atypical ductal hyperplasia and ductal carcinoma in situ lesions: improved accuracy with directional, vacuum-assisted biopsy. *Radiology* 1997;202:843–847.
3. Jackman RJ, Burbank F, Parker SH, et al. Atypical ductal hyperplasia diagnosed at stereotactic breast biopsy: improved reliability with 14-gauge, directional, vacuum-assisted biopsy. *Radiology* 1997;204:485–488.
4. Liberman L, Dershaw DD, Glassman JR, et al. Analysis of cancers not diagnosed at stereotactic core breast biopsy. *Radiology* 1997;203:151–157.
5. Liberman L, Smolkin JH, Dershaw DD, et al. Calcification retrieval at stereotactic, 11-gauge, directional, vacuum-assisted breast biopsy. *Radiology* 1998;208:251–260.

Case 90

Case History

A 40-year-old woman presents for her baseline mammogram.

Physical Examination

- normal exam

Mammogram

Calcifications (Figs. 90–1 and 90–2)

- type: amorphous/indistinct
- distribution: regional

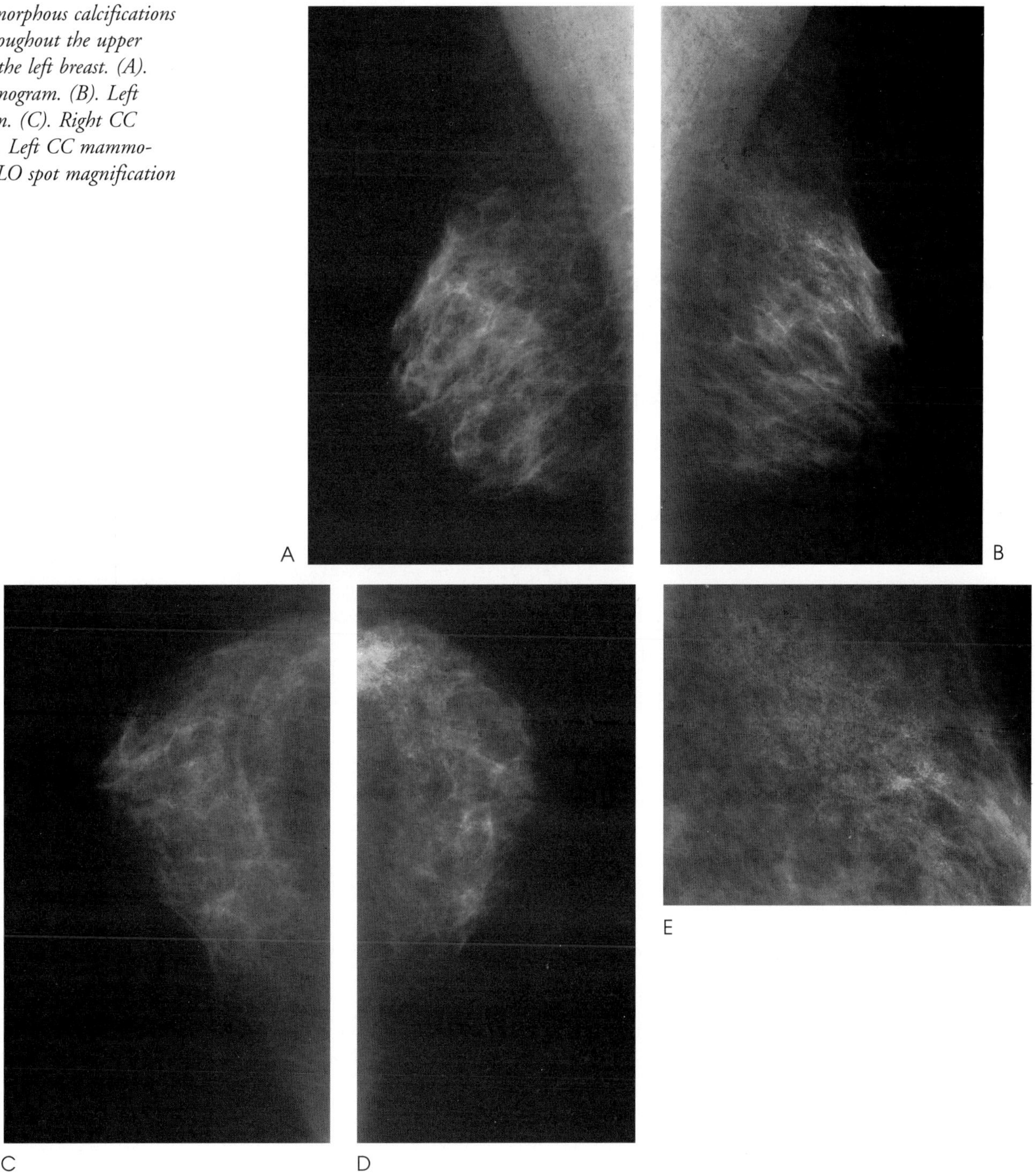

Figure 90–1. Amorphous calcifications are distributed throughout the upper outer quadrant of the left breast. (A). Right MLO mammogram. (B). Left MLO mammogram. (C). Right CC mammogram. (D). Left CC mammogram. (E). Left MLO spot magnification mammogram.

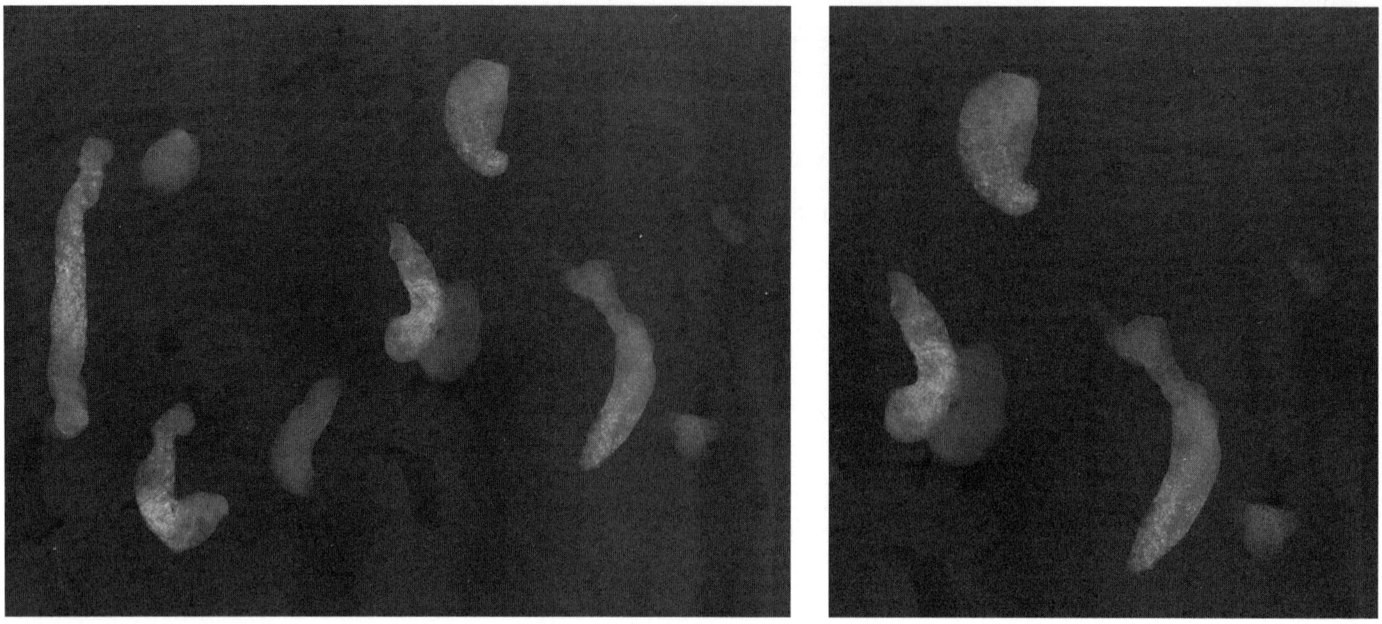

Figure 90–2. Specimen radiograph of percutaneous mammographically guided stereotactic core breast biopsy: The amorphous appearance of the calcifications is evident in all of the tissue cores.

Pathology

Lobular hyperplasia. Microscopically, the calcifications are within lobules.

Management

- BI-RADS Assessment Category 4, suspicious abnormality; biopsy should be considered

Pearls and Pitfalls

Microcalcifications within lobules may be either punctate or amorphous in appearance.

Suggested Readings

1. De Paredes ES. *Atlas of Film Screen Mammography*. 2nd ed. Baltimore: Williams & Wilkins; 1992:299–416.
2. Pope TL, Fechner RE, Wilhelm MC. Lobular carcinoma in situ of the breast: mammographic features. *Radiology* 1988;168:63–66.
3. Snyder RE. Mammography and lobular carcinoma in situ. *Surg Gynecol Obstet* 1966;255–260.

Case 91

Case History

A 74-year-old woman presents with a new cluster of calcifications in the area of her lumpectomy site.

Physical Examination

- right breast: stable scar in the right upper outer quadrant from previous lumpectomy
- left breast: normal exam

Mammogram

Calcifications (Fig. 91-1 and 91-2)

- type: amorphous/indistinct
- distribution: grouped/clustered

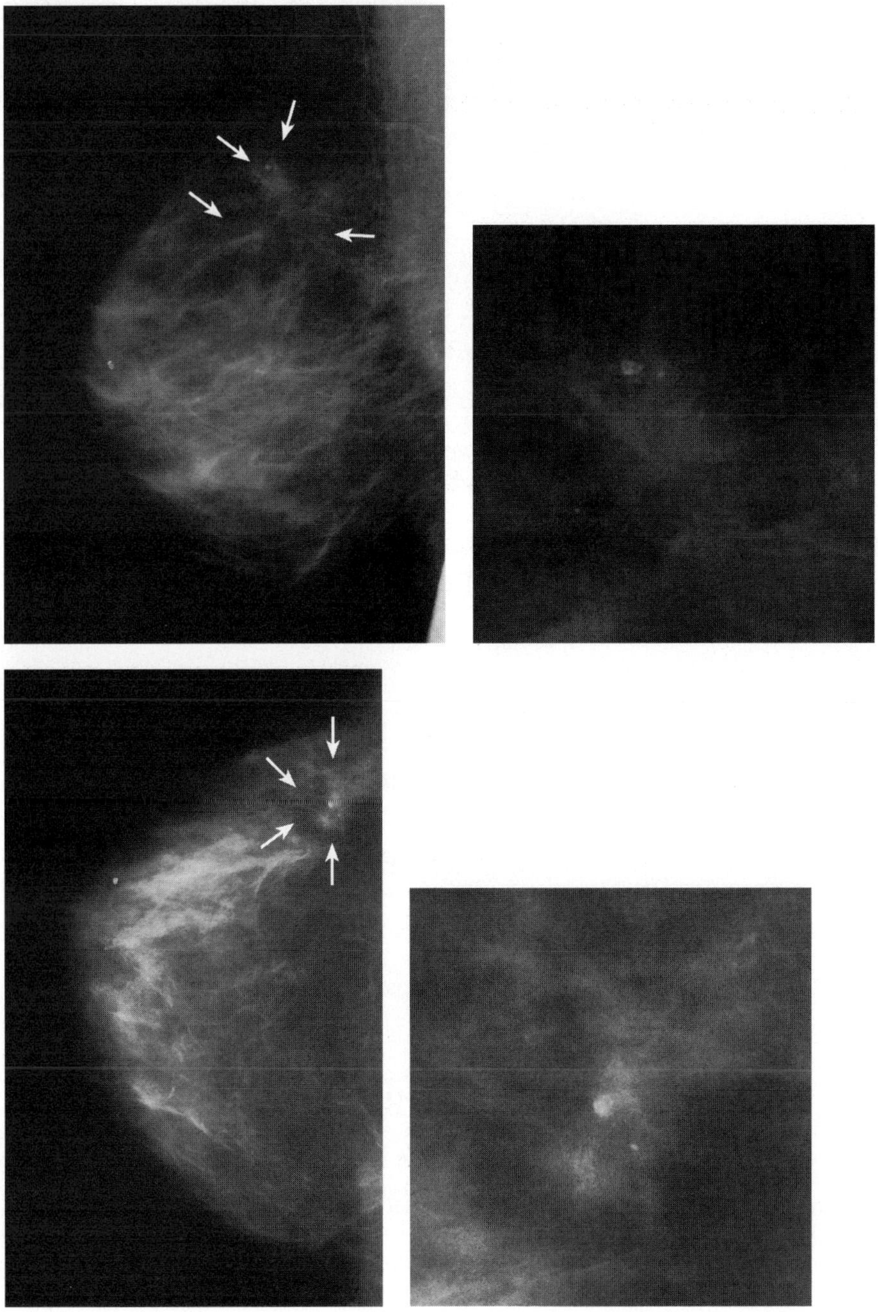

A

B

Figure 91-1. *In the right upper outer quadrant there are ill-defined density, architectural distortion, and calcification resulting from previous lumpectomy (arrows). (A). Right ML mammogram. (B). Right CC mammogram.*

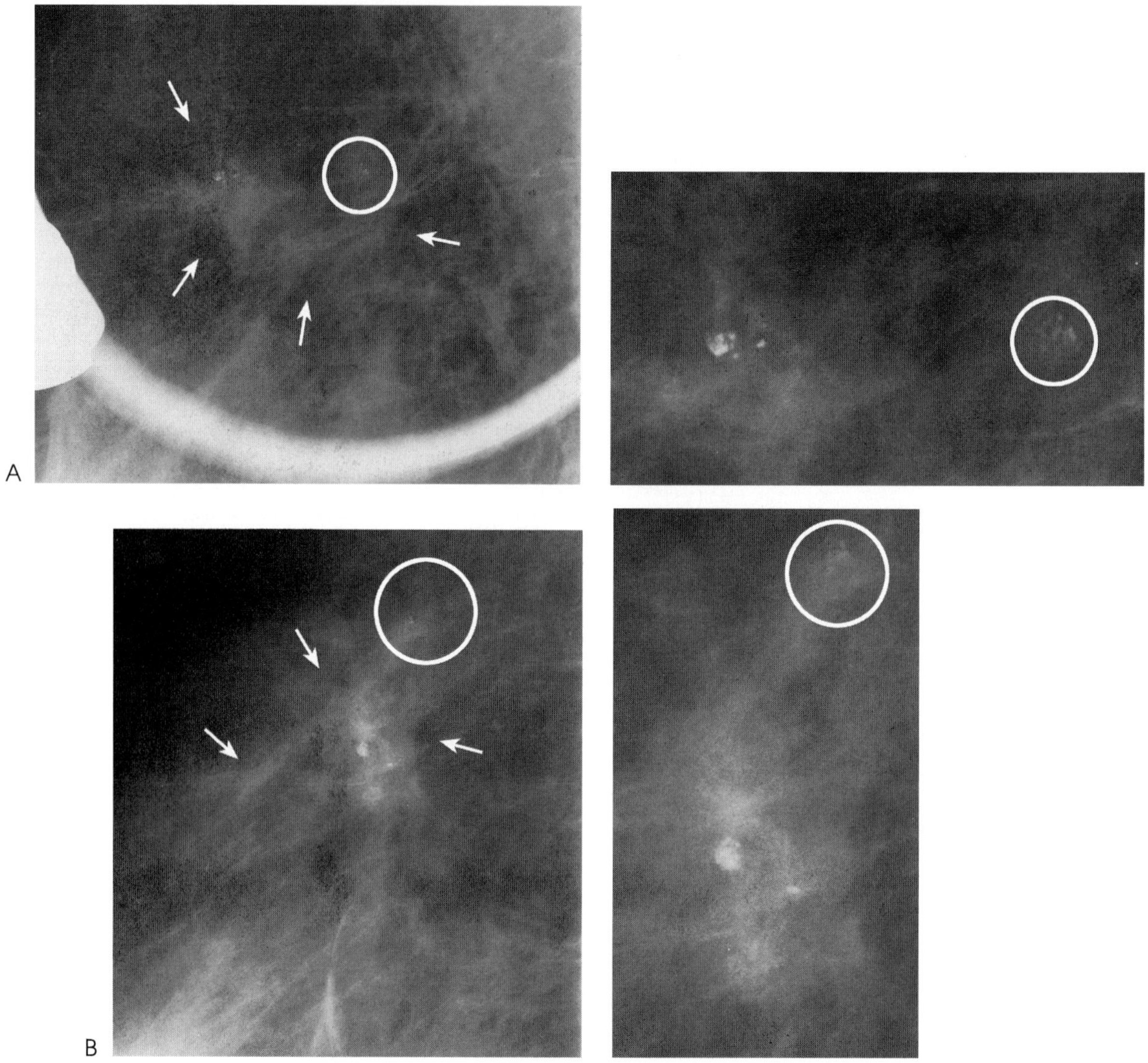

Figure 91–2. Magnification views demonstrate a new cluster of amorphous calcifications (circled) adjacent to the lumpectomy site (arrows). (A). Right MLO magnification mammogram. (B). Right CC magnification mammogram.

Pathology

- fat necrosis

Management

- BI-RADS Assessment Category 4, suspicious abnormality; biopsy should be considered

Pearls and Pitfalls

Amorphous calcifications may result from benign conditions such as fat necrosis, fibrocystic changes, or early vascular or fibroadenoma calcifications. However, these calcifications should be biopsied because, as in this patient, recurrent neoplasm may produce these calcifications.

Suggested Readings

1. Bassett LW, Gold RH, Cove HC. Mammographic spectrum of traumatic fat necrosis: the fallibility of "pathognomonic" signs of carcinoma. *AJR* 1998;130:119–122.
2. Liberman L, Van Zee KJ, Dershaw DD, et al. Mammographic features of local recurrance in women who have undergone breast-conserving therapy for ductal carcinoma in situ. *AJR* 1997;168:489–493.

Case 92

Case History

A 64-year-old woman with new right breast calcifications.

Physical Examination

- Normal exam

Mammogram

Calcifications (Figs. 92–1 and 92–2)

- type: amorphous/indistinct
- distribution: grouped/clustered

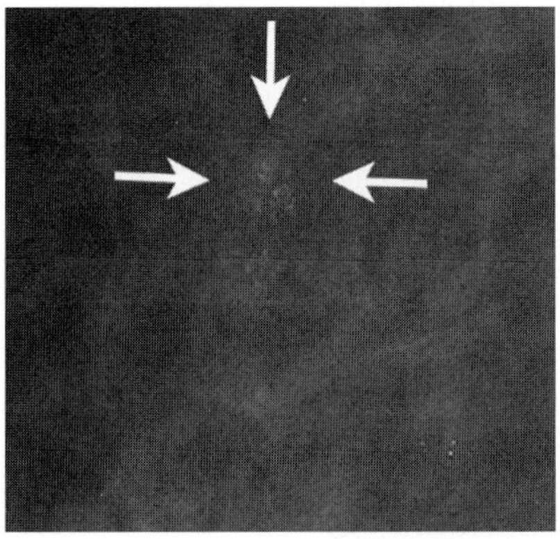

Figure 92–1. Right MLO magnification mammogram: Faint amorphous calcifications (arrows) are present in the upper breast.

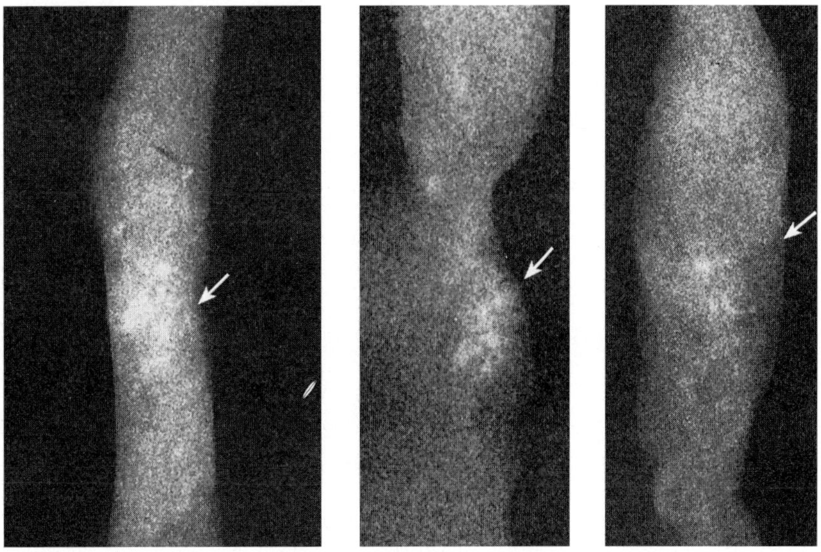

Figure 92–2. Specimen radiograph of percutaneous core right breast biopsy. Cores from the biopsy of the calcifications identified in Figure 92–1 confirm the amorphous appearance of the calcifications (arrows).

Pathology

- ductal carcinoma in situ, low nuclear grade, solid and cribiform type (Figs. 92–3 and 92–4)

Management

- BI-RADS Assessment Category 4, suspicious abnormality; biopsy should be considered

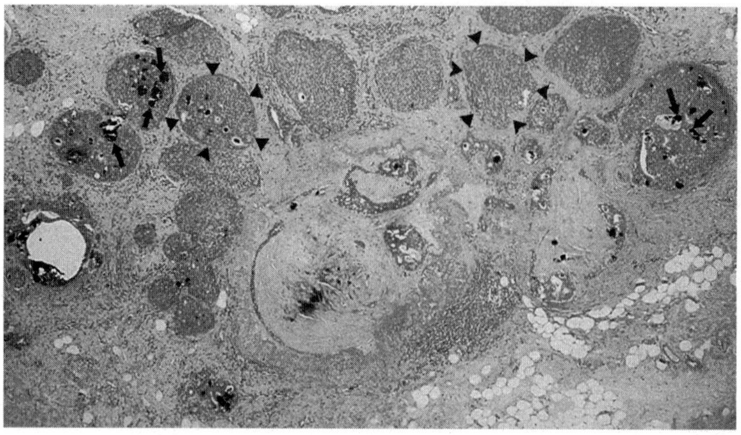

Figure 92–3. The lobules (arrowheads) are filled with malignant cells and calcifications (arrows). This type of malignant calcification results in a nonlinear pattern that is more typical of low-grade ductal carcinoma in situ (see Color Plate 92–3).

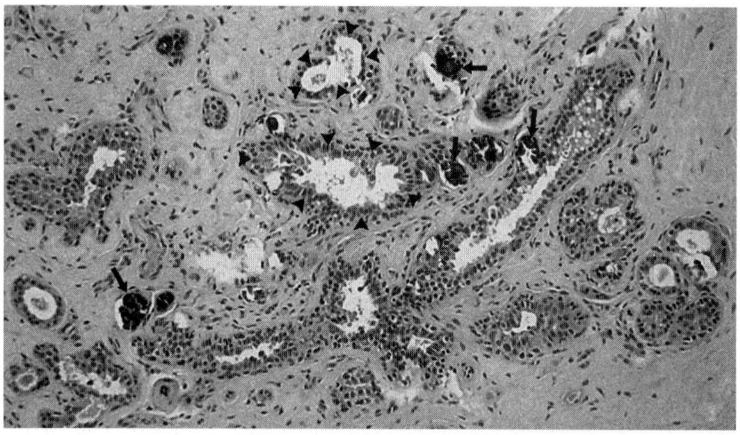

Figure 92–4. This is a different patient with calcifications (arrows) within normal lobules (arrowheads). Unless the calcifications are well defined, round, and have smooth borders, this type of nonlinear cluster of calcifications may be difficult to differentiate from the malignant cluster in Figure 92–3 (see Color Plate 92–4).

Pearls and Pitfalls

Ductal carcinoma in situ (DCIS) may present as either clustered or fine linear/branching calcifications. When DCIS is not associated with comedo necrosis, the tumor tends to form dystrophic calcifications within ductal debris or between cribiform spaces. This pattern produces a nonlinear cluster pattern, as illustrated in this case. This type of malignancy calcifies less than the necrotic type, so the size of the tumor may be larger than the area of the mammographic calcifications.

Suggested Readigns

1. Evans A, Pinder S, Wilson R, et al. Ductal carcinoma in situ of the breast: correlation between mammographic and pathologic findings. *AJR* 1994;162:1307–1311.
2. Holland R, Hendriks JHCL, Verbeek ALM, et al. Extent, distribution, and mammographic/histological correlations of breast ductal carcinoma in situ. *Lancet* 1990;335:519–522.

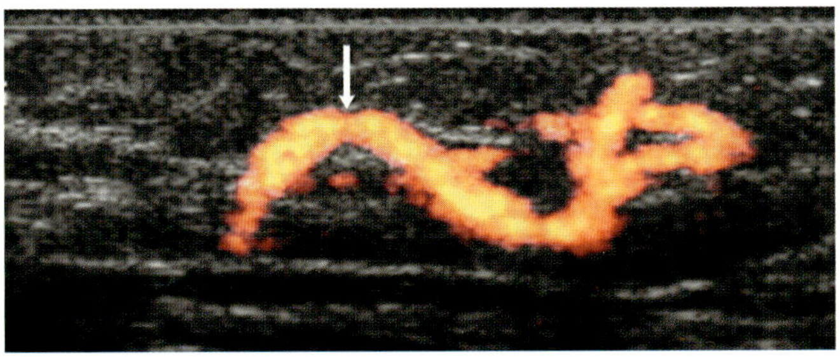

Color Plate 2-3D. Right radial breast sonogram: Color Doppler examination of the palpable lumps demonstrates that the lumps are due to the lateral blood vessels of the breast. Each lump corresponds to the superficial curve of the blood vessel (arrow). See figure 2-3D, page 24.

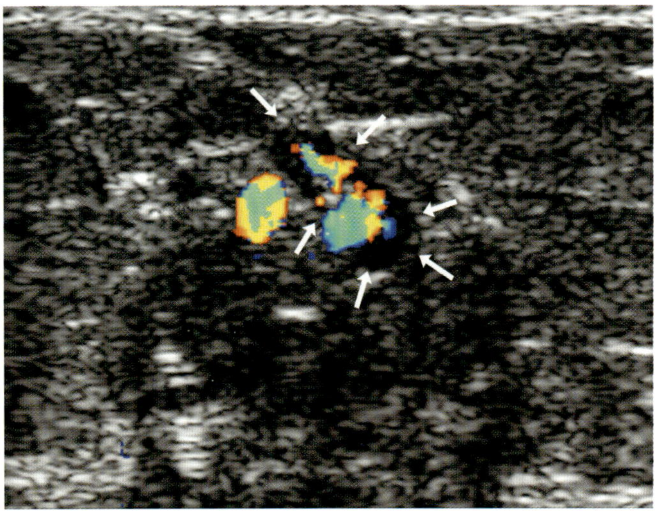

Color Plate 18-4. Left antiradial color Doppler breast sonogram: Color flow high-frequency images confirm the normal pattern of blood flow through the center of the lymph node (arrows). See figure 18-4, page 73.

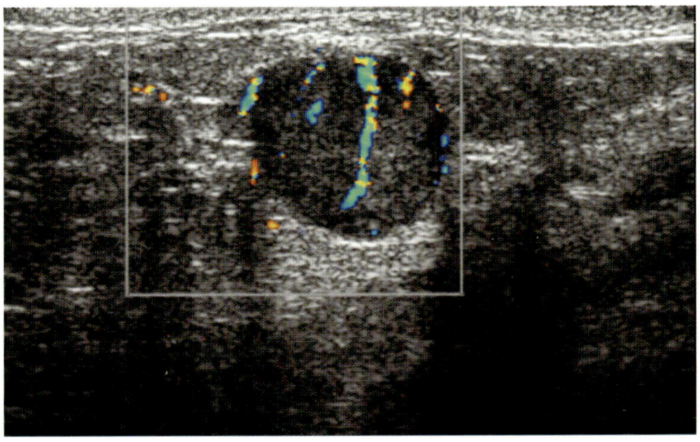

Color Plate 32-3. Left antiradial color Doppler breast sonogram: Color Doppler demonstrates blood flow throughout the mass indicating that this nodule is solid. See figure 32-3, page 104.

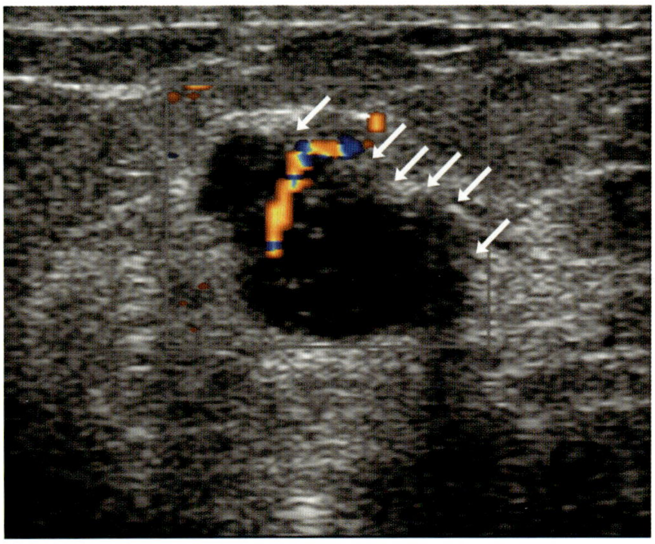

Color Plate 37-2. Left transverse color Doppler breast sonogram: At the 12:00 position, there is a lobulated multicystic mass. The septations within the mass have color flow and the edge of the mass consists of solid tissue that forms an ill-defined margin (arrows). See figure 37-2, page 116.

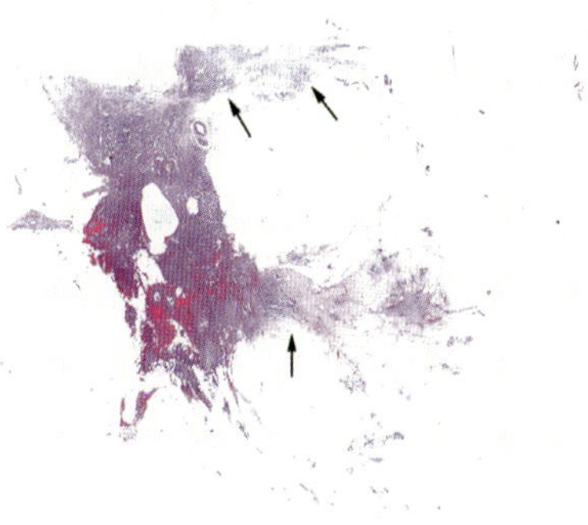

Color Plate 53-4. Low-power microscopic image of the malignancy demonstrates direct infiltration of tumor cells creating spiculation (arrows). See figure 53-4, page 157.

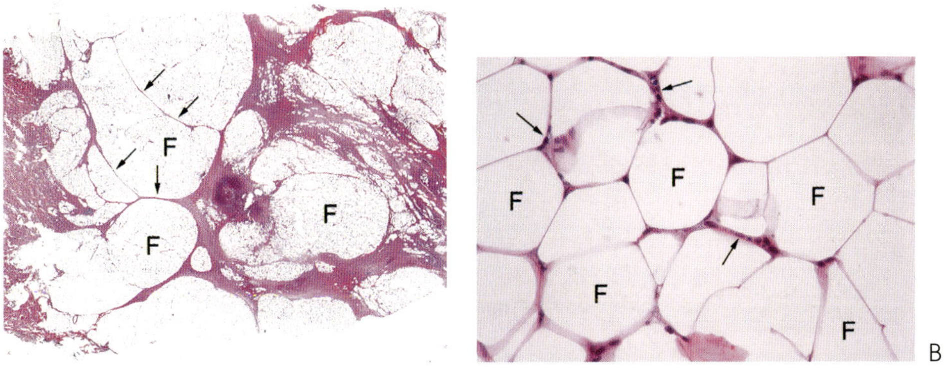

Color Plate 56-3A and B. Surgical specimen demonstrates that the malignant cells infiltrate the normal breast tissues without distorting the structure of the tissues. Normal fat cells (F) are distributed between thin collumns (arrows) of malignant cells and produce the low-density mammographic mass. (A) Low-power microscopic view. (B) High-power microscopic view. See figure 56-3, page 166.

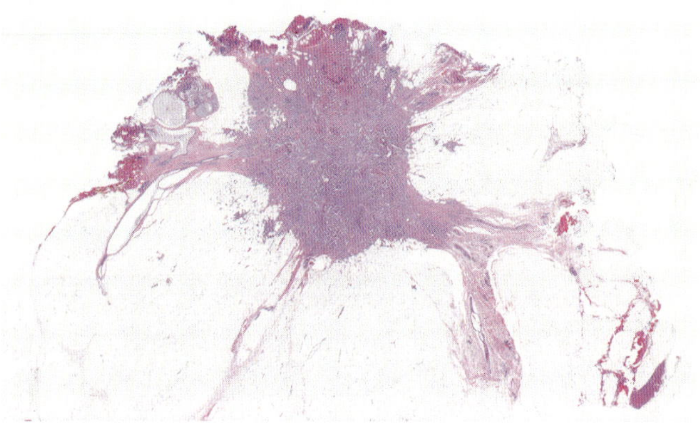

Color Plate 60-3. Low-power microscopic image: The irregular shape of the pathologic specimen corresponds to the mammographic spiculated mass. See figure 60-3, page 177.

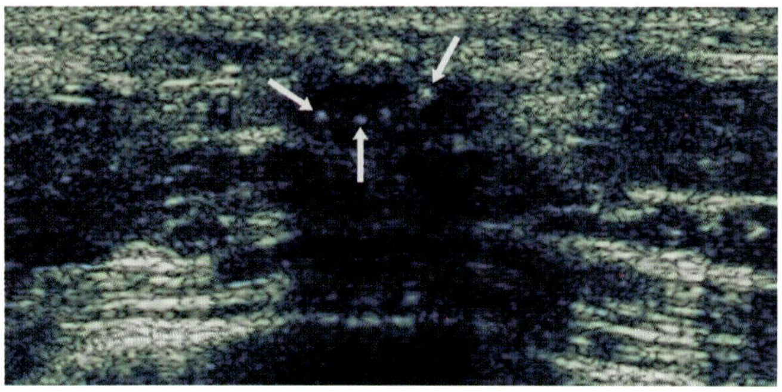

Color Plate 76-2. Right antiradial breast sonogram: In area of the lumpectomy scar, the sonographic findings include architectural distortion of the superficial tissue lines, calcifications (arrows), and an irregular hypoechoic mass with posterior acoustic shadowing. See figure 76-2, page 215.

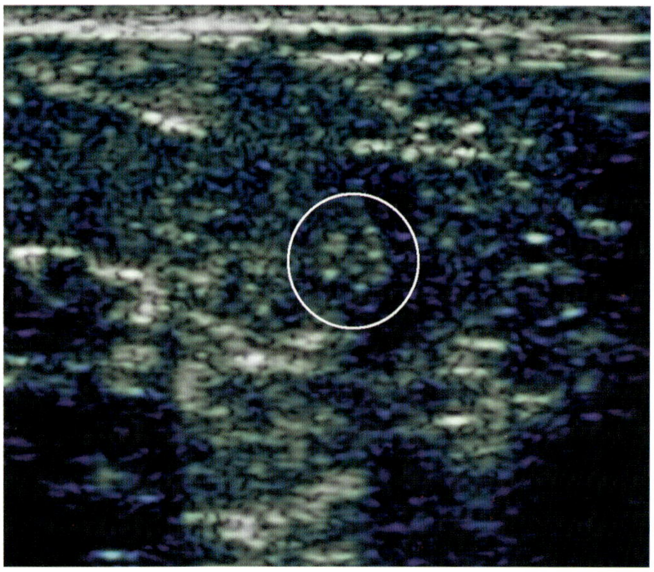

Color Plate 82-2. Left antiradial breast sonogram: The mammographic calcifications identified in Figures 82-1A and 1B correspond to a group of high acoustic intensity foci (circled). Sonographically, this group of calcifications were grouped in a cylindrical pattern that matched the linear pattern of the mammogram. No associated abnormal ducts or masses were present. See figure 82-2, page 228.

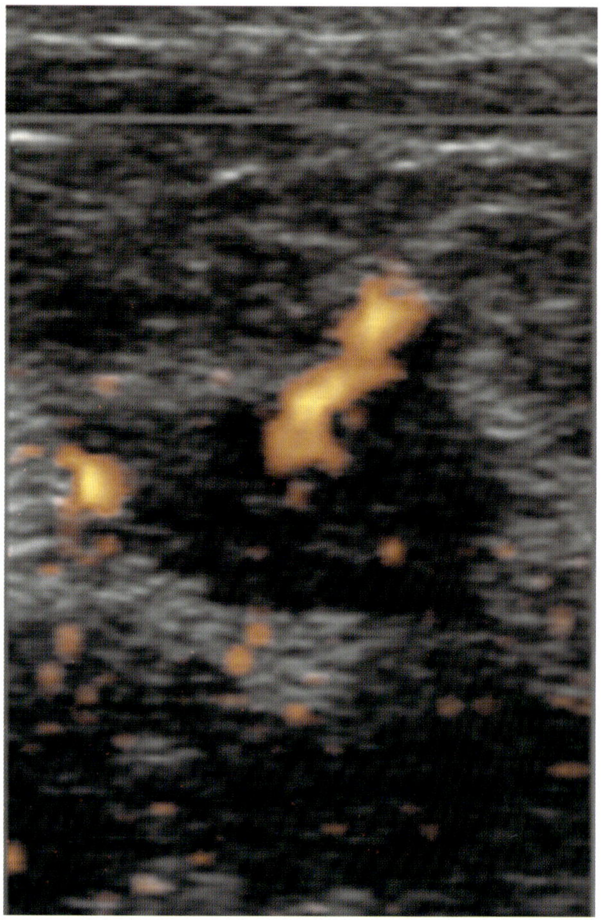

Color Plate 61-3. Left radial color Doppler breast sonogram: A second palpable lump corresponds to this smaller, irregular, spiculated mass, which is a satellite lesion of the dominant mass in Figure 61-2. See figure 61-3, page 180.

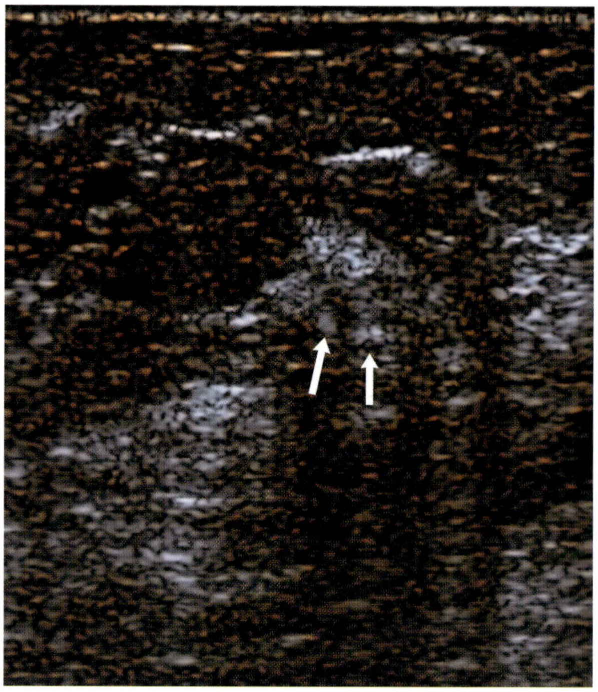

Color Plate 88-2. Right radial breast sonogram: The calcifications (arrows) identified in Figure 88-1 were localized sonographically. Lower-frequency sonography is generally more helpful when the breast tissue is extremely attenuating. In this case of fibroadenomatous hyperplasia, the lower frequency demonstrates that there is no mass in the area of the calcifications. Only benign-appearing hyperechoic tissue is present. See figure 88-2, page 241.

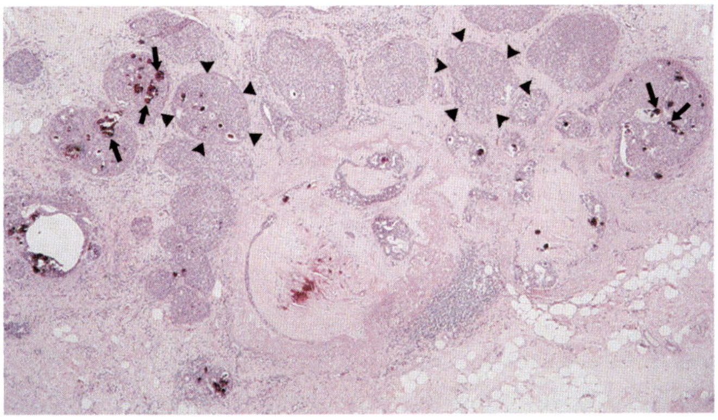

Color Plate 92-3. The lobules (arrowheads) are filled with malignant cells and calcifications (arrows). This type of malignant calcification results in a nonlinear pattern that is more typical of low-grade ductal carcinoma in situ. See figure 92-3, page 250.

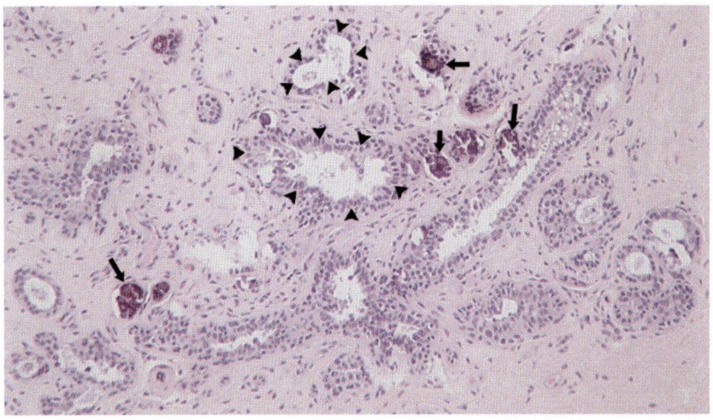

Color Plate 92-4. This is a different patient with calcifications (arrows) within normal lobules (arrowheads). Unless the calcifications are well defined, round, and have smooth borders, this type of nonlinear cluster of calcifications may be difficult to differentiate from the malignant cluster in Figure 92-3. See figure 92-4, page 250.

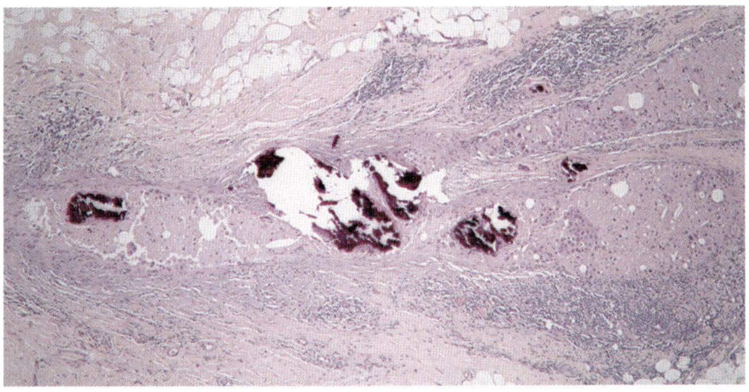

Color Plate 108-3. This malignancy is associated with extensive intraductal calcifications. The intraductal location of these calcifications results in the mammographically visible linear pattern. See figure 108-3, page 285.

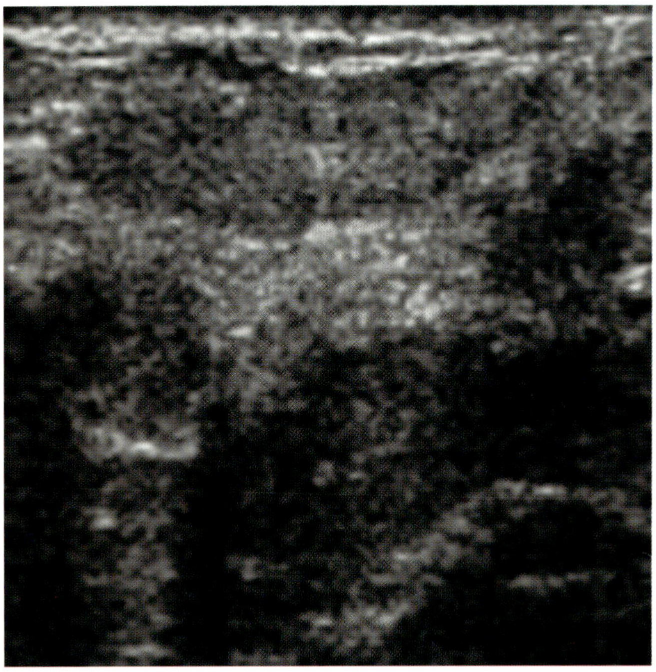

Color Plate 122-2. Right antiradial breast sonogram: No sonographic mass is identified in the area of the mammographic architectural distortion. Only normal hyperechoic tissue is present. See figure 122-2, page 327.

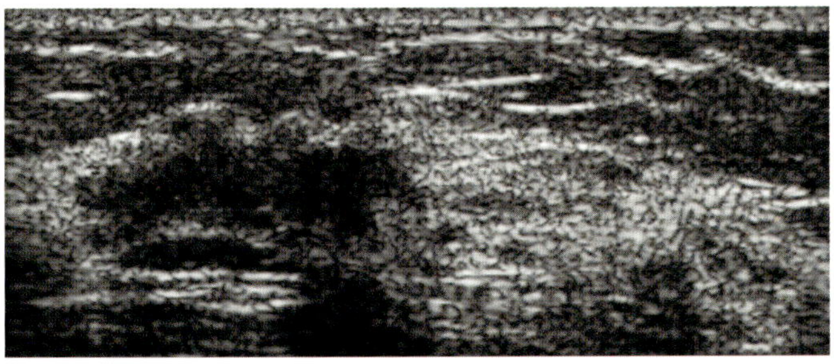

Color Plate 123-2. Right radial breast sonogram: In the upper outer quadrant, the mammographic architectural distortion corre sponds to an irregular hypoechoic mass. See figure 123-2, page 330.

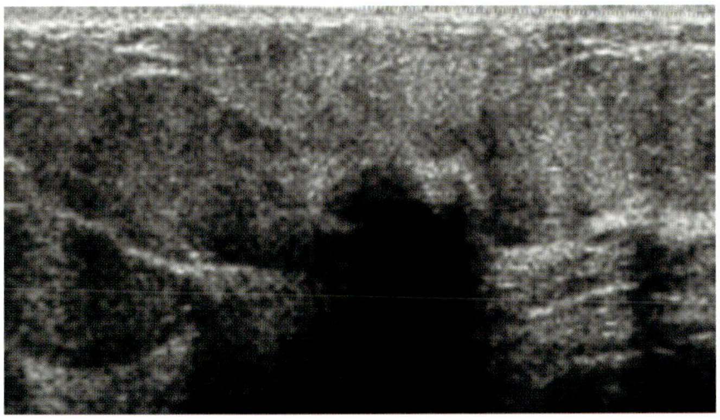

Color Plate 124-2. Right radial breast sonogram: The mammographic mass corresponds to a hypoechoic mass with severe shadowing. See figure 124-2, page 332.

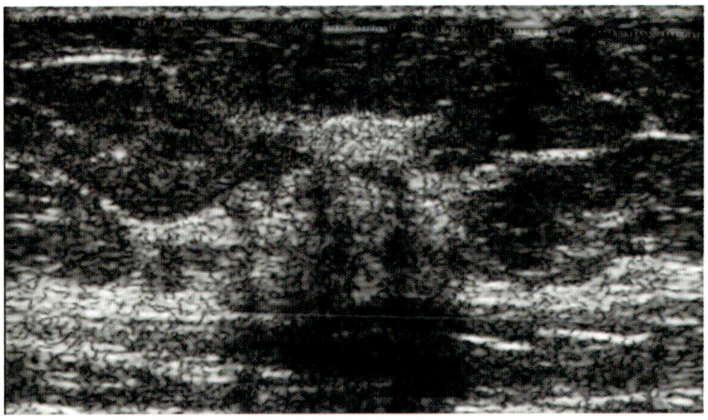

Color Plate 125-2. Right antiradial breast sonogram: The mammographic architectural distortion corresponds to an irregular, predominately hyperechoic mass with irregular shadowing. See figure 125-2, page 334.

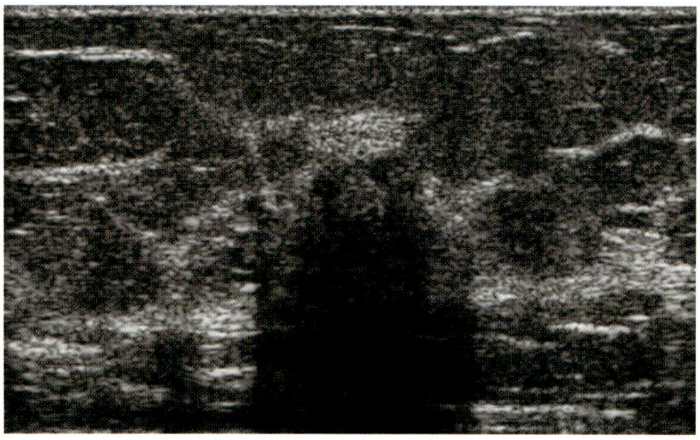

Color Plate 125-3. Right antiradial breast sonogram: With a higher frequency, the mass identified in Figure 125-2 appears as a focal area of severe acoustic shadowing. *See figure 125-3, page 334.*

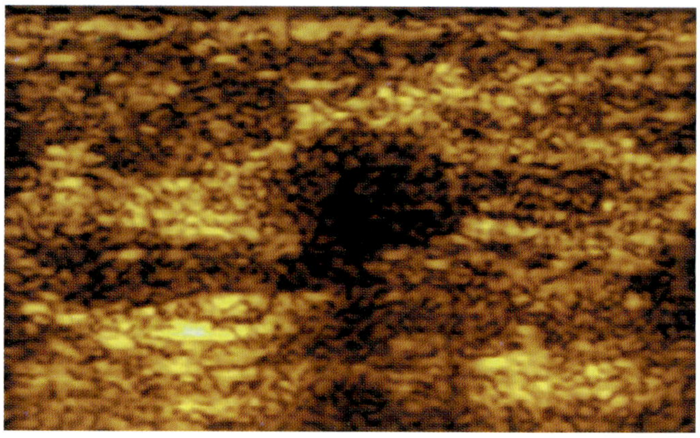

Color Plate 126-2. Right radial breast sonogram: The ill-defined mass identified in Figures 126-1A and 126-1C corresponds to an ill-defined hypoechoic solid mass with posterior acoustic shadowing. *See figure 126-2, page 337.*

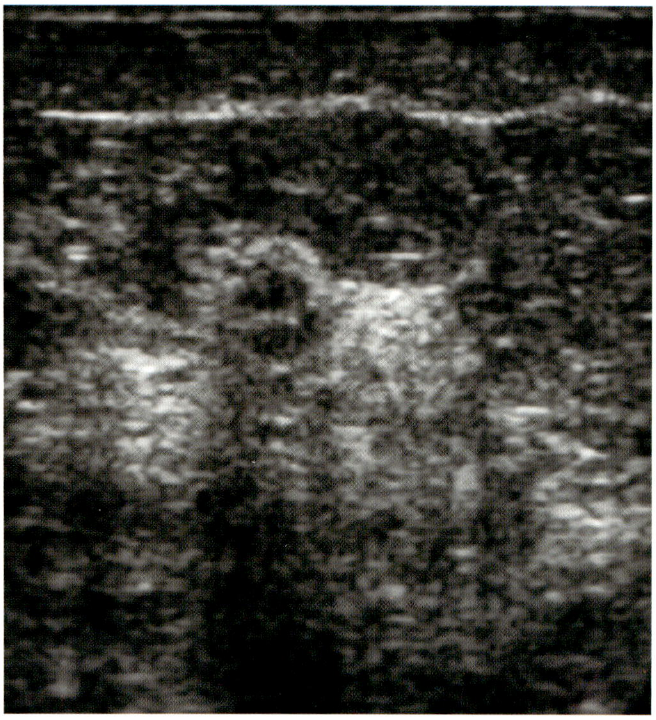

Color Plate 127-2. Right antiradial breast sonogram: With lower frequency, the mammographic architectural distortion is an irregular hypoechoic mass with posterior acoustic shadowing. *See figure 127-2, page 339.*

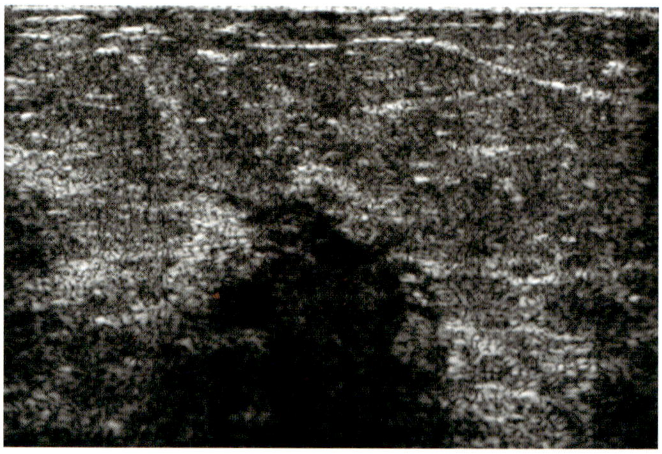

Color Plate 127-3. Right antiradial breast sonogram: Higher-frequency examination produces extensive shadowing. The mass identified in Figure 127-2 is hidden in the area of shadowing. *See figure 127-3, page 340.*

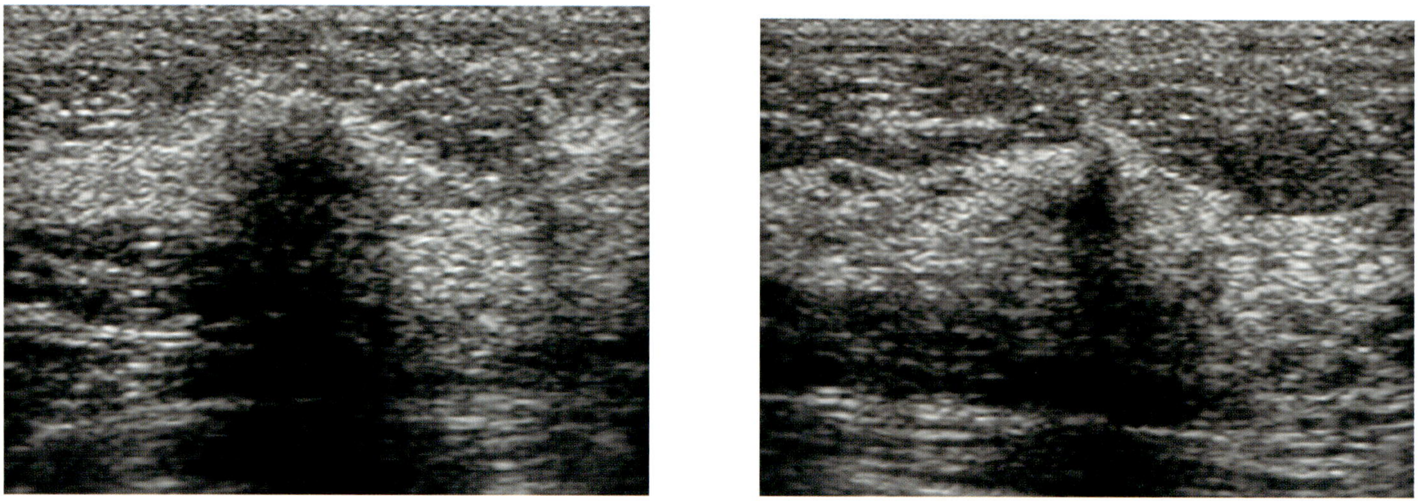

A B

Color Plate 128-2A and B. In the left upper outer quadrant, the mammographic architectural distortion corresponds to a lesion exhibiting severe shadowing. The lesion appears wide in the radial view (A) and narrow in the antiradial view (B). This extreme discrepancy in appearance is characteristic of either posttraumatic or radial scars. (A). Left radial breast sonogram. (B). Left antiradial breast sonogram. *See figure 128-2, page 342.*

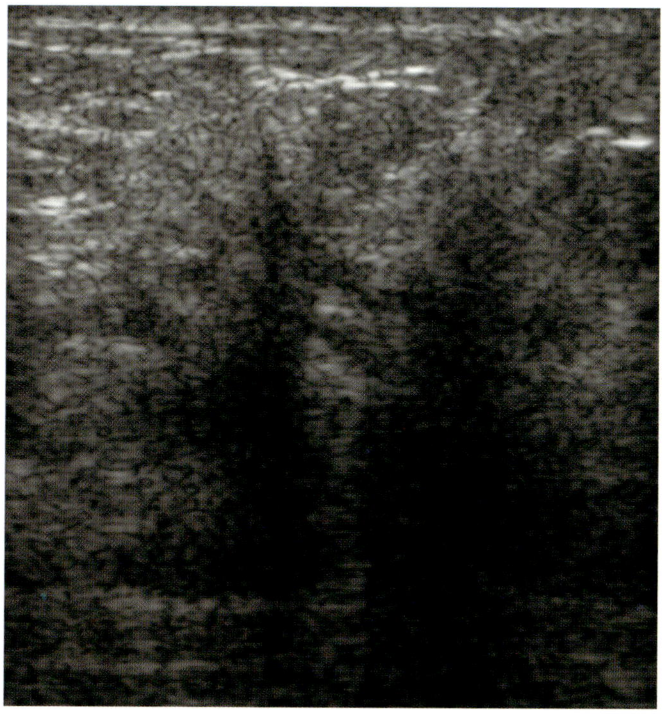

Color Plate 129-2. Left radial breast sonogram: The palpable lump in the upper outer quadrant is an ill-defined irregular hypoechoic solid mass. This mass corresponds to the spiculated mass on the left breast mammogram (Fig. 129-1). See figure 129-2, page 344.

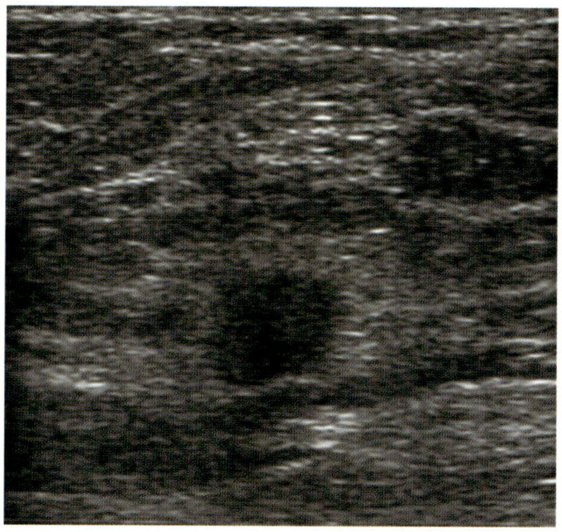

Color Plate 132-2. Right breast radial sonogram: The mammographic mass in Figure 132-1 corresponds to an ill-defined hypoechoic nodule with posterior acoustic shadowing. See figure 132-2, page 350.

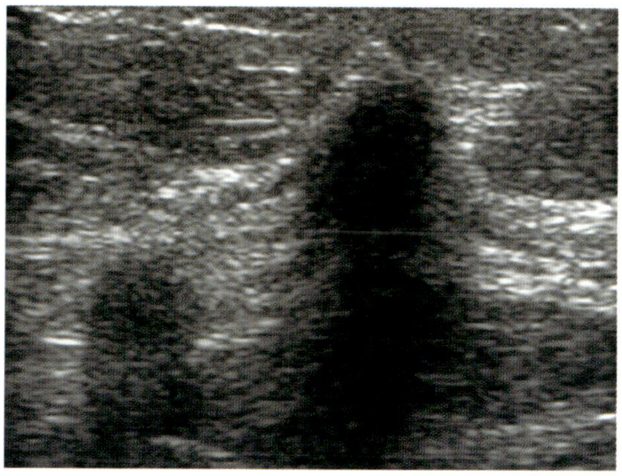

Color Plate 135-2. Right radial breast sonogram: In the upper breast, two hypoechoic, irregular shadowing masses are present. The larger mass is palpable. These masses correspond to the mammographic masses. See figure 135-2, page 357.

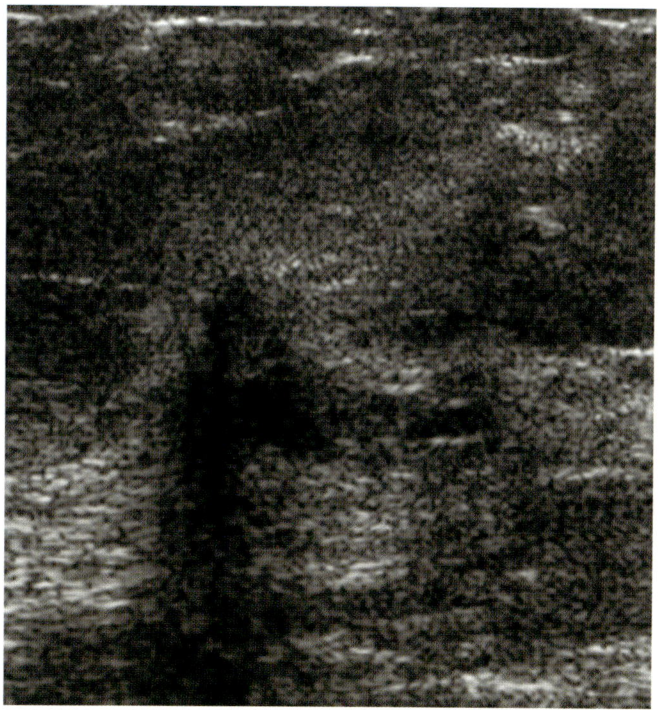

Color Plate 130-2. Right radial breast sonogram: In the right upper outer quadrant, there is an irregular hypoechoic mass that corresponds to the architectural distortion identified on Figure 130-1A. See figure 130-2, page 346.

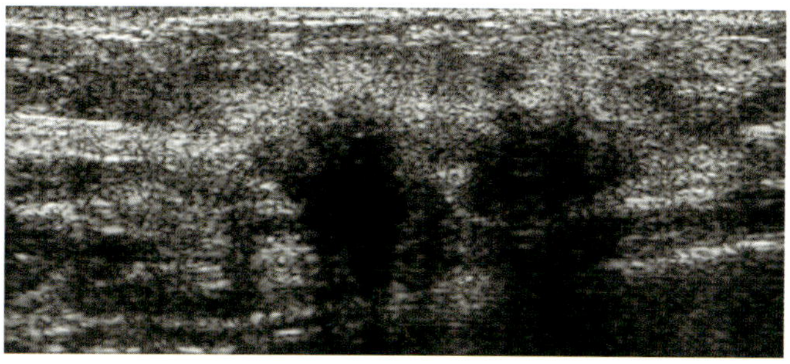

Color Plate 134-2. Left radial breast sonogram: The palpable lump is associated with a multilobulated, irregular, hypoechoic mass. This abnormality corresponds to the mammographic mass identified in Figure 134-1. See figure 134-2, page 354.

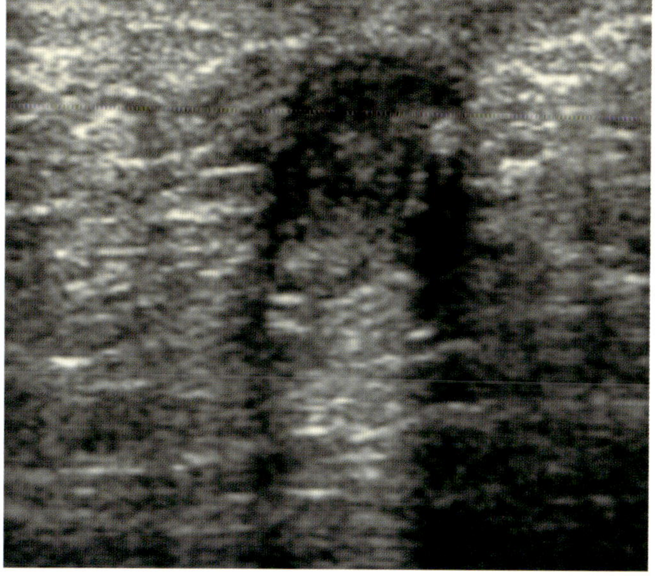

Color Plate 136-2. Left transverse breast sonogram: Under the nipple, there is a hypoechoic, well-defined fluid collection with mild posterior acoustic enhancement. See figure 136-2, page 361.

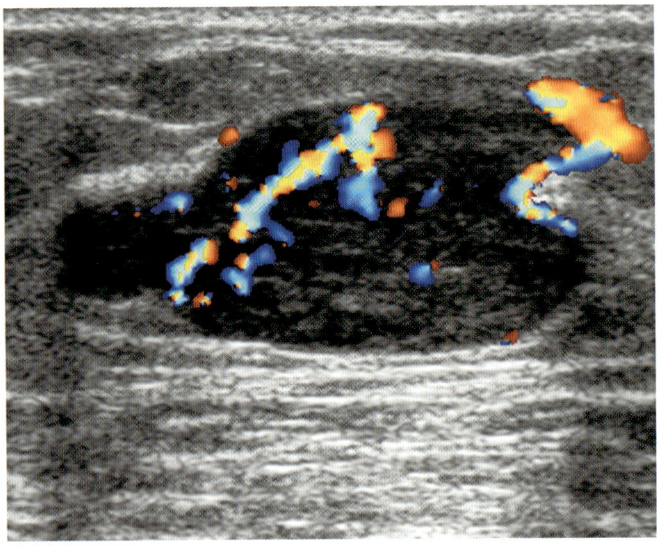

Color Plate 145–2B. The palpable firmness in the right upper outer quadrant corresponded to a well-defined, lobulated, hypoechoic mass. Right radial color Doppler breast sonogram. See figure 145–2, page 379.

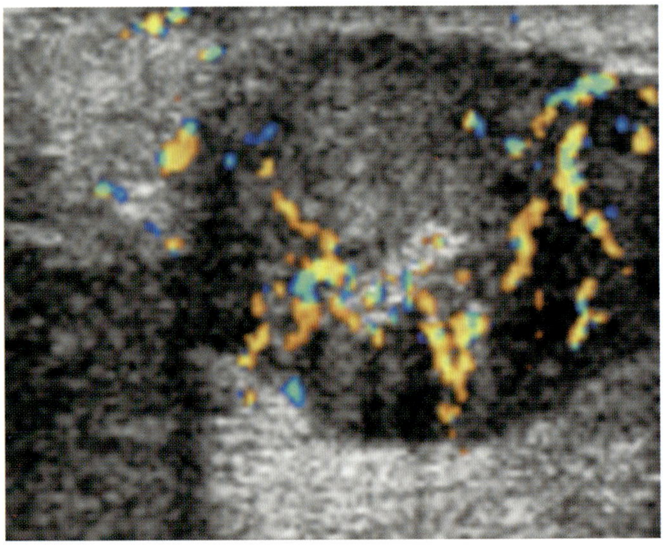

Color Plate 149–2B. In the right subareolar area, there is an oval, hypoechoic solid mass with calcifications. Although the margins are generally well defined, there is mild irregularity of the contour of the mass. Right radial color Doppler breast sonogram. See figure 149–2, page 388.

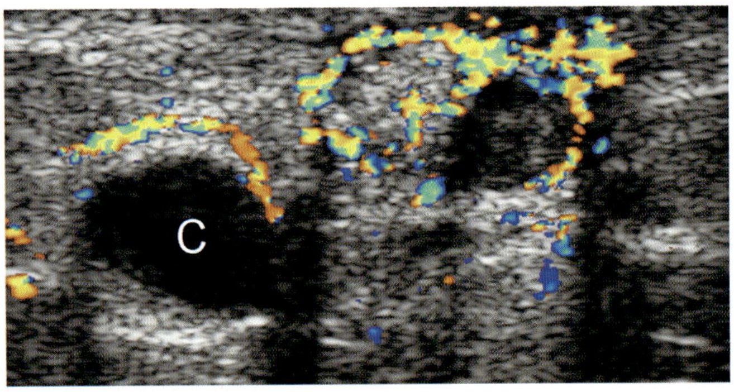

Color Plate 150–2B. The mammographic mass corresponds to an oval mass with heterogenous echogenicity. The mass has calcifications and is asymmetrically bordered by a cyst (C). Right transverse color doppler sonogram. See figure 150–2, page 391.

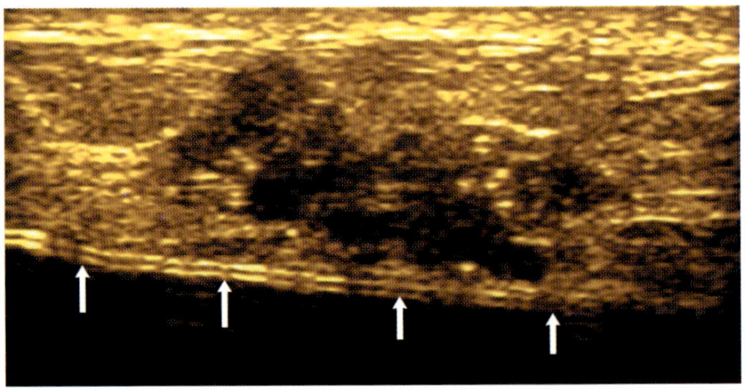

Color Plate 169–2. Left radial breast sonogram: The mammographic spiculated density and palpable mass correspond to an irregular hypoechoic mass with calcifications. With the lower frequency the mass does not shadow. No second mass is identified. Implant shell (arrows). See figure 169–2, page 434.

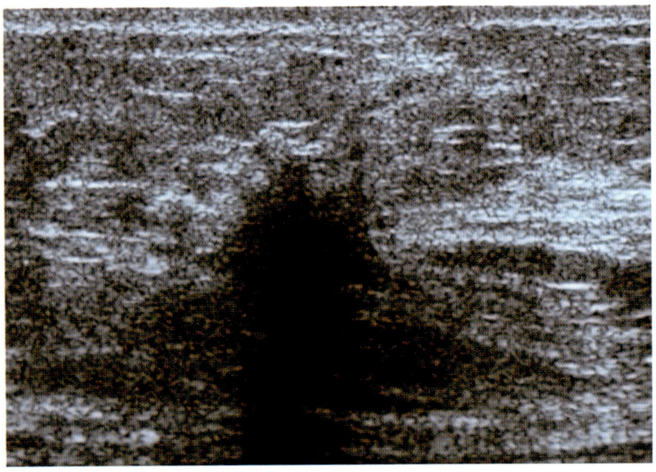

Color Plate 177–3. Right breast radial sonogram: With lower-frequency sonography, the lumpectomy site still exhibits an irregular, hypoechoic solid mass. See figure 177–3, page 453.

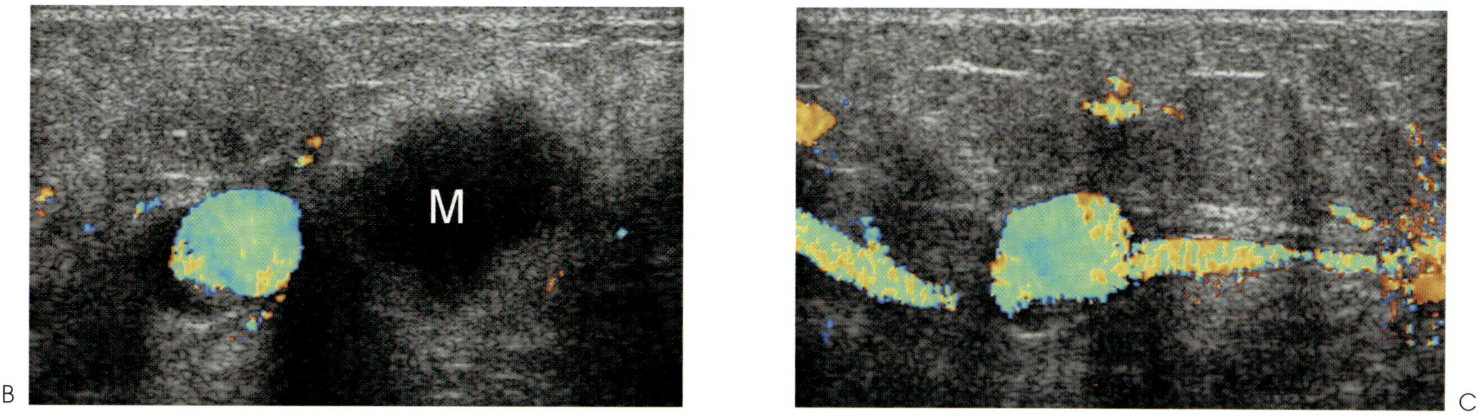

Color Plate 182-2B and C. *In the left upper outer quadrant, there was an ill-defined hypoechoic mass (M) that corresponded to the tumor (B). Adjacent to the tumor was an oval fluid collection, which was predominately anechoic except for its hypoechoic inferior rim (A). Color Doppler demonstrates that the hypoechoic lesion is filled with high-velocity swirling bloodflow characteristic of a pseudoaneurysm. (B). Left antiradial color Doppler breast sonogram: Pseudoaneurysm next to mass (M). (C). Left antiradial color Doppler breast sonogram: Pseudoaneurysm with feeding and draining vessels. See figure 182-2, page 466.*

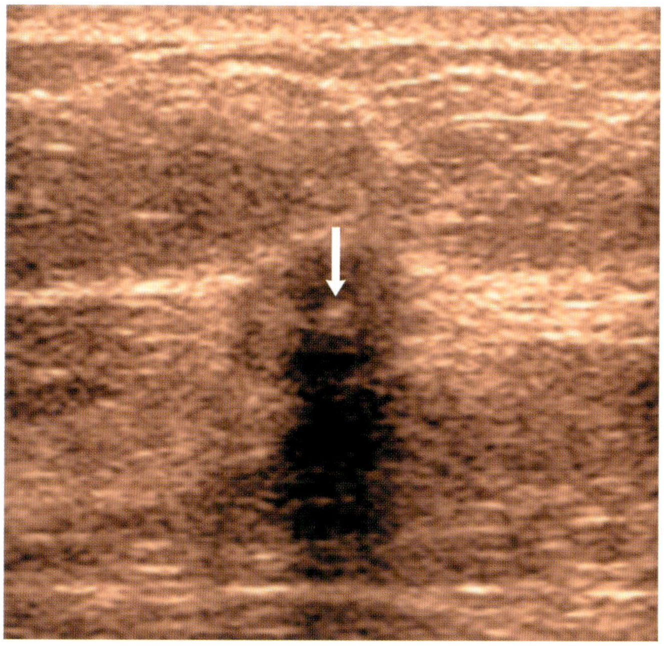

Color Plate 185-4. *Left transverse breast sonogram: At the 11:00 position, there is a hypoechoic ill-defined mass that corresponds to the mammographic lesion 1. In the center of the mass is a hyperechoic focus, which is a clip (arrow). See figure 185-4, page 473.*

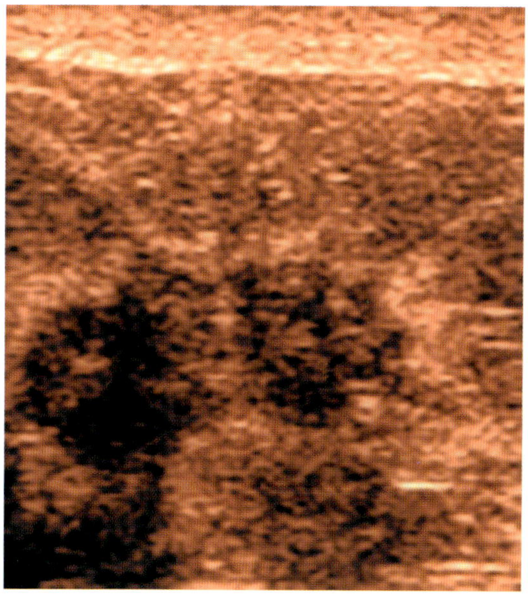

Color Plate 185-5. *Left transverse breast sonogram: In the subareolar area there is a hypoechoic, ill-defined lobular mass that corresponds to the mammographic lesion 2. See figure 185-5, page 473.*

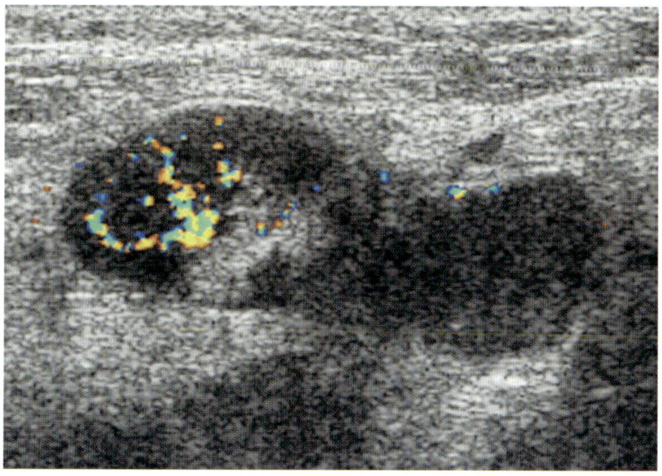

Color Plate 187-3. *Right longitudinal color Doppler breast sonogram: The palpable right axillary node exhibits abnormal architecture. The hilum is located in an asymmetric position compared to the nodal mass. See figure 187-3, page 479.*

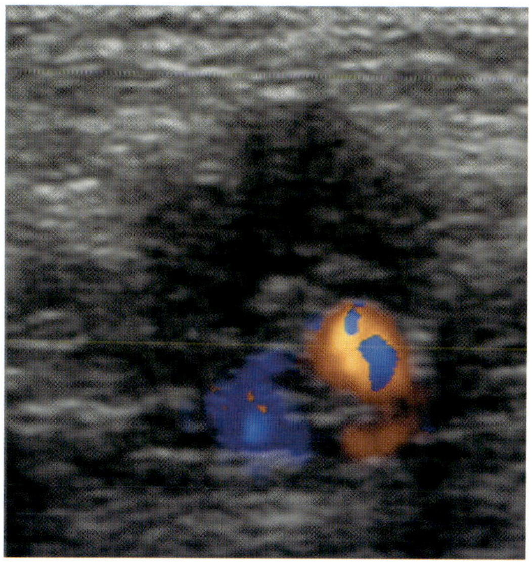

Color Plate 188-1B. *The palpable lump corresponds to a lobulated hypoechoic mass. Right radial color Doppler breast sonogram. See figure 188-1, page 482.*

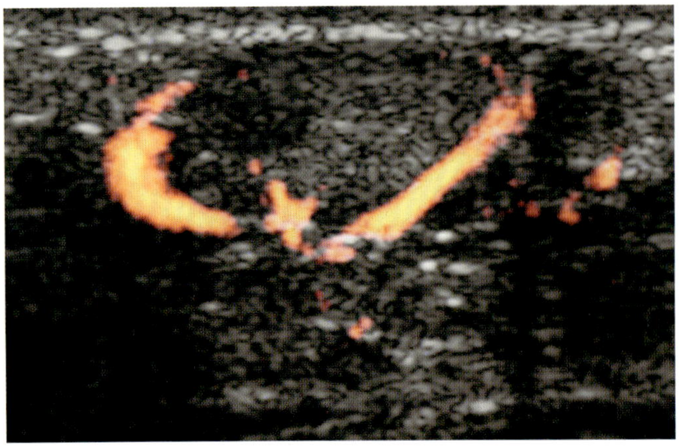

Color Plate 191–1C. The palpable lump corresponds to an well-defined, oval mass with heterogeneous echogencity. Right antiradial color power Doppler breast sonogram. See figure 191–1, page 489.

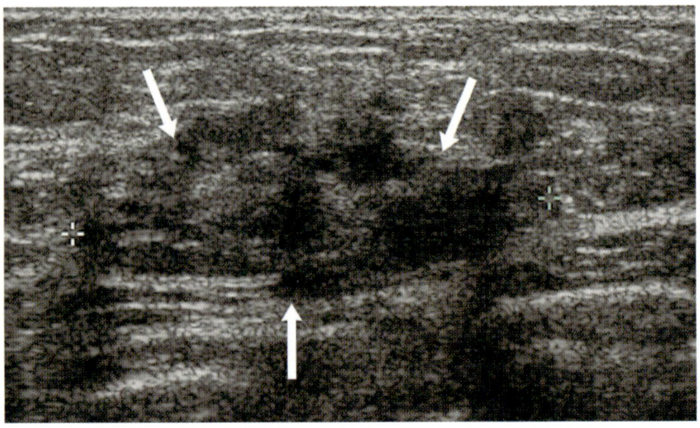

Color Plate 194–2. Left radial breast sonogram: The palpable thickening corresponded to an area of ill-defined hypoechogenicity (arrows). See figure 194–2, page 496.

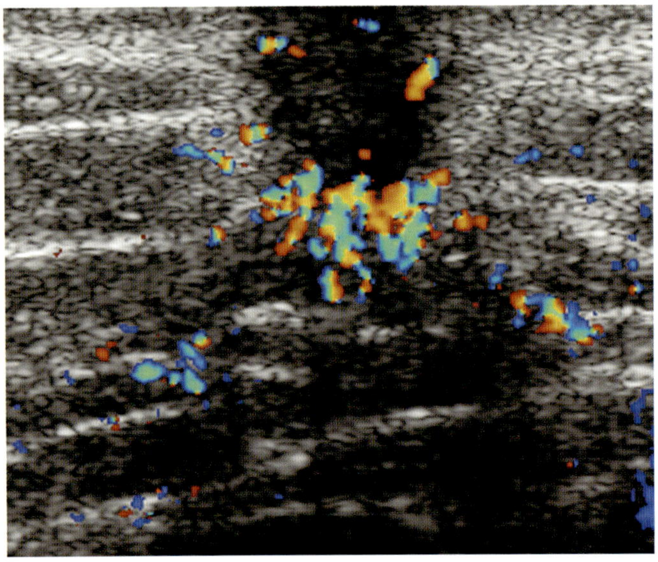

Color Plate 196–2B. The palpable mass corresponds to an irregular, hypoechoic mass. The mass extends into the hyperechoic skin. Right radial color Doppler breast sonogram. See figure 196–2, page 500.

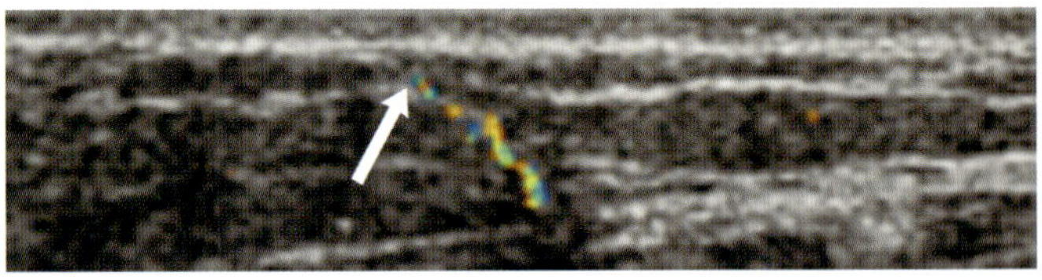

Color Plate 197–2. Left oblique breast color Doppler sonogram: The palpable lump corresponds to a Cooper's ligament attachment (arrow). See figure 197–2, page 502.

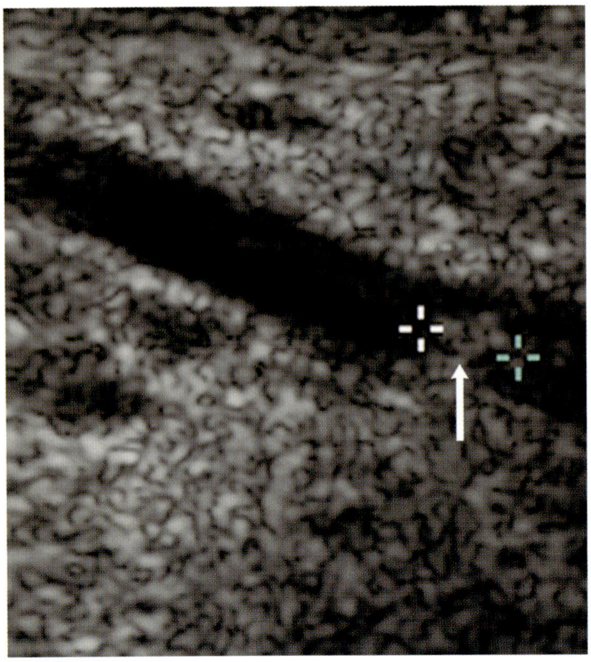

Color Plate 204–2. Right radial breast sonogram: At the 6:00 position of the nipple, there is a dilated duct. Within the duct is a small solid hypoechoic mass (arrow). See figure 204–2, page 517.

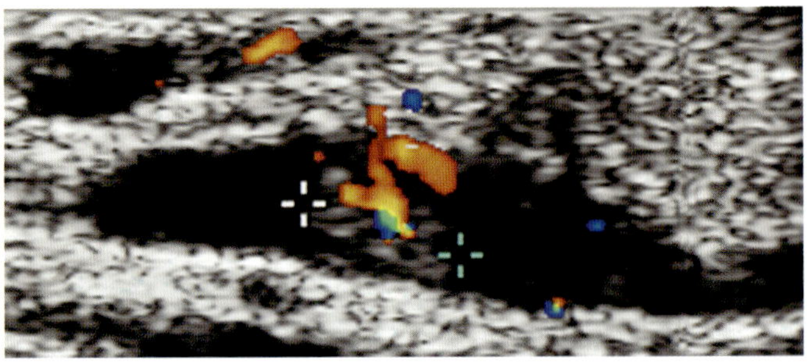

Color Plate 206–2C. At the 4:00 position of the left breast, there is a dilated duct containing a hypoechoic sausage-shaped solid mass. Left oblique color Doppler breast sonogram: Color Doppler demonstrates vessels within the mass. See figure 206–2, page 521.

Case 93

Case History

A 43-year-old woman initially presented at an outside institution with a pea-sized palpable mass near the right nipple and calcifications on her mammogram. The mass was biopsied at the outside institution.

Physical Examination

- right breast: biopsy ecchymosis near right nipple; original nodule no longer detectable
- left breast: normal exam

Mammogram

Calcifications (Fig. 93-1)

- type: amorphous/indistinct
- distribution: grouped/clustered

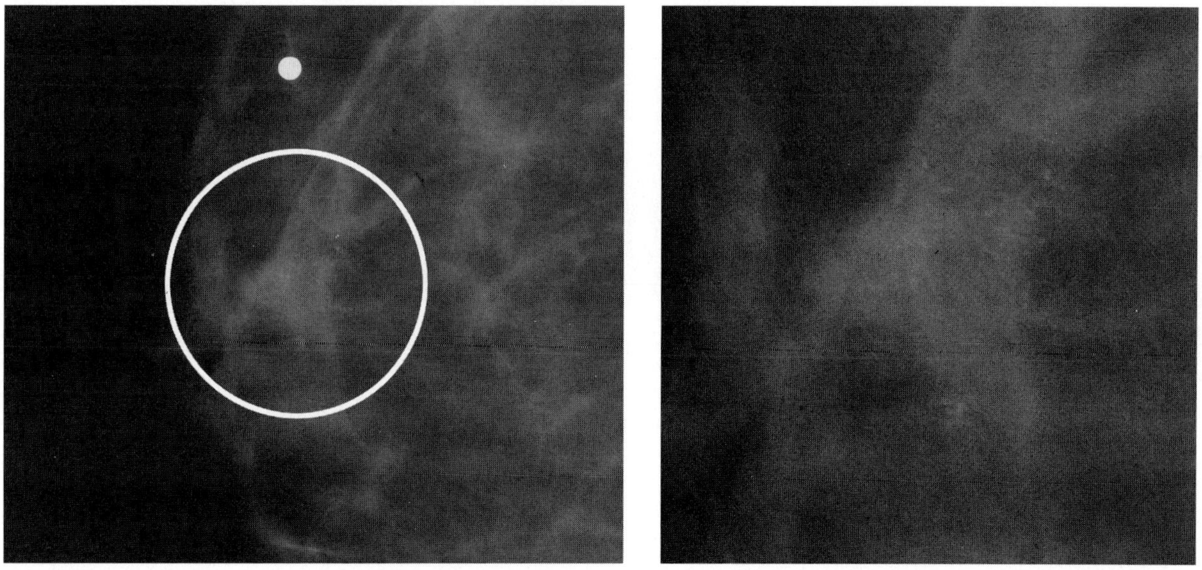

Figure 93-1. Right ML magnification mammogram: In the subareolar region there is a palpable lump marked by a radiopaque marker. The lump is associated with a cluster of amorphous calcifications (circled).

Ultrasound

Frequency

- 13 MHz

Mass

- margin: ill defined
- echogenicity: hypoechoic
- retrotumoral acoustic appearance: severe shadowing, mass completely obscured
- shape: irregular (Figs. 93-2 and 93-3)

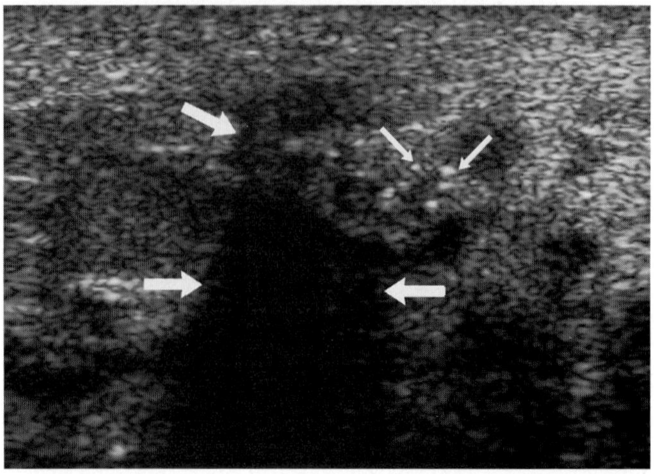

Figure 93-2. Right longitudinal breast sonogram: Associated with the subareolar calcifications (identified in Fig. 93-1) is a hypoechoic mass (large arrows) with severe shadowing. Some calcifications (small arrows) are associated with the mass.

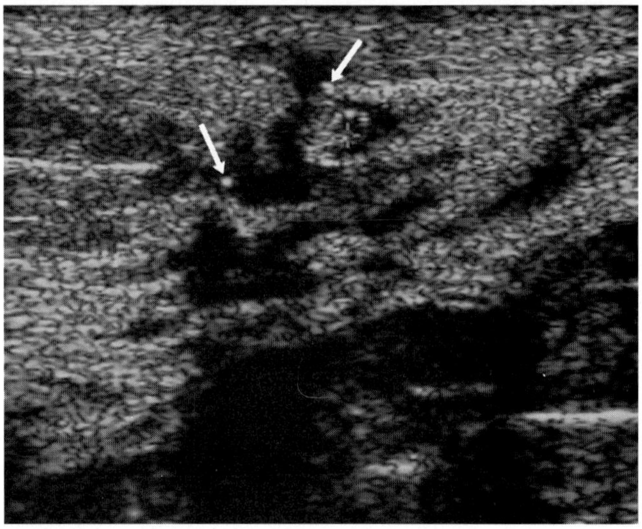

Figure 93-3. Right transverse breast sonogram: Adjacent to the subareolar mass in Figure 93-2 are abnormally dilated ducts with calcifications (arrows).

Pathology

Invasive ductal carcinoma with a predominant intraductal component. Final excisional specimen demonstrated 1 cm invasive ductal carcinoma with extensive intraductal component.

Management

- BI-RADS Assessment Category 4, suspicious abnormality; biopsy should be considered.

Pearls and Pitfalls

1. The assessment of this case is based upon the suspicious appearance of the calcifications alone. If one included the malignant-appearing sonographic mass then the assessment would be Category 5, highly suggestive of malignancy.
2. Because the site of the mass and calcifications were readily identifiable sonographically, the location of the lesion was marked on the skin sonographically. This site was reconfirmed intraoperatively and the surgeon made a direct incision into the lesion without preoperative wire localization.

Suggested Readings

1. Leucht D, Madjar H. Microcalcification in sonography. In: Leucht D, ed. *Teaching Atlas of Breast Ultrasound.* New York: Thieme; 1996:189-204.
2. Rickard MT. Ultrasound of malignant breast microcalcifications: role in evaluation and guided procedures. *Australas Radiol* 1996;40:26-31.
3. Yang WT, Suen M, Ahuja A, et al. In vivo demonstration of microcalcification in breast cancer using high resolution ultrasound. *Br J Radiol* 1997;70:685-690.

Case 94

Case History

A 46-year-old woman presents for her baseline mammogram.

Physical Examination

- normal exam

Mammogram

Calcifications (Fig. 94-1)

- type: amorphous/indistinct
- distribution: grouped/clustered

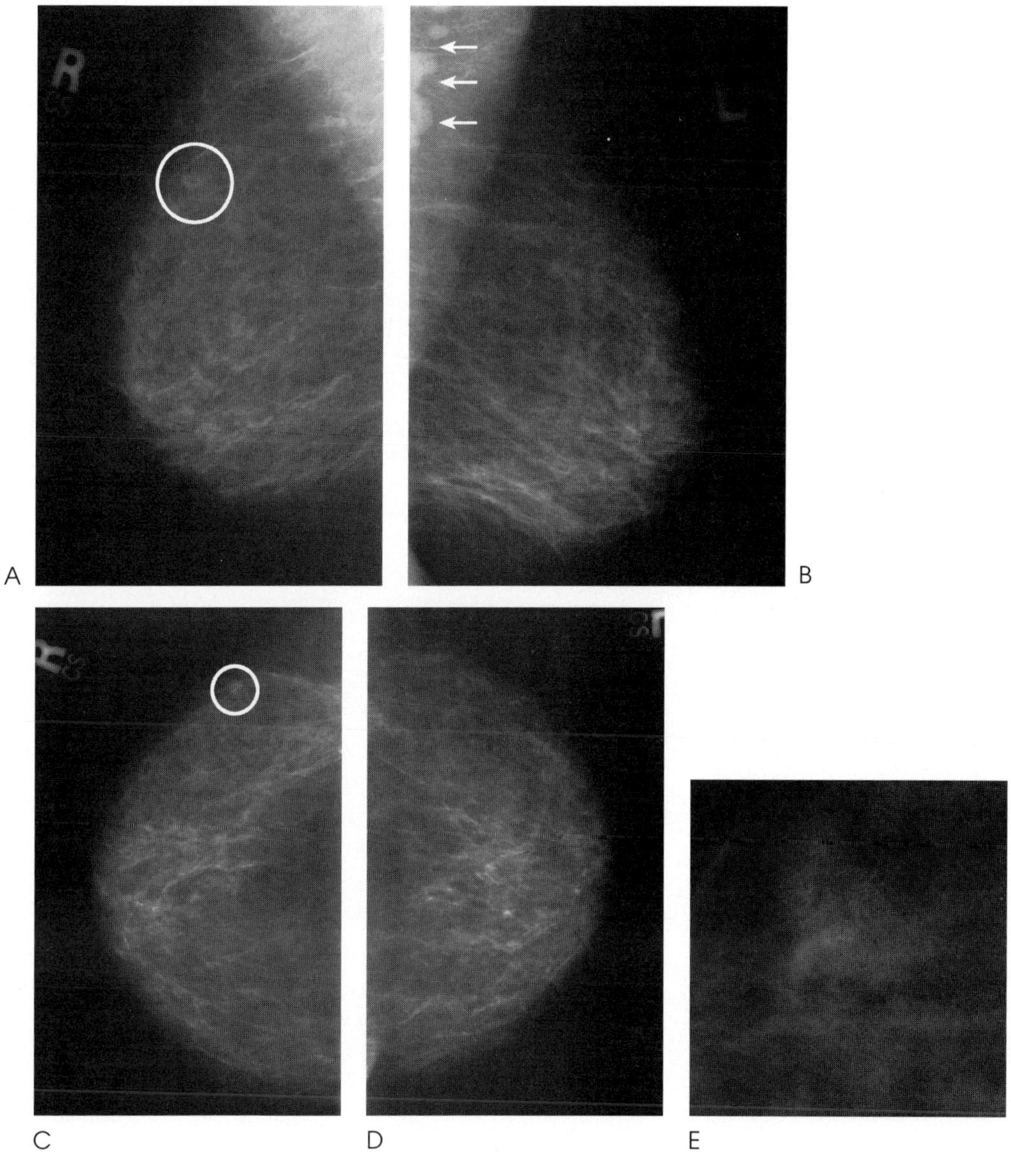

Figure 94-1. In the right upper outer breast, there is a 9 mm nodular density containing numerous amorphous microcalcifications (circle). In the left breast, there are multiple axillary nodes (arrows), which exhibit amorphous microcalcifications that are identical to the right breast nodule. (A). Right MLO mammogram. (B). Left MLO mammogram. (C). Right CC mammogram. (D). Left CC mammogram. (E). Right MLO magnification mammogram.

Pathology

Dermatopathic lymphangitis. The lymph node exhibits normal internal architecture, but there are many sinusoidal macrophages that contain melanin. The calcifications are associated with a giant foreign body reaction.

Management

- BI-RADS Assessment Category 4, suspicious; biopsy should be considered

Pearls and Pitfalls

Lymph nodes may be associated with amorphous or coarse calcifications in metastatic disease and granulomatous diseases such as histoplasmosis, tuberculosis, and sarcoidosis. In patients with rheumatoid arthritis, gold therapy may cause metallic deposition in the nodes, which simulate calcifications.

Suggested Readings

1. Aquel NM, Peters EE. Kikuchi's disease in axillary lymph nodes draining breast carcinoma. *Histolpathology* 2000;36:280–281.
2. Bassett LW, Jackson VP, Jahan R, Fu YS, Gold RH. *Diagnosis of Diseases of the Breast.* Philadelphia: WB Saunders; 1997:363–365.
3. Bruwer A, Nelson GW, Spark RP. Punctate intranodal gold deposits simulating microcalcifications on mammograms. *Radiology* 1987;16:87–88.
4. Chen SW, Bennett G, Price J. Axillary lymph nodes calcification due to metastatic papillary carcinoma. *Australasian Radiology* 1998;42:241–243.
5. Eisenkraft BL, Som PM. The spectrum of benign and malignant etiologies of cervical node calcification. *AJR* 1999;172:1433–1437.
6. Hooley R, Lee C, Tocino I, et. al. Calcifications in axillary lymph nodes caused by fat necrosis. *AJR* 1996;167:627–628.
7. Yang WT, Suen M, Metreweli C. Mammographic, sonographic and histopathological correlation of benign axillary masses. *Clin Radiol* 1997;52:130–135.

Case 95

Case History

A 44-year-old woman presents with new densities on her screening mammogram.

Physical Examination

- right breast: white Desitin cream
- left breast: normal exam

Mammogram

Calcifications (Figs. 95–1 and 95–2)

- type: pleomorphic/heterogeneous
- distribution: grouped/clustered

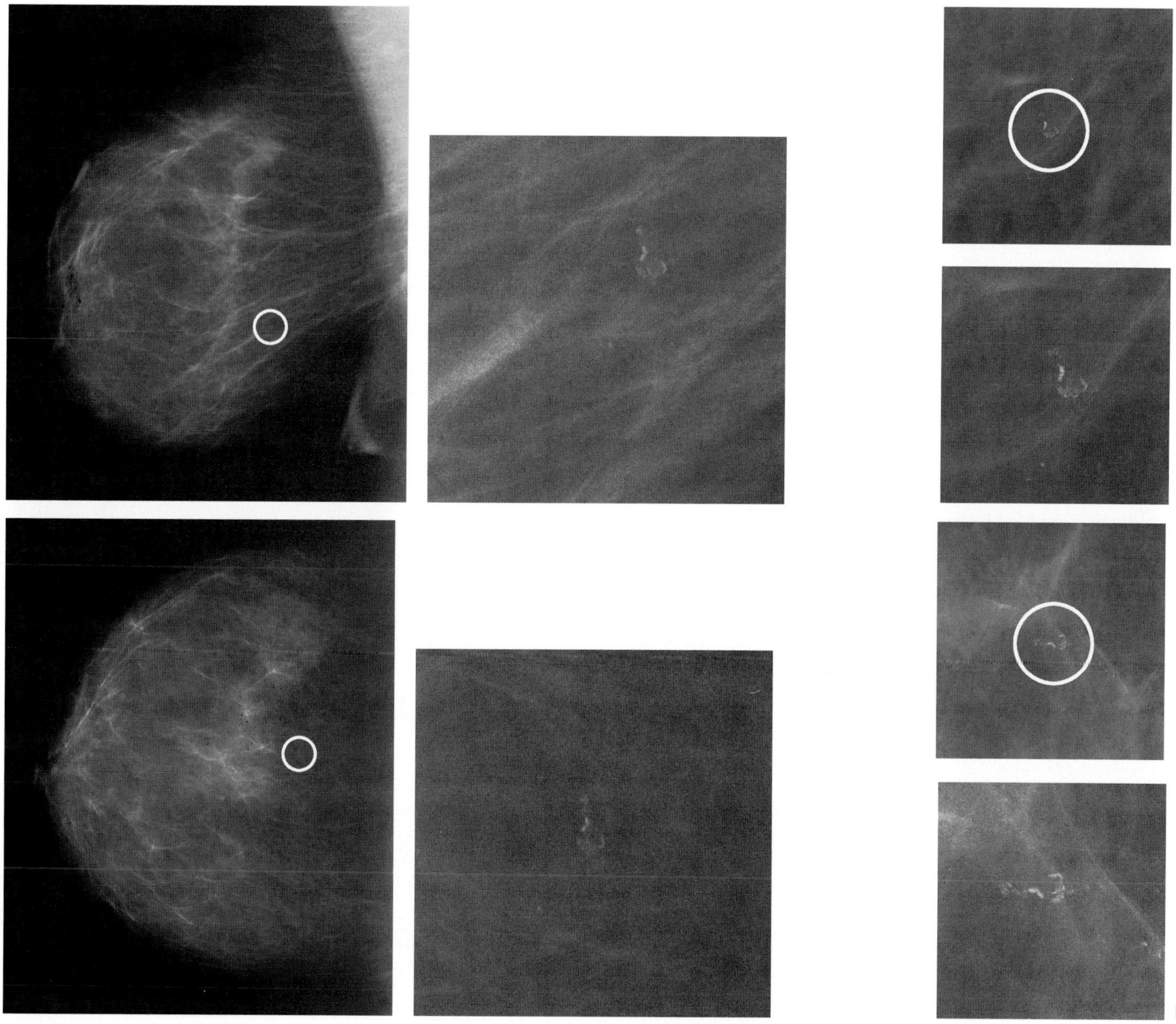

Figure 95–1. In the 6:00 position of the right breast there is a cluster of heterogeneous densities (circled). (A). Right MLO mammogram. (B). Right CC mammogram. (C). Right MLO spot magnification mammogram. (D). Right CC spot magnification mammogram.

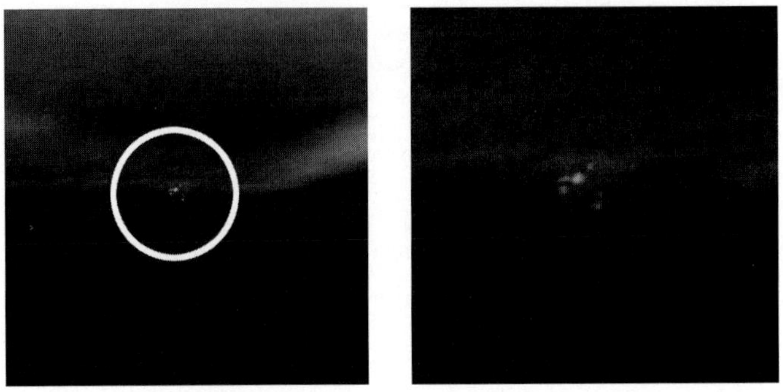

Figure 95-2. Right ML spot magnification mammogram: The heterogeneous densities are within the skin (circle).

Pathology

- Desitin ointment on skin

Management

- BI-RADS Assessment Category 2, benign finding

Pearls and Pitfalls

The cream could not be removed even after scrubbing with alcohol. She was advised to stop using the cream and return in 2 months. The mammogram 2 months later showed no abnormal densities. Skin powders and ointments may cause amorphous or heterogeneous densities, which are commonly faint, unusual in appearance, or only visible on one view.

Suggested Readings

1. Jackson VP, Jahan R, Fu YS. Benign breast lesions. In: Bassett LW, Jackson VP, Jahan R, Fu YS, Gold RH, eds. *Diagnosis of Diseases of the Breast.* Philadelphia: WB Saunders Company; 1997:357–443.

Case 96

Case History

A 68-year-old woman presents with increasing number of calcifications on her right breast screening mammogram.

Physical Examination

- normal exam

Mammogram

Calcifications (Fig. 96–1)

- type: pleomorphic/heterogeneous
- distribution: grouped/clustered

A

B

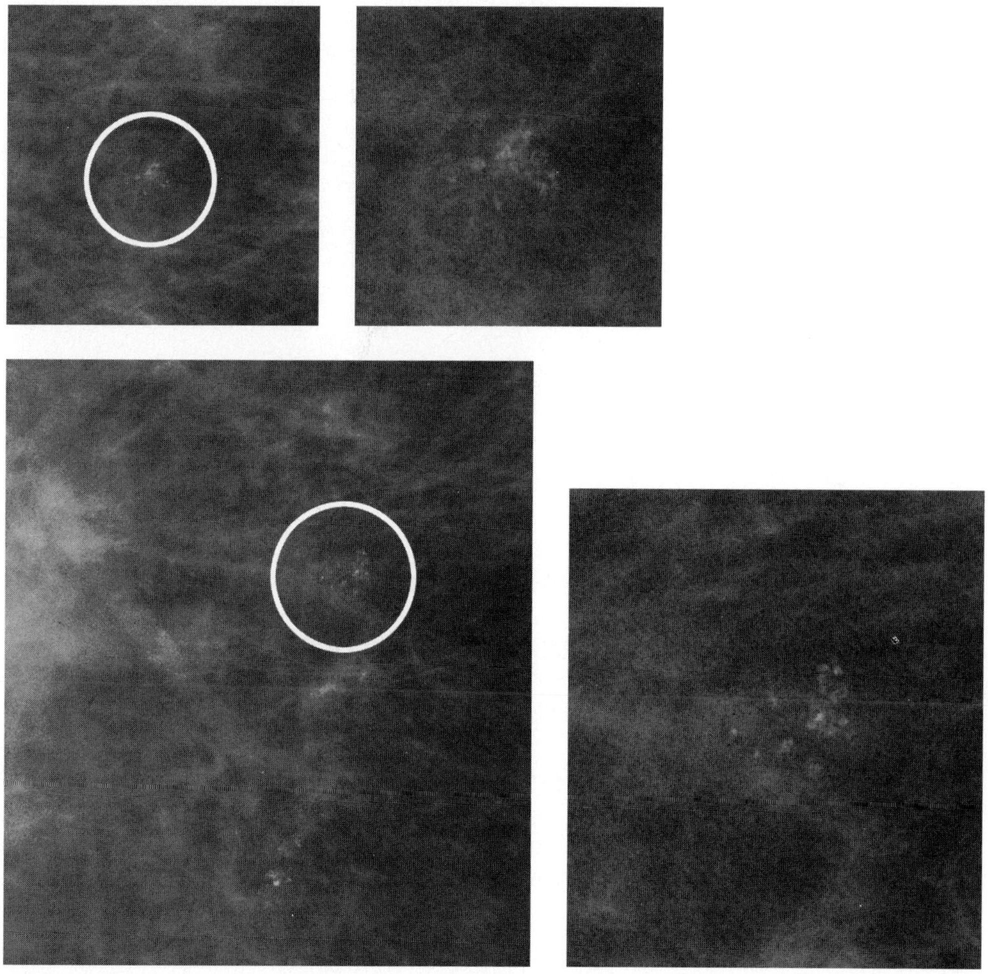

Figure 96–1. In the right upper outer breast there is a cluster of pleomorphic calcifications (circled). (A). Right ML magnification mammogram. (B). Right CC magnification mammogram.

Ultrasound

Frequency

- 11.5 MHz (Fig. 96–2)

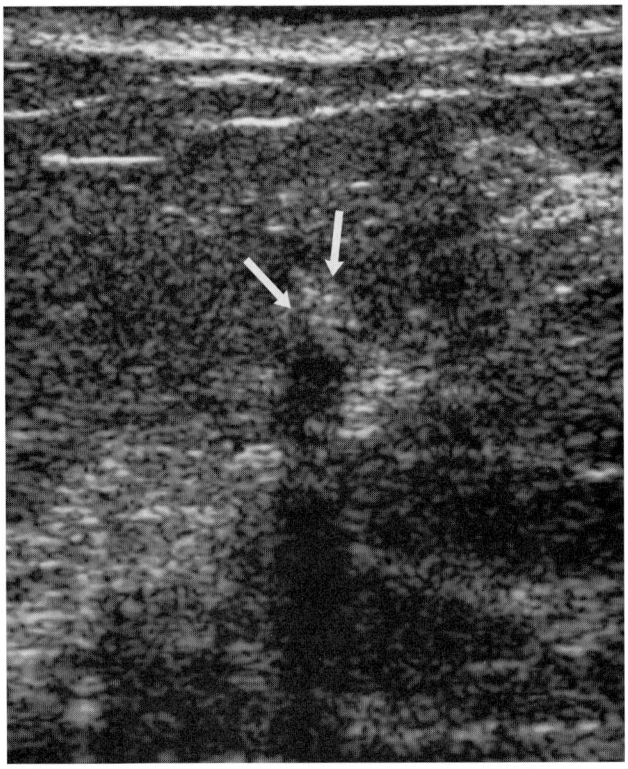

Figure 96–2. Right transverse breast sonogram: The mammographic calcifications correspond to multiple high-intensity foci (arrows) associated with posterior acoustic shadowing. No sonographic mass is present.

Pathology

- fibrocystic changes
- predominantly fatty tissue with benign calcifications in small area of stromal fibrosis and epithelial hyperplasia

Management

- BI-RADS Assessment Category 4, suspicious abnormality; biopsy should be considered

Pearls and Pitfalls

Clustered heterogeneous calcifications are due to both benign and malignant etiologies. Benign etiologies include early calcification of fibroadenomas or fat necrosis. Papillomas and fibrocystic changes may also produce these types of calcifications. Malignant causes include ductal carcinoma in situ and invasive ductal carcinoma.

Suggested Readings

1. Bird RE. Critical pathways in analyzing breast calcifications. *Radiographics* 1995;15:928–934.

Case 97

Case History

A 69-year-old woman presents with new left breast calcifications.

Physical Examination

- normal exam

Mammogram

Calcifications (Fig. 97–1)

- type: pleomorphic/heterogeneous
- distribution: grouped/clustered

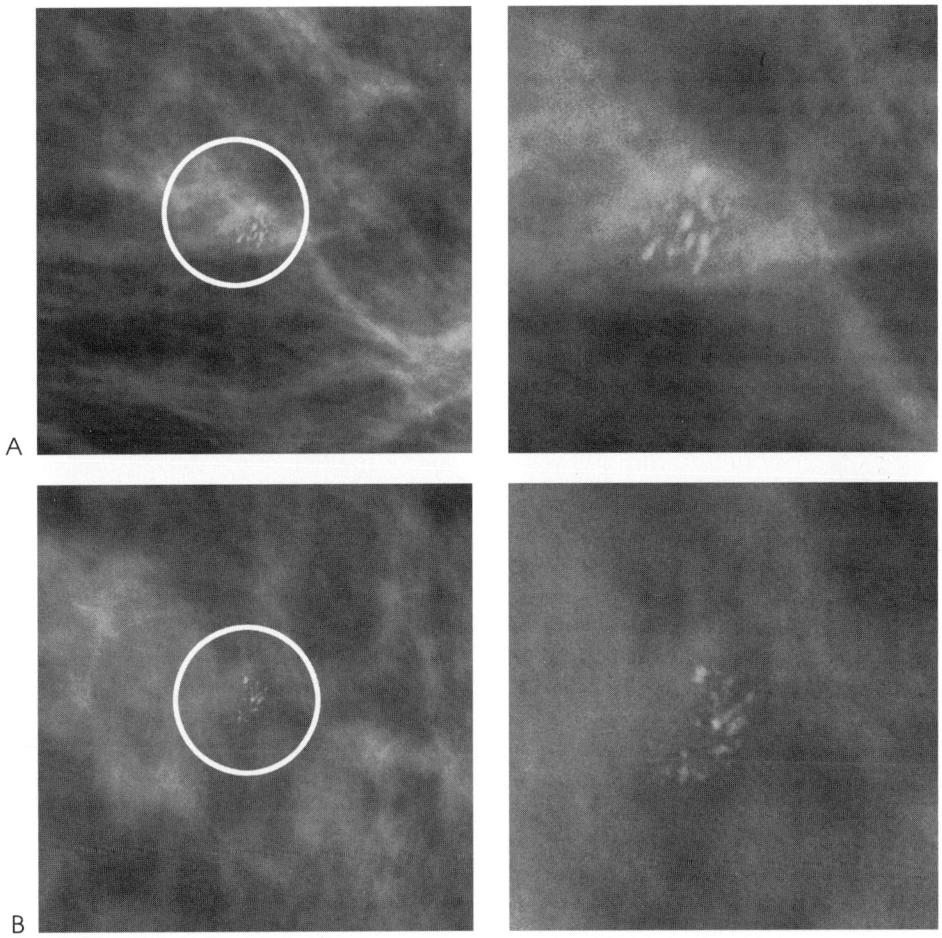

Figure 97–1. A cluster of pleomorphic calcifications (circled) is in the left outer inferior breast. (A). Left ML magnification view. (B). Left CC magnification view.

Pathology

- fibroadenomatoid hyperplasia

Management

- BI-RADS Assessment Category 4, suspicious abnormality; biopsy should be considered

Pearls and Pitfalls

Fibroadenomatous hyperplasia is an early stage of fibroadenoma formation. Calcifications formed during this process may be indistinguishable from malignant calcifications.

Suggested Readings

1. Kamal M, Evans AJ, Denley H, et al. Fibroadenomatoid hyperplasia: a cause of suspicious microcalcification on mammographic screening. *AJR* 1998;171:1331–1334.
2. Tavassoli FA, Fattaneh A. *Pathology of the Breast.* 2nd ed. Stamford: Appleton and Lange; 1999:590–597.

Case 98

Case History

An 80-year-old woman presents with new calcifications on her screening mammogram.

Physical Examination

- normal exam

Mammogram

Calcifications (Fig. 98–1)

- type: pleomorphic/heterogeneous
- distribution: grouped/clustered

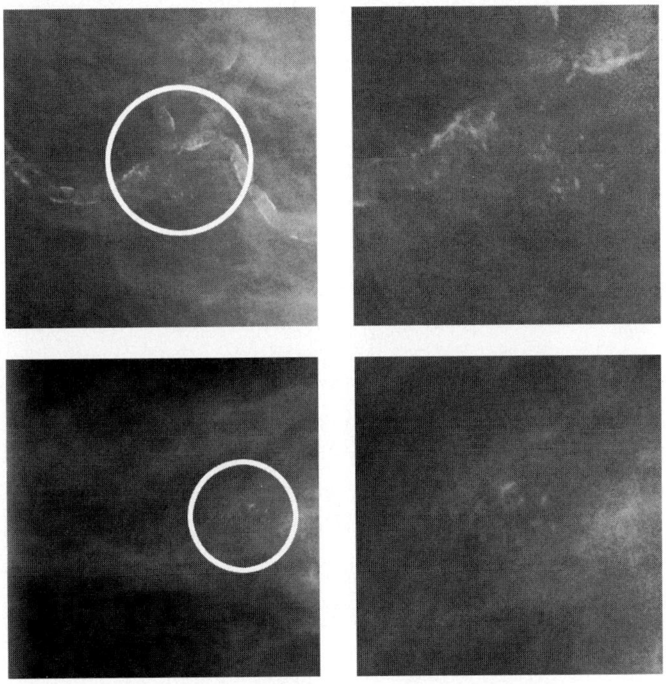

A

B

Figure 98–1. In the left upper outer quadrant, there is a cluster of calcifications (circled). (A). Left LM magnification mammogram. (B). Left CC magnification mammogram.

Ultrasound

Low Frequency

Frequency

- 7 MHz

Mass

- margin: well defined, oval/round
- echogenicity: hypoechoic
- retrotumoral acoustic appearance: no shadowing
- shape: ellipsoid (Fig. 98–2)

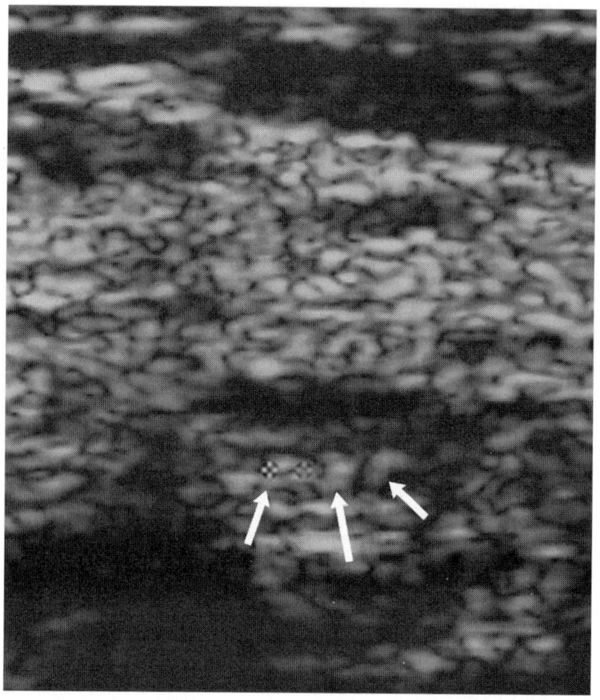

Figure 98–2. Left radial breast sonogram: The calcifications (arrow) identified in Figure 98–1 are associated with a hypoechoic mass. With this lower frequency, the hypoechoic mass is not well identified.

High Frequency

Frequency

- 11.5 MHz (Fig. 98–3)

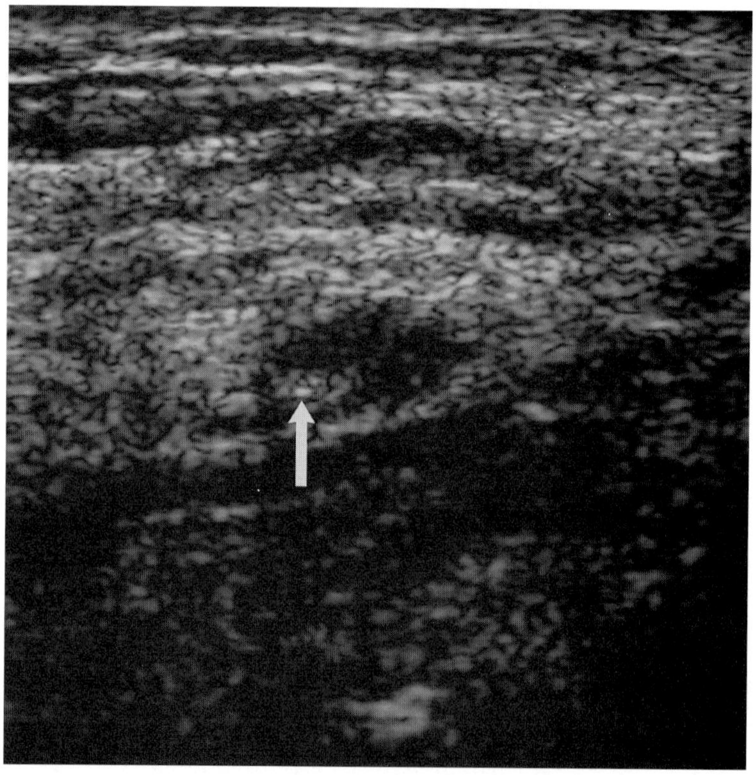

Figure 98–3. Left radial breast sonogram: The calcifications (arrow) are within a well-defined oval hypoechoic mass. The mass is more clearly identified with this high-frequency technique compared to the low-frequency exam.

Pathology

- fibroadenoma (not otherwise specified)

Management

- BI-RADS Assessment Category 4, suspicious abnormality; biopsy should be considered

Pearls and Pitfalls

Although the mass has a more benign appearance on the higher-frequency sonographic exam, the small size prevents confident definition of the margins. This limitation and the presence of suspicious mammographic calcifications result in a suspicious, Category 4 assessment.

Suggested Readings

1. Bassett LW. Mammographic analysis of calcifications. *Radiol Clin North Am* 1992;30:93–105.
2. Gershon-Cohen J, Ingleby H. Roentgenography of fibroadenoma of the breast. *Radiology* 1952;59:77–86.
3. Kopans DB. *Breast Imaging.* 2nd ed. Philadelphia: Lippincott-Raven; 1998:511–615.

Case 99

Case History

A 64-year-old woman, 6 months after right breast lumpectomy and radiation therapy, has new calcifications adjacent to her lumpectomy site.

Physical Examination

- right breast: scar in upper outer quadrant of right breast from previous lumpectomy; no new masses
- left breast: normal exam

Mammogram

Calcifications (Fig. 99–1)

- type: pleomorphic/heterogeneous
- distribution: grouped/clustered

A

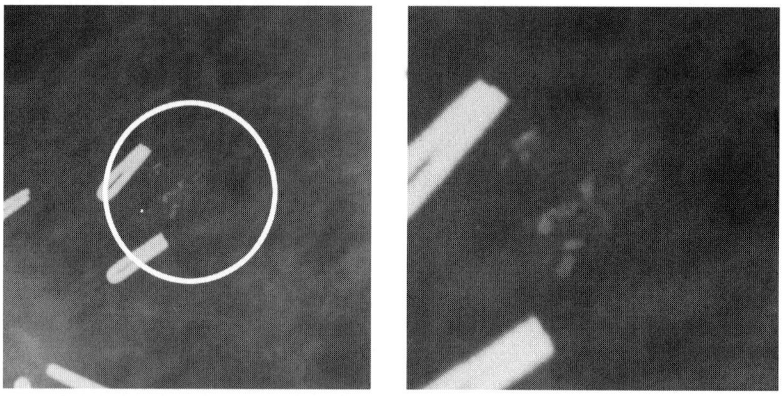

B

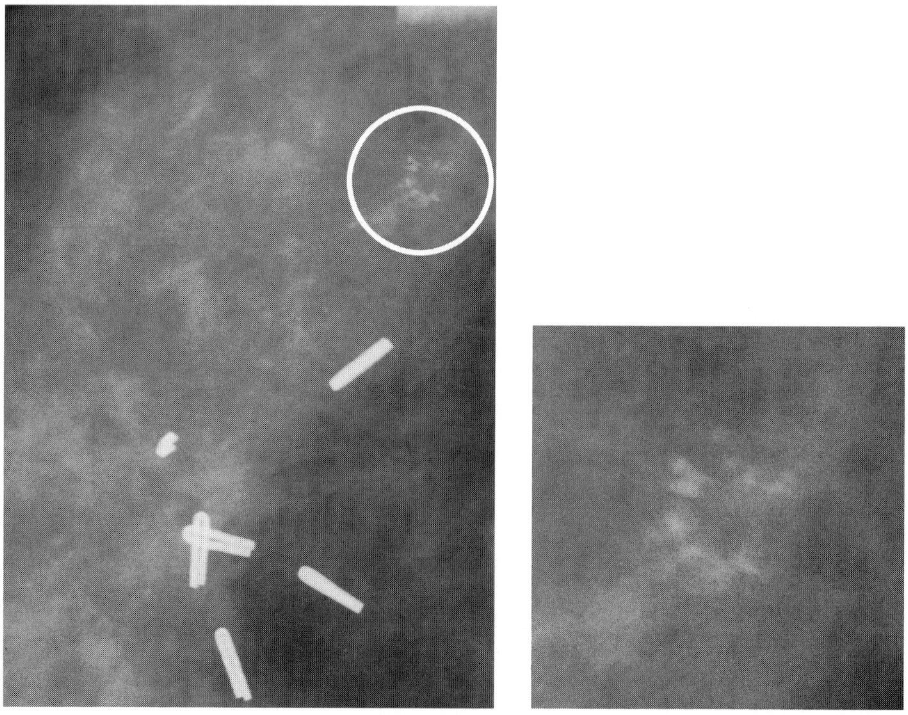

Figure 99–1. In the right upper outer quadrant there are clips associated with architectural distortion from previous lumpectomy. Adjacent to the clips is a group of new heterogeneous calcifications (circled). (A). Right MLO magnification mammogram. (B). Right CC magnification mammogram.

Ultrasound

Frequency

- 5 MHz

Mass

- margin: spiculation/architectural distortion
- echogenicity: hypoechoic
- retrotumoral acoustic appearance: severe shadowing, mass completely obscured
- shape: irregular (Fig. 99–2)

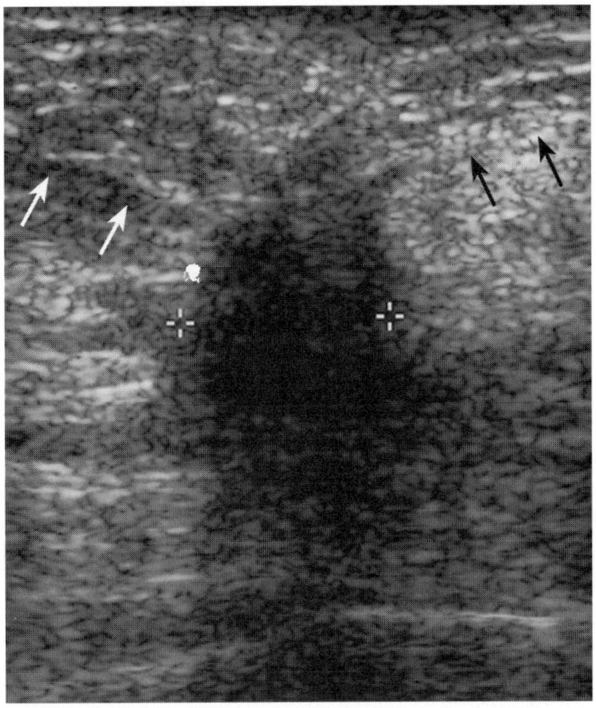

Figure 99–2. Right longitudinal breast sonogram: The patient's lumpectomy scar is an irregular, hypoechoic, spiculated abnormality with severe posterior acoustic shadowing. The superficial tissue lines exhibit architectural distortion.

Pathology

- scar

Management

- BI-RADS Assessment Category 4, suspicious abnormality; biopsy should be considered

Pearls and Pitfalls

1. Differential diagnosis for etiology of these calcifications is either fat necrosis from lumpectomy or malignancy.
2. Sonographically, scars are hypoechoic areas with severe acoustic shadowing. Scars are associated with architectural distortion and spiculation.

Suggested Readings

1. Dershaw DD, Giess CS, McCormick B, et al. Patterns of mammographically detected calcifications after breast-conserving therapy associated with tumor recurrence. *Cancer* 1997;79:1355–1361.
2. Liberman L, Van Zee KJ, Dershaw DD, et al. Mammographic features of local recurrence in women who have undergone breast-conserving therapy for ductal carcinoma in situ. *AJR* 1997;168:489–493.
3. Rissanen TJ, Makarainen HP, Mattila SI, et al. Breast cancer recurrence after mastectomy: diagnosis with mammography and US. *Radiology* 1993;188:463–467.
4. Vora SA, Wazer DE, Homer MJ. Management of microcalcifications that develop at the lumpectomy site after breast-conserving therapy. *Radiology* 1997;203:667–671.

Case 100

Case History

A 42-year-old woman presents with increasing calcifications.

Physical Examination

- normal exam

Mammogram

Calcifications (Fig. 100-1)

- type: pleomorphic/heterogeneous
- distribution: segmental

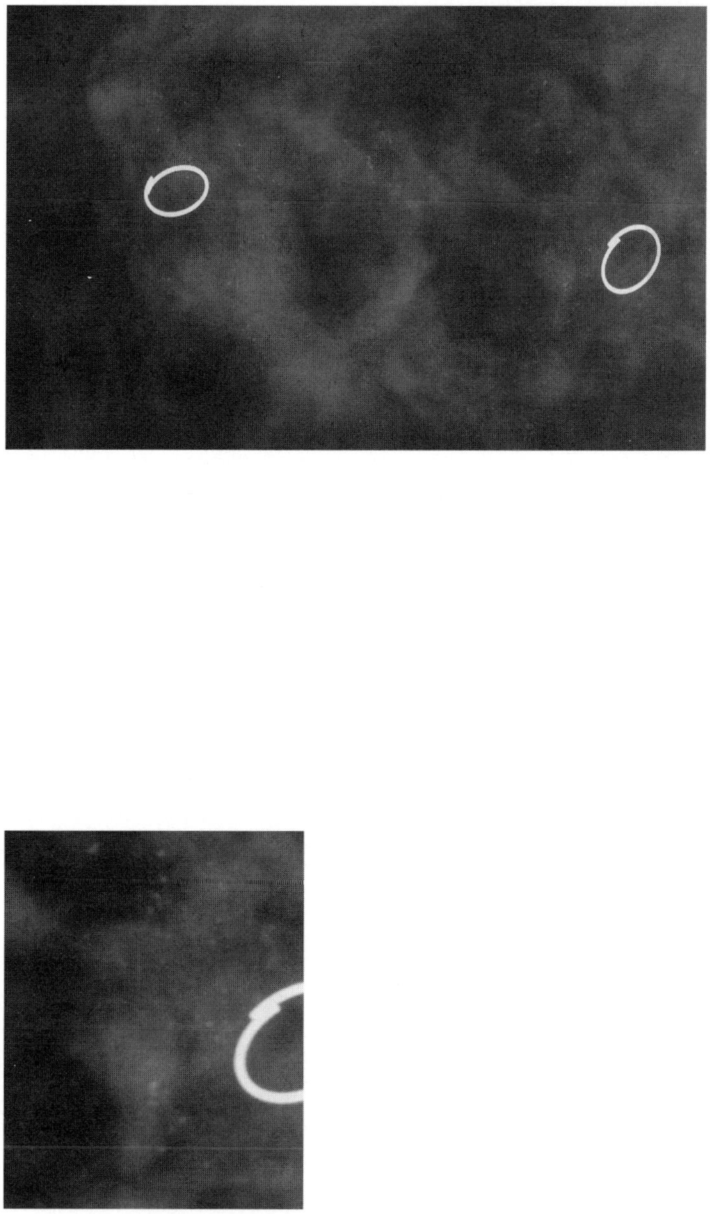

A

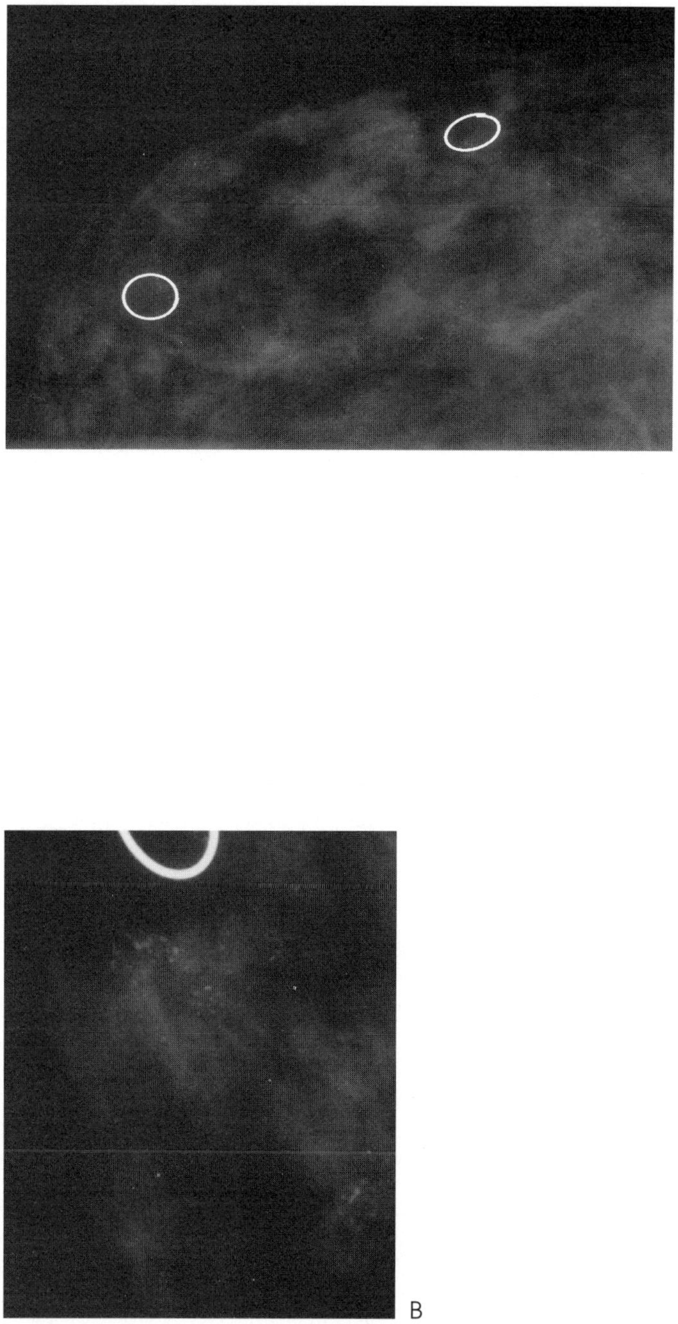

B

Figure 100-1. In the inner breast there are numerous clusters of heterogeneous calcifications. (A). Right ML magnification mammogram. (B). Right CC magnification mammogram.

Ultrasound

Frequency

- 13 MHz (Fig. 100–2)

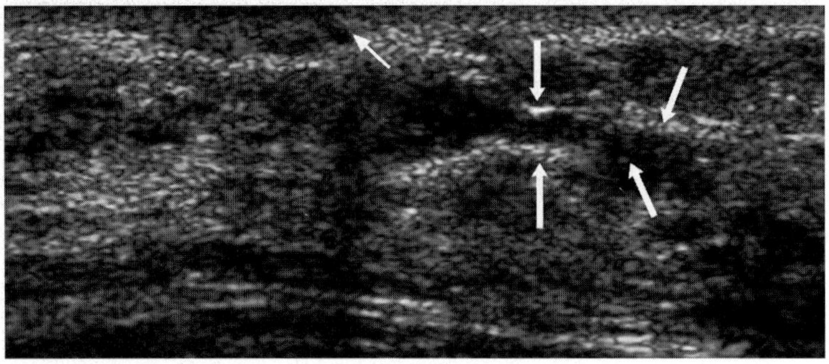

Figure 100–2. Right radial breast sonogram: Abnormally dilated duct (large arrows) filled with punctate echogenic foci are present in the area associated with mammographic calcifications. Nipple (small white arrow).

Pathology

- ductal carcinoma in situ

Management

- BI-RADS Assessment Category 4, suspicious abnormality; biopsy should be considered

Pearls and Pitfalls

Songraphically, DCIS may appear as isolated calcifications, dilated ducts containing calcifications, an irregular solid mass, or a diffuse area of hypoechogenicity. This case illustrates the second of these appearances.

Suggested Readings

1. Tohno E, Cosgrove DO. Malignant diseases-primary carcinomas. In: Tohno D, Cosgrove DO, Sloane JP, eds. *Ultrasound Diagnosis of Breast Diseases*. New York: Churchill Livingston; 1994:158–180.

Case 101

Case History

A 71-year-old woman presents with new calcifications on her screening mammogram.

Physical Examination

- normal exam

Mammogram

Calcifications (Fig. 101-1)

- type: pleomorphic/heterogeneous
- distribution: grouped/clustered

A

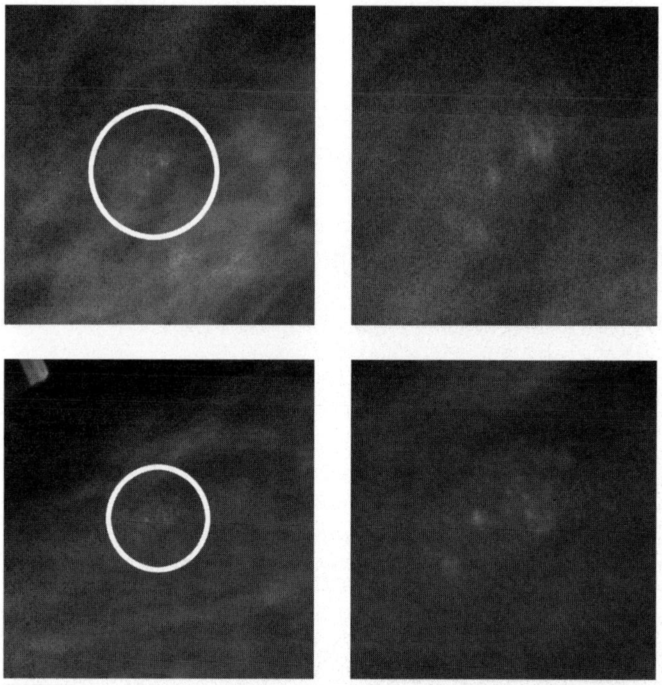

B

Figure 101-1. In the lower outer right breast, there is a cluster of heterogeneous calcifications (circle). (A). Right MLO magnification view. (B). Right CC magnification view.

Ultrasound

Frequency

- 10 MHz

Mass

- margin: ill defined
- echogenicity: hypoechoic
- retrotumoral acoustic appearance: severe shadowing, mass partially obscured
- shape: irregular (Fig. 101-2)

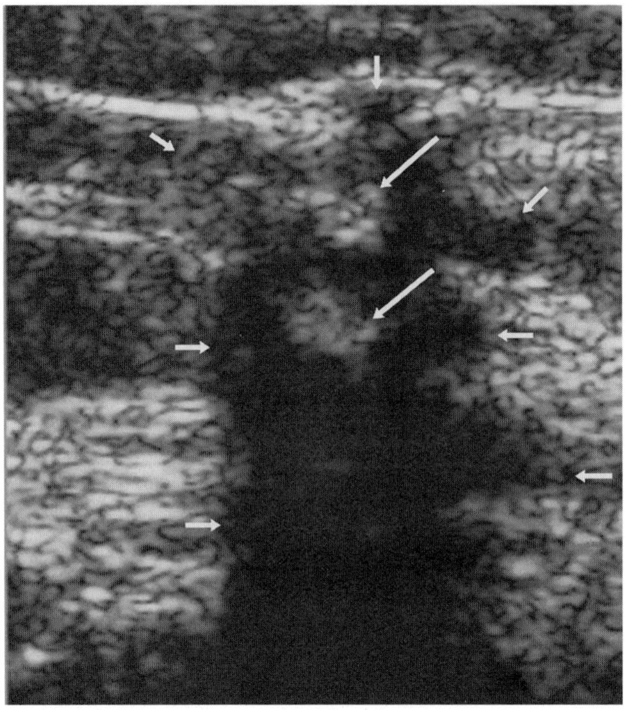

Figure 101–2. Right longitudinal breast sonogram: In the area of the cluster of calcifications identified in Figure 101–1, there is a hypoechoic, irregular mass (short arrows) with calcifications (long arrows) and severe posterior acoustic shadowing.

Pathology

- ductal carcinoma in situ

Management

- BI-RADS Assessment Category 4, suspicious abnormality; biopsy should be considered

Pearls and Pitfalls

Because sonographic examination is not part of the standard assessment of calcifications, clinical assessment is based upon the appearance of the mammographic calcifications alone. If one also used the sonographic information, then the assessment category would be Category 5, highly suspicious for malignancy.

Suggested Readings

1. Ranieri E, D'Andrea MR, D'Alessio A, et al. Ultrasound in the detection of breast cancer associated with isolated clustered microcalcifications, mammographically identified. *Anticancer Res* 1997;17:2831–2836.

Case 102

Case History

A 39-year-old woman presents with a right breast palpable lump. She is 6 months postpartum and is still breast-feeding. She was initially studied with lower-frequency sonography (Fig. 102–2). Her sonogram was interpreted as BI-RADS Category 3 (probably benign lesion, short-term follow-up recommended). After 1 month, because symptoms persisted, she was examined with high-frequency sonography (Fig. 102–3). As a result of her high-frequency sonogram, mammograms were performed (Fig. 102–1).

Physical Examination

- right breast: palpable lump at the 6:00 position
- left breast: normal exam

Mammogram

Calcifications (Fig. 102–1)

- type: pleomorphic/heterogeneous
- distribution: grouped/clustered

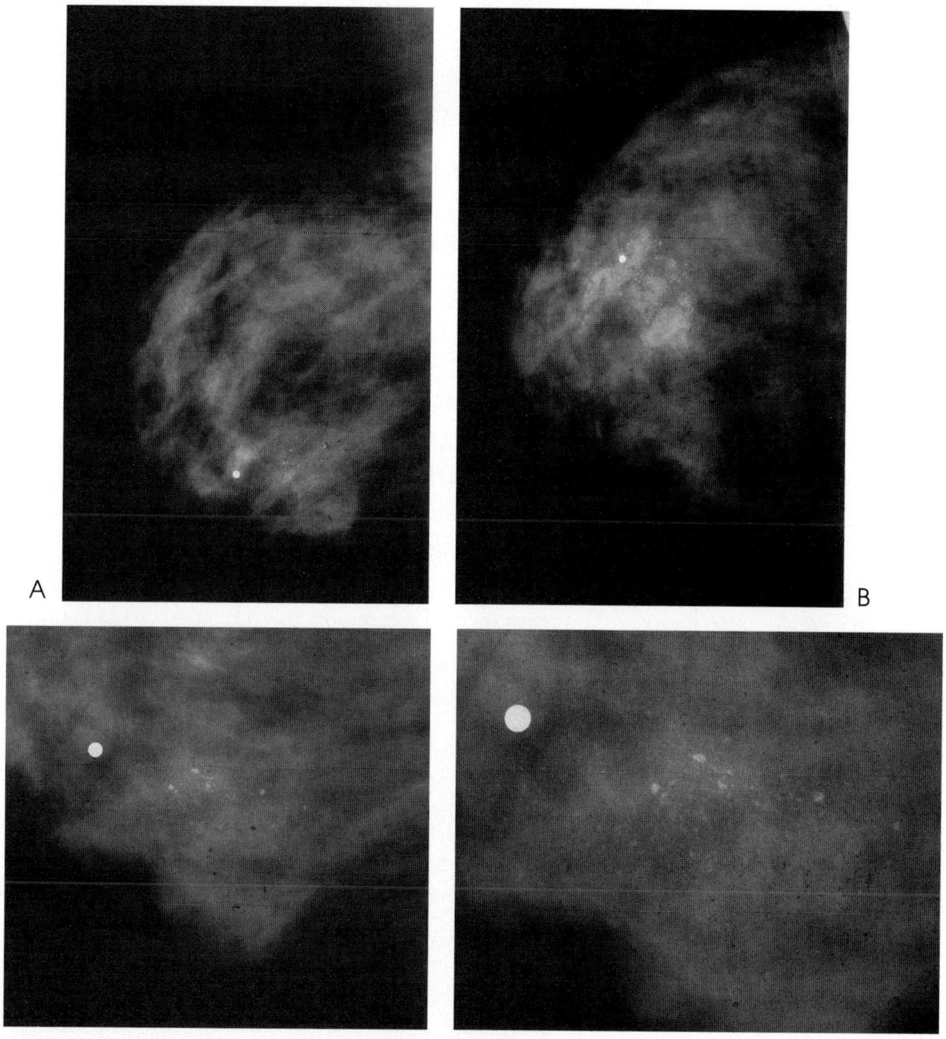

Figure 102–1. Near the right 6:00 position, there is a cluster of heterogeneous calcifications that corresponds to a palpable lump, which is marked with a radiopaque marker. (A). Right MLO mammogram. (B). Right CC mammogram. (C). Right MLO magnification mammogram.

Ultrasound

Low Frequency

Frequency

- 7 MHz

Mass

- margin: well defined, lobulated
- echogenicity: hypoechoic
- retrotumoral acoustic appearance: bilateral edge shadowing
- shape: lobulated (Fig. 102–2)

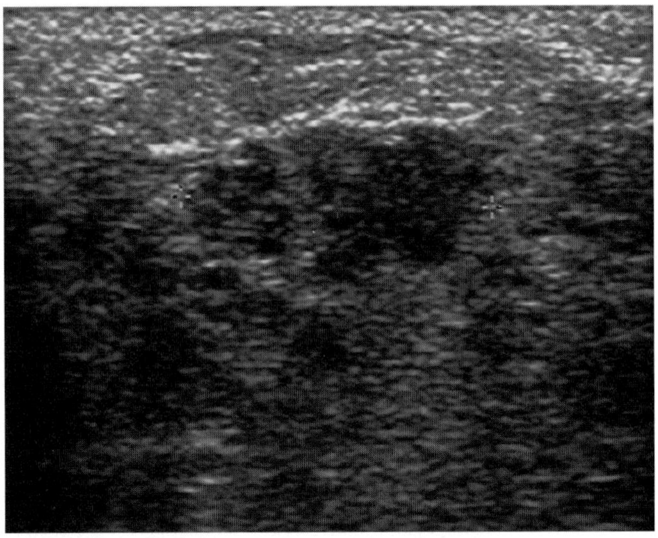

Figure 102–2. Right radial breast sonogram: A palpable lump corresponded to a lobulated hypoechoic mass.

High Frequency

Frequency

- 13 MHz

Associated Findings

High frequency (Fig. 102–3) better displays the irregularity of the margins of the mass. Furthermore, the high-frequency examination demonstrates calcifications that were not visible on the lower-frequency study. Mammography confirmed the presence of malignant calcifications (Fig. 102–1).

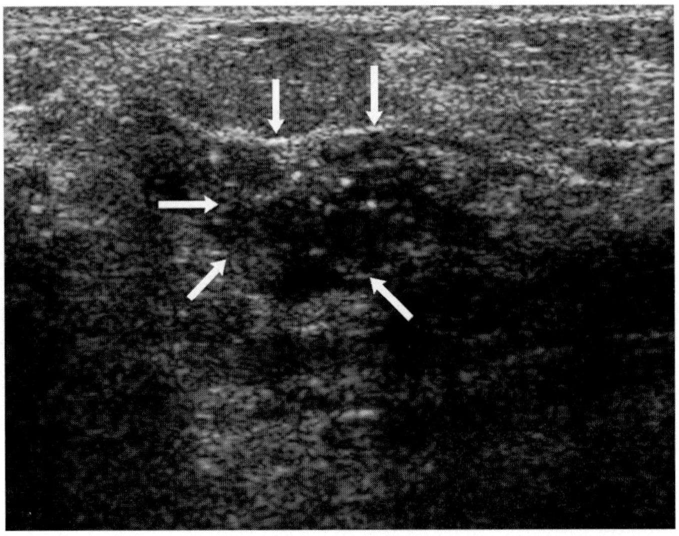

Figure 102–3. Right radial breast sonogram: With higher frequency, the margins of the mass (arrows) are ill defined and irregular. High-intensity foci consistent with calcifications are also evident in this examination.

Other Modalities

Findings

Lymphoscintigraphy for sentinel node biopsy demonstrated one sentinel axillary node. This node was histologically benign (Fig. 102-4).

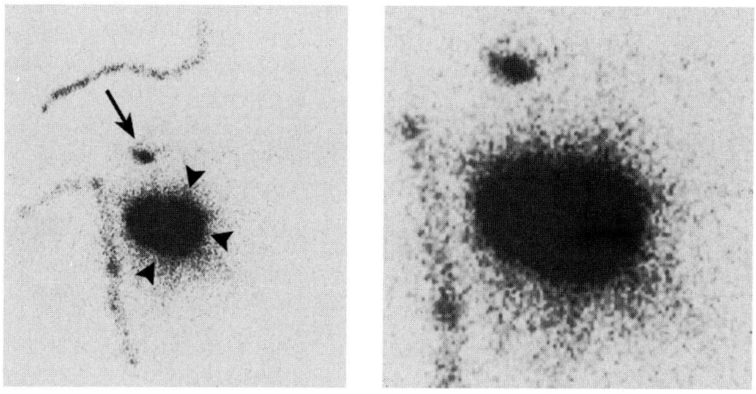

Figure 102-4. Tc-99m sulfur colloid lymphoscintigraphy for sentinel node biopsy: Radionuclide activity is evident in the malignant mass (arrowheads) as well as in a single (sentinel) axillary node (arrow).

Pathology

- 3 cm invasive ductal carcinoma with a predominant intraductal component

Management

- BI-RADS Assessment Category 5, highly suggestive of malignancy

Pearls and Pitfalls

1. High-frequency sonography demonstrates irregularity of the margins of this mass, which increases the suspicious characterization of the lesion.
2. When lymphoscintigraphy is used to stage for breast nodal metastasis the sentinel node is positive in 5% of patients with DCIS, 25% of those with invasive tumors less than 2 cm, and 41% of cases in which tumors are 2 to 5 cm.

Suggested Readings

1. Alazraki NP, Eshima D, Eshima LA, et al. Lymphoscintigraphy, the sentinel node concept, and the intraoperative gamma probe in melanoma, breast cancer, and other potential cancers. *Semin Nucl Med* 1997;27:55-67.
2. Cox CE, Pandas S, Cox JM, et al. Guidelines for sentinel node biopsy and lymphatic mapping of patients with breast cancer. *Ann Surg* 1998;227:645-653.
3. Giuliano AE. Sentinel lymphadenectomy in primary breast carcinoma: an alternative to routine axillary dissection. *J Surg Oncol* 1996;62:75-77.
4. Giuliano AE, Dale PS, Turner RR, et al. Improved axillary staging of breast cancer with sentinel lymphadenectomy. *Ann Surg* 1995;222:394-401.
5. Kelley MC, Giuliano AE. Lymphatic mapping and sentinel lymphadenectomy for breast cancer. In: Bland KI, ed. *The Breast: Comprehensive Management of Benign and Malignant Diseases*. Philadelphia: WB Saunders; 1998:1100-1111.
6. Stavros AT, Thickman D, Rapp CL, Dennis MA, Parker SH, Sisney GA. Solid breast nodules: use of sonography to distinguish between benign and malignant lesions. *Radiology* 1995;196:123-134.

Case 103

Case History

A 51-year-old woman presents with new left breast calcifications on her screening mammogram.

Physical Examination

- normal exam

Mammogram

Calcifications (Fig. 103–1)

- type: pleomorphic/heterogeneous
- distribution: grouped/clustered

Figure 103–1. Left CC magnification mammogram: A cluster of heterogeneous calcifications is present in the outer breast.

Ultrasound

Frequency

- 10 MHz

Mass

- margin: ill defined
- echogenicity: hypoechoic
- retrotumoral acoustic appearance: severe shadowing, mass partially obscured
- shape: irregular (Fig. 103–2)

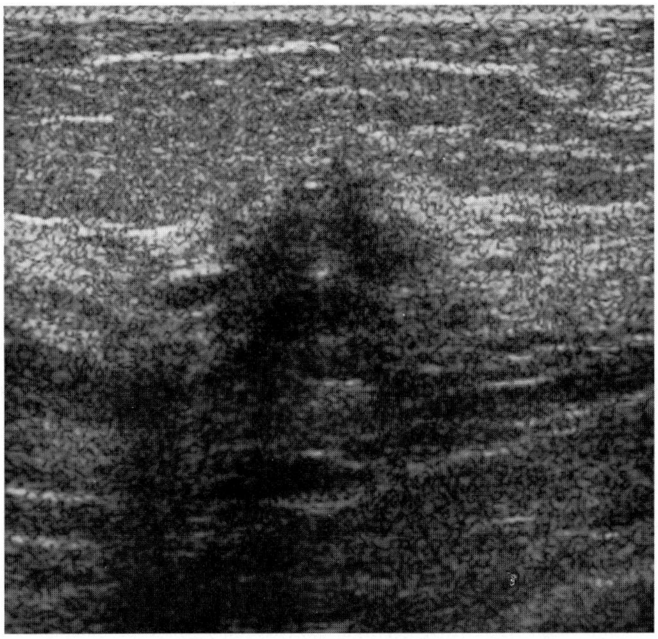

Figure 103–2. Left antiradial breast sonogram: The calcifications identified in Figure 103–1 corresponded to an irregular, hypoechoic mass with calcifications.

Pathology

- invasive ductal carcinoma with a predominant intraductal component

Management

- BI-RADS Assessment Category 4, suspicious abnormality; biopsy should be considered

Pearls and Pitfalls

Because the calcifications were easily identified with high-frequency sonography, sonography was used to localize the injection of the radioactive tracer for sentinel node lymphoscintigraphy and to guide a direct surgical cutdown and removal of the mass.

Suggested Readings

1. Fornage BD, Coan JD, David CL. Ultrasound-guided needle biopsy of the breast and other interventional procedures. *Radiol Clin North Am* 1992;30:167–185.
2. Leucht D, Madjar H. Microcalcification in sonography. In: Leucht D, ed. *Teaching Atlas of Breast Ultrasound.* New York: Thieme; 1996:189–204.
3. Rickard MT. Ultrasound of malignant breast microcalcifications: role in evaluation and guided procedures. *Australas Radiol* 1996;40:26–31.
4. Yang WT, Suen M, Ahuja A, et al. In vivo demonstration of microcalcification in breast cancer using high resolution ultrasound. *Br J Radiol* 1997;70:685–690.

Case 104

Case History

A 72-year-old woman presents with new calcifications on her right screening mammogram.

Physical Examination

- right breast: two palpable cysts at the 10:00 and 6:00 position; a third palpable nodule adjacent to the cyst at 10:00, corresponding to a solid mass
- left breast: one palpable cyst

Mammogram

Calcifications (Figs. 104–1 and 104–2)

- type: pleomorphic/heterogeneous
- distribution: grouped/clustered

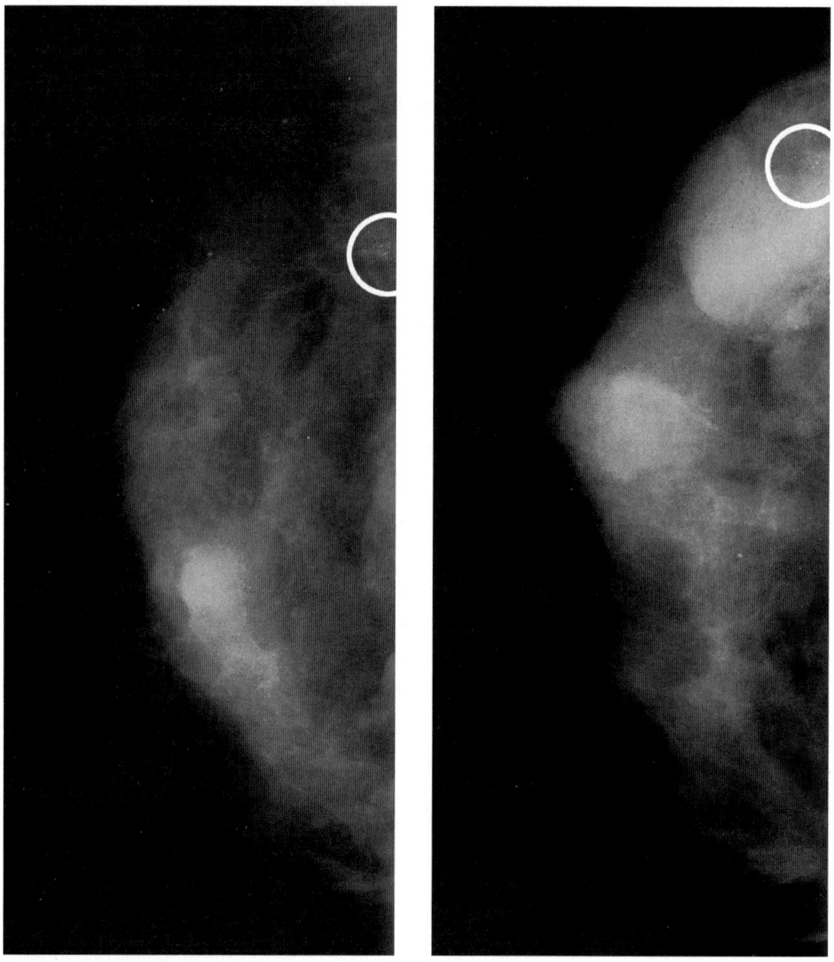

A B

Figure 104–1. The breast is extremely dense and contains multiple round masses that sonographically correspond to cysts. In the upper outer breast there is a cluster of calcifications (circled), which corresponds to a sonographically solid mass. (A). Right MLO mammogram. (B). Right CC mammogram.

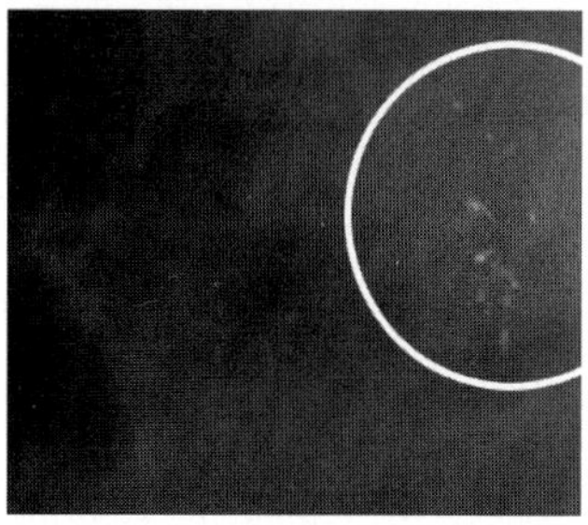

Figure 104–2. Right MLO magnification mammogram: The cluster of calcifications (circled) identified in Figure 104–1 consists of numerous punctate and linear heterogeneous calcifications.

Ultrasound

Frequency

- 11.5 MHz

Mass

- margin: ill defined
- echogenicity: hypoechoic
- retrotumoral acoustic appearance: posterior shadowing distal to mass
- shape: irregular (Fig. 104-3)

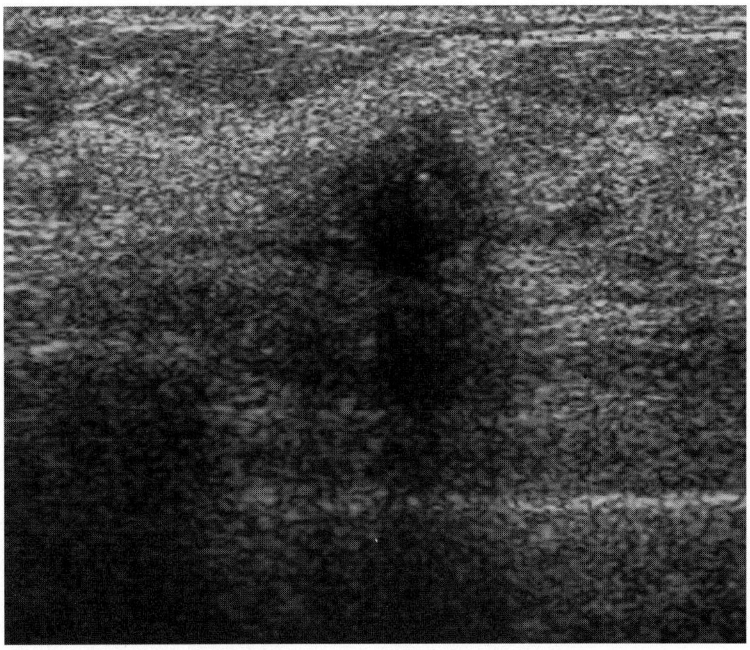

Figure 104-3. Right breast radial breast sonogram: The calcifications identified in Figures 104-1 and 104-2 correspond to an ill-defined hypoechoic mass with posterior acoustic shadowing. Calcification is present within the mass.

Pathology

- apocrine carcinoma

Management

- BI-RADS Assessment Category 4, suspicious abnormality; biopsy should be considered

Pearls and Pitfalls

Apocrine carcinoma is a variant of ductal carcinoma that represents <1% of ductal malignancies. Since this tumor is rare, imaging information is limited. These malignancies have been reported to present as mammographic masses, usually with ill-defined margins. However, sometimes these masses are well defined. Calcifications have also been associated with these masses. The sonographic features would be expected to be similar to other ductal malignancies. Like this case, these masses would be solid, hypoechoic, with varying degrees of shadowing. Clinically these tumors behave in a manner similar to ductal carcinoma.

Suggested Readings

1. Giles R, Lesnik A, Guinebretiere J, et al. Apocrine carcinoma: clinical and mammographic features. *Radiology* 1994;190:495-497.

Case 105

Case History

A 79-year-old woman presents with new left breast calcifications.

Physical Examination

- normal exam

Mammogram

Calcifications (Fig. 105–1)

- type: pleomorphic/heterogeneous
- distribution: grouped/clustered

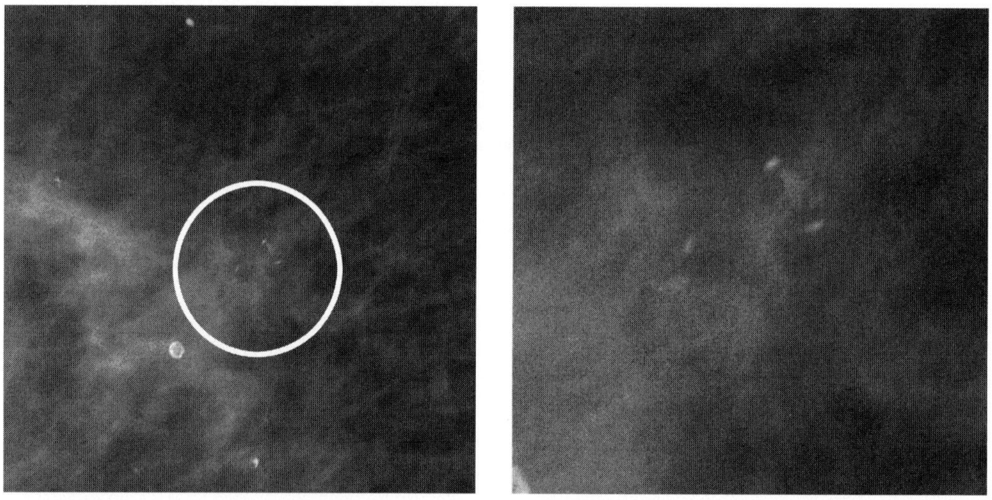

A

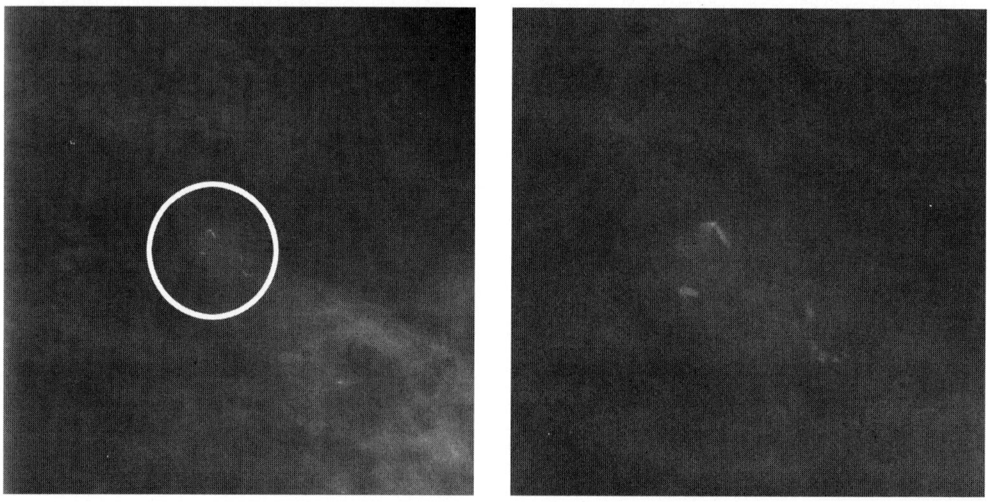

B

Figure 105–1. *In the left upper outer breast there is a cluster of heterogeneous calcifications (circled). (A). Left LM magnification mammogram. (B). Left CC magnification mammogram.*

Pathology

- papilloma

Management

- BI-RADS Assessment Category 4, suspicious abnormality; biopsy should be considered

Pearls and Pitfalls

1. There are three types of papillomas: solitary central papilloma, multiple papillomas, juvenile papillomatosis.
2. This case is an example of solitary papilloma. Although this papilloma is peripheral, these masses are usually within a major duct in the subareolar region. Mammographically, they present as circumscribed masses or cluster of calcifications.

Suggested Readings

1. De Paredes ES. *Atlas of Film Screen Mammography*. 2nd ed. Baltimore: Williams & Wilkins; 1992:299–416.
2. Jackson VP, Jahan R, Fu YS. Benign breast lesions. In: Bassett LW, Jackson VP, Jahan R, Fu YS, Gold RH, eds. *Diagnosis of Diseases of the Breast*. Philadelphia: WB Saunders Company; 1997:357–443.
3. Tabar L, Dean PB. *Teaching Atlas of Mammography.* 3rd ed. New York: Thieme; 2001 220–221.

Case 106

Case History

A 70-year-old woman presents with new right breast calcifications on her screening mammogram.

Physical Examination

- normal exam

Mammogram

Calcifications (Fig. 106–1)

- type: fine linear/branching
- distribution: grouped/clustered

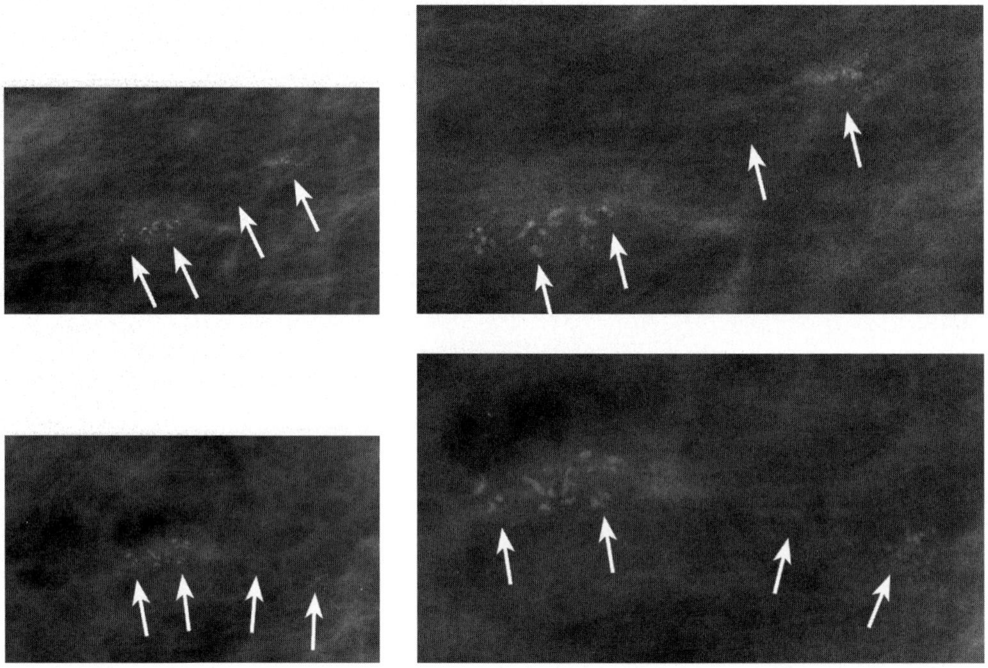

A

B

Figure 106–1. In the inferior outer breast there is a cluster of heterogeneous calcifications that are arranged in a linear pattern (arrows). (A). Right MLO magnification mammogram. (B). Right exaggerated CC magnification mammogram.

Pathology

- ductal carcinoma in situ
- solid type with high nuclear grade and high mitotic rate and with comedo necrosis and dystrophic calcifications

Management

- BI-RADS Assessment Category 4, suspicious abnormality; biopsy should be considered

Pearls and Pitfalls

Calcification in DCIS with comedo necrosis usually occurs in the center of the necrotic tumor debris within the ducts. As a result, the mammographic calcification pattern of this histology is commonly fine linear or branching. However, there is considerable mammographic overlap between the different DCIS subtypes so histologic subtype cannot be mammographically predicted with great accuracy.

Suggested Readings

1. Hermann, G, Keller RJ, Drossman S, et al. Mammographic pattern of microcalcifications in the preoperative diagnosis of comedo ductal carcinoma in situ: histopathologic correlation. *Can Assoc Radiol J* 1999;50:235–240.
2. Stomper PC, Connolly JL. Ductal carcinoma in situ of the breast: correlation between mammographic calcification and tumor subtype. *AJR* 1992;159:483–485.

Case 107

Case History

A 43-year-old woman presents with new calcifications on her screening mammogram.

Physical Examination

- normal exam

Mammogram

Calcifications (Fig. 107-1)

- type: fine linear/branching
- distribution: grouped/clustered

A 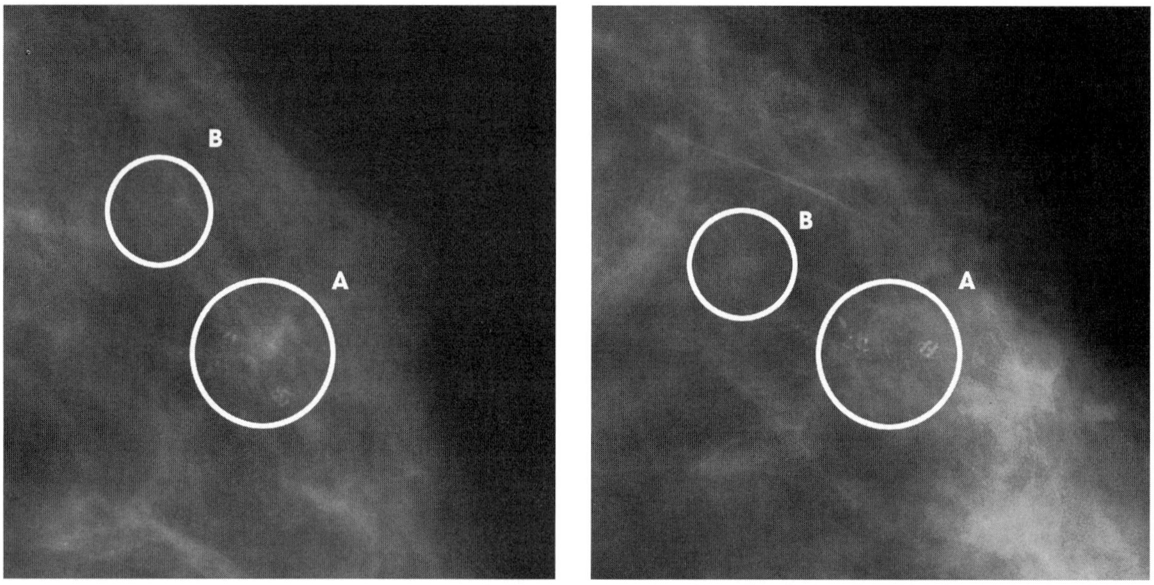 B

Figure 107-1. In the left upper outer quadrant there are two groups of calcifications (labeled A and B). Cluster A is a group of fine linear branching calcifications. Cluster B is a group of amorphous, punctate calcifications. (A). Left ML magnification mammogram. (B). Left CC magnification mammogram.

Pathology

- Cluster A is an intermediate-grade ductal carcinoma in situ with prominent necrosis. At lumpectomy the maximum diameter of the lesion was 10 mm.
- Cluster B is an intralobular calcification associated with epithelial hyperplasia without atypia.

Management

- BI-RADS Assessment Category 4, suspicious abnormality; biopsy should be considered

Pearls and Pitfalls

This case illustrates that the configuration of calcifications reflects the type of pathology. The linear configuration of cluster A suggests that these calcifications result from a ductal process (DCIS) and the round, punctate appearance of cluster B calcifications is consistent with an intralobular process.

Suggested Readings

1. De Paredes ES, Abbitt PL, Tabbarah S, et al. Mammographic and histologic correlations of microcalcifications. *Radiographics* 1990;10:577–589.

Case 108

Case History

A 42-year-old woman presents with left breast calcifications identified on screening mammogram.

Physical Examination

- normal exam

Mammogram

Calcifications (Figs. 108–1 and 108–2)

- type: fine linear/branching
- distribution: segmental

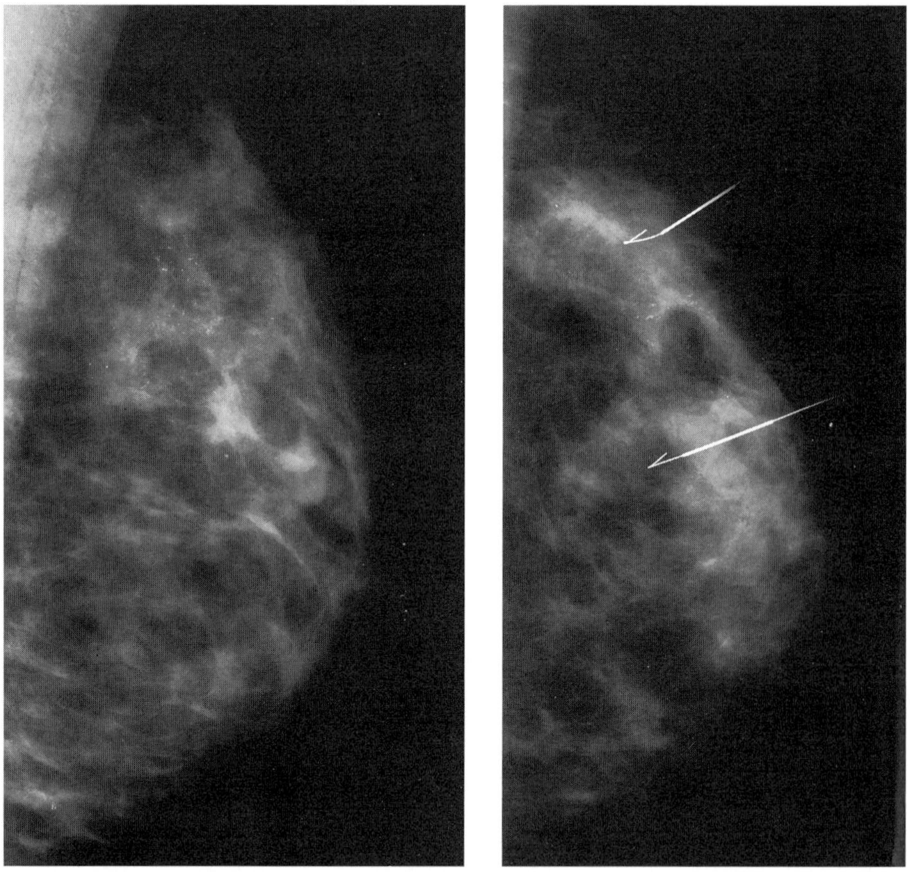

A B

Figure 108–1. In the upper outer left breast there are fine linear branching calcifications. (A). Left ML mammogram. (B). Left CC mammogram.

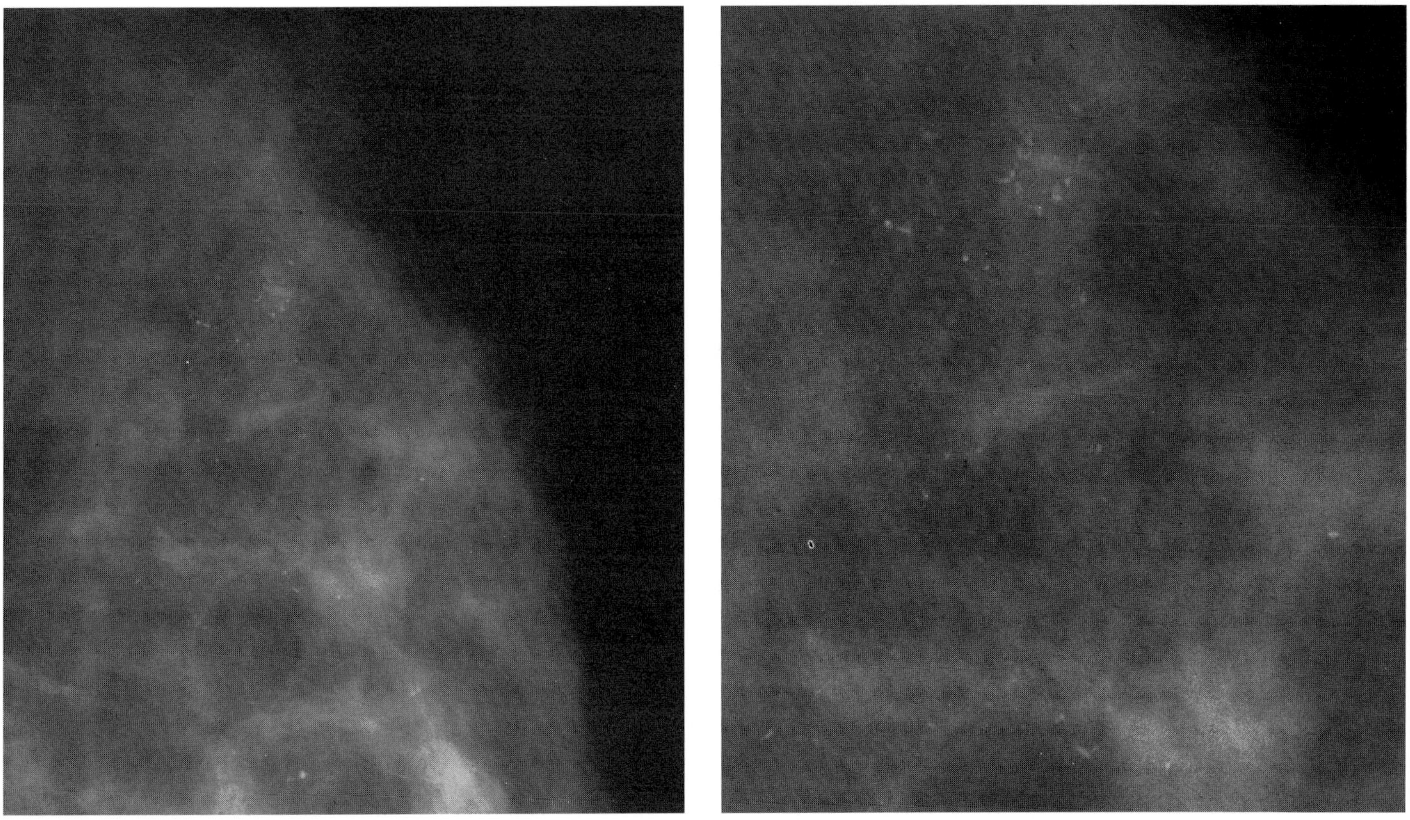

Figure 108-2. Left ML magnification view mammogram: The calcifications form a branching linear pattern.

Pathology

- ductal carcinoma in situ
- high nuclear grade, solid to focal cribiform growth with comedo type necrosis and microcalcifications (Fig. 108-3)

Management

- BI-RADS Assessment Category 5, highly suggestive of malignancy

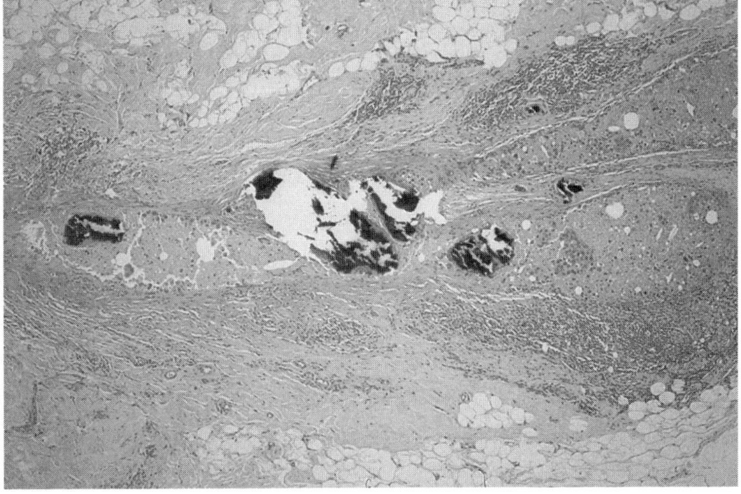

Figure 108-3. This malignancy is associated with extensive intraductal calcifications. The intraductal location of these calcifications results in the mammographically visible linear pattern (see Color Plate 108-3).

Pearls and Pitfalls

About 75% of cases of DCIS appear as isolated mammographic calcifications. In 10%, both calcifications and soft tissue mass are mammographically demonstrated, and in another 10% only a soft tissue mass is evident. In 5%, the DCIS is incidentially discovered adjacent to a benign mammographic lesion.

Suggested Readings

1. Stomper PC, Connolly JL, Meyer JE, et al. Clinically occult ductal carcinoma in situ detected with mammography: analysis of 100 cases with radiologic-pathologic correlation. *Radiology* 1989;172:235–241.
2. Stomper PC, Margolin FR. Ductal carcinoma in situ: the mammographer's perspective. *AJR* 1994;162:585–591.

Case 109

Case History

A 43-year-old woman presents with left breast calcifications identified on screening mammogram.

Physical Examination

- normal exam

Mammogram

Calcifications (Fig. 109–1)

- type: fine linear/branching
- distribution: segmental

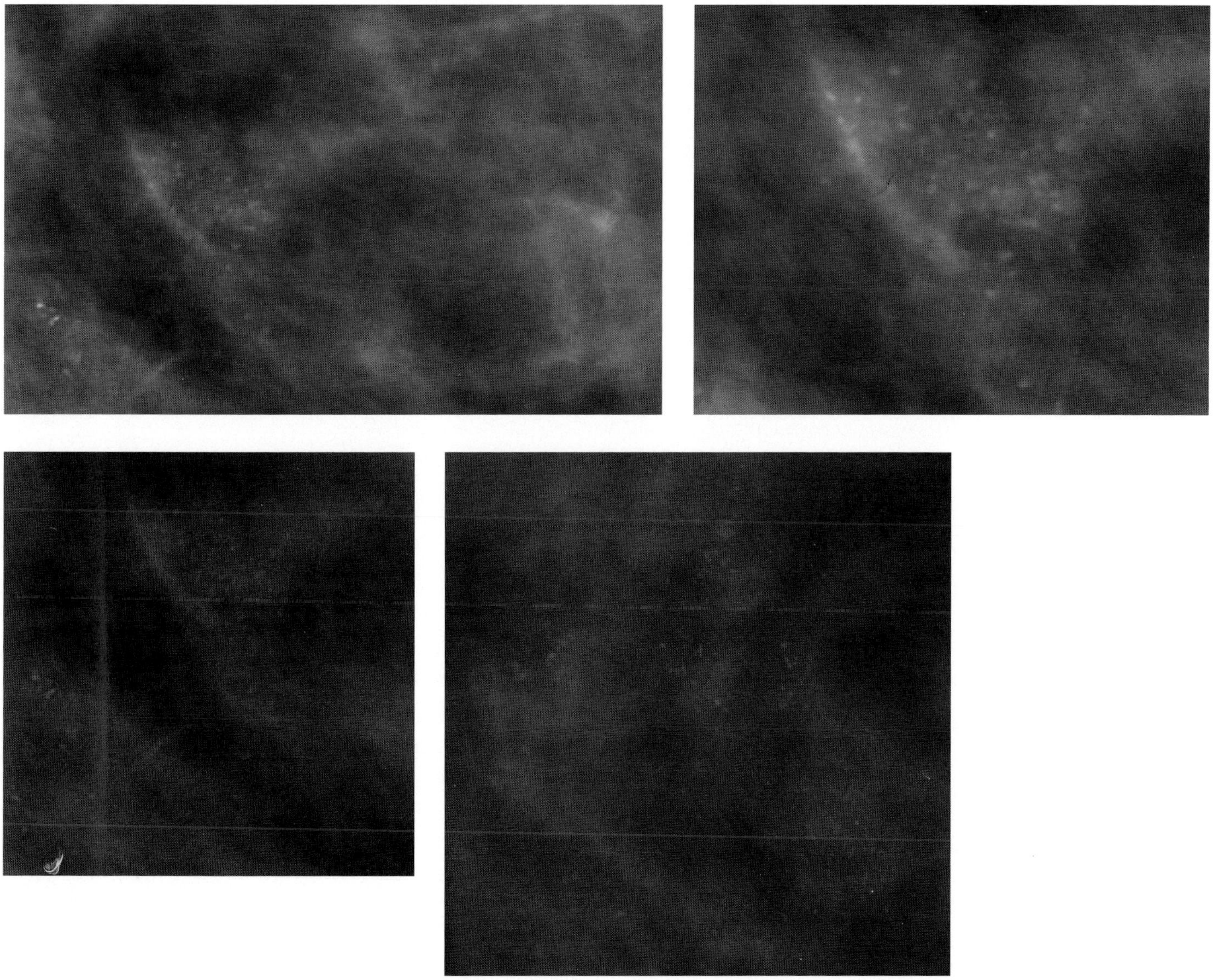

A

B

Figure 109–1. In the left outer inferior breast there are numerous clusters of heterogeneous linear-shaped calcifications. (A). Left MLO magnification view. (B). Left exaggerated CC magnification view.

Pathology

- invasive ductal carcinoma with a predominant intraductal component

Management

- BI-RADS Assessment Category 5, highly suggestive of malignancy

Pearls and Pitfalls

Invasive tumor with an extensive intraductal component is associated with greater incidence of recurrence after surgical excision and radiotherapy. (Five-year recurrence rate with extensive intraductal component is 25% vs. 6% without extensive intraductal component.) This increase in recurrence appears to be related to a higher rate of inadequate surgical margins, resulting in leaving residual neoplasm in the breast. Therefore, it is important that pathologic margins are clean and radiographic examination of the remaining breast be free of suspicious calcifications.

Suggested Readings

1. Fowble B, Rosser C, Hanlon A. Conservative surgery and radiation for stages I and II breast cancer. In: Bland KI, ed. *The Breast: Comprehensive Management of Benign and Malignant Diseases*. Philadelphia: WB Saunders Company; 1998:1172–1178.
2. Holland R, Connolly JL, Gelman R, et al. The presence of an extensive intraductal component following a limited excision correlates with prominent residual disease in the remainder of the breast. *J Clin Oncol* 1990;8:113–118.
3. Stomper PC, Connolly JL. Mammographic features predicting an extensive intraductal component in early-stage infiltrating duct carcinoma. *AJR* 1992;158:269–272.

Case 110

Case History

A 40-year-old woman presents with a palpable breast lump. Mammographically, the lump is associated with abnormal calcifications. Sonographically, the lump corresponds to a hypoechoic ill-defined mass. Biopsy of the lump demonstrates infiltrating ductal carcinoma. Sestamibi study demonstrates abnormal activity in both the breast and the axilla. She is treated with preoperative chemotherapy and the palpable lump disappears. However, the mammographic calcifications remain stable. The sonographic mass shrinks but is still visible. The sestamibi exam shows reduction of breast activity and disappearance of the activity in the axilla.

Physical Examination

- right breast: palpable lump at the 11:00 position
- left breast: normal

Mammogram

Calcifications (Fig. 110–1)

- type: fine linear/branching
- distribution: segmental

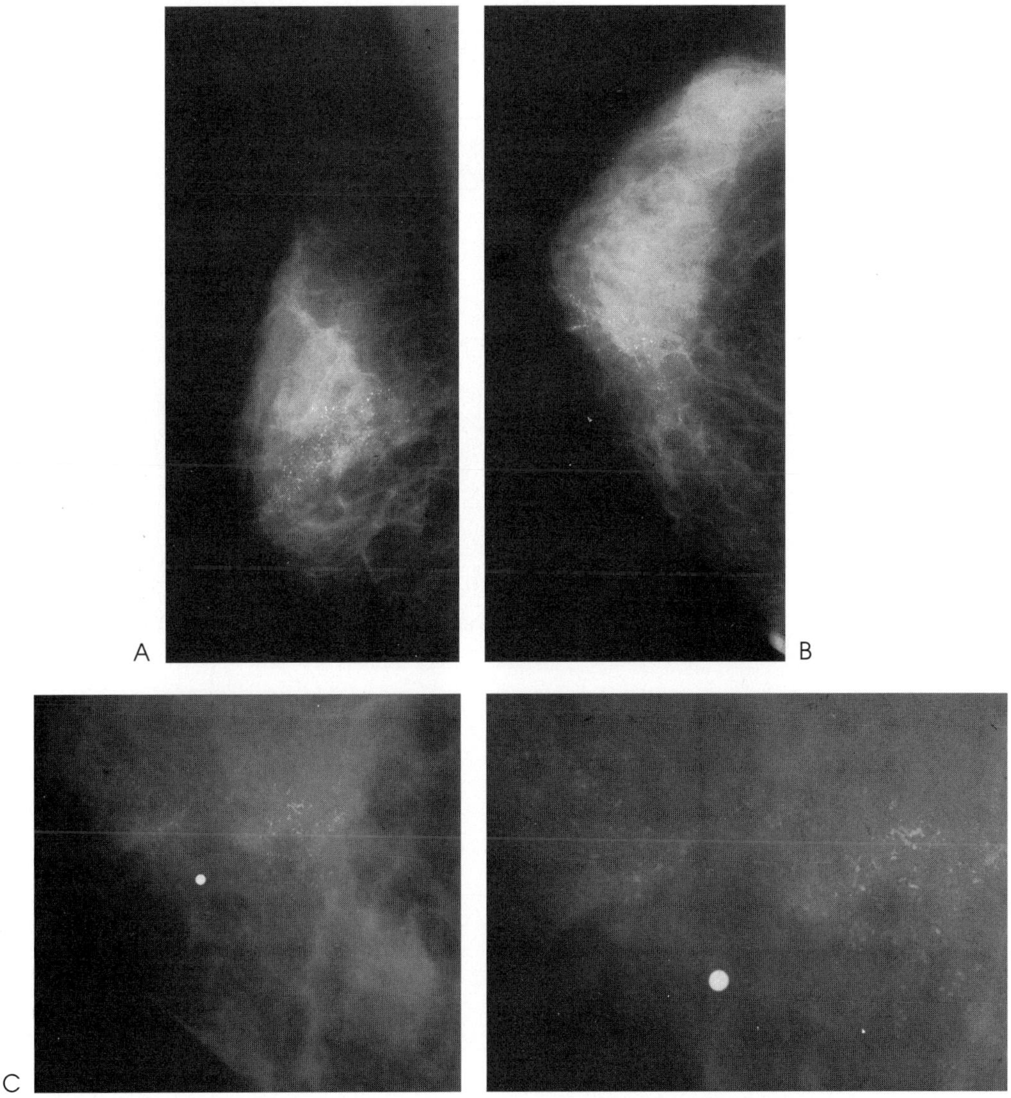

Figure 110–1. In the upper medial breast, there is a segmental group of fine linear branching calcifications. (A). Right ML mammogram. (B). Right CC mammogram. (C). Right CC magnification mammogram.

Ultrasound

Frequency

- 7.5 MHz

Mass

- margin: ill defined
- echogenicity: hypoechoic
- retrotumoral acoustic appearance: increased acoustic transmission
- shape: irregular (Figs. 110-2 and 110-3)

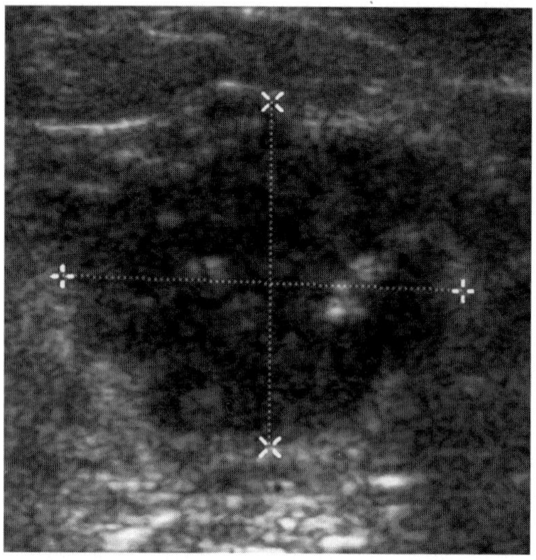

Figure 110-2. Right radial breast sonogram: The palpable lump located within the segment of abnormal calcifications identified in Figure 110-1 corresponds to an ill-defined hypoechoic solid mass with calcifications.

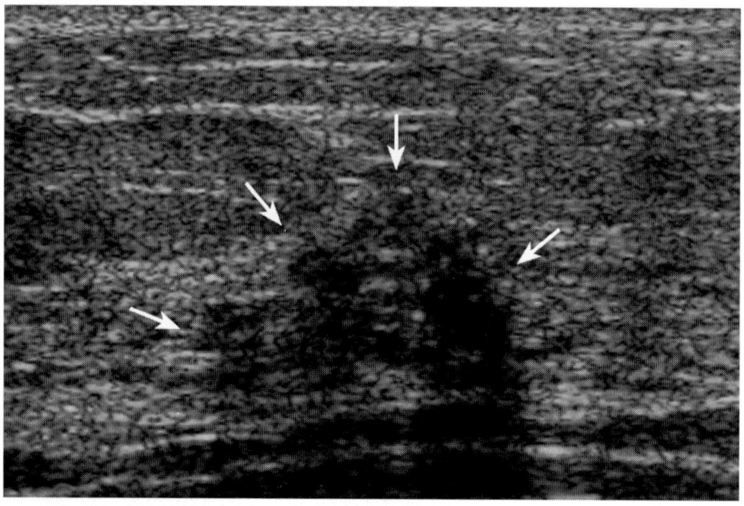

Figure 110-3. Right radial breast sonogram: After chemotherapy, the hypoechoic mass shrank from 18 to 12 mm and was no longer palpable.

Other Modalities (Figs. 110-4 and 110-5)

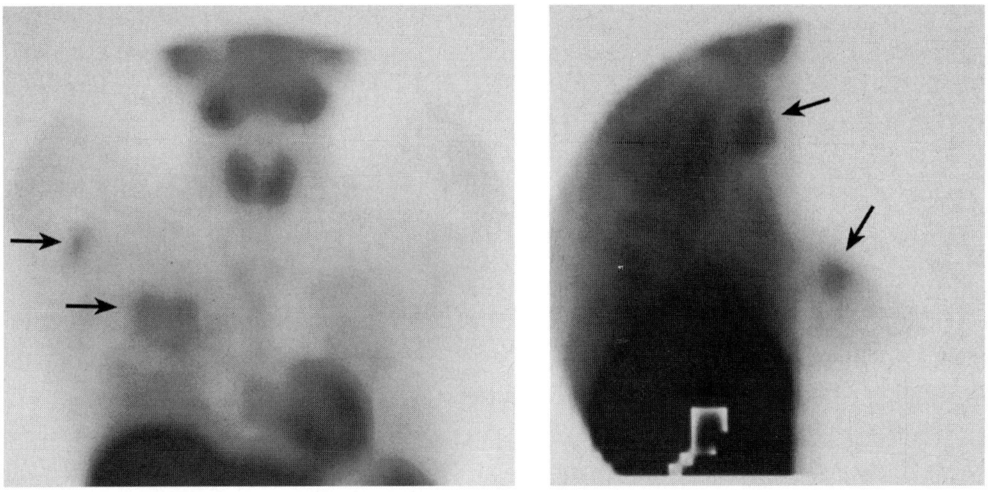

A B

Figure 110-4. *Breast sestamibi scan prior to preoperative chemotherapy demonstrates abnormal activity consistent with a primary right breast malignancy associated with metastatic adenopathy (arrows). (A). Breast sestamibi scan: Right anteroposterior position. (B). Breast sestamibi scan: Right lateral position.*

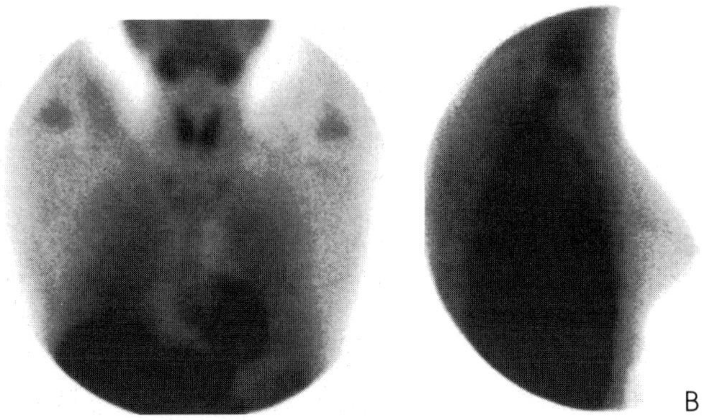

A B

Figure 110-5. *Breast sestamibi scan performed after preoperative chemotherapy shows that the abnormal activity in the right breast and axilla has resolved. (A). Breast sestamibi scan: Anteroposterior position. (B). Breast sestamibi scan: Right lateral position.*

Pathology

Invasive ductal carcinoma with a predominant intraductal component. Mastectomy specimen obtained after chemotherapy demonstrated extensive fibrosis with residual ductal carcinoma in situ measuring 3 × 2.5 cm with 1 mm focus of infiltrating ductal carcinoma. Four axillary nodes were negative.

Management

- BI-RADS Assessment Category 5, highly suggestive of malignancy

Pearls and Pitfalls

1. In patients undergoing preoperative chemotherapy, clinical and mammographic information is in agreement in 79% of cases. In this case they were discordant, but the mammographic information reflected the pathologic findings more accurately.
2. Technetium-labeled sestamibi imaging is useful in following these patients. This technique has a sensitivity of 92%, specificity of 89%, positive predictive value of 81%, and negative predictive value of 96%. However, false-negative findings increase with malignancies <1 cm. Metastatic lymph nodes can be detected with a sensitivity of 84% and specificity of 91%.
3. Some studies have shown that the sonographic tumor size correlates closer to the pathologic size and that sonography correlates better with tumor shrinkage than mammography.

Suggested Readings

1. Fornage BD, Toubas O, Morel M. Clinical mammographic and sonographic determination of preoperative breast cancer size. *Cancer* 1987;60:765–771.
2. Khalkali I, Cutrone JA, Mena IG, et al. Scintimammography: the complementary role of technetium-99 sestamibi prone breast imaging for the diagnosis of breast cancer. *Radiology* 1995;196:421–426.
3. Moskovic EC, Mansi JL, King DM, et al. Mammography in the assessment of response to medical treatment of large primary breast cancer. *Clin Radiol* 1993;47:339–344.
4. Powles TJ, Hickish TF, Makris A, et al. Randomized trial of chemoendocrine therapy started before or after surgery for treatment of primary breast cancer. *J Clin Oncol* 1995;13:547–552.
5. Taillefer R, Robidoux A, Lambert R, et al. Technetium-99 m sestamibi prone scintimammography to detect primary breast cancer and axillary lymph node involvement. *J Nucl Med* 1995;36:1758–1765.

Case 111

Case History

A 68-year-old woman has increasing calcifications on her screening mammogram. She has past history of lung cancer and bladder cancer. Stereotactic core needle biopsy of the calcifications was not conclusive so a needle localization and excisional biopsy were performed. Patient was unable to maintain an upright position for the needle localization, so sonographic guidance of the wire localization was performed.

Physical Examination

- normal exam

Mammogram

Calcifications (Figs. 111-1 and 111-2)

- type: fine linear/branching
- distribution: linear

Figure 111-1. In the 6:00 position of the left breast, there is a nodular density associated with linear calcifications (circled). (A). Left MLO mammogram. (B). Left CC mammogram. (C). Left CC magnification mammogram.

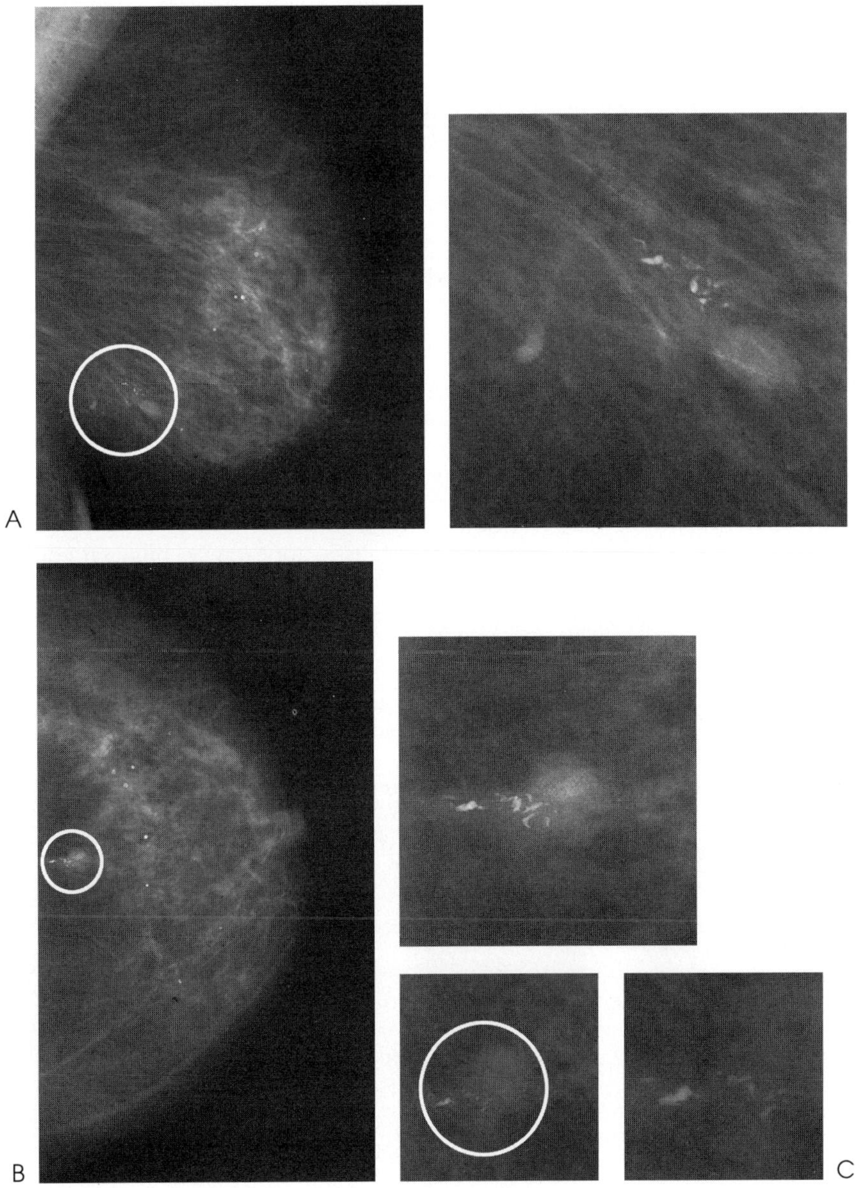

A

B

C

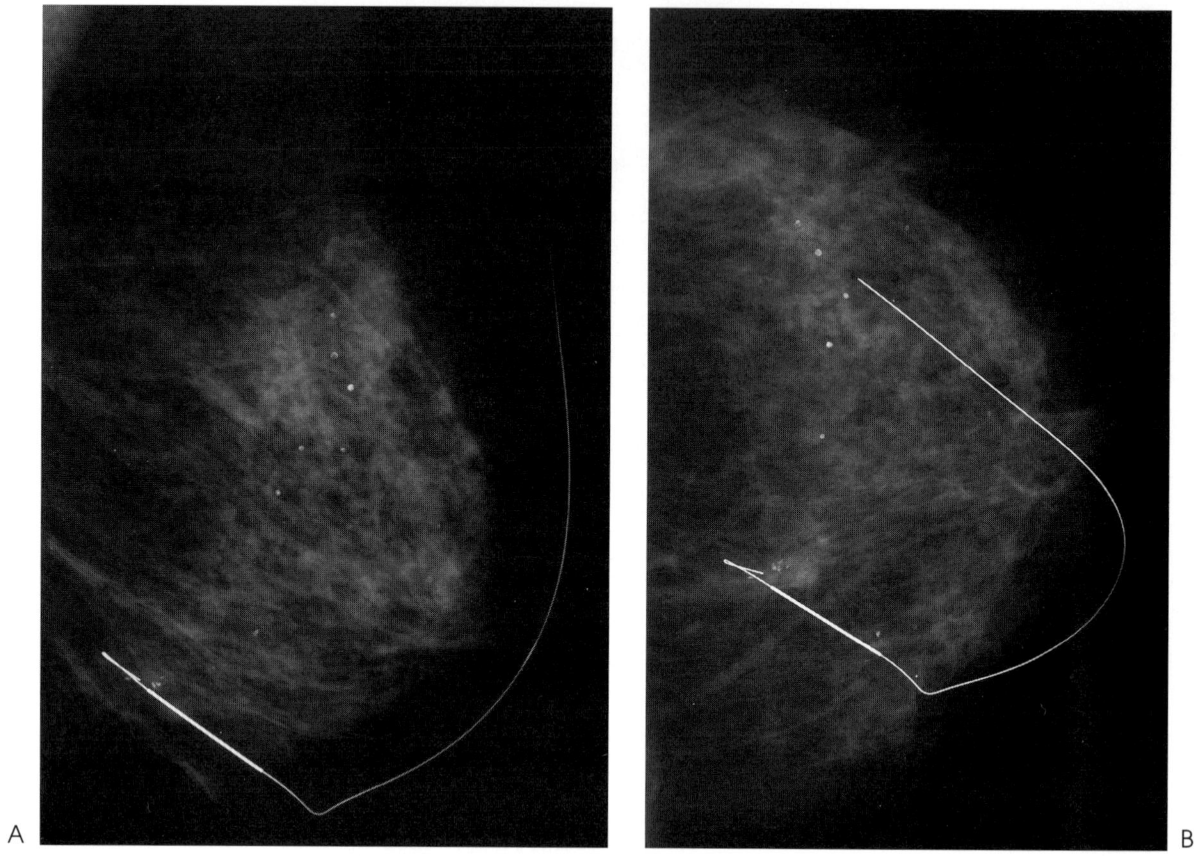

Figure 111–2. *Mammograms performed after sonographic guidance of needle localization demonstrate that the wire is in excellent position with respect to the calcifications. (A). Left ML mammogram after needle localization. (B). Left CC mammogram after needle localization.*

Ultrasound

Frequency

- 13 MHz

Mass

- margin: ill defined
- echogenicity: hypoechoic
- retrotumoral acoustic appearance: bilateral edge shadowing
- shape: ellipsoid (Fig. 111–3)

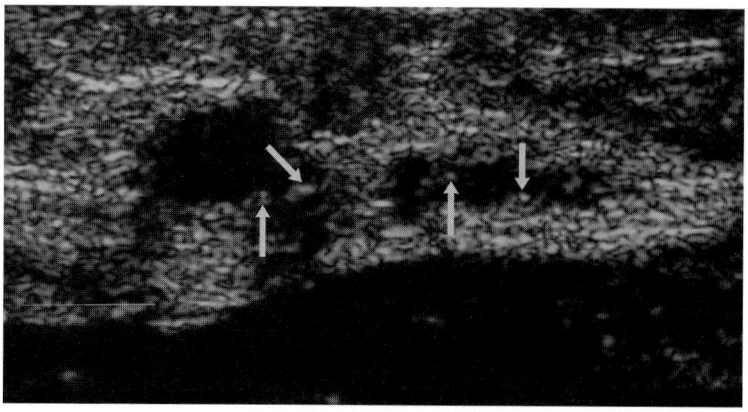

Figure 111–3. *Left radial breast sonogram: The calcifications identified in Figure 111–1 corresponded to a focally dilated tubular structure associated with a solid nodule. Both the tubular structure and the nodule contained multiple calcifications (arrows). Sonographic needle localization was performed using this image. After localization, mammographic images were taken to confirm the wire position (see Fig. 111–2).*

Pathology

- adenomyoepithelioma

Management

- BI-RADS Assessment Category 4, suspicious abnormality; biopsy should be considered

Pearls and Pitfalls

1. Adenomyoepithelioma is an unusual breast tumor that is generally benign but may recur after local excision. Occasionally, carcinoma or malignant myoepithelioma will arise within an adenomyoepithelioma.
2. Sonographic guidance for needle localization of calcifications is rarely necessary. To perform this procedure, it is critical that one is confident in locating the calcifications. High-frequency sonography is generally a necessity in this situation.

Suggested Readings

1. Leucht D, Madjar H. Microcalcification in sonography. In: Leucht D, ed. *Teaching Atlas of Breast Ultrasound.* New York: Thieme; 1996:189–204.
2. Tavassoli FA, Fattaneh A. *Pathology of the Breast.* 2nd ed. Stamford: Appleton and Lange; 1999:763–791.

Section VI

Increased Density

I. Increased density should first be categorized into the following categories:

A. Generalized increased density: either the entire breast or both breasts exhibit increased density
B. Large area of increased density: generally greater or equal to 5 cm or about 25% of the breast
C. Focal asymmetric density: generally less than 5 cm

II. Differential diagnosis of generalized increased density

A. Lymphatic spread of breast cancer
B. Lymphedema (i.e., secondary to obstruction of axillary lymphatic drainage from lymphoproliferative disease, or lymphatic metastases from breast gynecologic, bronchial, or esophageal malignancies)
C. Radiation therapy to the breast
D. Infection or inflammation (e.g., mastitis)
E. Right heart failure
F. Increased estrogen (e.g., hormonal replacement therapy, pregnancy)

III. Differential diagnosis of large area of increased density

A. Increased estrogen
B. Fibrocystic change
C. Diabetic fibrous mastopathy
D. Infection and inflammation (including abscess)
E. Trauma (including fat necrosis and hematoma)
F. Primary breast malignancy (especially lobular and infiltrating ductal carcinomas)
G. Lymphoproliferative disease

IV. Differential diagnosis of focal asymmetric density

A. Overlap of benign parenchymal density
B. Fibrocystic change
C. Diabetic fibrous mastopathy
D. Infection and inflammation
E. Trauma (e.g., fat necrosis, hematoma, scar)
F. Radial scar
G. Benign breast tumor
H. Primary breast malignancy

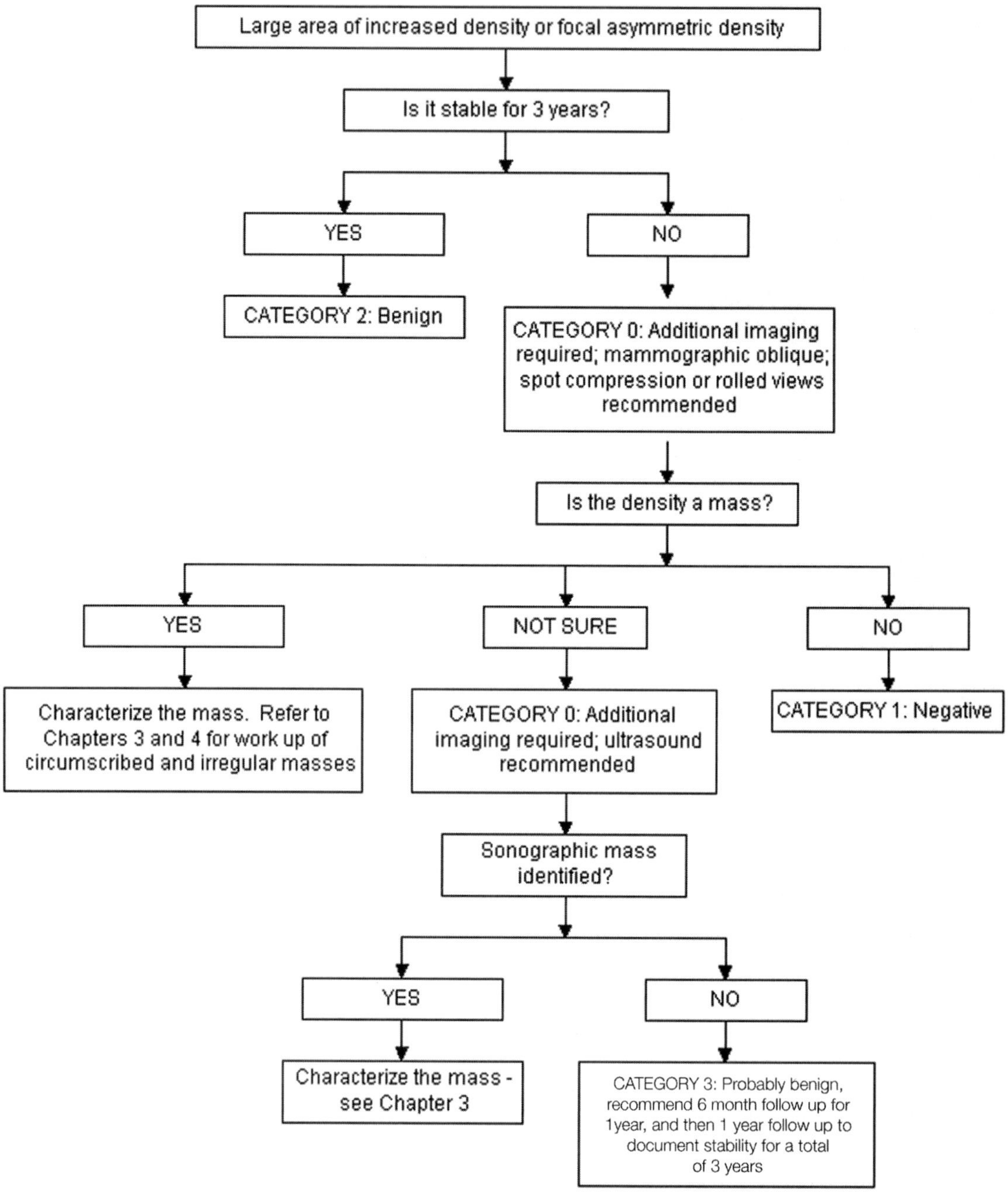
Large area of increased density or focal asymmetric density
Is it stable for 3 years?
YES
NO
CATEGORY 2: Benign
CATEGORY 0: Additional imaging required; mammographic oblique; spot compression or rolled views recommended
Is the density a mass?
YES
NOT SURE
NO
Characterize the mass. Refer to Chapters 3 and 4 for work up of circumscribed and irregular masses
CATEGORY 0: Additional imaging required; ultrasound recommended
CATEGORY 1: Negative
Sonographic mass identified?
YES
NO
Characterize the mass - see Chapter 3
CATEGORY 3: Probably benign, recommend 6 month follow up for 1year, and then 1 year follow up to document stability for a total of 3 years

Case 112

Case History

An 84-year-old woman presents 2 years after left axillary dissection for left arm melanoma and right lumpectomy for breast cancer.

Physical Examination

- right breast: well-healed scar in the upper outer breast
- left breast: diffuse swelling without redness

Mammogram

- diffuse increased density (Fig. 112–1)

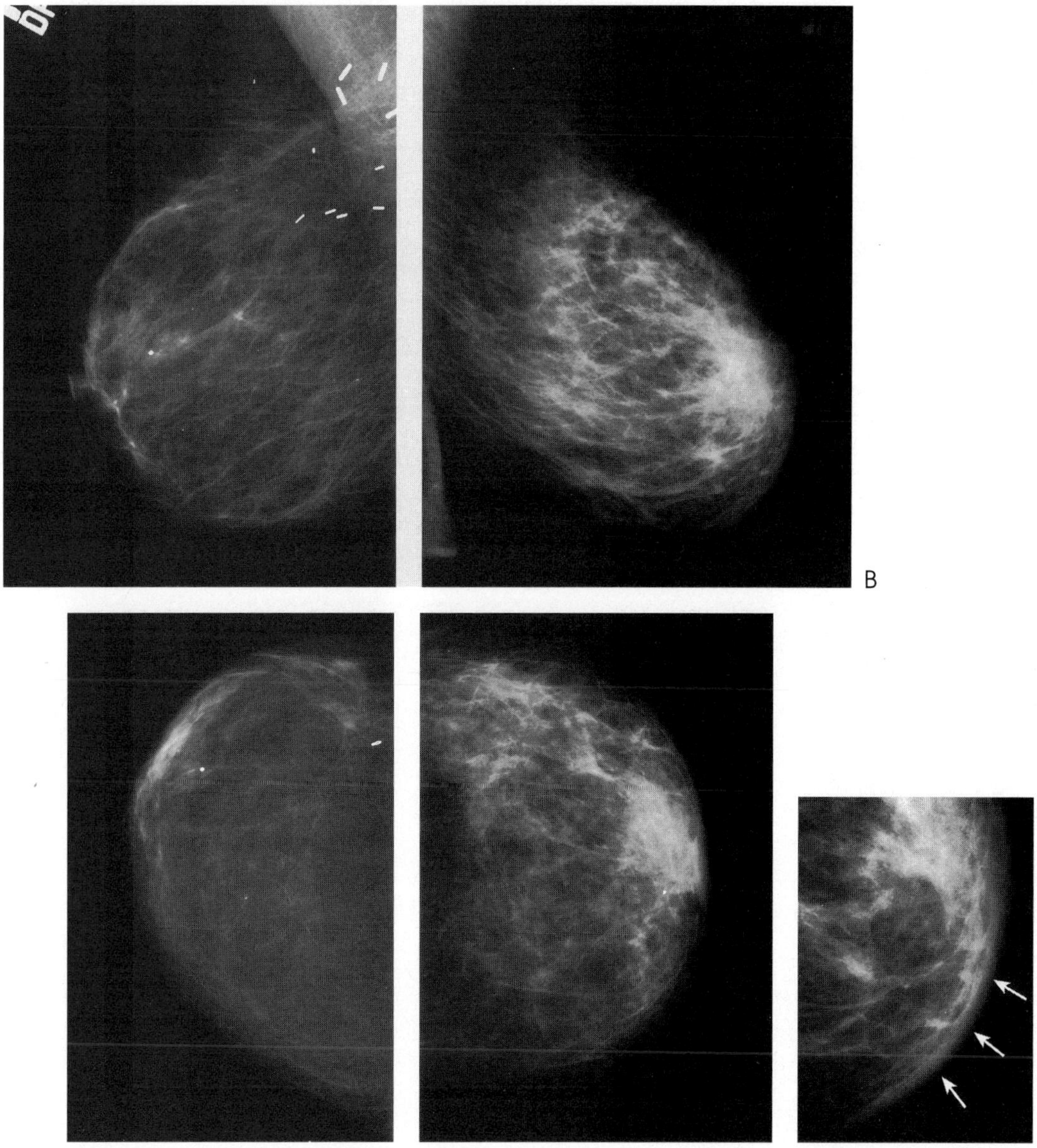

A B C D E

Figure 112–1. The left breast exhibits diffuse increased density with skin thickening (skin thickening highlighted by arrows in E). Clips in the right upper outer quadrant are from previous lumpectomy. (A). Right MLO mammogram. (B). Left MLO mammogram. (C). Right CC mammogram. (D). Left CC mammogram. (E). Left MLO mammogram (close-up).

Pathology

- lymphedema

Management

- BI-RADS Assessment Category 2, benign finding

Pearls and Pitfalls

Lymphedema is due to five main etiologies: (1) obstruction of axillary nodes (either due to malignant involvement or surgical removal of nodes); (2) general lymphatic obstruction from contralateral breast cancer; (3) inflammation; (4) postradiation effect; (5) systemic fluid overload (e.g., from congestive heart failure or renal failure). In this case, the patient's lymphedema resulted from an axillary dissection performed for melanoma staging.

Suggested Readings

1. Tabar L, Dean PB. Thickened skin syndrome of the breast. In: Tabar L, Dean PB. *Teaching Atlas of Mammography.* 3rd ed. New York: Thieme; 2001:239–247.

Case 113

Case History

Two weeks after a normal vaginal delivery, this 34-year-old woman develops severe left breast pain and erythema. Clinically, she appears to have mastitis and is started on antibiotics.

Physical Examination

- left breast: diffusely tender and erythematous
- right breast: normal exam

Mammogram

- diffuse increased density (Figs. 113-1 and 113-2)

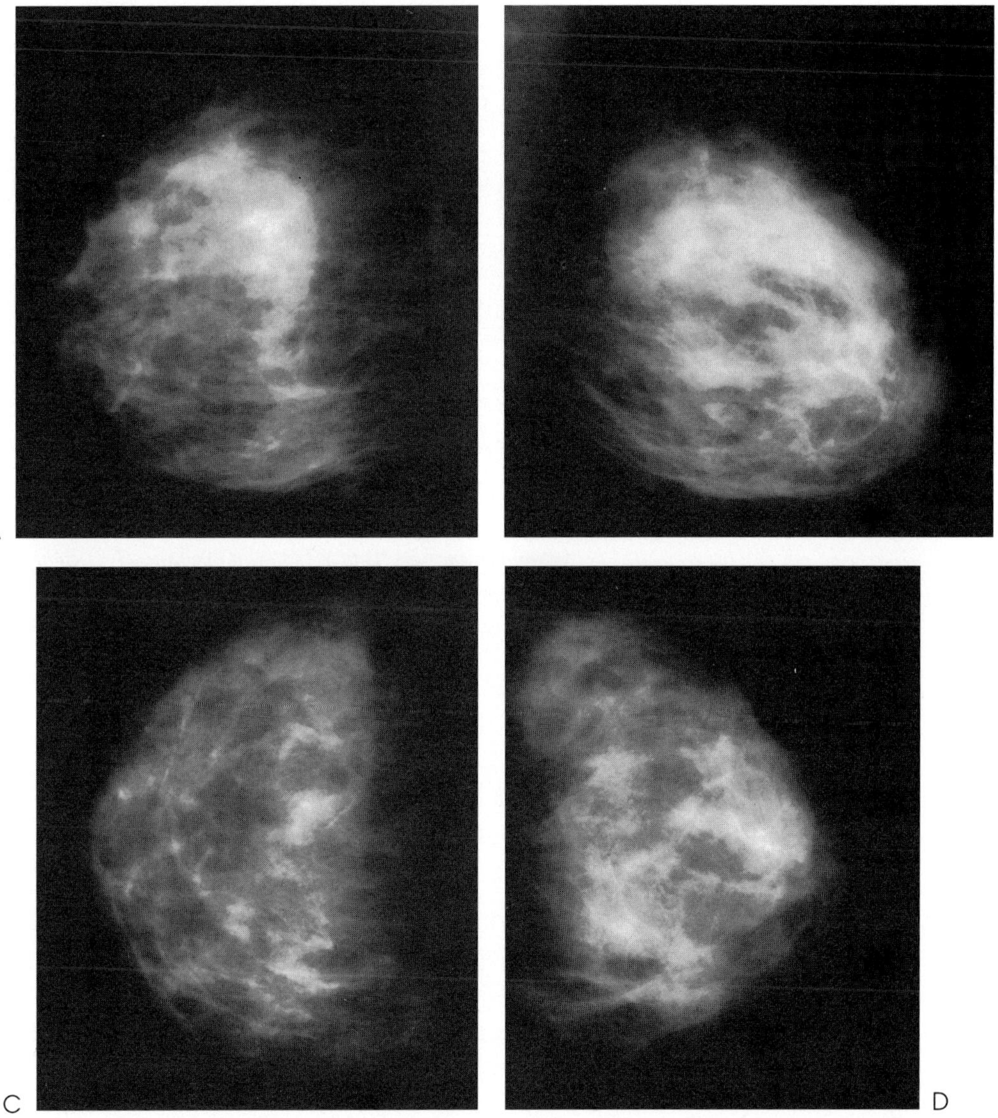

A B C D

Figure 113-1. Although both breasts exhibit diffuse increased density, the left breast is more dense than the right breast. (A). Right MLO mammogram. (B). Left MLO mammogram. (C). Right CC mammogram. (D). Left CC mammogram.

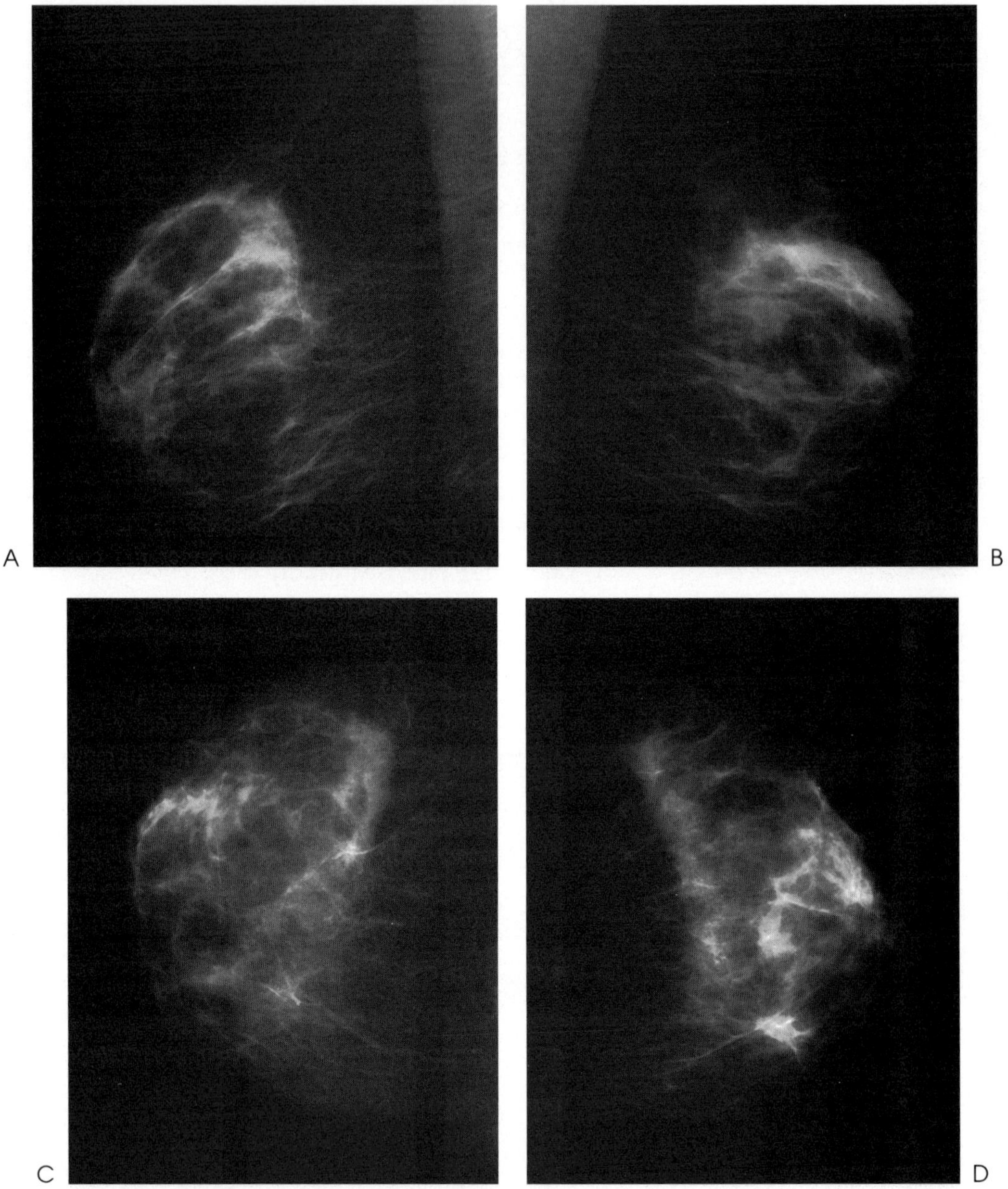

Figure 113–2. *Nine months after the examination in Figure 113–1, bilateral mammograms demonstrate reduction in overall density. The density is now relatively symmetric. (A). Right MLO mammogram. (B). Left MLO mammogram. (C). Right CC mammogram. (D). Left CC mammogram.*

Ultrasound

Frequency

- 7.5 MHz (Fig. 113-3)

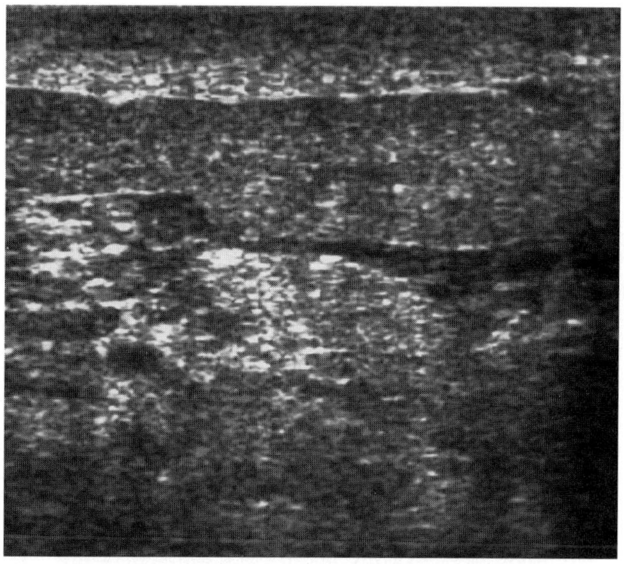

Figure 113-3. Left radial breast sonogram: Sonography is performed at the same time as Figure 113-1 to identify a possible abscess. No abscess is identified. There is skin thickening and multiple linear fluid collections thoughout the parenchyma.

Pathology

- mastitis

Management

- BI-RADS Assessment Category 3, probably benign; short-interval follow-up

Pearls and Pitfalls

1. This case illustrates bilateral increased density due to prominent postpartum glandular tissue. The asymmetric increased left breast density is due to mastitis.
2. Sonographically, mastitis produces thickening of the skin, subcutaneous fat, and glandular tissue. The interface between the fat and glandular tissue is indistinct. Numerous thin linear fluid collections are present. With progression of inflammation, an abscess may form. Abscesses are generally hypoechoic round or oval masses. The margins may either be smooth or irregular. Commonly, abscesses contain solid material, septations, or movable internal echoes. Sonography is useful to identify and drain abscesses.

Suggested Readings

1. Heywang-Kobrunner SH, Schreer I, Dershaw DD. *Diagnostic Breast Imaging.* New York: Thieme; 1997:194–201.
2. Tohno D, Cosgrove DO, Sloane JP, eds. *Ultrasound Diagnosis of Breast Diseases.* New York: Churchill Livingston; 1994:136–138.

Case 114

Case History

A 63-year-old woman presents with right breast swelling.

Physical Examination

- right breast: mild diffuse erythema and peau d'orange; no focal palpable mass
- left breast: normal exam

Mammogram

- diffuse increased density (Fig. 114–1)

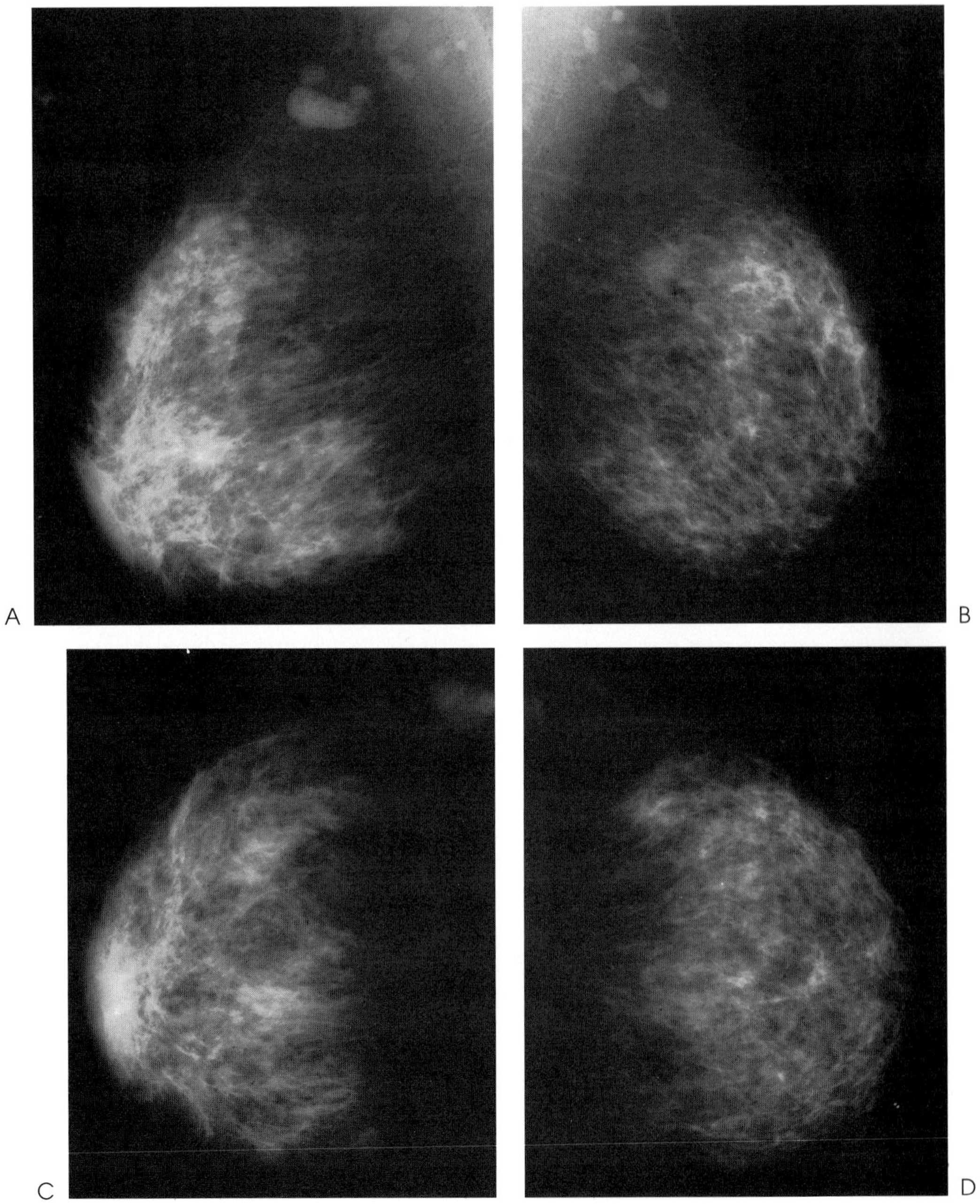

Figure 114–1. *The right breast exhibits diffuse increased density, trabecular thickening, and periareolar skin thickening. Multiple enlarged right axillary nodes are present. (A). Right MLO mammogram. (B). Left MLO mammogram. (C). Right CC mammogram. (D). Left CC mammogram.*

Pathology

Infiltrating ductal carcinoma. Patient was treated with chemotherapy prior to mastectomy. Residual tumor was 1.5 cm. No dermal lymphatic invasion was present, but lack of involvement may be due to tumor response to chemotherapy. Six of 14 axillary nodes had metastatic disease.

Management

- BI-RADS Assessment Category 5, highly suggestive of malignancy

Pearls and Pitfalls

The definition of inflammatory carcinoma is mildly controversial. Some have defined this entity clinically (i.e., skin erythema, edema, and warmth) and others insist on microscopic confirmation of metastatic involvement of the dermal lymphatics. Some patients do not fit these criteria. Only 80% of women with skin changes have dermal lymphatic involvement, and 4% with dermal lymphatic tumor do not have skin abnormalities.

Suggested Readings

1. Cardenosa G. *Breast Imaging Companion.* Philadelphia: Lippincott-Raven; 1997:166–167.

Case 115

Case History

A 74-year-old woman presents for screening mammogram.

Physical Examination

- normal exam

Mammogram

- diffuse increased density (Figs. 115–1 and 115–2)

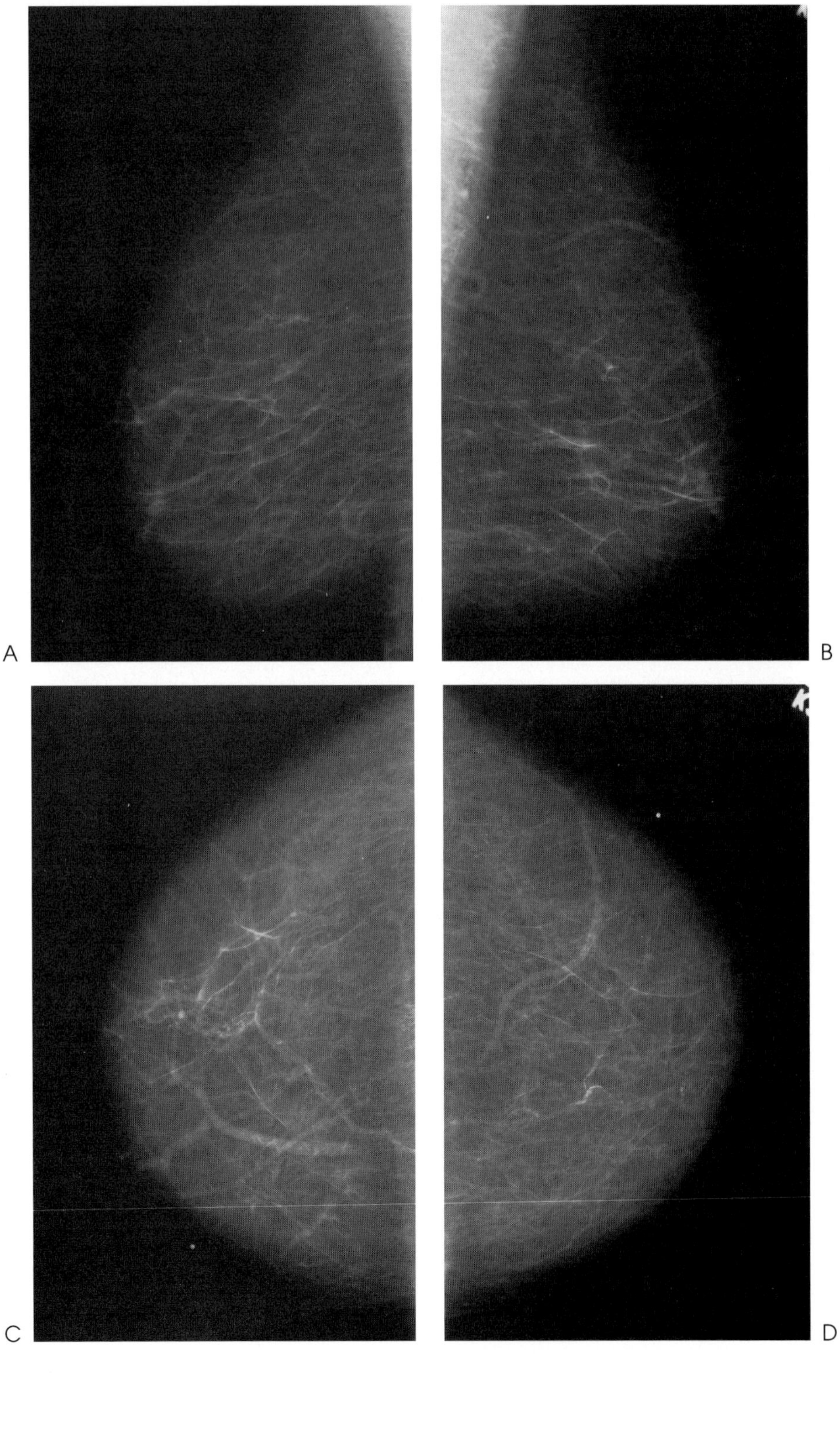

Figure 115–1. Normal fatty breast pattern. (A). Right MLO mammogram. (B). Left MLO mammogram. (C). Right CC mammogram. (D). Left CC mammogram.

Figure 115–2. This bilateral mammographic examination was performed 2 years later on the same patient as Figure 115–1. (A). Right MLO mammogram. (B). Left MLO mammogram. (C). Right CC mammogram. (D). Left CC mammogram.

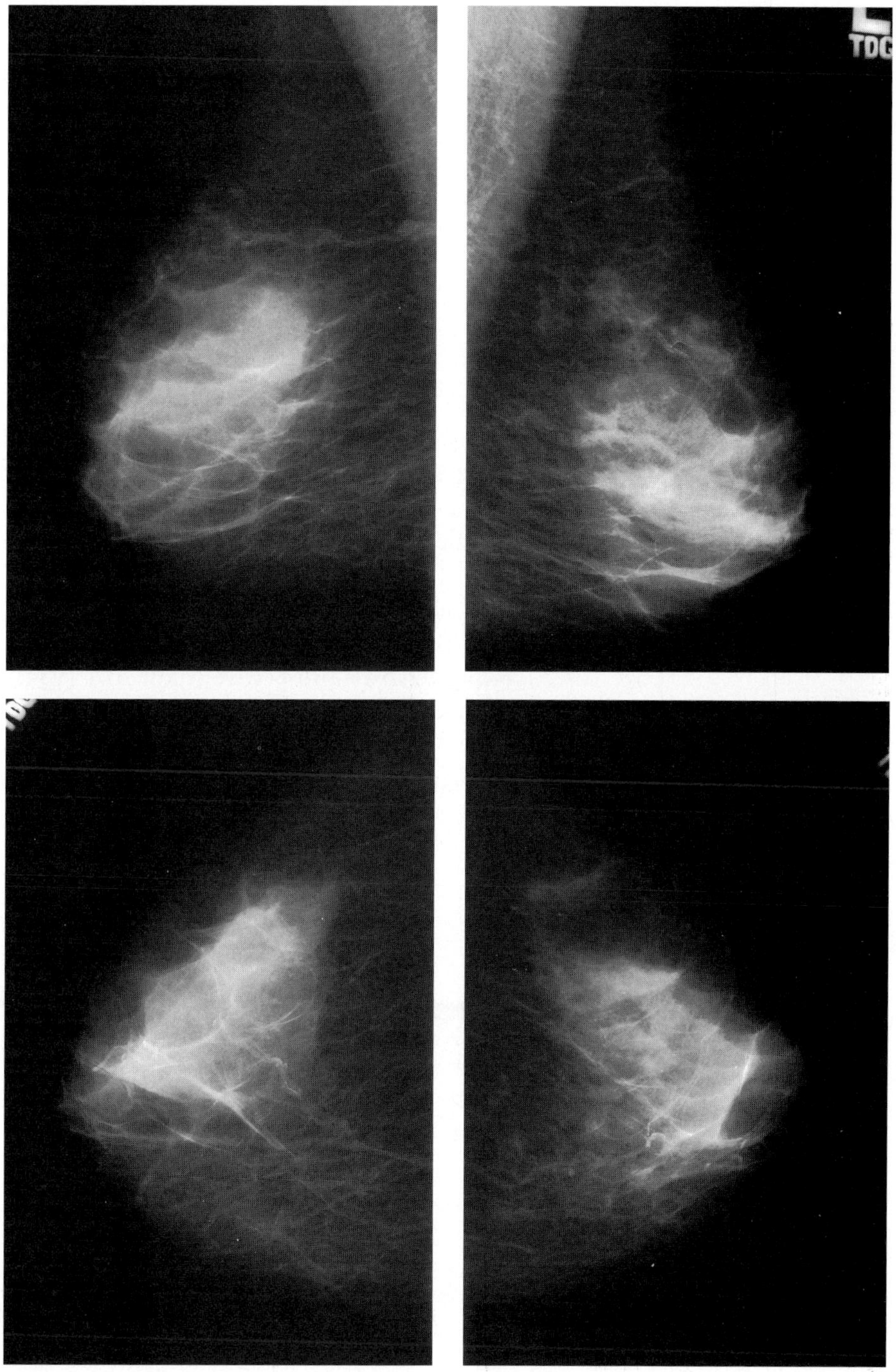

A B C D

Pathology

- normal breast tissue

Management

- BI-RADS Assessment Category 1, negative

Pearls and Pitfalls

1. The patient started hormone replacement therapy (HRT) just after the earlier mammographic examination (Fig. 115–1). Studies have shown that about 24% of women develop increased mammographic density after starting HRT. Estrogen stimulates growth of ductal epithelium and periductal connective tissue. Although progesterone is an antagonist to these proliferative effects, progesterone enhances the effect of estrogen by encouraging distal ductal development.
2. Besides causing diffuse increased density, HRT will also cause asymmetric densities and cystic formation.

Suggested Readings

1. Cyrlak D, Wong CH. Mammographic changes in postmenopausal women undergoing hormonal replacement therapy. *AJR* 1993;161:1177–1183.
2. Laya MB, Gallagher JC, Schreiman JS, Larson EB, Watson P, Weinstein L. Effect of postmenopausal hormonal replacement therapy on mammographic density and parenchymal pattern. *Radiology* 1995;196:433–437.
3. McNicholas MMJ, Heneghan JP, Milner MH, Tunney T, Hourihane JB, MacErlaine DP. Pain and increased mammographic density in women receiving hormone replacement therapy: a prospective study. *AJR* 1994;163:311–315.
4. Stomper PC, Van Vorrhis BJ, Ravnikar VA, Meyer JE. Mammographic changes associated with postmenopausal hormone replacement therapy: a longitudinal study. *Radiology* 1990;174:487–490.

Case 116

Case History

A 70-year-old woman, who sustained severe right breast injury during a fall 1 year ago, presents with right breast lump in area of previous trauma.

Physical Examination

- right breast: palpable lump in the upper outer quadrant
- left breast: normal exam

Mammogram

- asymmetric density (Figs. 116–1 and 116–2)

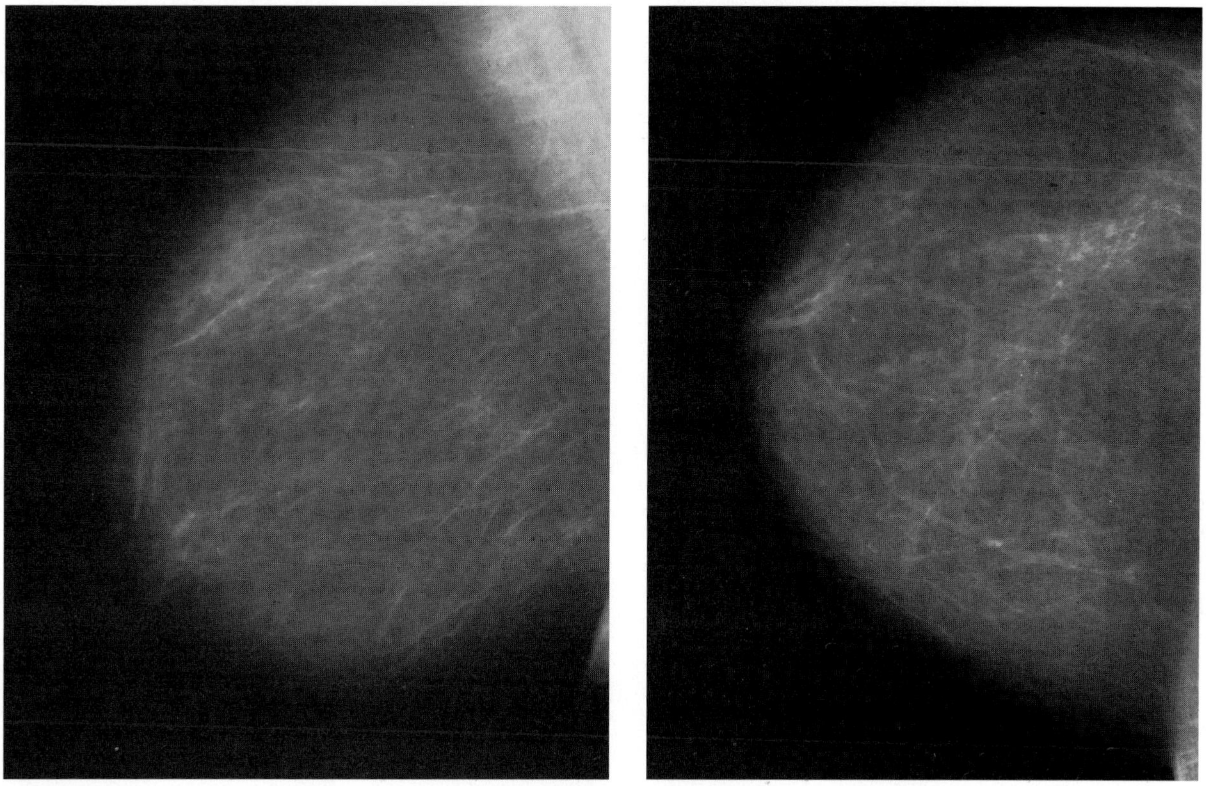

A B

Figure 116–1. Prior to the injury, the patient's right breast mammogram was normal. (A). Right MLO mammogram. (B). Right CC mammogram.

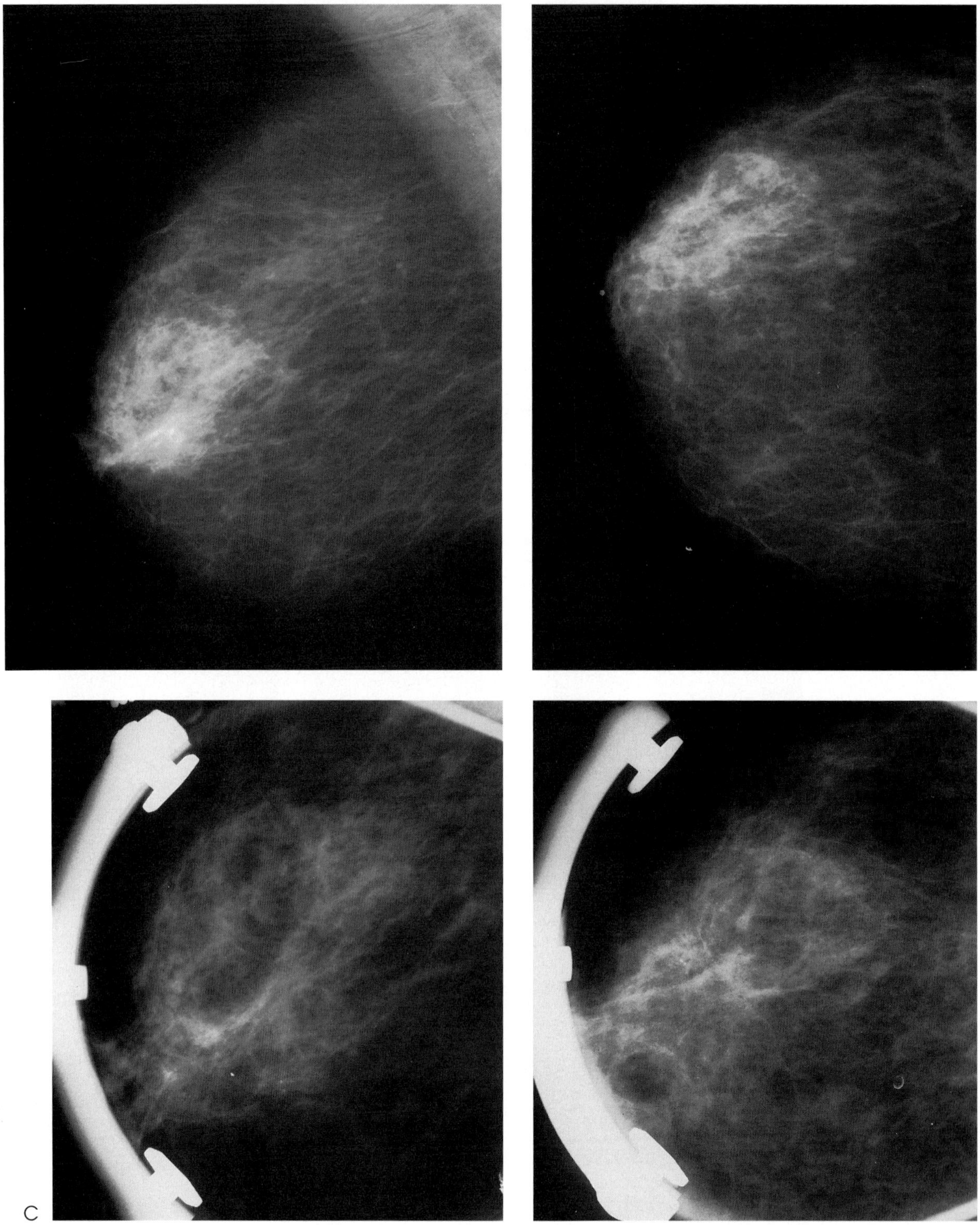

Figure 116–2. *One year after the injury, there is a new asymmetric density in the right upper outer quadrant. (A). Right MLO mammogram. (B). Right CC mammogram. (C). Right MLO spot compression. (D). Right CC spot compression.*

Ultrasound

Frequency

- 8 MHz

Mass

- margin: ill defined
- echogenicity: hypoechoic
- retrotumoral acoustic appearance: posterior shadowing distal to mass
- shape: irregular (Fig. 116–3)

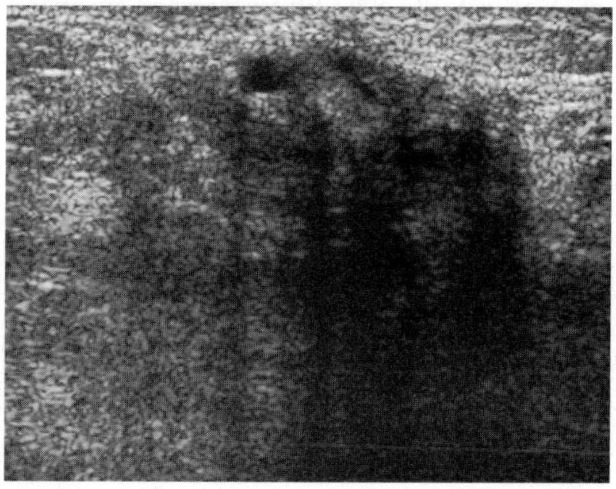

Figure 116–3. Right radial breast sonogram: In the right upper outer quadrant, the palpable mass corresponds to an irregular hypoechoic mass. This mass corresponds to the mammographic asymmetric density.

Pathology

- fat necrosis

Management

- BI-RADS Assessment Category 4, suspicious; biopsy should be considered

Pearls and Pitfalls

1. Trauma (such as this case), infection or inflammation, hormonal replacement therapy, and malignancy will produce large areas of increased mammographic density.
2. In cases of infection or trauma, sonographic examination is useful to identify abscess or hematoma.
3. If the asymmetric density is stable for longer than 3 years, then one should recommend routine mammographic screening. For densities that have been stable for 1 to 3 years, one may proceed with short-term follow-up. For new asymmetries or those increasing in size or density, biopsy is recommended.

Suggested Readings

1. Heywang-Kobrunner SH, Schreer I, Dershaw DD. *Diagnostic Breast Imaging.* New York: Thieme; 1997:353–357.

Case 117

Case History

A 65-year-old woman presents with left breast lump. This is her first mammographic examination.

Physical Examination

- left breast: 10 cm hard mass in the superior breast
- right breast: normal exam

Mammogram

- asymmetric density (Fig. 117–1)

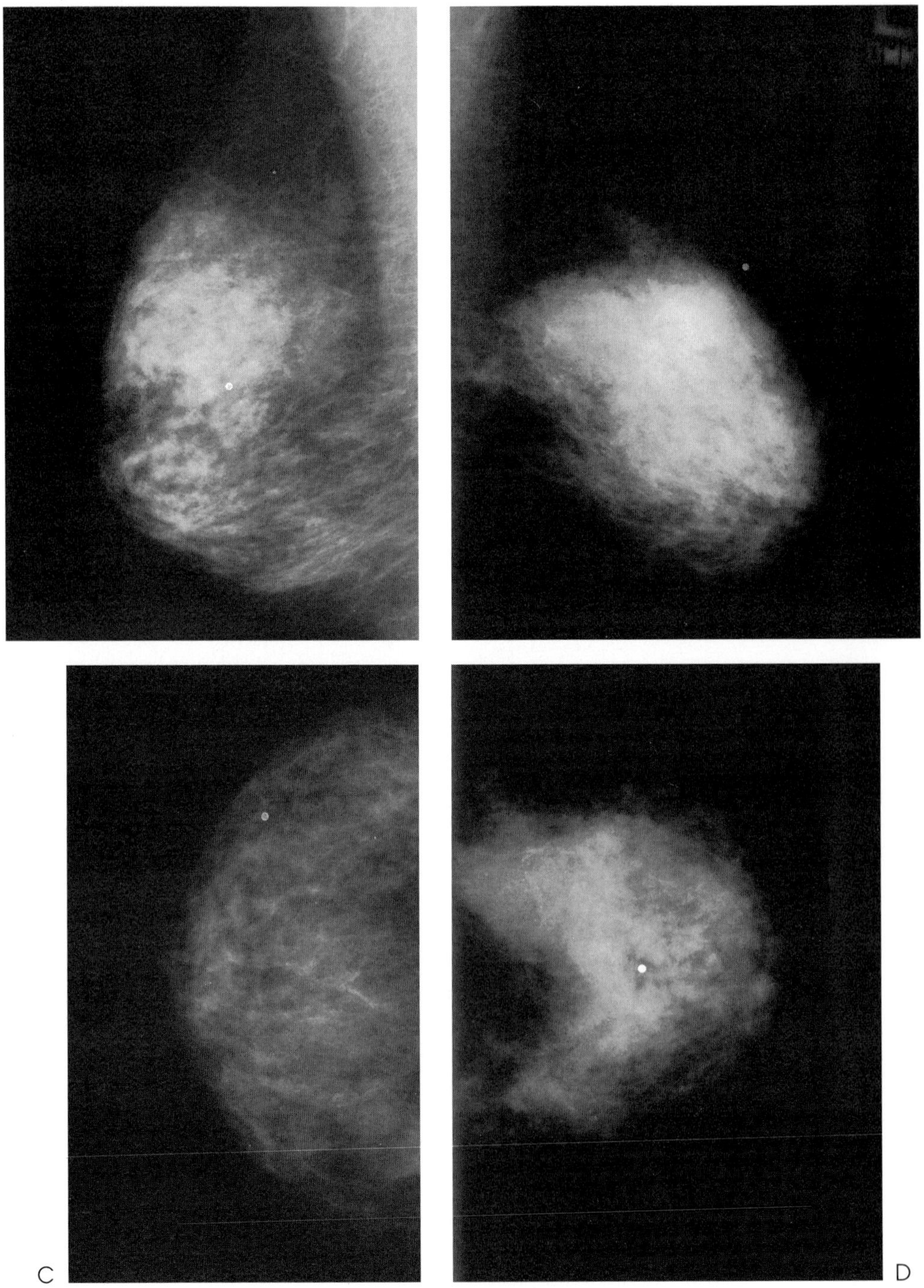

Figure 117–1. There is asymmetric increased density in the left upper breast, which is associated with a palpable mass (palpable mass marked with a radiopaque marker). (A). Right MLO mammogram. (B). Left MLO mammogram. (C). Right CC mammogram. (D). Left CC mammogram.

Pathology

Ductal carcinoma in situ with small area of invasion. The left mastectomy specimen demonstrated a 9 cm mass that predominantly consisted of ductal carcinoma in situ of low to intermediate grade. Only 0.1 cm of infiltrating ductal carcinoma was identified within the mass.

Management

- BI-RADS Assessment Category 5, highly suggestive of malignancy

Pearls and Pitfalls

This case differs from inflammatory carcinoma because the patient did not have any skin changes. Any large malignancy may produce an increase in mammographic density. Besides ductal carcinoma in situ or infiltrating ductal carcinoma, invasive lobular carcinoma may also cause generalized increased breast density.

Suggested Readings

1. Harvey JA, Fechner RE, Moore MM. Apparent ipsilateral decrease in breast size at mammography: a sign of infiltrating lobular carcinoma. *Radiology* 2000;214:883–889.

Case 118

Case History

A 36-year-old woman felt two left breast lumps. Histology from biopsy of both lumps was infiltrating ductal carcinoma. The patient's mammograms were interpreted as normal and the surgeon recommended a lumpectomy. The patient was seen at our institution for a second opinion.

Physical Examination

- left breast: two healing biopsy incisions at the 1:30 position about 5 cm apart; no other palpable masses
- right breast: normal exam

Mammogram

- asymmetric density (Fig. 118–1)

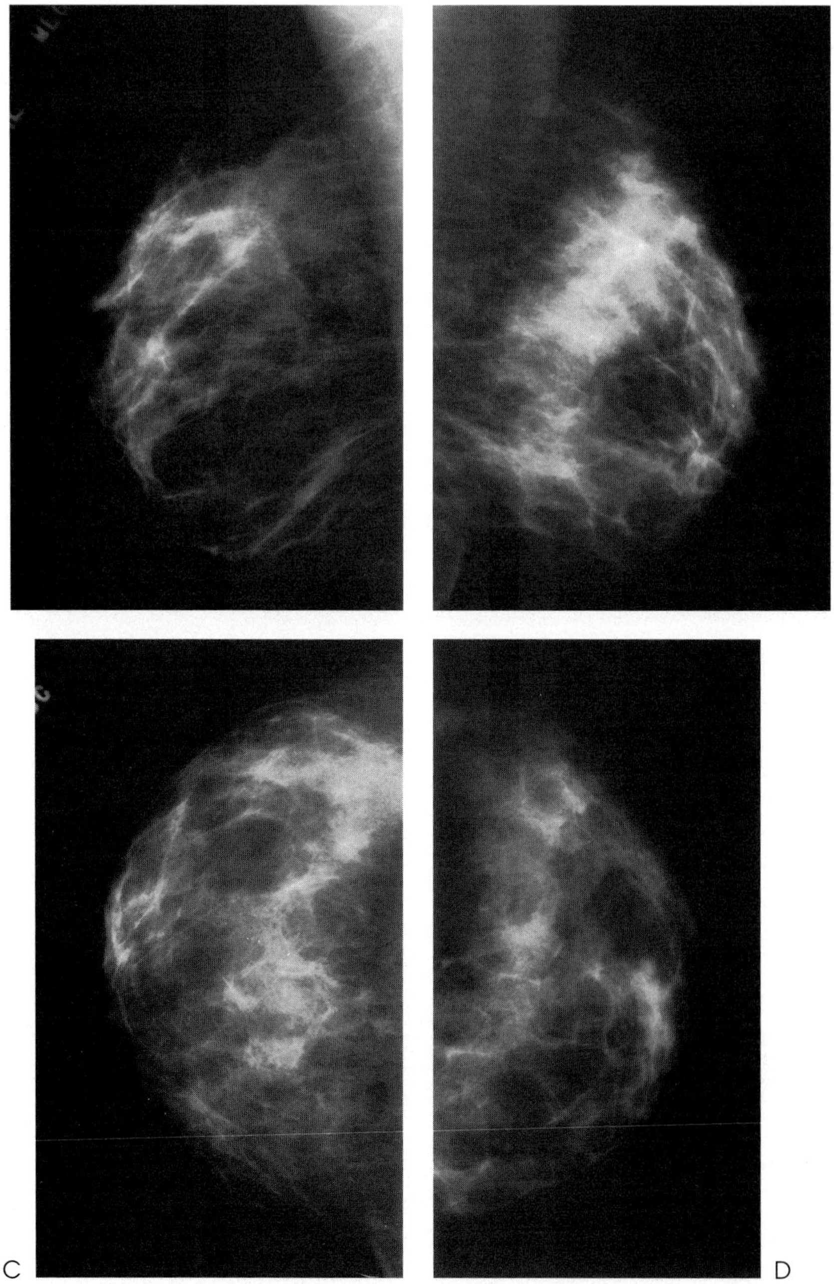

A B C D

Figure 118–1. There is a band of asymmetric increased density in the posterior third of the left breast on the MLO view. This asymmetry is not evident on the left CC view. (A). Right MLO mammogram. (B). Left MLO mammogram. (C). Right CC mammogram. (D). Left CC mammogram.

Ultrasound

Frequency

- 10 MHz

Mass

- margin: ill defined
- echogenicity: hypoechoic
- retrotumoral acoustic appearance: bilateral edge shadowing
- shape: irregular (Figs. 118–2 and 118–3)

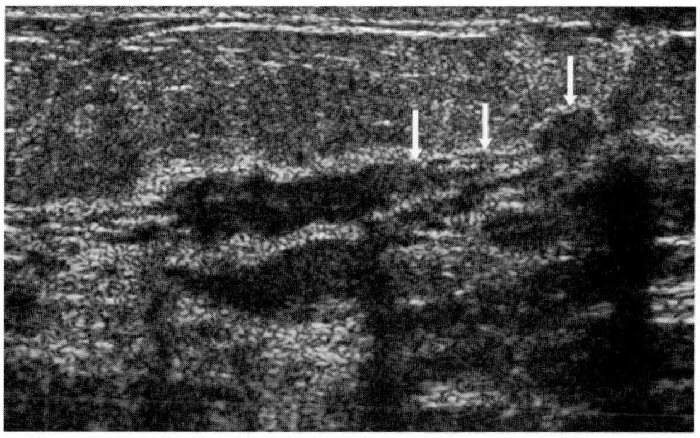

Figure 118–2. Left radial breast sonogram at 1:30: Sonographically, the patient had numerous (too many to count) masses between the 12:00 and 5:00 positions of the left breast. These masses had a variety of appearances. At the 1:30 position (area of original palpable lumps), there is a large hypoechoic mass that was responsible for both lumps. The mass exhibited ductal extension toward the nipple (arrows).

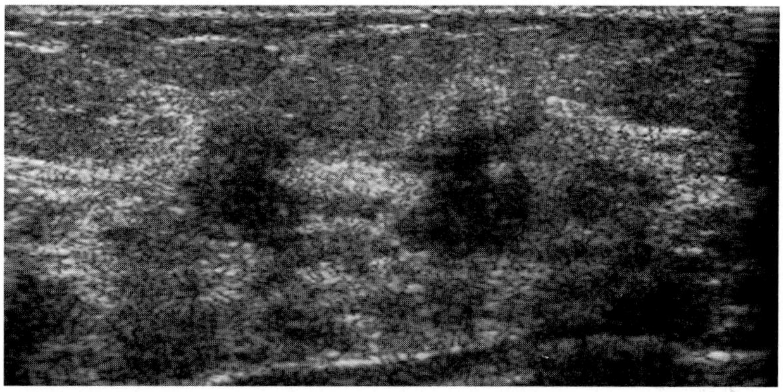

Figure 118–3. Left radial breast sonogram at 3:00: In this area, there is a series of spiculated masses that follow the ductal system.

Other Modalities (Fig. 118–4)

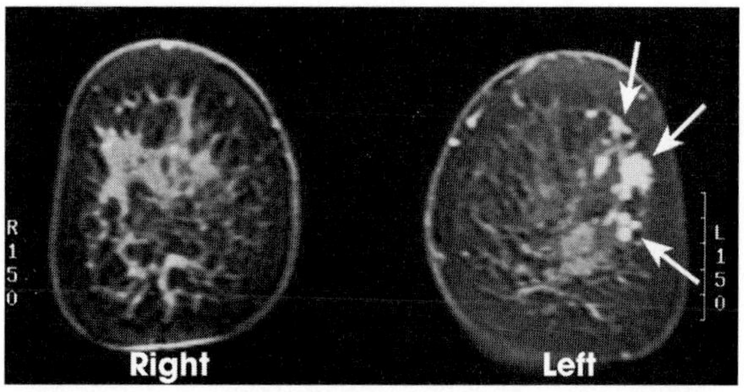

Figure 118–4. Bilateral coronal dynamic bolus three-dimensional (3-D) volume gradient breast magnetic resonance imaging (MRI): There is abnormal contrast enhancement in the left breast (arrows) indicating extensive neoplastic involvement.

Pathology

Invasive ductal carcinoma with a predominate intraductal component. The mastectomy specimen demonstrated multifocal infiltrating ductal carcinoma with 40% in situ carcinoma. Over 10 nodules were identified during gross inspection.

Management

- BI-RADS Assessment Category 5, highly suggestive of malignancy

Pearls and Pitfalls

In cases when multicentric neoplasm is suspected and there are no discrete mammographic masses or abnormal calcifications, sonography and MRI are useful methods to identify multiple malignant foci. Therefore, the mammographic assessment in this case would be Category 0. The final assessment of imaging for this case (Category 5) is based upon the sonographic and MRI findings. Findings from either of these modalities and the clinical information should lead one to conclude that the patient has multicentric disease. Although most cases of multicentric disease are treated with mastectomy, in certain cases a partial mastectomy may be preferred. MRI provides a better global image for surgical planning. However, sonography is useful for biopsy and needle localization guidance.

Suggested Readings

1. Berg WA, Gilbreath PL. Multicentric and multifocal cancer: whole breast US in preoperative evaluation. *Radiology* 2000;214:59–66.
2. Heywang-Kobrunner SH, Schreer I, Dershaw DD. *Diagnostic Breast Imaging*. New York: Thieme; 1997:224–225.
3. Rosenblatt R, Fineberg SA, Sparano JA, Kaleya RN. Stereotactic core needle biopsy of multiple sites in the breast: efficacy and effect on patient care. *Radiology* 1996;201:67–70.

Case 119

Case History

A 48-year-old woman presents for screening mammogram.

Physical Examination

- normal exam

Mammogram

- focal asymmetric density (Fig. 119–1)

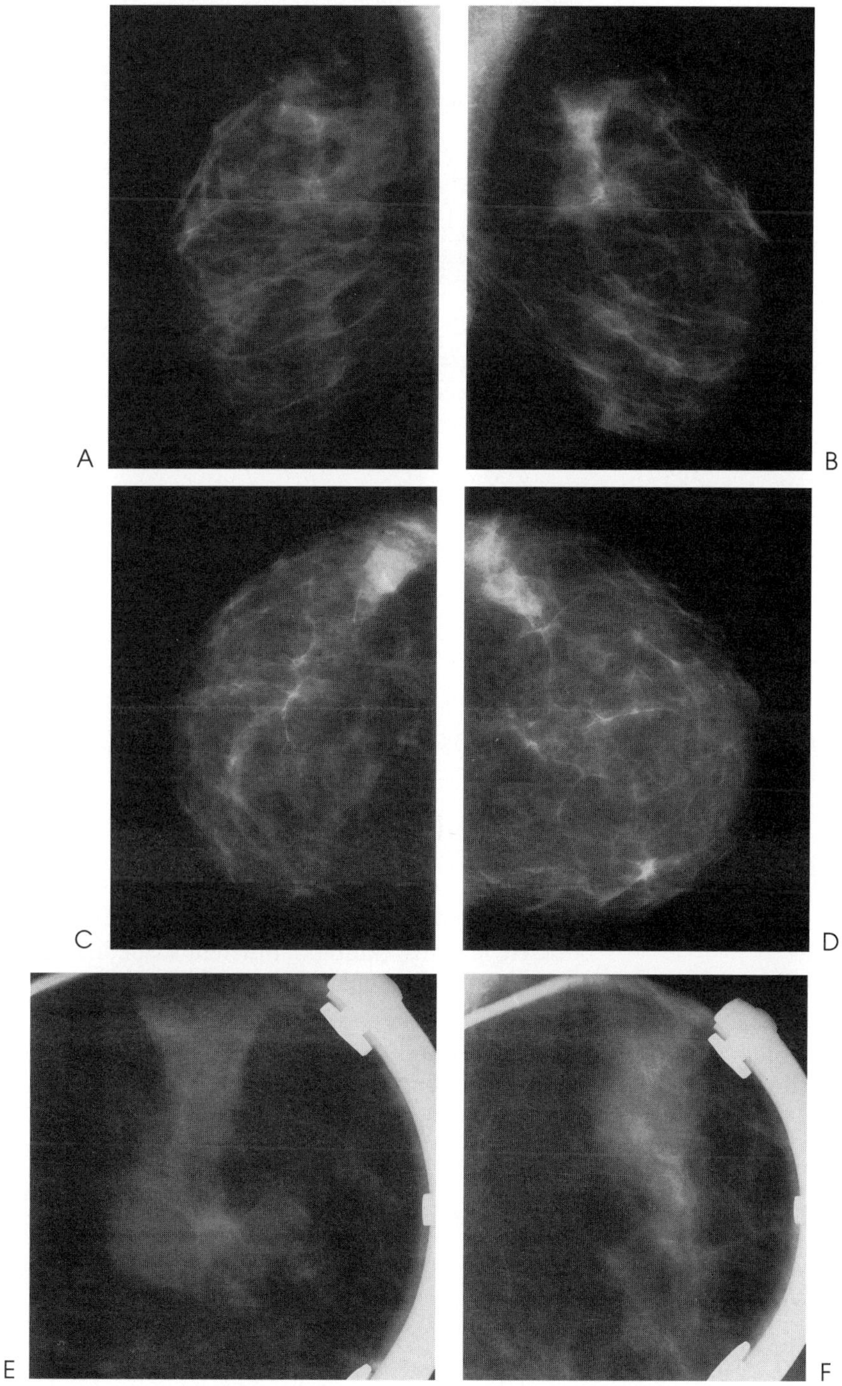

Figure 119–1. *In the left upper outer breast, there is a focal asymmetric density, which is better identified on the MLO view. The density not visible in the CC and exaggerated cranio-caudal (XCCL) views. The density is new since the patient's previous exam 3 years ago. (A). Right MLO mammogram. (B). Left MLO mammogram. (C). Right CC mammogram. (D). Left CC mammogram. (E). Left MLO spot compression mammogram. (F). Left XCCL spot compression mammogram.*

Ultrasound

Frequency

- 10 MHz

Mass

- margin: well defined
- echogenicity: echogenic
- retrotumoral acoustic appearance: bilateral edge shadowing
- shape: ellipsoid (Fig. 119–2)

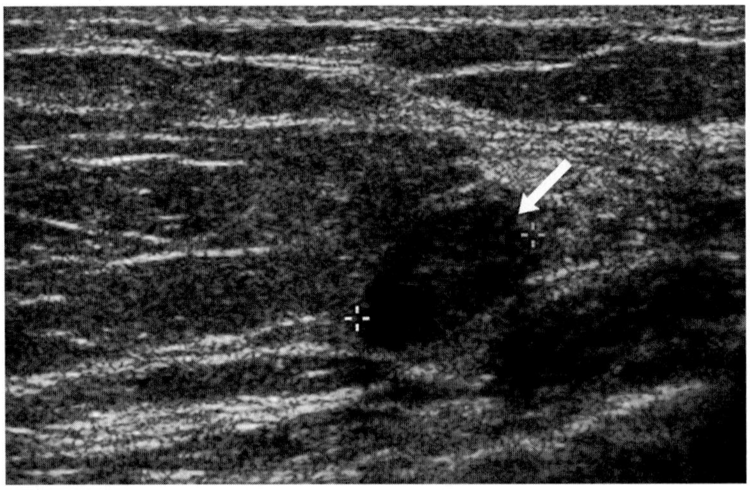

Figure 119–2. Left radial breast sonogram: In the upper outer quadrant, the mammographic focal asymmetric density corresponds to an oval hypoechoic solid mass. Although most of the margins are well defined, part of the edge is irregular and ill defined (arrow).

Pathology

- fibroadenoma

Management

- BI-RADS Assessment Category 4, suspicious; biopsy should be considered

Pearls and Pitfalls

An area of focal asymmetric density that is classified as asymmetric fibroglandular tissue is probably benign (malignancy rate 0.4%). Benign asymmetric parenchymal tissue has no discrete margins, exhibits a different shape in different views, and generally has small areas of fat interspersed within it. Unfortunately, some focal asymmetric densities cannot be optimally characterized by mammography alone. In these cases, sonography is useful to confirm that the density is a solid mass and to provide biopsy guidance.

Suggested Readings

1. Kopans DB. *Breast Imaging.* 2nd ed. Philadelphia: Lippincott-Raven; 1998:400.
2. Sickles EA. Periodic mammographic follow-up of probably benign lesions: results in 3,184 consecutive cases. *Radiology* 1991;179:463–468.

Case 120

Case History

- A 51-year-old woman presents for screening mammogram.

Physical Examination

- left breast: ill-defined, firm area in left upper outer breast
- right breast: normal exam

Mammogram

- focal asymmetric density (Figs. 120–1 and 120–2)

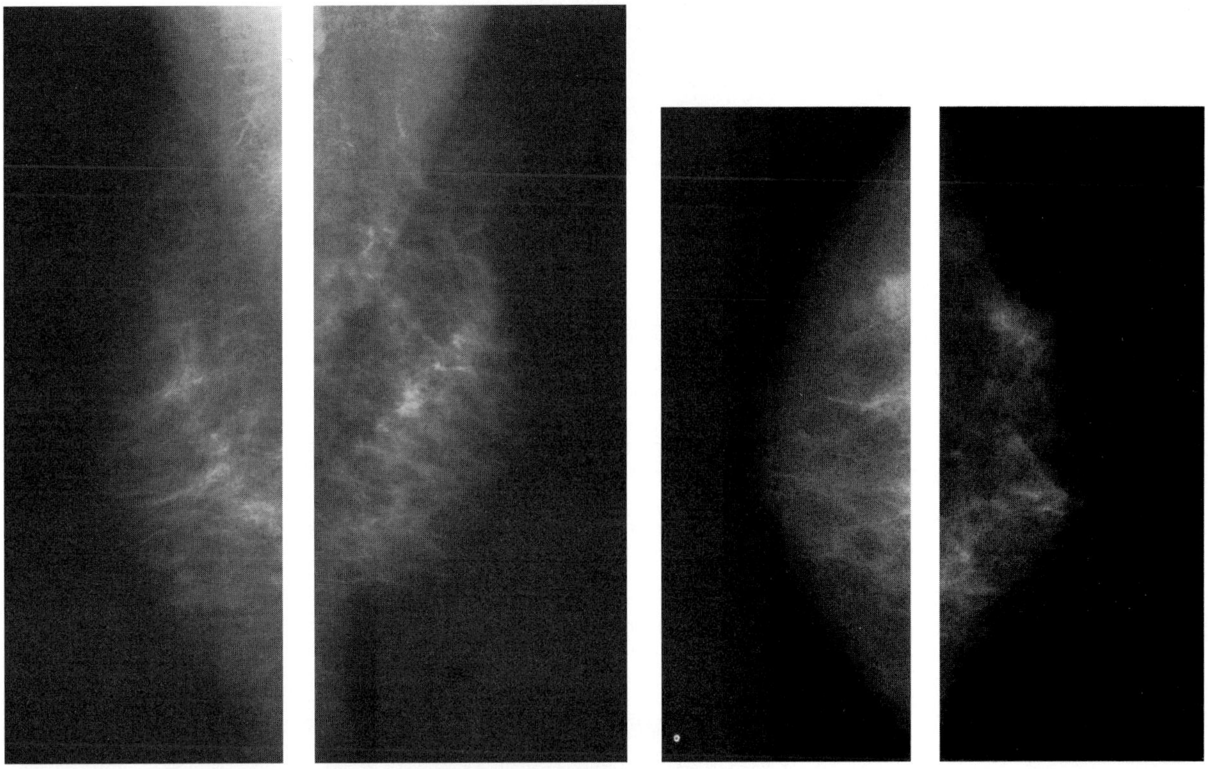

A B C D

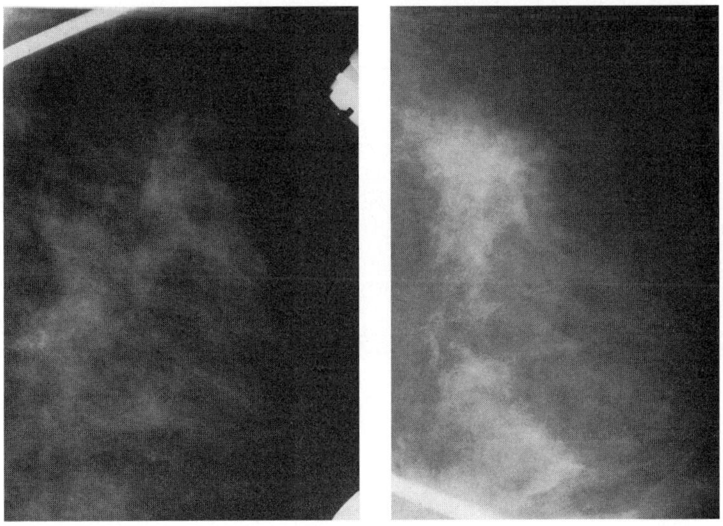

E F

Figure 120–1. There is a focal asymmetric density in the left outer breast only visible on the CC views. (A). Right MLO mammogram. (B). Left MLO mammogram. (C). Right CC mammogram. (D). Left CC mammogram. (E). Left MLO spot compression mammogram. (F). Left CC spot compression mammogram.

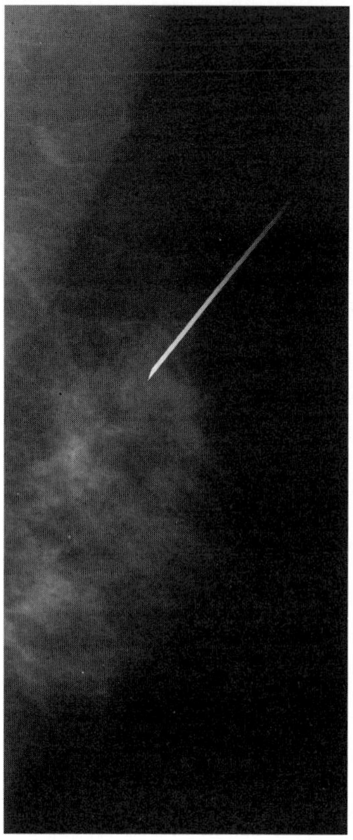

Figure 120–2. Left MLO after sonographically guided needle localization: This mammogram illustrates that the mass is not visible in this view even when the location of the mass is marked with a needle.

Ultrasound

Frequency

- 7 MHz

Mass

- margin: spiculation/architectural distortion
- echogenicity: heterogeneous (mixed)
- retrotumoral acoustic appearance: posterior shadowing distal to mass
- shape: irregular (Fig. 120–3)

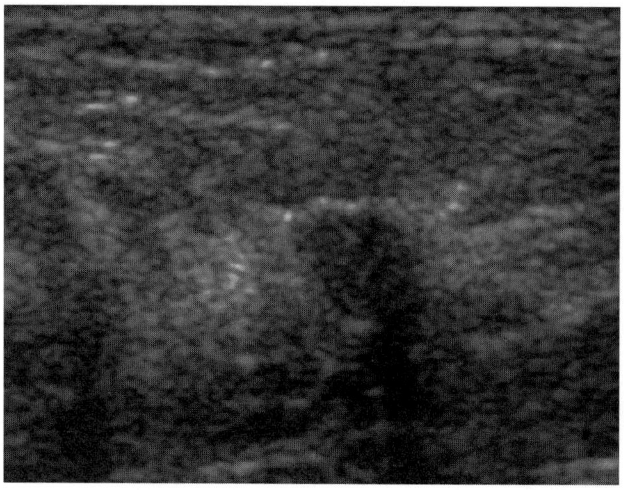

Figure 120–3. Left breast longitudinal sonogram: At the 3:00 position there is a spiculated irregular mass with heterogeneous echogenicity and posterior acoustic shadowing. This mass corresponds to the mammographic density.

Pathology

- invasive lobular carcinoma

Management

- BI-RADS Assessment Category 4, suspicious abnormality; biopsy should be considered

Pearls and Pitfalls

1. Lobular carcinoma is sometimes difficult to identify mammographically because it may appear as an asymmetric density that is visible on only one view. To localize this abnormality, shallow mammographic obliques may be more useful than spot compression views. Lobular carcinoma is commonly easily compressible and may blend into the surrounding parenchymal density.
2. Ultrasound is useful to localize suspicious mammographic densities that are only visible on one view.

Suggested Readings

1. Butler RS, Venta LA, Wiley EL, Ellis RL, Dempsey PJ, Rubin E. Sonographic evaluation of infiltrating lobular carcinoma. *AJR* 1999;172:325–330.
2. Evans N, Lyons K. The use of ultrasound in the diagnosis of invasive lobular carcinoma of the breast less than 10 mm in size. *Clin Radiol* 2000;55:261–263.

Case 121

Case History

A 67-year-old female, transferred from another medical facility, was evaluated for abdominal pain. Abdominal computed tomography (CT) demonstrated multiple low-density liver masses. Liver biopsy indicated metastatic adenocarcinoma.

Physical Examination

- normal exam

Mammogram

- focal asymmetric density (Fig. 121–1)

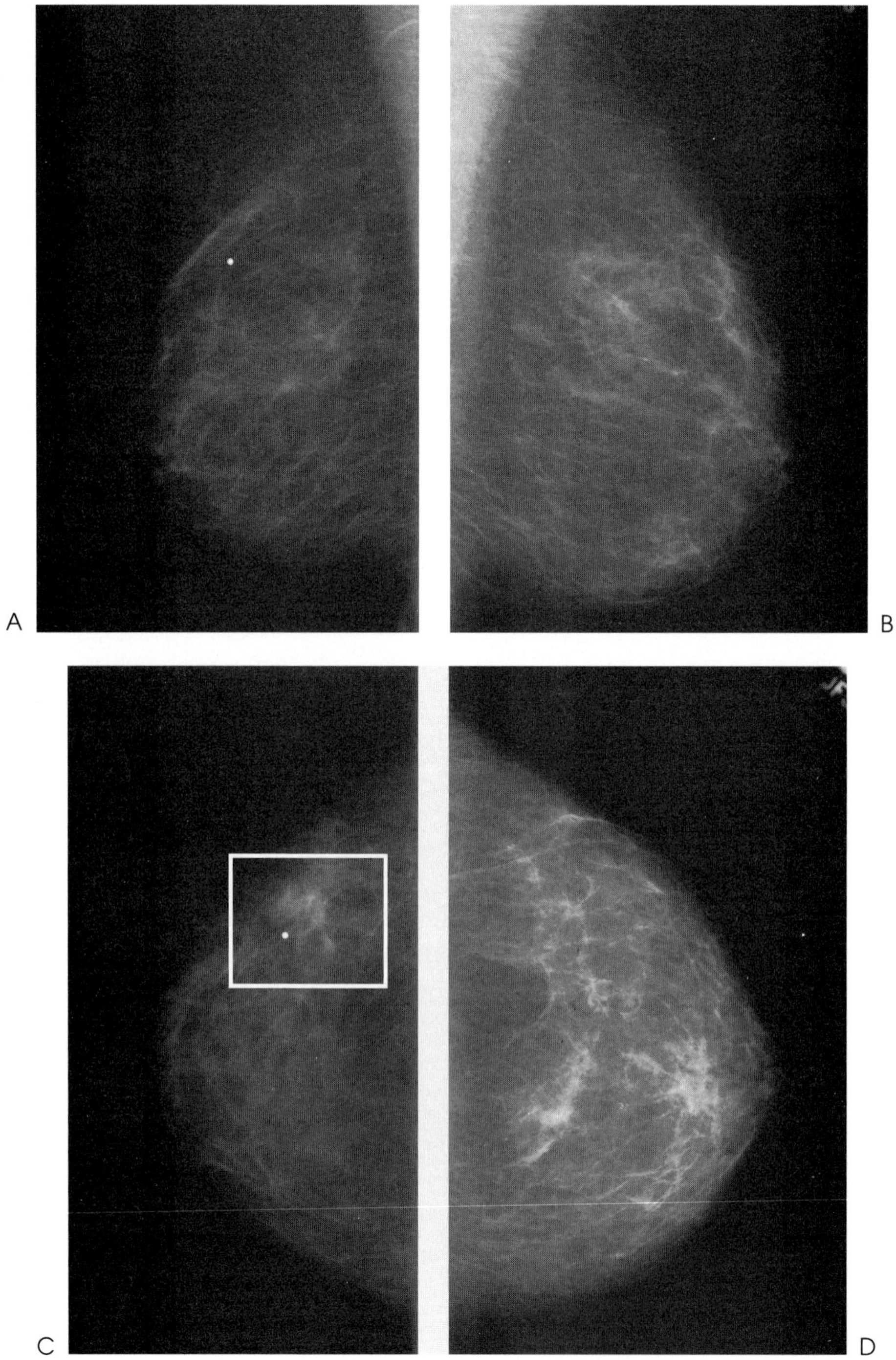

Figure 121–1. A focal asymmetric density (square) in the right outer breast is visible only on the CC view. This density has been unchanged for 5 years. (Radiopaque marker has been placed on skin to aid locating the density on other views.) (A). Right MLO mammogram. (B). Left MLO mammogram. (C). Right CC mammogram. (D). Left CC mammogram.

Ultrasound

Low Frequency

Frequency

- 7 MHz

Mass

- margin: ill defined
- echogenicity: hypoechoic
- retrotumoral acoustic appearance: severe shadowing, mass partially obscured
- shape: irregular (Fig. 121–2)

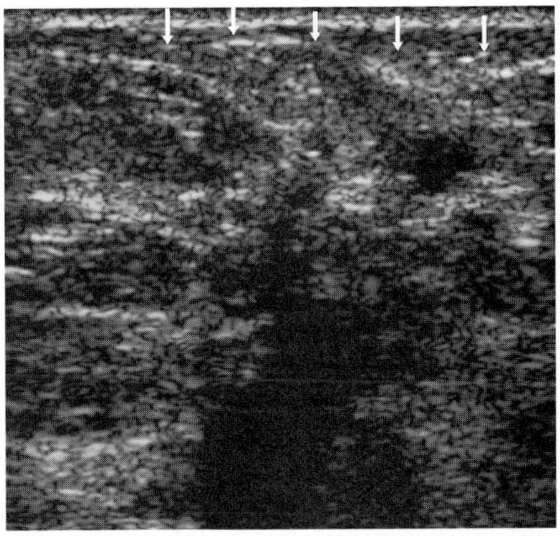

Figure 121–2. Right radial breast sonogram: Mammographic asymmetric density demonstrated in Figure 121–1 corresponds to an ill-defined hypoechoic mass associated with architectural distortion due to retraction of Cooper's ligaments and the anterior fascial line (arrows).

High Frequency

Frequency

- 10 MHz (Fig. 121–3)

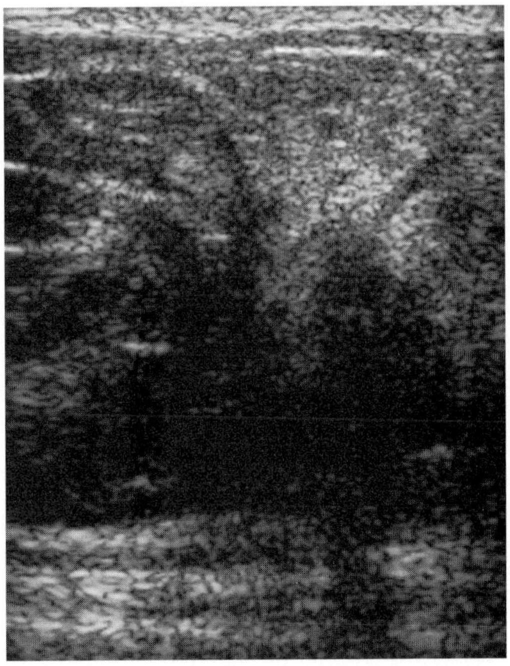

Figure 121–3. Right radial breast sonogram: Sonographic examination of same mass as Figure 121–2. The architectural distortion, spiculation, and hyperechoic haziness are better defined by this higher-frequency exam compared to the lower-frequency examination (Fig. 121–2).

Other Modalities (Fig. 121-4)

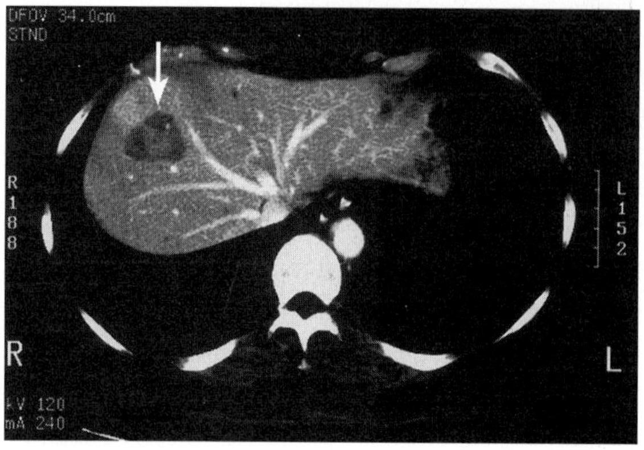

Figure 121-4. Abdominal CT scan with intravenous contrast: Because the patient's initial chief complaint was abdominal pain, an abdominal CT was the first imaging test performed. In the liver there are multiple low-density solid masses. The largest mass (arrow) is in the right lobe of the liver. These masses are metastases from the patient's occult breast cancer.

Pathology

- invasive lobular carcinoma

Management

- BI-RADS Assessment Category 4, suspicious abnormality; biopsy should be considered

Pearls and Pitfalls

Sonography is useful to identify masses that may be mammographically subtle. Higher-frequency examination improves the conspicuity of malignancies by enhancing visibility of architectural distortion. Sometimes lobular carcinoma is difficult to sonographically identify because the mass is hidden by severe acoustic shadowing. In these cases, architectural distortion is the main clue that differentiates the neoplasm from adjacent dense fibrous tissue.

Suggested Readings

1. Skaane P, Skjorten F. Ultrasonographic evaluation of invasive lobular carcinoma. *Acta Radiologica* 1999;40:369–375.

Section VII

Architectural Distortion

Signs of Architectural Distortion

1. Contour abnormality: The contour may exhibit retraction (e.g., tent sign), straightening, or bulging.
2. Trabecular thickening: The lines that point to the nipple are focally denser or thicker.
3. Trabecular disorganization: The lines, which normally point to the nipple, lose their uniform directional pattern. The lines may point to one center or may point in many directions. This finding is commonly associated with trabecular thickening.

Because architectural distortion may be subtle, this finding is best confirmed by comparing the study with mammograms that are at least 3 years old.

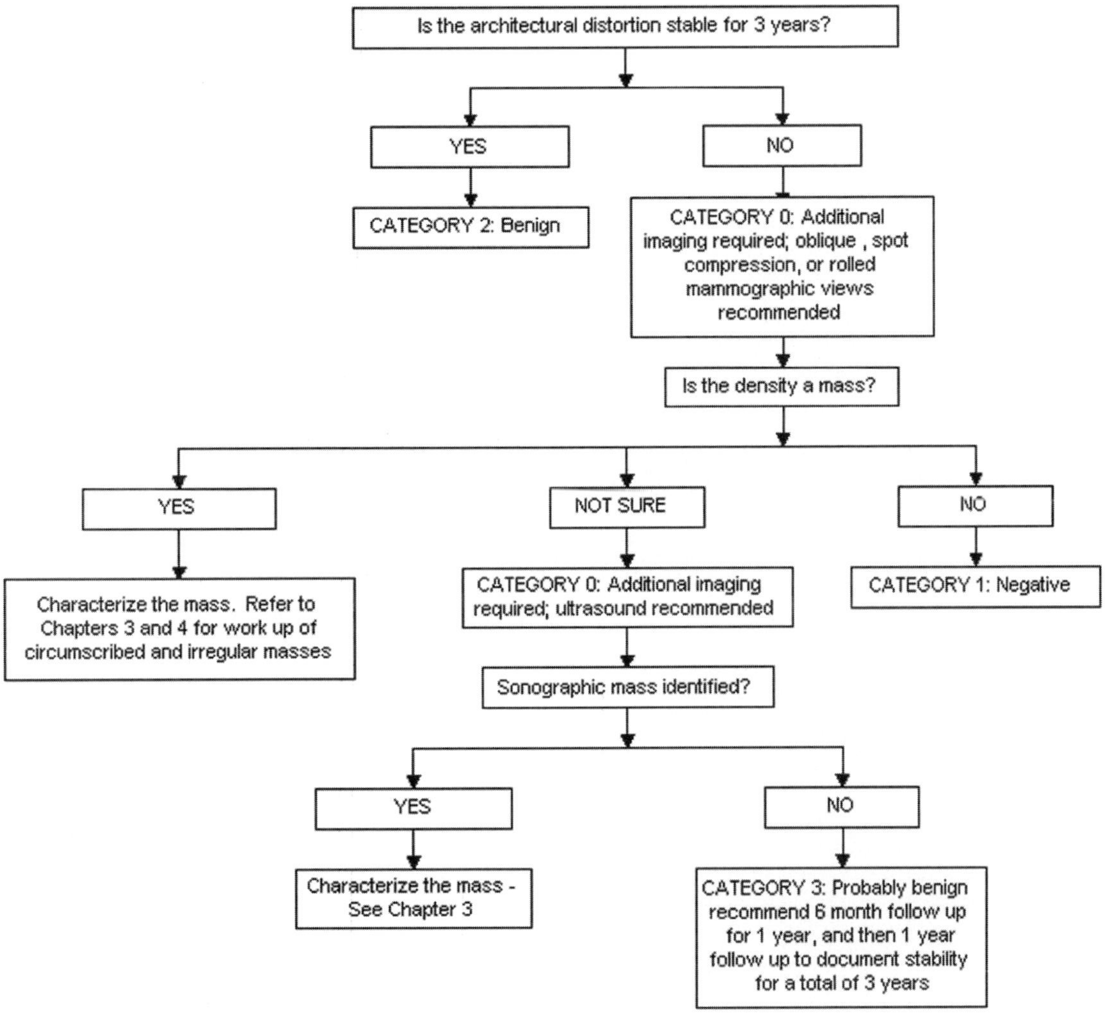

Case 122

Case History

A 62-year-old woman presents for screening mammogram.

Physical Examination

- normal exam

Mammogram

- architectural distortion (Fig. 122–1)

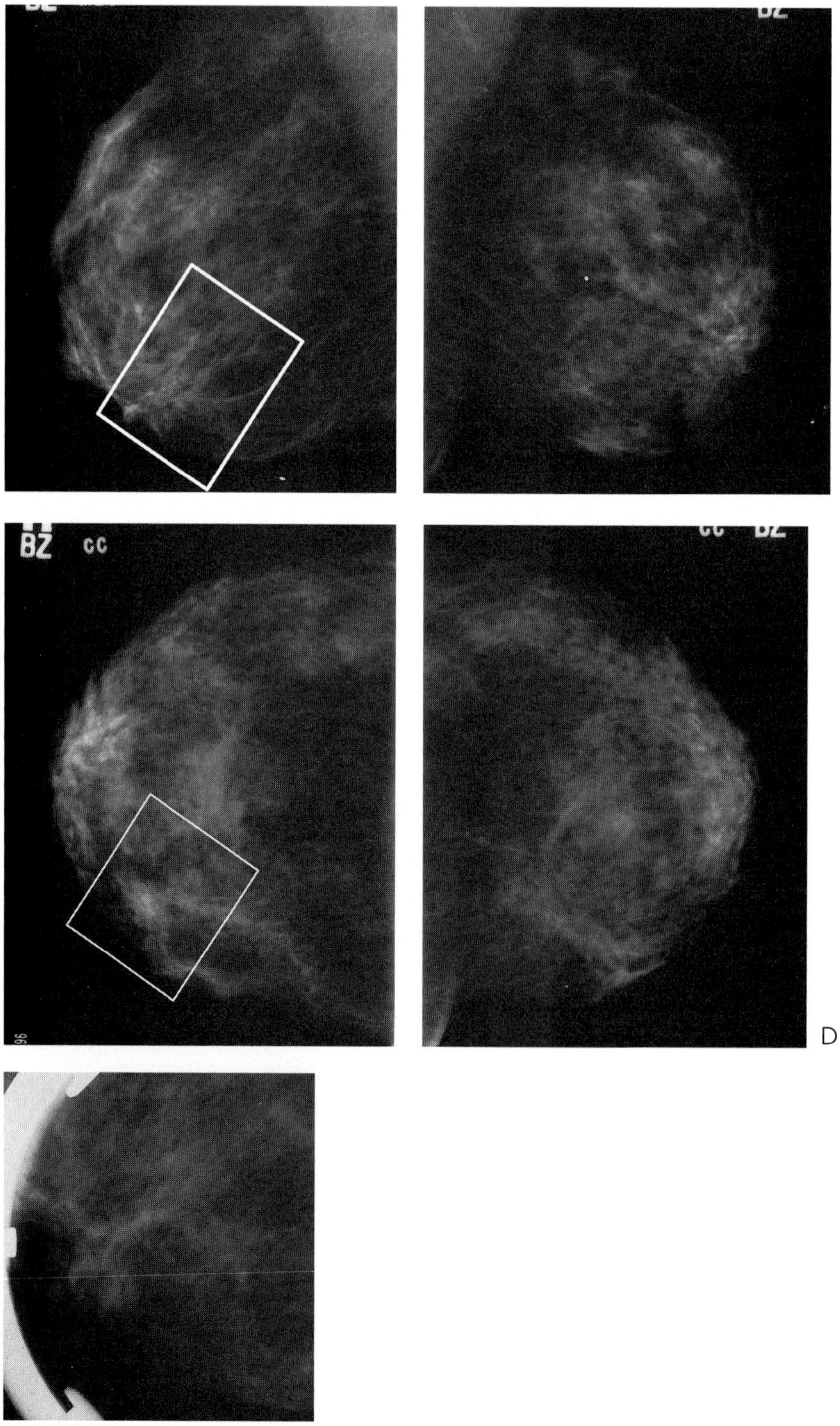

Figure 122–1. In the right inferior inner breast there is an area of architectural distortion (surrounded by a square). (A). Right MLO mammogram. (B). Left MLO mammogram. (C). Right CC mammogram. (D). Left CC mammogram. (E). Right MLO spot compression mammogram.

Ultrasound

Frequency

- 13 MHz (Fig. 122-2)

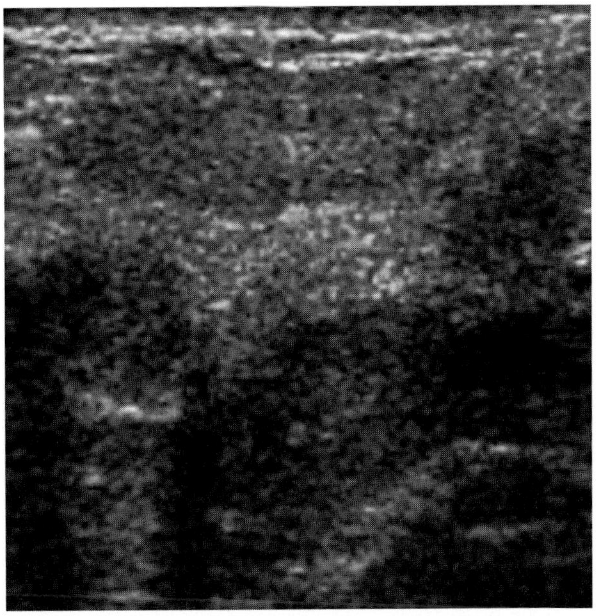

Figure 122-2. Right antiradial breast sonogram: No sonographic mass is identified in the area of the mammographic architectural distortion. Only normal hyperechoic tissue is present (see Color Plate 122-2).

Other Modalities (Fig. 122-3)

Findings

Although magnetic resonance imaging (MRI) demonstrates architectural distortion and skin thickening, the lack of contrast enhancement suggests that the architectural distortion is benign.

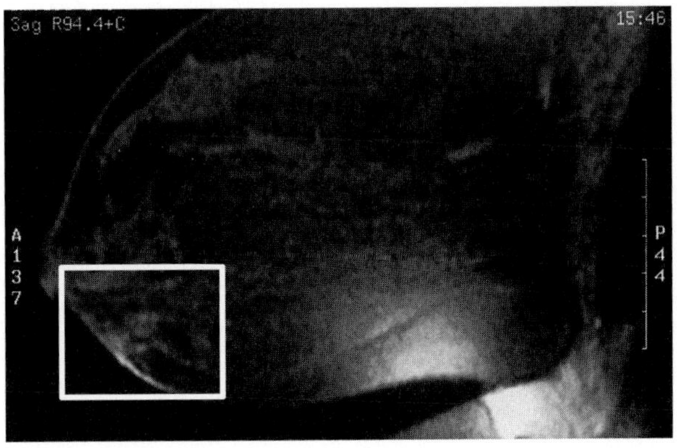

Figure 122-3. Right sagittal dynamic bolus three-dimensional (3-D) volume gradient series breast MRI: In the area of the mammographic architectural distortion, MRI also demonstrates architectural distortion and skin thickening (marked by square). However, there is no associated contrast enhancement of the area.

Pathology

- fibroadenomatoid hyperplasia

Management

- BI-RADS Assessment Category 4, suspicious; biopsy should be considered

Pearls and Pitfalls

1. This case illustrates peripheral architectural distortion. The spot compression emphasizes the retraction of the edge of the parenchyma associated with abnormal deviation of the parenchymal lines. Normally, the axis of the parenchymal lines should be toward the nipple. In this case, they are pointing toward the skin away from the nipple.
2. The etiologies of architectural distortion are similar to the causes of irregular masses. Benign entities include scar, mastitis, fibrocystic changes, adenosis, and mesenchymal lesions (fat necrosis, fibromatosis), and benign neoplasms (e.g., sclerosing papillomas, myofibroblastomas). Malignant entities include infiltrating ductal, invasive lobular, tubular, and occasionally lymphoma.

Suggested Readings

1. Jones MK. *Atlas of Breast Imaging.* Madden: Blackwell Science; 1996:108–112.

Case 123

Case History

A 54-year-old woman presents for screening mammogram.

Physical Examination

- normal exam

Mammogram

- architectural distortion (Fig. 123–1)

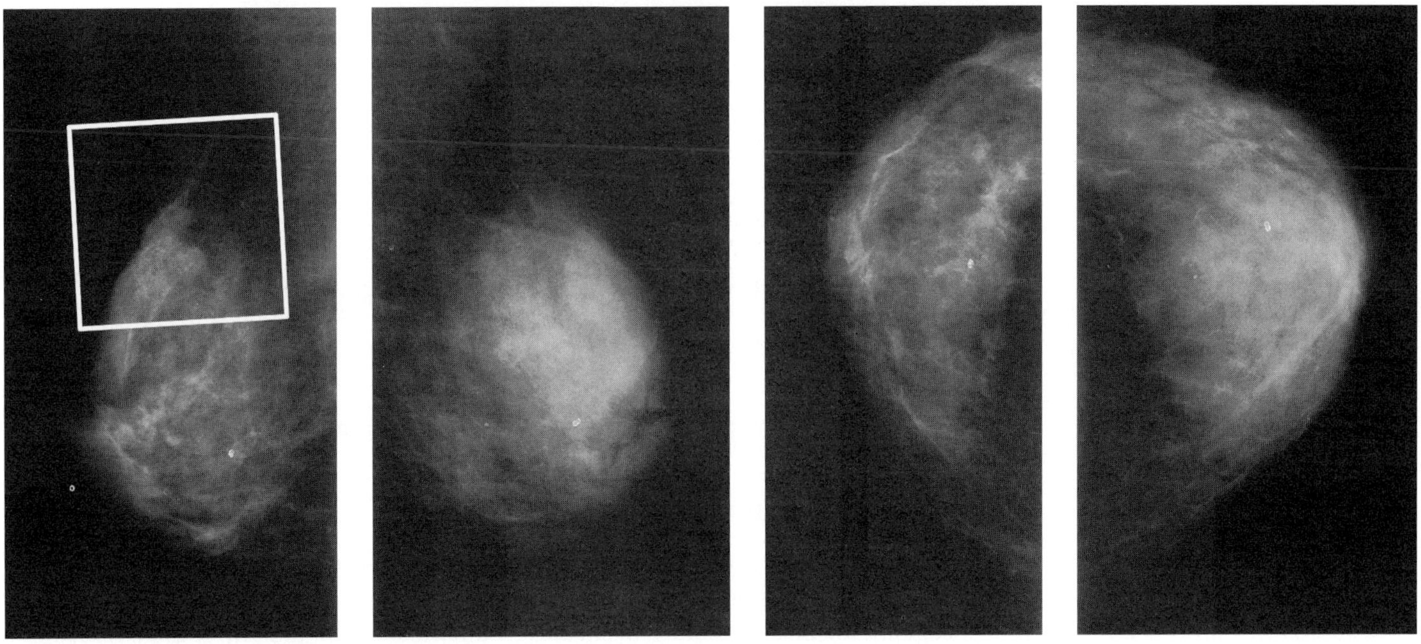

A B C D

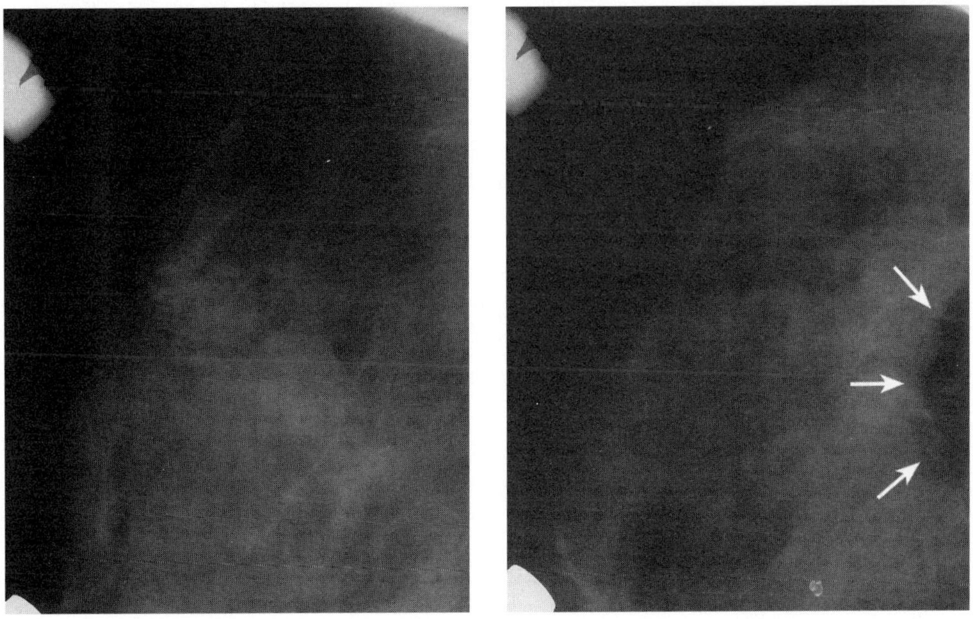

E F

Figure 123–1. There is architectural distortion of the superior edge of the right breast on the MLO view (outlined by square in A). Posterior parenchymal retraction is present on the right XCCL spot magnification view (outlined by arrows in F). (A). Right MLO mammogram. (B). Left MLO mammogram. (C). Right CC mammogram. (D). Left CC mammogram. (E). Right MLO spot magnification mammogram. (F). Right XCCL spot magnification mammogram.

Ultrasound

Frequency

- 10 MHz

Mass

- margin: ill defined
- echogenicity: hypoechoic
- retrotumoral acoustic appearance: single edge shadowing
- shape: irregular (Fig. 123–2)

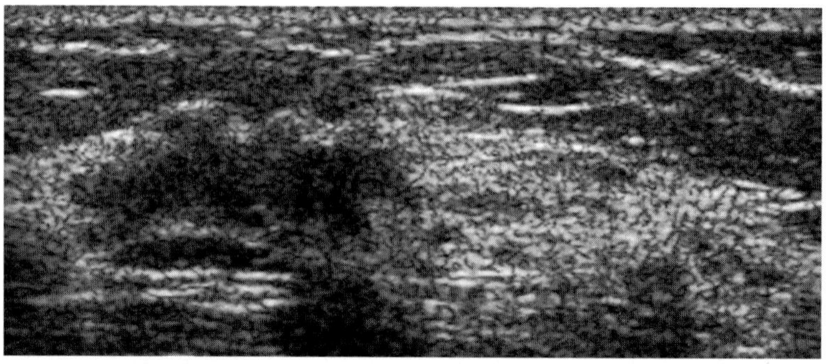

Figure 123–2. Right radial breast sonogram: In the upper outer quadrant, the mammographic architectural distortion corresponds to an irregular hypoechoic mass (see Color Plate 123–2).

Pathology

- radial sclerosing lesion (radial scar)
- ductal carcinoma in situ
- 0.8 cm ductal carcinoma in situ was within the 2.2 cm radial scar

Management

- BI-RADS Assessment Category 4, suspicious; biopsy should be considered

Pearls and Pitfalls

1. This case illustrates two common areas of architectural distortion in denser breasts: parenchymal retraction of the superior and posterior parenchymal edges. The superior edges of the breast should generally be symmetric in configuration. If there is asymmetry, the superior edge should have a curved or lobulated contour. The parenchymal density should gradually decrease until it blends into the axilla. When a mass produces parenchymal retraction, the superior edge loses the curved or lobular contour and forms a sharp triangular appearance. There is a greater difference between the density of the parenchymal edge and the axillary fat on the abnormal side compared with the normal side.
2. When a mass causes retraction of the posterior edge of the breast, the abnormal density forms a "V" and has been termed the *tent sign.*

Suggested Readings

1. Tabar L, Dean PB. *Teaching Atlas of Mammography.* 3rd ed. New York: Thieme; 2001:12–13, 119, 137.

Case 124

Case History

A 78-year-old woman presents for screening mammogram.

Physical Examination

- right breast: vague thickening in the 3:00 to 4:00 position
- left breast: normal exam

Mammogram

Mass

- margin: spiculated
- shape: irregular
- density: equal density
- architectural distortion (Fig. 124–1)

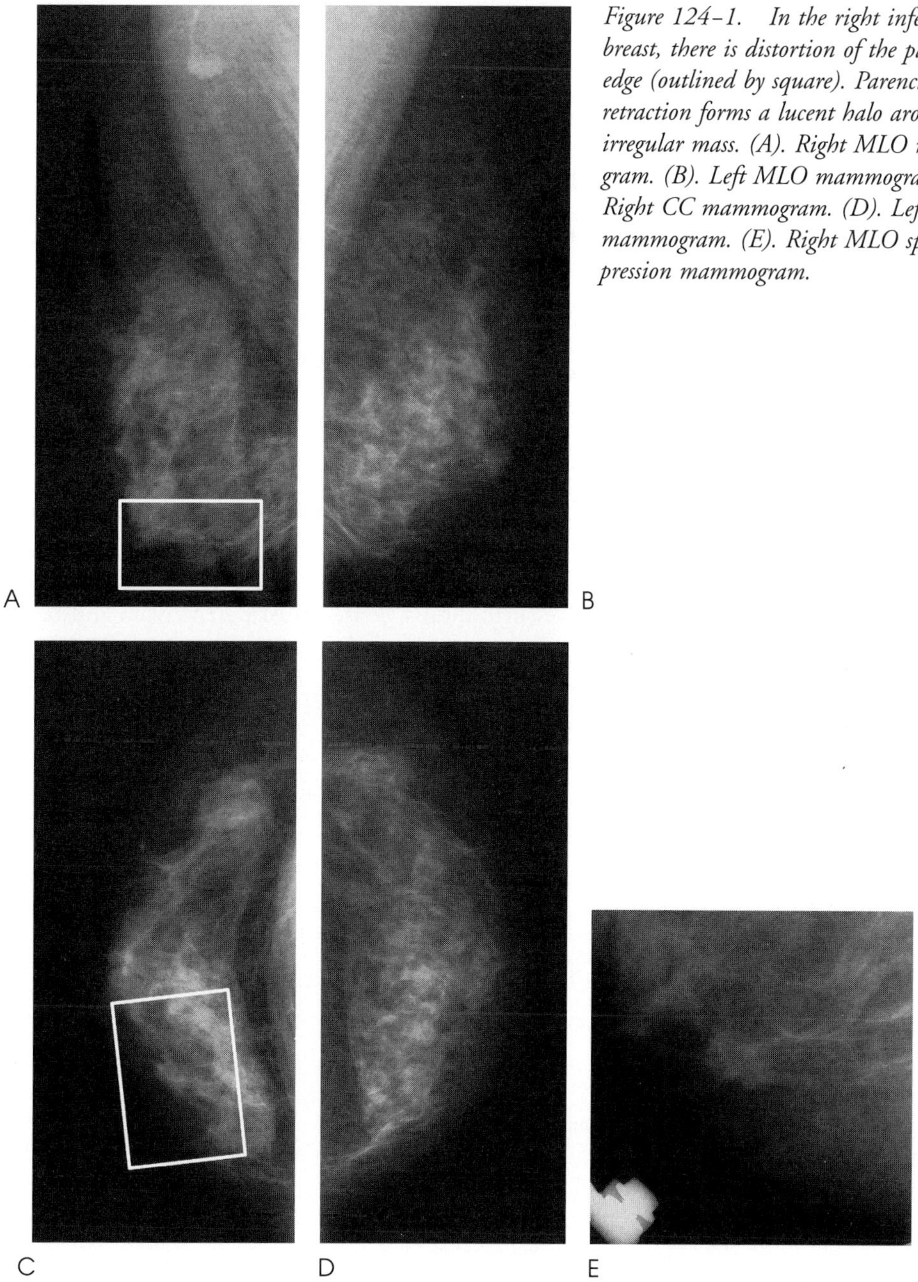

Figure 124–1. In the right inferior inner breast, there is distortion of the parenchyma edge (outlined by square). Parenchymal retraction forms a lucent halo around an irregular mass. (A). Right MLO mammogram. (B). Left MLO mammogram. (C). Right CC mammogram. (D). Left CC mammogram. (E). Right MLO spot compression mammogram.

Ultrasound

Frequency

- 13 MHz

Mass

- margin: ill defined
- echogenicity: hypoechoic
- retrotumoral acoustic appearance: severe shadowing, mass completely obscured
- shape: irregular (Fig. 124–2)

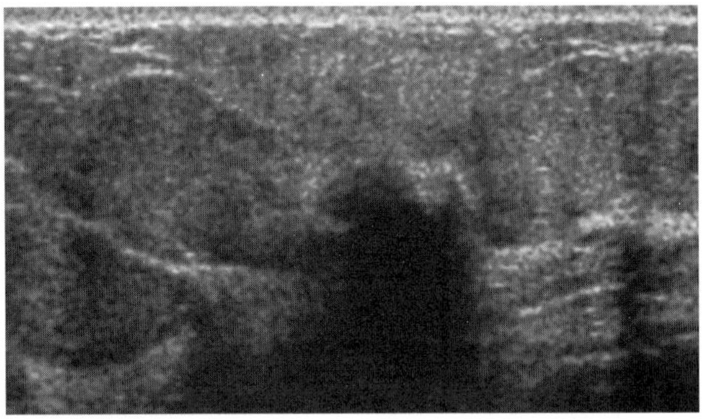

Figure 124–2. Right radial breast sonogram: The mammographic mass corresponds to a hypoechoic mass with severe shadowing (see Color Plate 124–2).

Pathology

- infiltrating ductal carcinoma

Management

- BI-RADS Assessment Category 4, suspicious; biopsy should be considered

Pearls and Pitfalls

In a dense breast, peripheral architectural distortion is an important sign of malignancy. In this case, the lucency created by the abnormal parenchymal retraction highlights the presence of a malignant mass. Without the architectural distortion, this mass would blend into the surrounding dense breast parenchyma and be poorly visible.

Suggested Readings

1. Bassett LW, Jackson VP, Jahan R, Fu YS, Gold RH. *Diagnosis of Diseases of the Breast.* Philadelphia: WB Saunders; 1997:469–473.

Case 125

Case History

An 81-year-old woman presents for screening mammogram.

Physical Examination

- normal exam

Mammogram

- architectural distortion (Fig. 125–1)

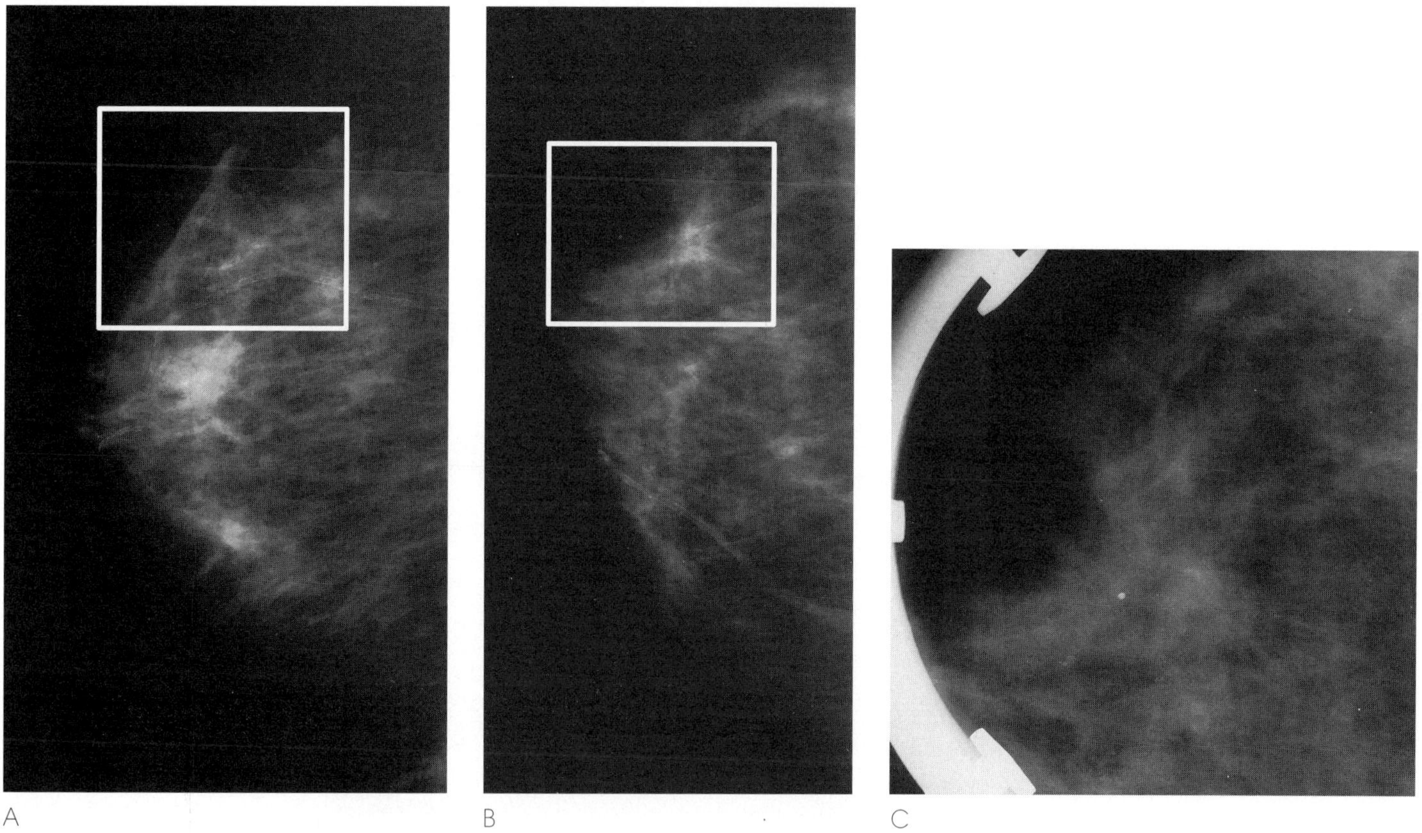

Figure 125–1. In the right upper outer quadrant there is peripheral architectural distortion (outlined by squares). In the ML view, the superior parenchymal contour is abnormally triangular (A) and in the CC view the anterior parenchymal line is retracted (B). (A). Right ML mammogram. (B). Right CC mammogram. (C). Right CC spot compression.

Ultrasound

Low Frequency

Frequency

- 8 MHz

Mass

- margin: ill defined
- echogenicity: hypoechoic
- retrotumoral acoustic appearance: posterior shadowing distal to mass
- shape: irregular (Fig. 125–2)

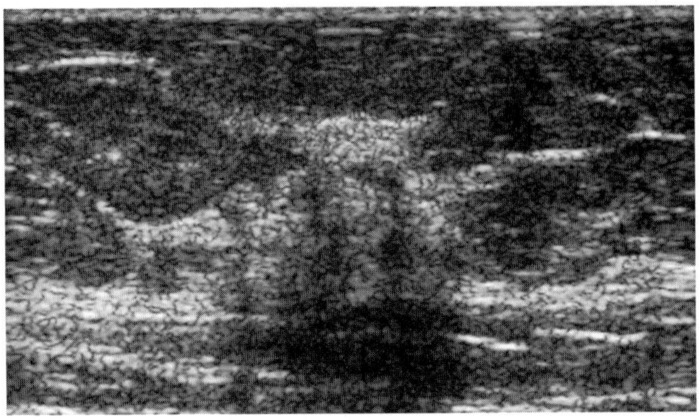

Figure 125-2. Right antiradial breast sonogram: The mammographic architectural distortion corresponds to an irregular, predominately hyperechoic mass with irregular shadowing (see Color Plate 125–2).

High Frequency

Frequency

- 11.5 MHz

Associated Findings

The higher frequency improves the conspicuity of the mass. With higher frequency, the heavily shadowing mass is easily separated from the surrounding hyperechoic parenchyma. (See Fig. 125-3.)

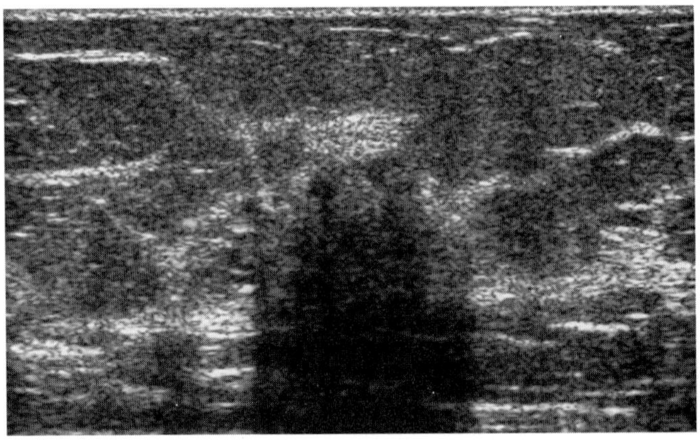

Figure 125-3. Right antiradial breast sonogram: With a higher frequency, the mass identified in Figure 125-2 appears as a focal area of severe acoustic shadowing (see Color Plate 125–3).

Pathology

- mixed invasive lobular and ductal carcinoma

Management

- BI-RADS Assessment Category 4, suspicious; biopsy should be considered

Pearls and Pitfalls

1. This case illustrates a malignant mass producing triangular distortion of the superior parenchymal contour and retraction of the anterior contour.
2. For cases of mammographic architectural distortion, sonography is useful to increase diagnostic confidence, clarify the location of the mass, and provide biopsy guidance. However, sonographically identifying the etiology of mammographic architectural distortion is commonly difficult, so sonographic cross correlation with mammographic anatomy and utilization of high-frequency sonography are important to optimize diagnostic accuracy.

Suggested Readings

1. Kopans DB. *Breast Imaging.* 2nd ed. Philadelphia: Lippincott-Raven; 1998:298–302, 384–386.

Case 126

Case History

A 70-year-old woman presents for screening mammogram.

Physical Examination

- normal exam

Mammogram

Mass

- margin: indistinct
- shape: irregular
- density: equal density
- architectural distortion (Fig. 126–1)

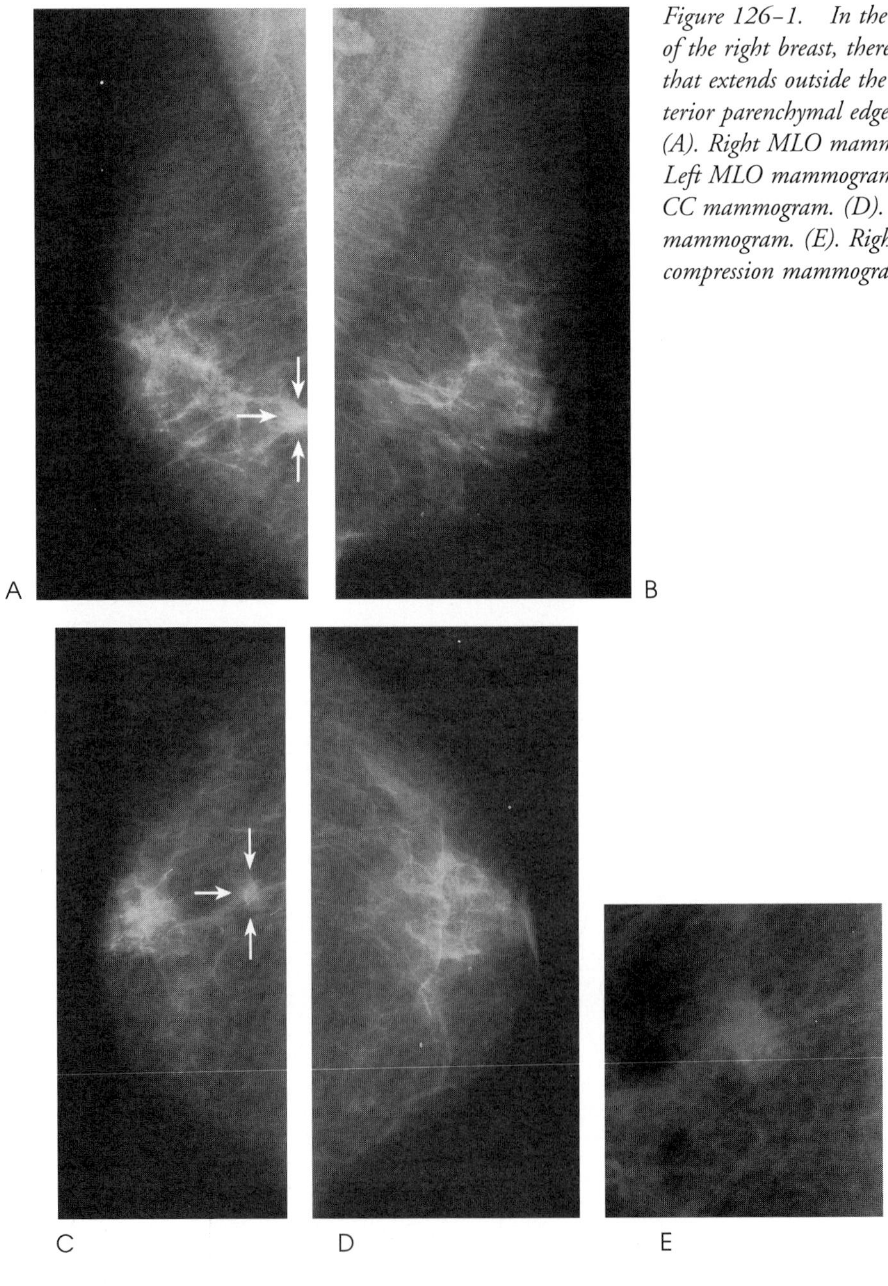

Figure 126–1. In the 7:00 position of the right breast, there is a mass that extends outside the normal posterior parenchymal edge (arrows). (A). Right MLO mammogram. (B). Left MLO mammogram. (C). Right CC mammogram. (D). Left CC mammogram. (E). Right CC spot compression mammogram.

Ultrasound

Low Frequency

Frequency

- 7 MHz

Mass (Fig. 126-2)

- margin: ill defined
- echogenicity: hypoechoic
- retrotumoral acoustic appearance: posterior shadowing distal to mass
- shape: irregular

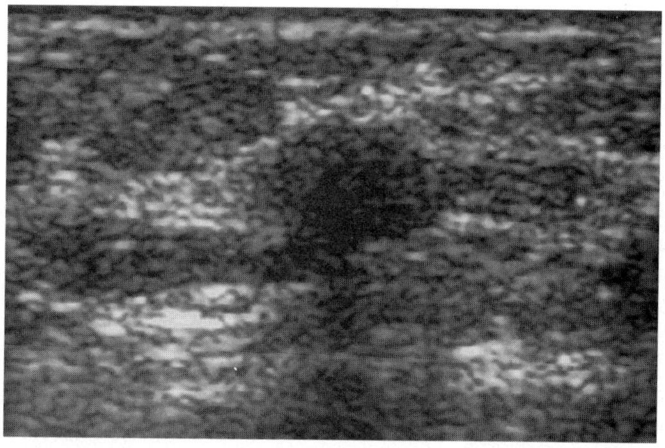

Figure 126-2. Right radial breast sonogram: The ill-defined mass identified in Figures 126-1A and 126-1C corresponds to an ill-defined hypoechoic solid mass with posterior acoustic shadowing (see Color Plate 126–2).

Pathology

- tubular carcinoma

Management

- BI-RADS Assessment Category 4, suspicious; biopsy should be considered

Pearls and Pitfalls

Besides creating retraction of the parenchymal edge, masses also protrude beyond the normal edge. Tubular carcinoma commonly presents mammographically as a small irregular mass with architectural distortion.

Suggested Readings

1. Evans AJ, Wilson ARM, Blamey RW, Robertson JFR, Ellis IO, Elston CW. *Atlas of Breast Disease Management.* Philadelphia: WB Saunders; 1998:98–100.
2. Tabar L, Dean PB. *Teaching Atlas of Mammography.* 3rd ed. New York: Thieme; 2001:5–9.

Case 127

Case History

A 71-year-old woman presents for screening mammogram.

Physical Examination

- normal exam

Mammogram

- architectural distortion (Fig. 127–1)

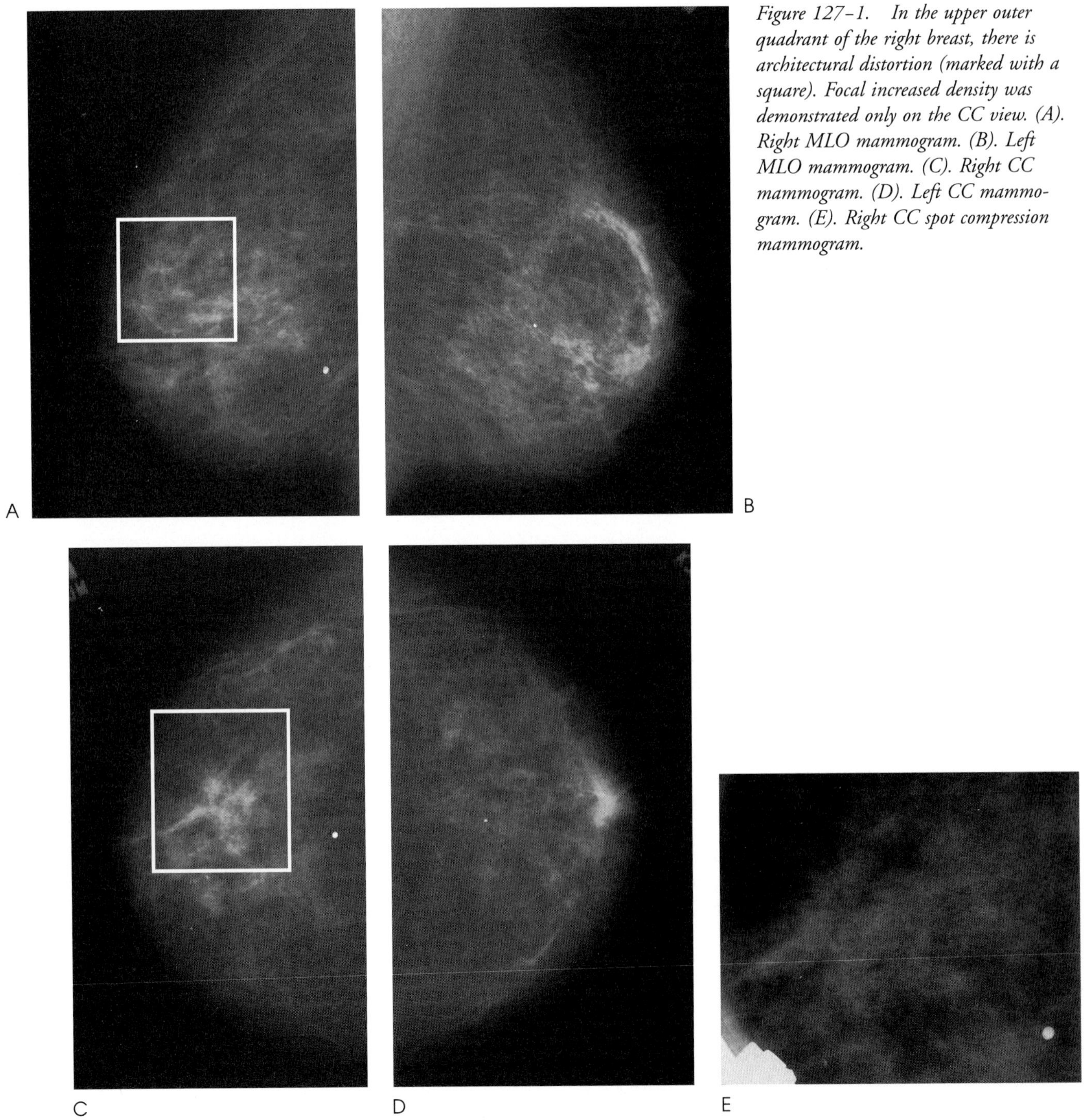

Figure 127–1. In the upper outer quadrant of the right breast, there is architectural distortion (marked with a square). Focal increased density was demonstrated only on the CC view. (A). Right MLO mammogram. (B). Left MLO mammogram. (C). Right CC mammogram. (D). Left CC mammogram. (E). Right CC spot compression mammogram.

Ultrasound

Low Frequency

Frequency

- 7 MHz

Mass

- margin: ill defined
- echogenicity: hypoechoic
- retrotumoral acoustic appearance: posterior shadowing distal to mass
- shape: irregular (Fig. 127–2)

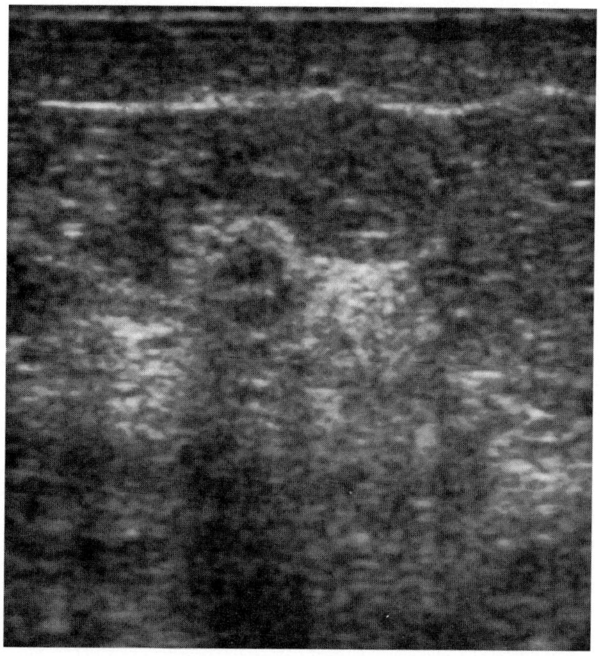

Figure 127–2. Right antiradial breast sonogram: With lower frequency, the mammographic architectural distortion is an irregular hypoechoic mass with posterior acoustic shadowing (see Color Plate 127–2).

High Frequency

Frequency

- 10 MHz

Associated Findings

This case illustrates that weaker penetration with higher frequency causes increased shadowing with benign masses as well as malignant ones. In this case, lower frequency is more useful than high frequency to identify the location of the mass. (See Fig. 127–3.)

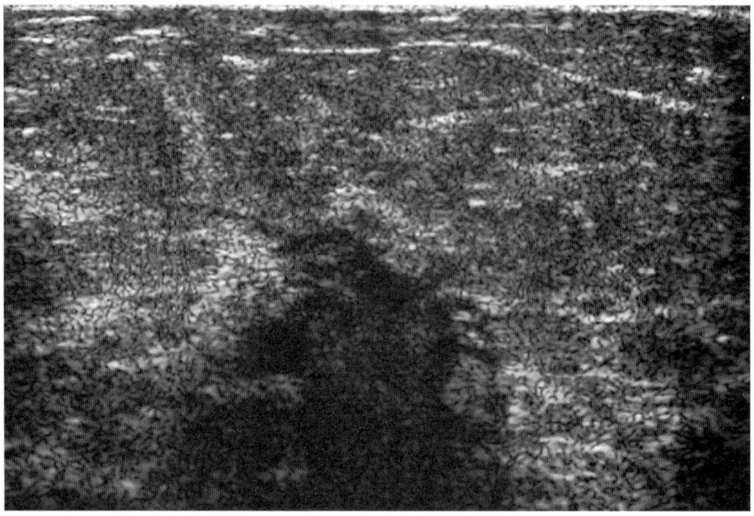

Figure 127–3. Right antiradial breast sonogram: Higher-frequency examination produces extensive shadowing. The mass identified in Figure 127–2 is hidden in the area of shadowing (see Color Plate 127–3).

Pathology

- sclerosing adenosis

Management

- BI-RADS Assessment Category 4, suspicious; biopsy should be considered

Pearls and Pitfalls

1. Sclerosing adenosis is present in 3.1% of breasts. This lesion may present as a palpable mass and is occasionally associated with tenderness.
2. Mammographically, sclerosing adenosis produces architectural distortion with or without a focal mass and may simulate malignancy.
3. Sonographically, sclerosing adenosis is an irregular hypoechoic mass that cannot be differentiated from malignancy.

Suggested Readings

1. Tabar L, Dean PB. *Teaching Atlas of Mammography.* 3rd ed. New York: Thieme; 2001:2–3, 197.
2. Tavassoli FA. *Pathology of the Breast.* 2nd ed. Stamford: Appleton and Lange; 1999:130–133.

Case 128

Case History

A 58-year-old woman presents for screening mammogram.

Physical Examination

- normal exam

Mammogram

- architectural distortion (Fig. 128–1)

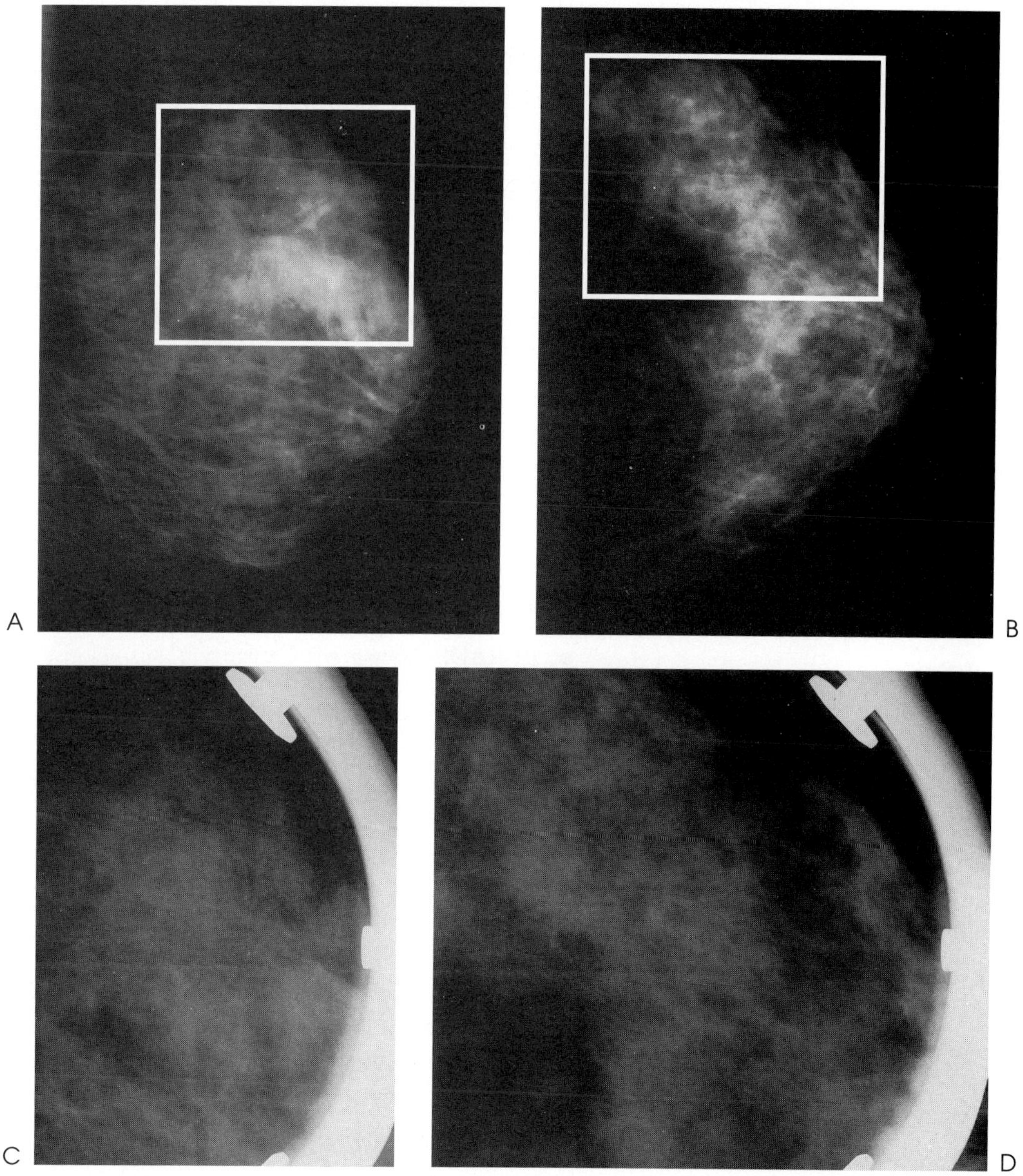

Figure 128–1. In the left upper outer quadrant, there is a spiculated density on the MLO view, which is less apparent on the CC view. Area of architectural distortion is surrounded by a square. (A). Left MLO mammogram. (B). Left CC mammogram. (C). Left MLO spot compression mammogram. (D). Left CC spot compression mammogram.

Ultrasound

Frequency

- 7 MHz

Mass

- margin: ill defined
- echogenicity: hypoechoic
- retrotumoral acoustic appearance: severe shadowing, mass partially obscured
- shape: irregular (Fig. 128–2)

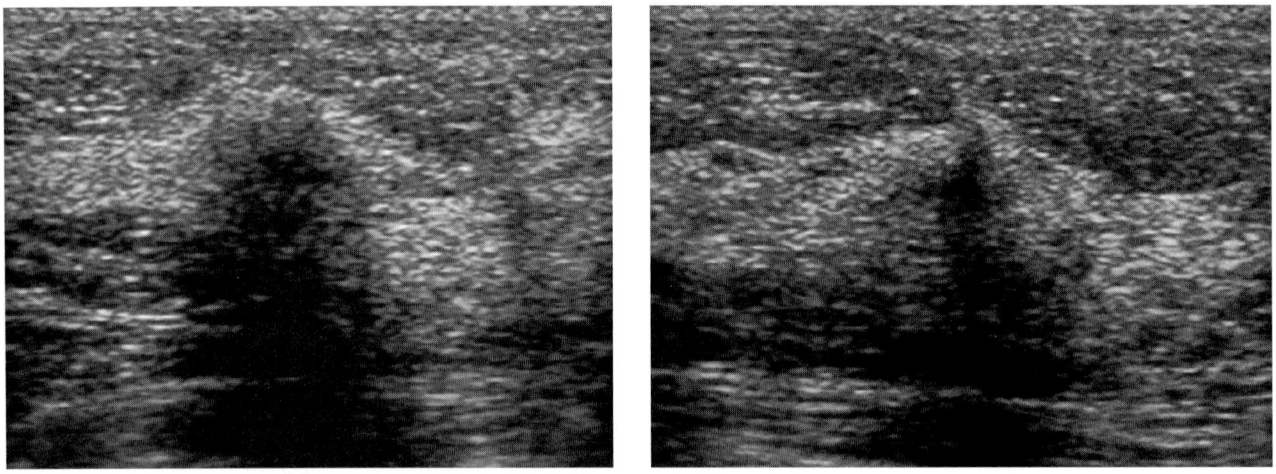

A B

Figure 128–2. In the left upper outer quadrant, the mammographic architectural distortion corresponds to a lesion exhibiting severe shadowing. The lesion appears wide in the radial view (A) and narrow in the antiradial view (B). This extreme discrepancy in appearance is characteristic of either posttraumatic or radial scars. (A). Left radial breast sonogram. (B). Left antiradial breast sonogram (see Color Plate 128–2A and B).

Pathology

- radial sclerosing lesion (radial scar)

Management

- BI-RADS Assessment Category 4, suspicious; biopsy should be considered

Pearls and Pitfalls

1. Clinically, radial scars are generally not palpable.
2. Mammographically, radial scars commonly exhibit thin radiating lines without a central dense mass. The abnormality commonly changes appearance from one projection to another.
3. Sonographically, radial scars are similar in appearance to surgically produced scars. Radial scars exhibit a large hypoechoic or shadowing area in one view and a thin abnormality in the orthogonal view. The sonographic appearance should not prevent biopsy and excision of this lesion since about one third of radial scars are associated with ductal carcinoma in situ or tubular carcinoma.

Suggested Readings

1. Evans AJ, Wilson ARM, Blamey RW, Robertson JFR, Ellis IO, Elston CW. *Atlas of Breast Disease Management.* Philadelphia: WB Saunders; 1998:94–97.
2. Tabar L, Dean PB. *Teaching Atlas of Mammography.* 3rd ed. New York: Thieme; 2001:93–96, 102–106.

Case 129

Case History

A 63-year-old woman presents with a palpable lump in the left breast.

Physical Examination

- right breast: normal
- left breast: palpable mass in upper outer quadrant

Mammogram

Mass

- margin: spiculated
- shape: irregular
- density: equal density
- architectural distortion (Fig. 129–1)

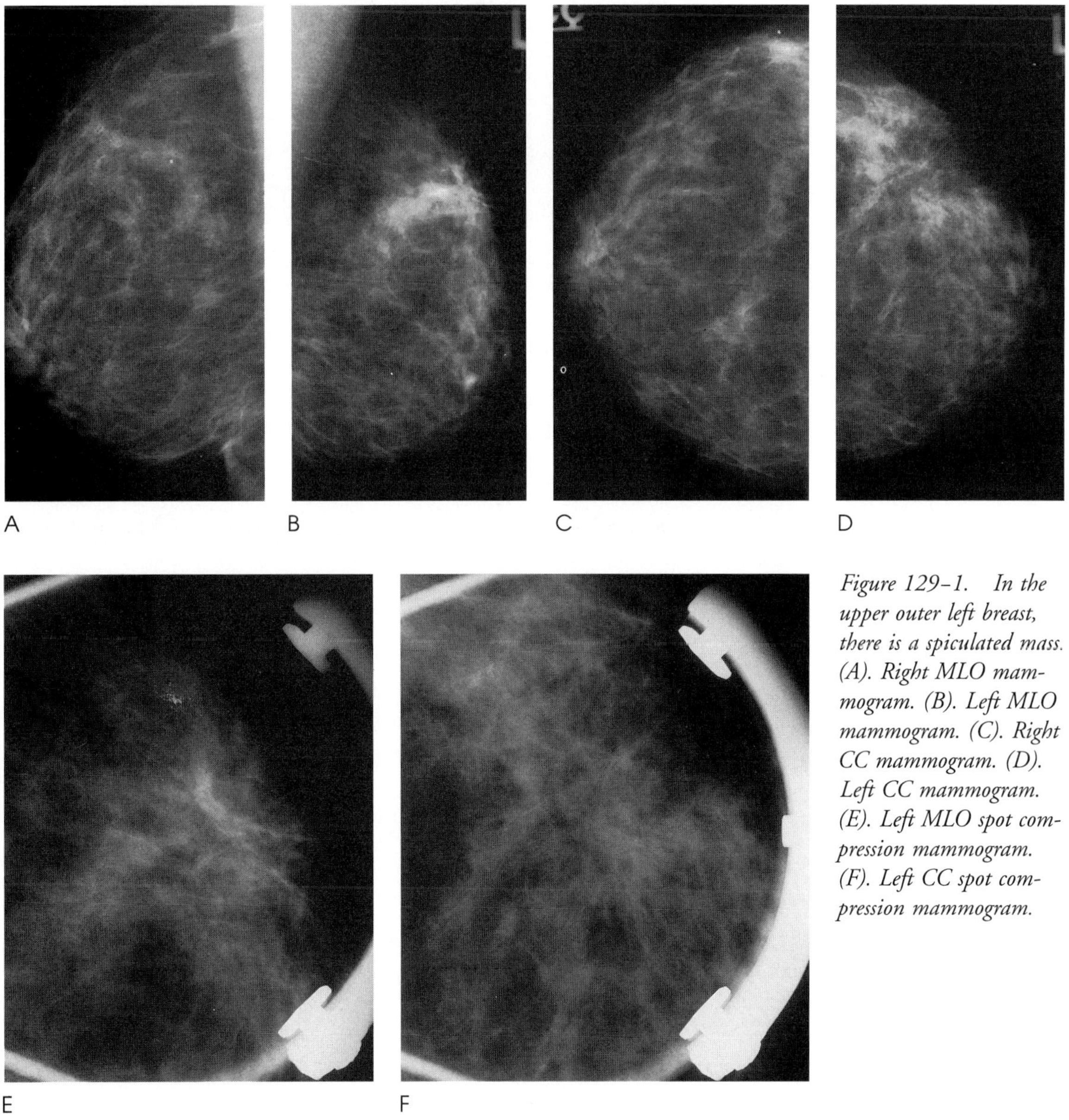

Figure 129–1. *In the upper outer left breast, there is a spiculated mass. (A). Right MLO mammogram. (B). Left MLO mammogram. (C). Right CC mammogram. (D). Left CC mammogram. (E). Left MLO spot compression mammogram. (F). Left CC spot compression mammogram.*

Ultrasound

Frequency

- 7 MHz

Mass

- margin: ill defined
- echogenicity: hypoechoic
- retrotumoral acoustic appearance: severe shadowing, mass partially obscured
- shape: irregular (Fig. 129-2)

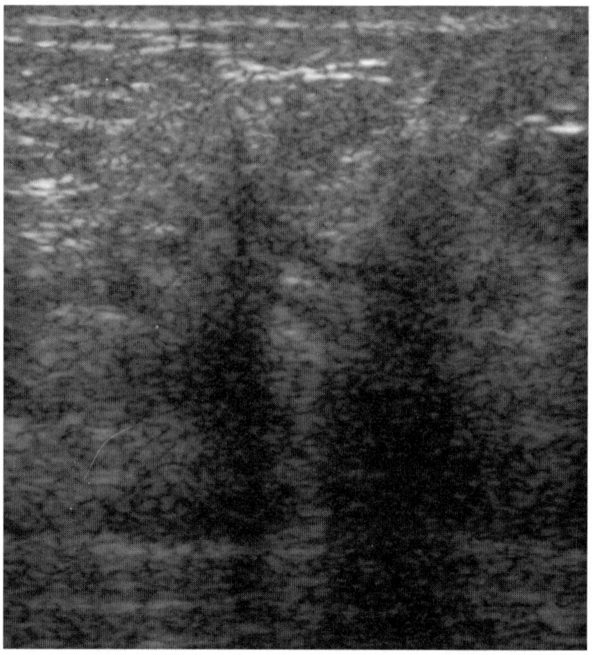

Figure 129-2. Left radial breast sonogram: The palpable lump in the upper outer quadrant is an ill-defined irregular hypoechoic solid mass. This mass corresponds to the >spiculated mass on the left breast mammogram (Fig. 129-1) (see Color Plate 129–2).

Pathology

- invasive ductal carcinoma

Management

- BI-RADS Assessment Category 4, suspicious; biopsy should be considered

Pearls and Pitfalls

1. Although malignancies commmonly produce radiating spiculations, this mass is unusual because it appears more dense on the MLO view compared to the CC view. However, persistent architectural distortion in both views is a suspicous finding if there is no history of trauma or surgery.
2. Sonography is useful in this case to confirm that the palpable abnormality corresponds to the mammographic mass and to guide for biopsy.

Suggested Readings

1. Heywang-Kobrunner SH, Schreer I, Dershaw DD. *Diagnostic Breast Imaging.* New York: Thieme; 1997:347-357.

Case 130

Case History

A 74-year-old woman presents for screening mammogram.

Physical Examination

- normal exam

Mammogram

- architectural distortion (Fig. 130–1)

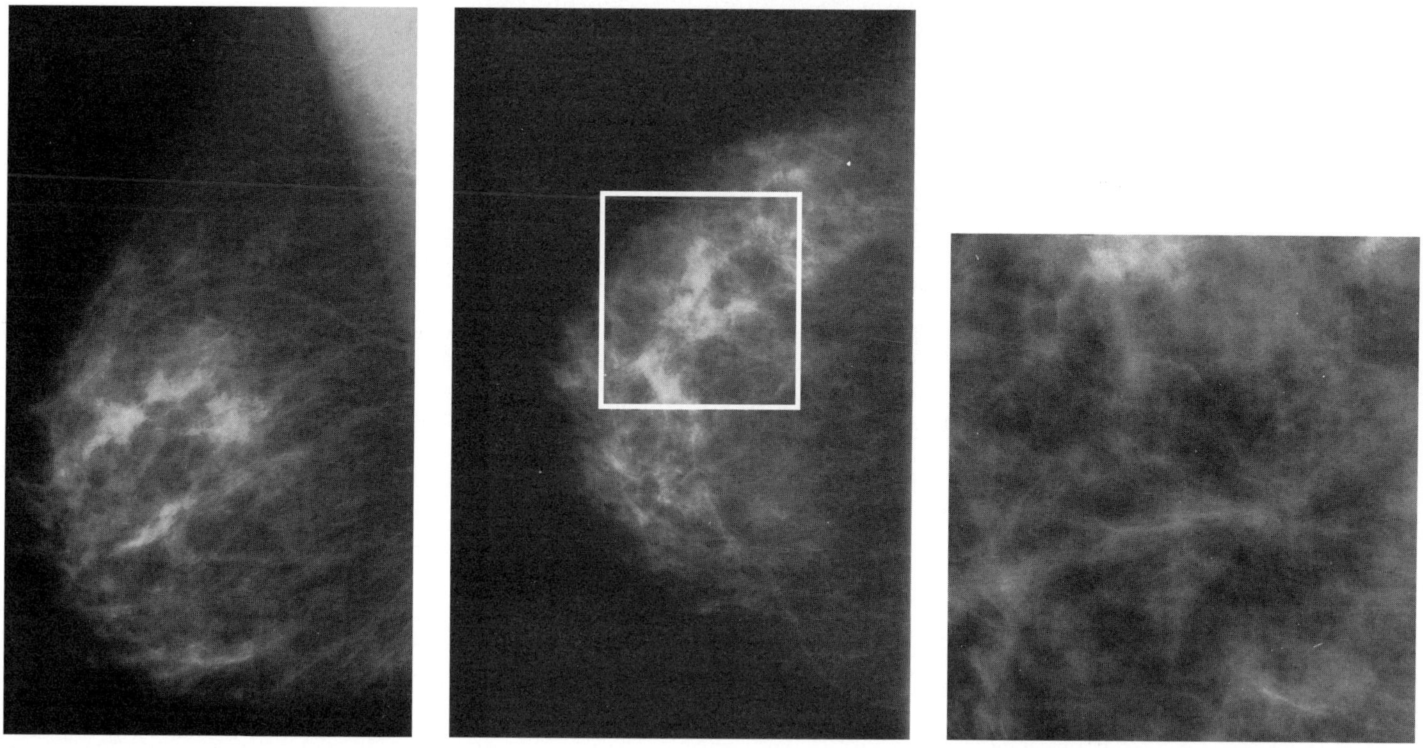

A B C

Figure 130–1. In the outer right breast on the CC view, there is an area of architectural distortion. The lesion consists of radiating lines. No mass or architectural distortion is identified in any other mammographic view. (A). Right MLO mammogram. (B). Right CC mammogram. (C). Right CC spot magnification mammogram.

Ultrasound

Frequency

- 12 MHz

Mass

- margin: ill defined
- echogenicity: hypoechoic
- retrotumoral acoustic appearance: posterior shadowing distal to mass
- shape: irregular (Fig. 130–2)

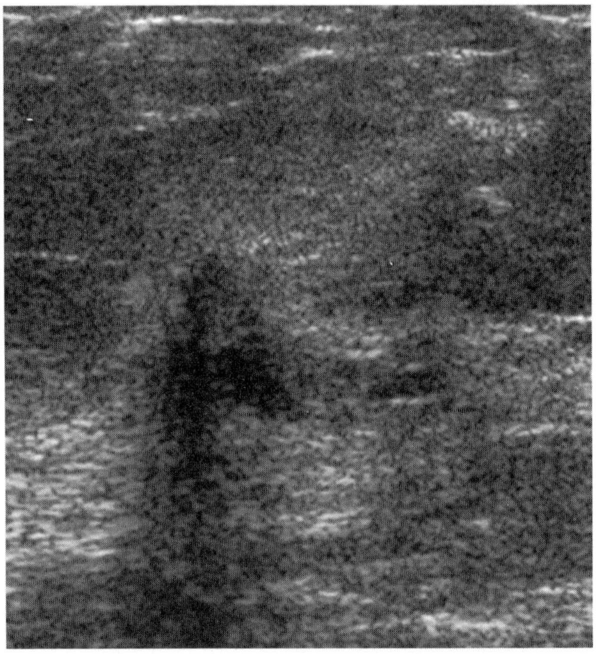

Figure 130–2. Right radial breast sonogram: In the right upper outer quadrant, there is an irregular hypoechoic mass that corresponds to the architectural distortion identified on Figure 130–1A (see Color Plate 130–2).

Pathology

- infiltrating ductal carcinoma

Management

- BI-RADS Assessment Category 4, suspicious; biopsy should be considered

Pearls and Pitfalls

Occasionally, architectural distortion is only clearly identified on one view. Sonography is useful to identify the location of the mass as well as provide biopsy guidance.

Suggested Readings

1. Bassett LW, Jackson VP, Jahan R, Fu YS, Gold RH. *Diagnosis of Diseases of the Breast.* Philadelphia: WB Saunders; 1997:116, 169–472.

Case 131

Case History

An 86-year-old woman presents for screening mammogram.

Physical Examination

- normal exam

Mammogram

Mass

- margin: indistinct
- shape: irregular
- density: high density
- architectural distortion (Fig. 131–1)

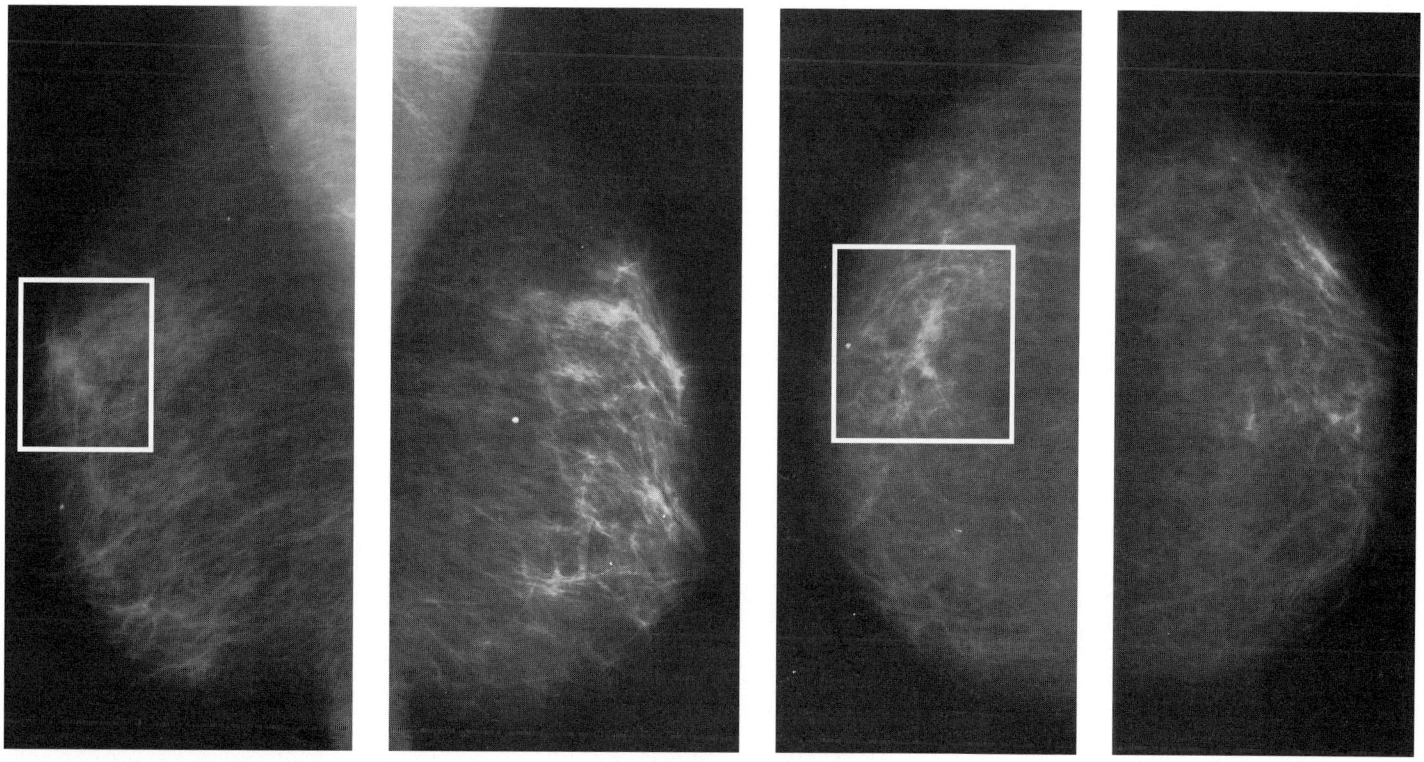

A B C D

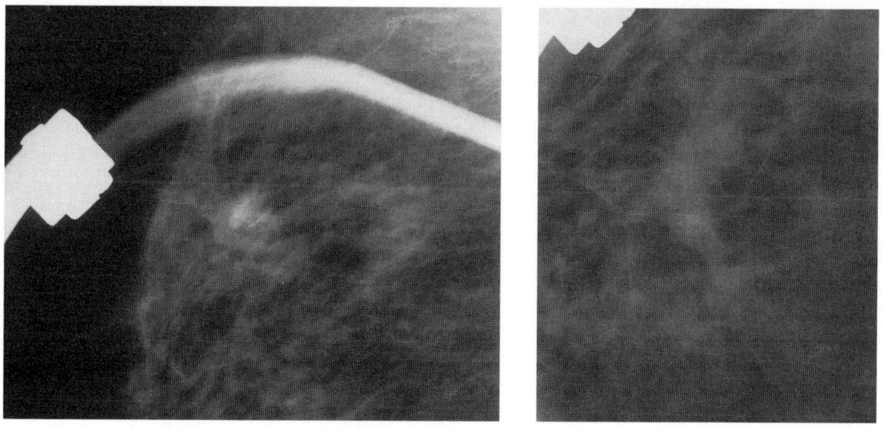

E F

Figure 131–1. In the right upper outer quadrant, there is an ill-defined irregular density associated with trabecular thickening. (Square encloses abnormal area.) (A). Right MLO mammogram. (B). Left MLO mammogram. (C). Right CC mammogram. (D). Left CC mammogram. (E). Right MLO spot compression mammogram. (F). Right CC spot compression mammogram.

Pathology

- invasive ductal carcinoma

Management

- BI-RADS Assessment Category 4, suspicious; biopsy should be considered

Pearls and Pitfalls

The normal trabecular pattern of the breast is a combination of densities created by Cooper's ligaments and lactiferous ducts. Benign conditions such as infection or inflammation and malignant abnormalities may cause trabecular thickening. In this case, the focal nature of the thickening is suspicious for malignancy.

Suggested Readings

1. Kopans DB. *Breast Imaging.* 2nd ed. Philadelphia: Lippincott-Raven; 1998:342, 405.

Case 132

Case History

A 77-year-old woman presents for screening mammogram.

Physical Examination

- normal exam

Mammogram

Mass

- margin: indistinct
- shape: oval
- density: equal
- architectural distortion (Fig. 132–1)

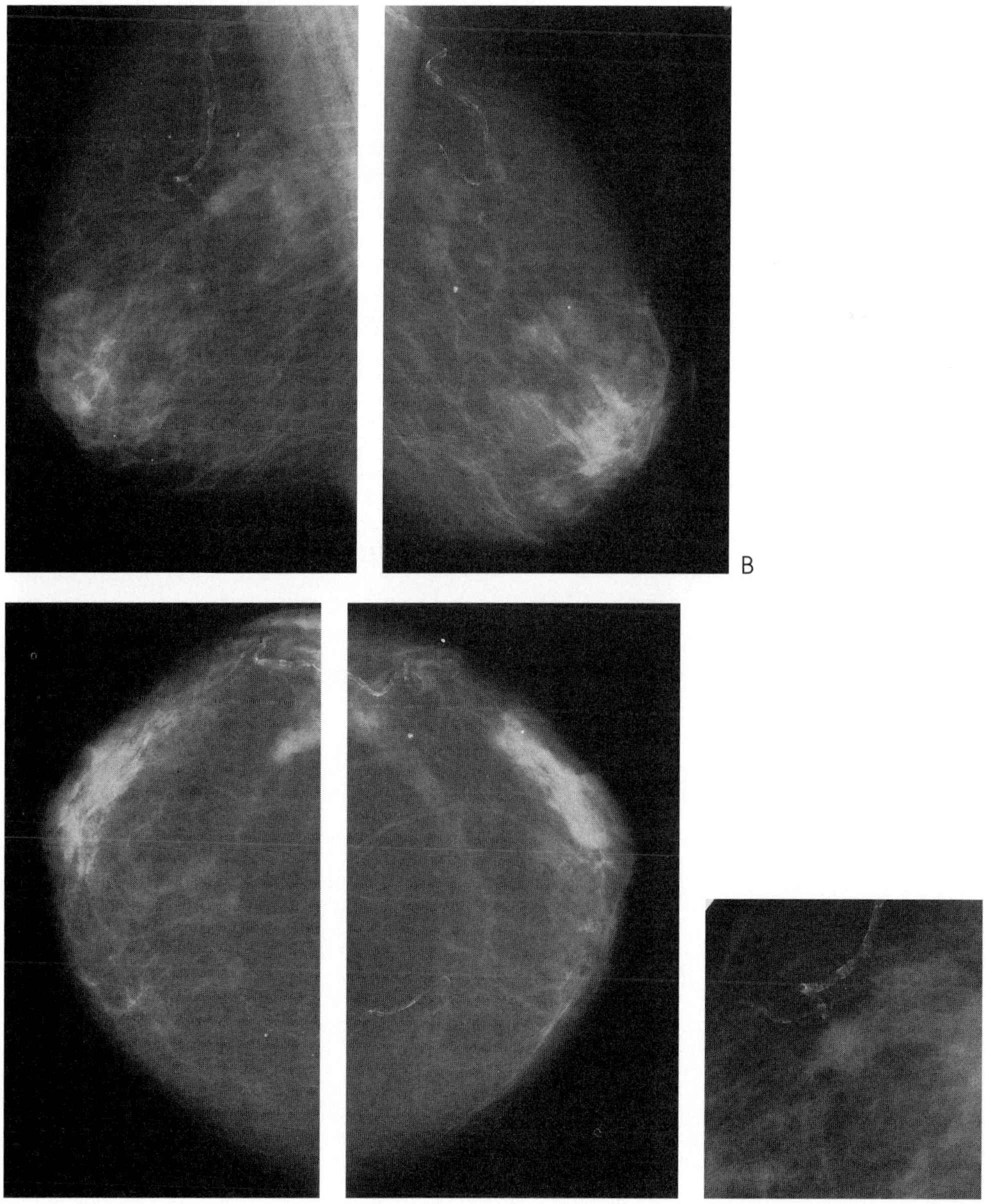

A B C D E

Figure 132–1. In the right upper outer quadrant there is a partially obscured oval mass associated with architectural distortion. (A). Right MLO mammogram. (B). Left MLO mammogram. (C). Right CC mammogram. (D). Left CC mammogram. (E). Right MLO spot compression mammogram.

Ultrasound

Frequency

- 7 MHz

Mass

- margin: ill defined
- echogenicity: hypoechoic
- retrotumoral acoustic appearance: single edge shadowing
- shape: ellipsoid (Fig. 132–2)

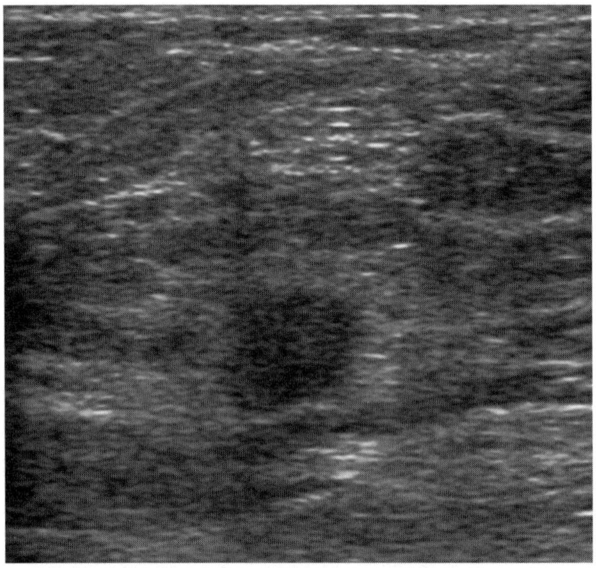

Figure 132–2. Right breast radial sonogram: The mammographic mass in Figure 132–1 corresponds to an ill-defined hypoechoic nodule with posterior acoustic shadowing (see Color Plate 132–2).

Pathology

- infiltrating ductal carcinoma

Management

- BI-RADS Assessment Category 4, suspicious; biopsy should be considered

Pearls and Pitfalls

This case demonstrates central architectural distortion due to a malignancy. The tumor is causing retraction of the surrounding density toward the mass. The resulting distorted pattern is readily identified by comparing the abnormal area to the opposite side.

Suggested Readings

1. Egan RL. *Breast Imaging: Diagnosis and Morphology of Breast Diseases*. Philadelphia: WB Saunders; 1988:226–240.
2. Kopans DB. *Breast Imaging.* 2nd ed. Philadelphia: Lippincott-Raven; 1998:382–389.

Case 133

Case History

A 57-year-old woman presents with an inverted nipple.

Physical Examination

- right breast: inverted right nipple and an 8 cm palpable subareolar mass
- left breast: normal exam

Mammogram

Mass

- margin: spiculated
- shape: irregular
- density: high
- architectural distortion (Fig. 133–1)

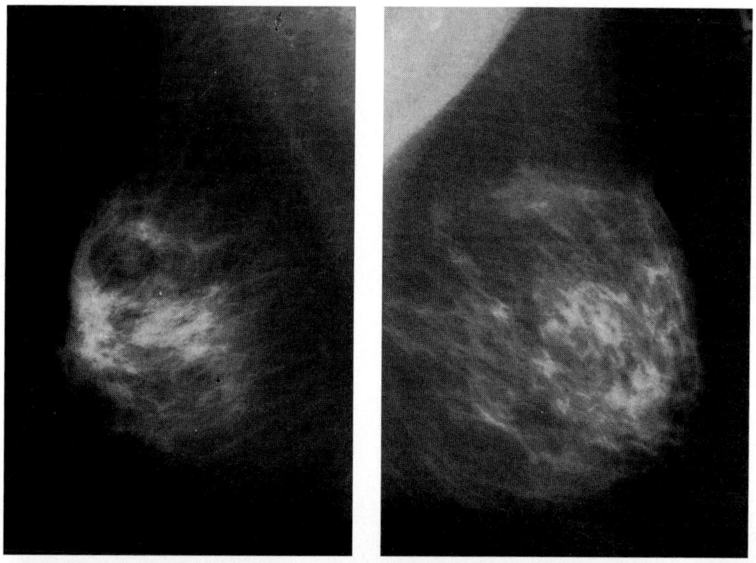

Figure 133–1. There is a right subareolar spiculated mass associated with nipple retraction and trabecular thickening. (A). Right MLO mammogram. (B). Left MLO mammogram. (C). Right CC mammogram. (D). Left CC mammogram. (E). Right CC spot compression mammogram.

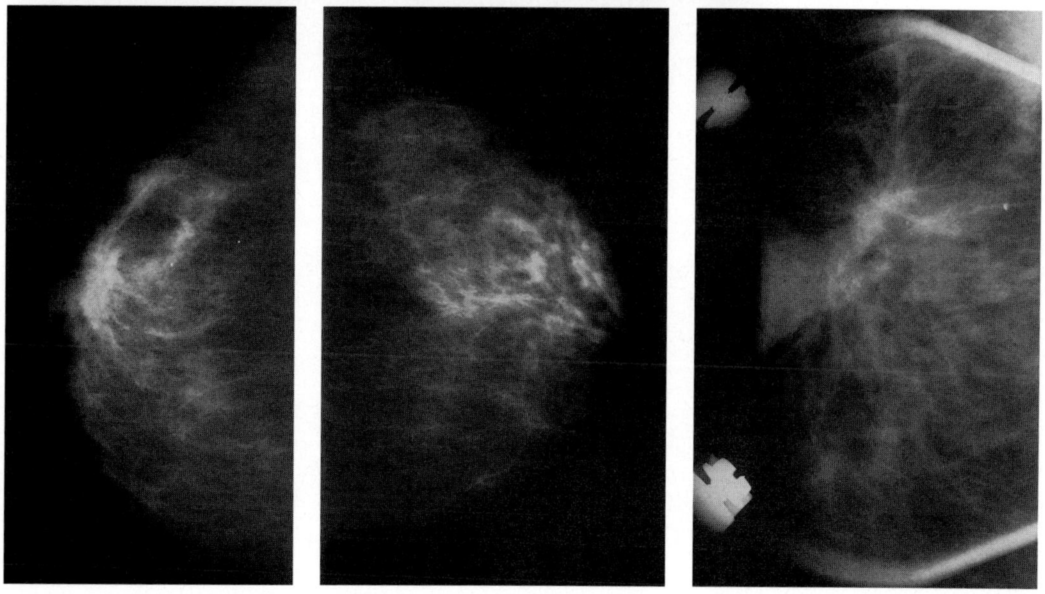

Pathology

- invasive ductal carcinoma

Management

- BI-RADS Assessment Category 5, highly suggestive of malignancy

Pearls and Pitfalls

Subareaolar architectural distortion is sometimes difficult to identify. Even in predominantly fatty breasts this region may be fairly dense. Spiculations from a subareolar mass may blend into the normal ductal lines that meet at the nipple. Therefore, one should spend extra attention on this region to avoid missing subtle masses or architectural distortion.

Suggested Readings

1. Heywang-Kobrunner SH, Schreer I, Dershaw DD. *Diagnostic Breast Imaging.* New York: Thieme; 1997:134–135, 370.

Case 134

Case History

A 57-year-old woman presents with new left breast lump.

Physical Examination

- left breast: 4 cm mass extending from 2:00 to 4:00
- right breast: normal exam

Mammogram

Mass

- margin: indistinct
- shape: irregular
- density: high density
- architectural distortion (Fig. 134–1)

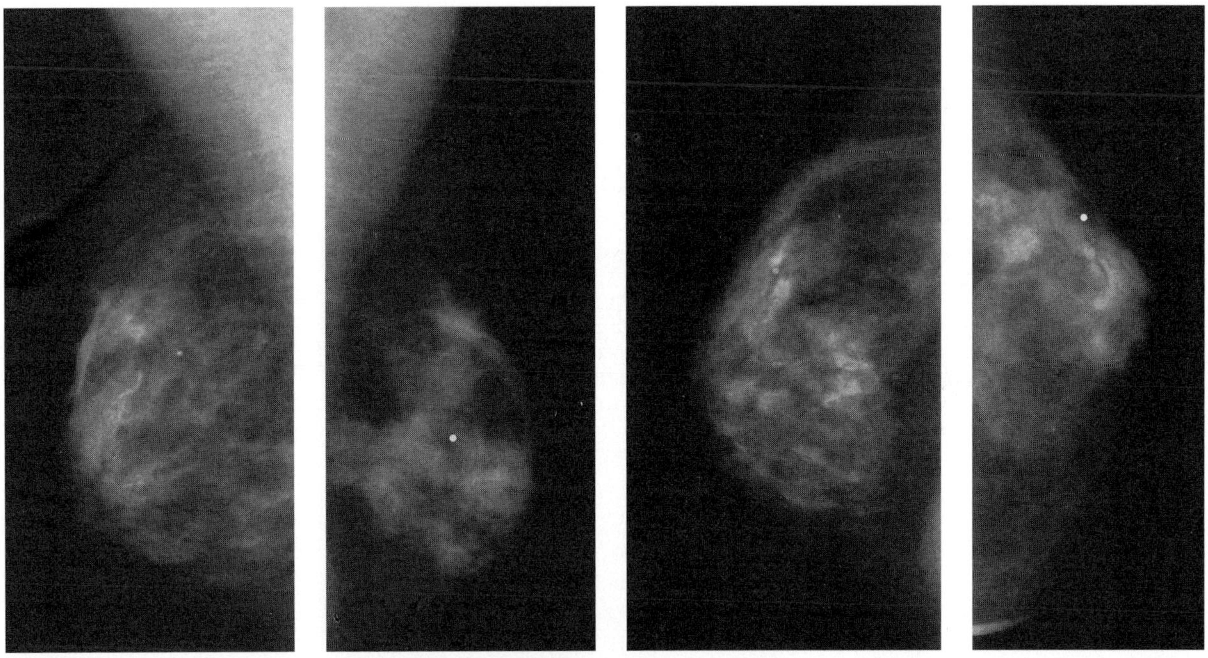

A B C D

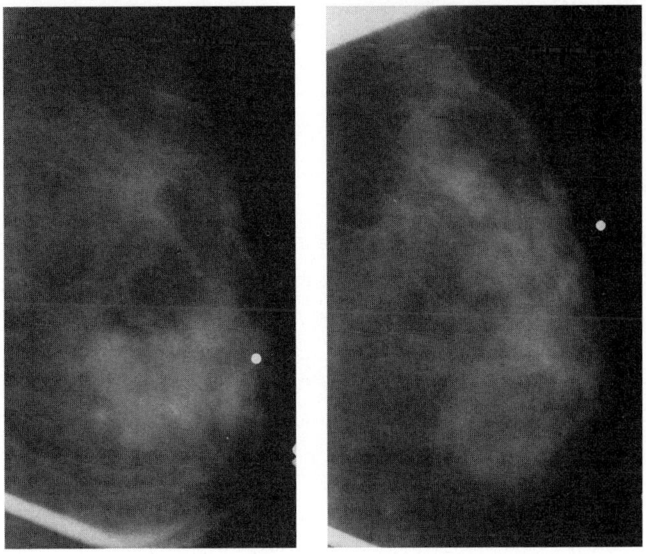

E F

Figure 134–1. In the left breast there is an ill-defined mass in the left outer breast. (A). Right MLO mammogram. (B). Left MLO mammogram. (C). Right CC mammogram. (D). Left CC mammogram. (E). Left MLO spot compression mammogram. (F). Left CC spot compression mammogram.

Ultrasound

Frequency

- 10 MHz

Mass

- margin: ill defined
- echogenicity: hypoechoic
- retrotumoral acoustic appearance: posterior shadowing distal to mass
- shape: irregular (Fig. 134–2)

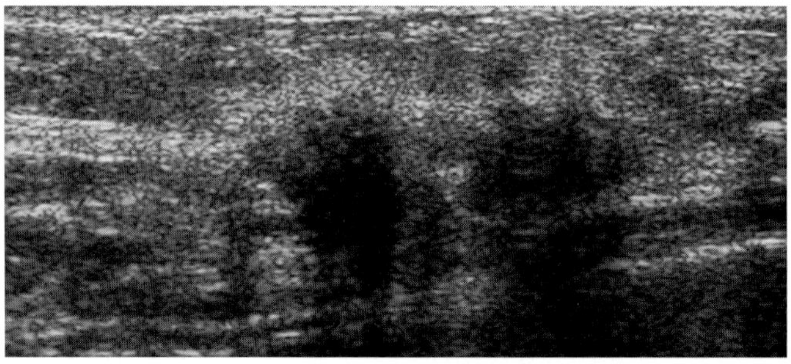

Figure 134–2. Left radial breast sonogram: The palpable lump is associated with a multilobulated, irregular, hypoechoic mass. This abnormality corresponds to the mammographic mass identified in Figure 134–1 (see Color Plate 134–2).

Other Modalities (Fig. 134–3)

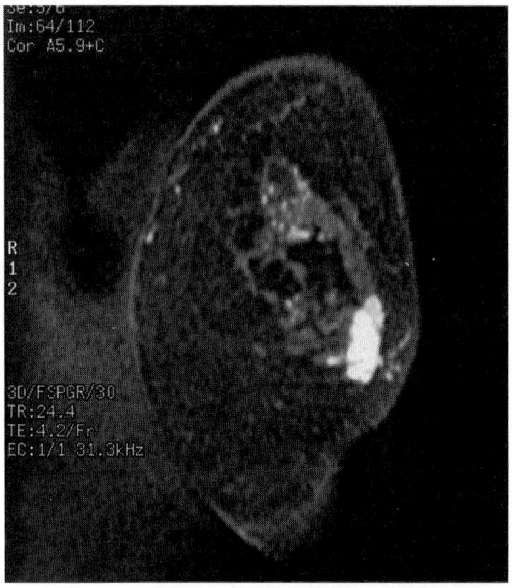

Figure 134–3. Left coronal dynamic bolus 3-D volume gradient breast MRI: In the outer breast, there is an enhancing mildly irregular, lobulated mass that corresponds to the mammographic and sonographic mass.

Pathology

- infiltrating ductal carcinoma

Management

- BI-RADS Assessment Category 4, suspicious; biopsy should be considered

Pearls and Pitfalls

1. Architectural distortion is a particularly useful sign in denser breasts as masses are more difficult to identify in these breasts. In this case, the neoplasm causes retraction of the surrounding normal density. This retraction produces a distorted asymmetric parenchymal pattern.
2. In this case, sonography was used to correlate the palpable lump with the mammographic abnormality and to provide biopsy guidance. Because of the density of the breast, both sonography and MRI provide better definition of lesion size and location compared with mammography.

Suggested Readings

1. Bassett LW, Jackson VP, Jahan R, Fu YS, Gold RH. *Diagnosis of Diseases of the Breast.* Philadelphia: WB Saunders; 1997:116.

Case 135

Case History

A 55-year-old woman presents with a new right breast lump.

Physical Examination

- right breast: palpable mass at 12:00
- left breast: normal exam

Mammogram

Mass

- margin: spiculated
- shape: irregular
- density: high density
- architectural distortion (Fig. 135–1)

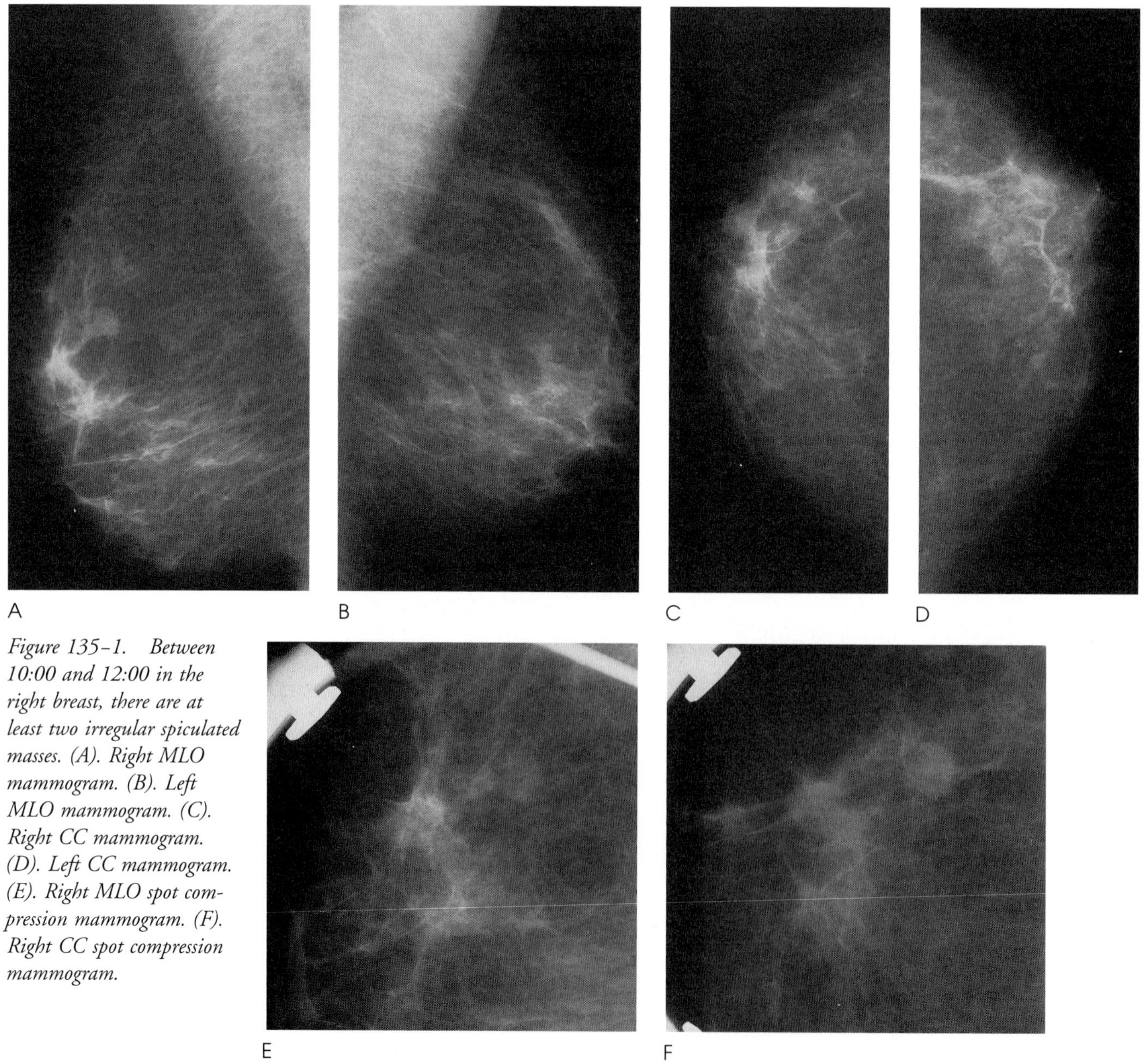

Figure 135–1. Between 10:00 and 12:00 in the right breast, there are at least two irregular spiculated masses. (A). Right MLO mammogram. (B). Left MLO mammogram. (C). Right CC mammogram. (D). Left CC mammogram. (E). Right MLO spot compression mammogram. (F). Right CC spot compression mammogram.

Ultrasound

Frequency

- 7 MHz

Mass

- margin: ill defined
- echogenicity: hypoechoic
- retrotumoral acoustic appearance: posterior shadowing distal to mass
- shape: irregular (Fig. 135–2)

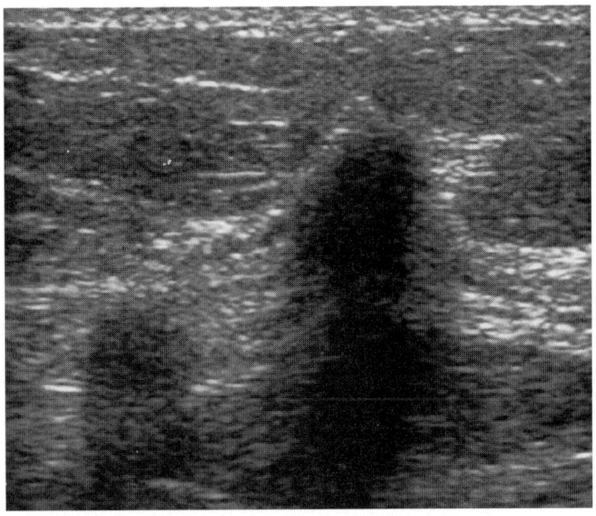

Figure 135–2. Right radial breast sonogram: In the upper breast, two hypoechoic, irregular shadowing masses are present. The larger mass is palpable. These masses correspond to the mammographic masses (see Color Plate 135–2).

Pathology

Infiltrating ductal carcinoma. Both sonographic masses were found to be infiltrating ductal carcinoma so this is a multifocal neoplasm.

Management

- BI-RADS Assessment Category 4, suspicious; biopsy should be considered

Pearls and Pitfalls

1. For surgical planning, it is important to define the size of the neoplasm within the breast. Architectural distortion of the parenchymal pattern may provide evidence that multifocal disease (multiple lesions within the same quadrant or within 5 cm) is present. With multifocal disease, the parenchymal pattern appears clumped into closely packed irregular or spiculated densities. For small lesions or masses spaced farther apart, magnification views may be useful to identify spiculations connecting the masses.
2. Sonography is useful to further confirm the presence of multiple masses and to provide biopsy guidance.

Suggested Readings

1. Berg WA, Gilbreath PL. Multicentric and multifocal cancer: whole breast us in preoperative evaluation. *Radiology* 2000;214:59–66.
2. Gump FE, Habif DV, Logergo P, et al. The extent and distribution of cancer in breasts with palpable primary tumors. *Ann Surg* 1986;204:384–388.

Section VIII

Male Breast

Imaging Characteristics of Gynecomastia

The assessment of male breast calcifications is the same as the female breast (see Introduction to Section V). The approach to solid male breast masses is also similar to the female breast except for the inclusion of gynecomastia.

I. Mammography

A. There are three mammographic types of gynecomastia:
1. Nodular: subareolar, fanlike density; may be nodular and simulate a mass
2. Dendritic: wispy, flame-shaped subareolar densities
3. Glandular: large, severe increased density that simulates a female heterogeneously or severely dense fibroglandular pattern

B. Pseudogynecomastia: excess fatty breast tissue usually associated with obesity

II. Ultrasound: Gynecomastia has three main patterns. A patient may exhibit any combination of these patterns.

A. Mass: may either be oval or irregular in shape with either well-defined or ill-defined margins. This finding most commonly seen with nodular gynecomastia.

B. Diffuse hyperechoic or heterogeneous tissue: This appearance is similar to normal female fibroglandular tissue. No focal hypoechoic mass is present. Random, intermittent shadowing may be present.

C. Diffusely dilated ducts: similar to female ductal ectasia.

D. Ultrasound Pearls: to differentiate gynecomastia from another mass:
1. In gynecomastia, the pattern of dilated ducts will not be distorted by the hypoechoic tissue.
2. Shadowing from gynecomastia will be random and the pattern will change with transducer position.

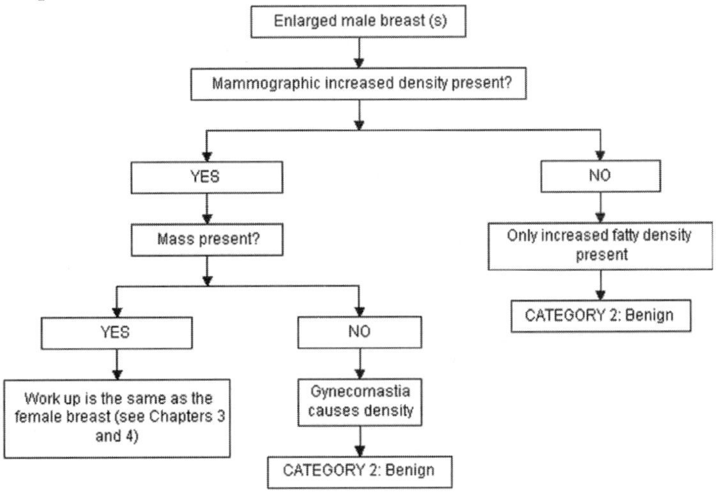

Case 136

Case History

A 64-year-old man presents with chronic, draining sinus tract in the left breast. Two years prior he had a hypophysectomy for Cushing's disease, and he has chronic pituitary insufficiency.

Physical Examination

- left breast: ulcerated nipple with a subareolar mass
- right breast: enlarged but otherwise normal

Mammogram (Fig. 136–1)

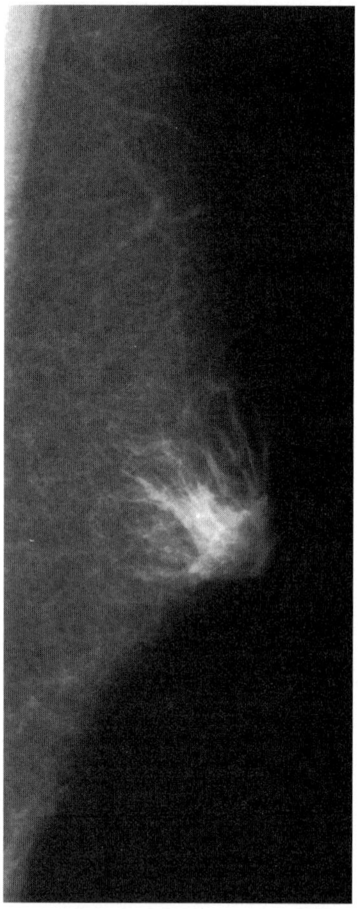

A

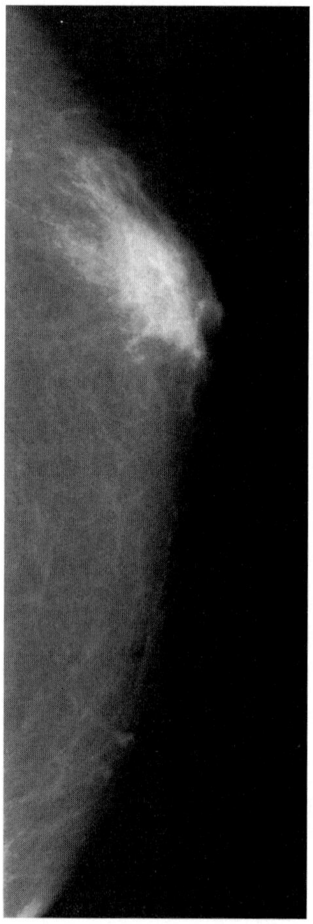

B

Figure 136–1. There is ill-defined left subareolar density with coarse linear densities extending into the surrounding fat. (A). Left MLO mammogram. (B). Left CC mammogram.

Ultrasound

Frequency

- 7.5 MHz

Mass

- margin: well defined
- echogenicity: hypoechoic
- retrotumoral acoustic appearance: mild acoustic enhancement
- shape: ellipsoid (Fig. 136–2)

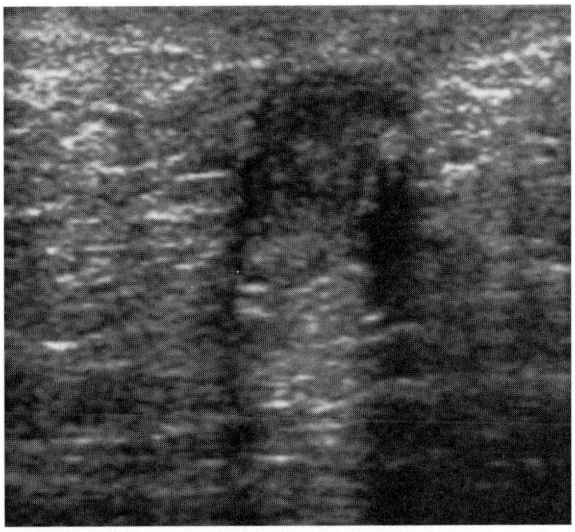

Figure 136–2. Left transverse breast sonogram: Under the nipple, there is a hypoechoic, well-defined fluid collection with mild posterior acoustic enhancement (see Color Plate 136–2).

Pathology

- abscess
- nipple discharge cultures positive for *Staphylococcus aureus*

Management

- BI-RADS Assessment Category 3, probably benign; short-interval follow-up

Pearls and Pitfalls

1. Because subareolar abscess is a rare lesion of the male breast, there is little previous clinical and radiographic information. In women, the most common infecting organism is *Staphylococcus aureus*. These lesions are commonly recurrent and require excision. This patient failed antibiotic therapy and eventually was treated with excision.
2. In females, mammographically, these abscesses produce an ill-defined subareolar mass. Sonographically, there is a hypoechoic fluid collection, which may be mistaken for a solid mass.

Suggested Readings

1. Appelbaum AH, Evans GFF, Evans MB, Levy KR, Amirkhan RH, Schumpert TD. Mammographic appearances of male breast disease. *Radiographics* 1999;19:559–568.
2. Tavassoli FA. *Pathology of the Breast.* 2nd ed. Stamford: Appleton and Lange; 1999:792.

Case 137

Case History

A 75-year-old man presents with a new left breast mass.

Physical Examination

- left breast: palpable, firm, nontender lump at 9:00 position
- right breast: normal exam

Mammogram

Mass

- margin: indistinct
- shape: irregular
- density: fat-containing (Fig. 137–1)

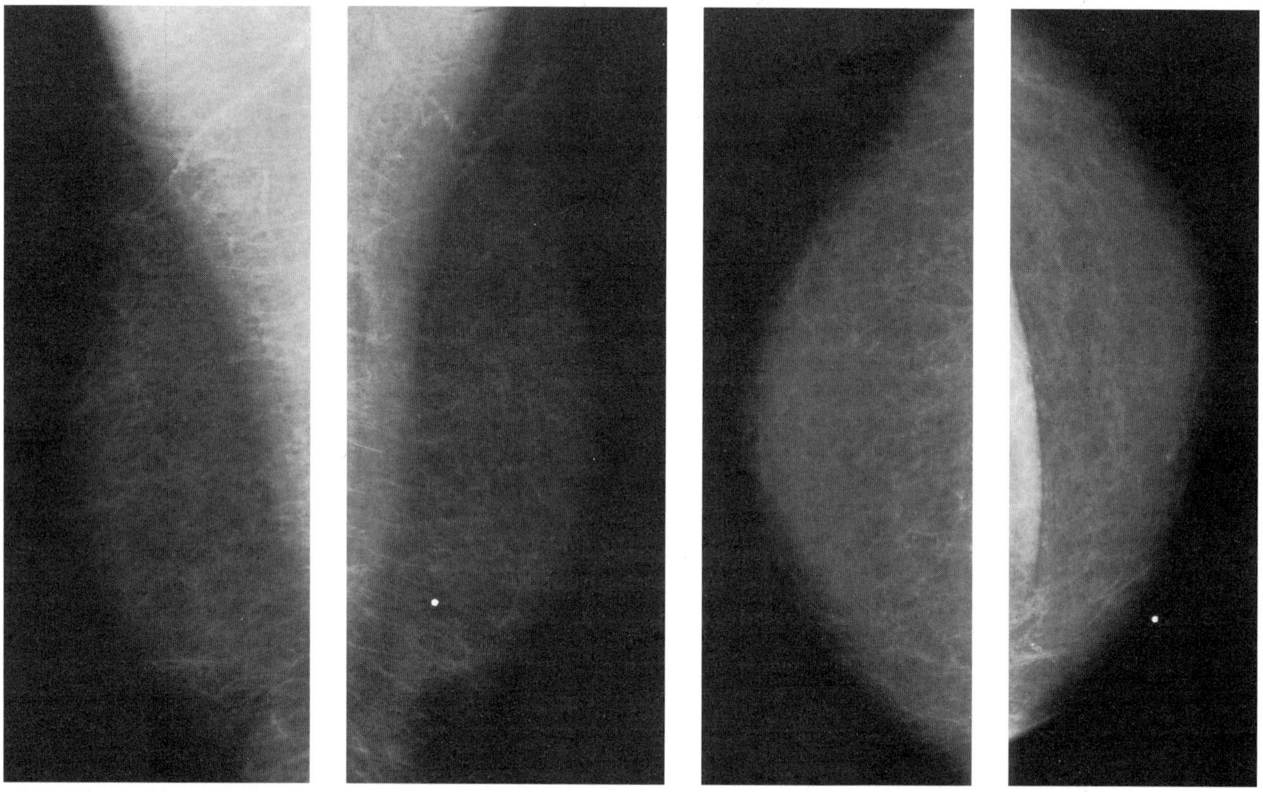

A B C D

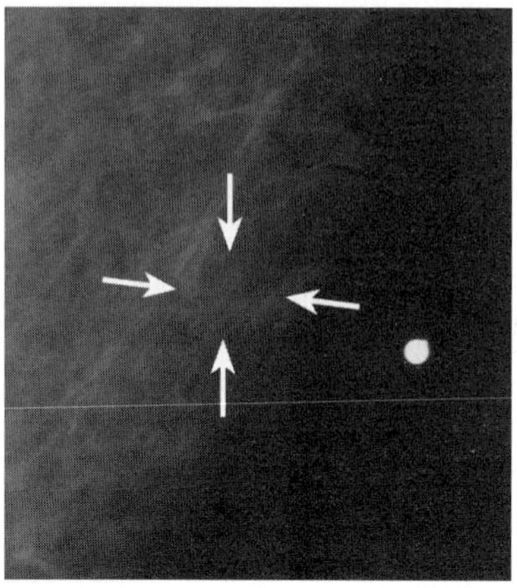

E

Figure 137–1. *In the left inner breast, the palpable lump corresponds to a small, faint, ill-defined opacity that is partially fat density (arrows). (A). Right MLO mammogram. (B). Left MLO mammogram. (C). Right CC mammograms. (D). Left CC mammograms. (E). Left CC spot magnification mammogram.*

Pathology

- angiolipoma

Management

- BI-RADS Assessment Category 2, benign finding

Pearls and Pitfalls

1. Angiolipomas resemble lipomas. They are encapsulated masses of mature lipocytes with a prominent vascular network. Angiolipomas are commonly found in males. An Armed Forces Institute of Pathology (AFIP) series reported that 17 (24%) of 70 breast angiolipomas were found in males.
2. Mammographically, angiolipomas commonly have a benign, fat density appearance.

Suggested Readings

1. Tavassoli FA. *Pathology of the Breast.* 2nd ed. Stamford: Appleton and Lange; 1999:695-697.

Case 138

Case History

A 51-year-old man presents with new left breast lumps.

Physical Examination

- left breast: two firm nodules between 12:00 and 1:00
- right breast: normal exam

Mammogram

Mass

- margin: indistinct
- shape: oval
- density: equal density (Fig. 138–1)

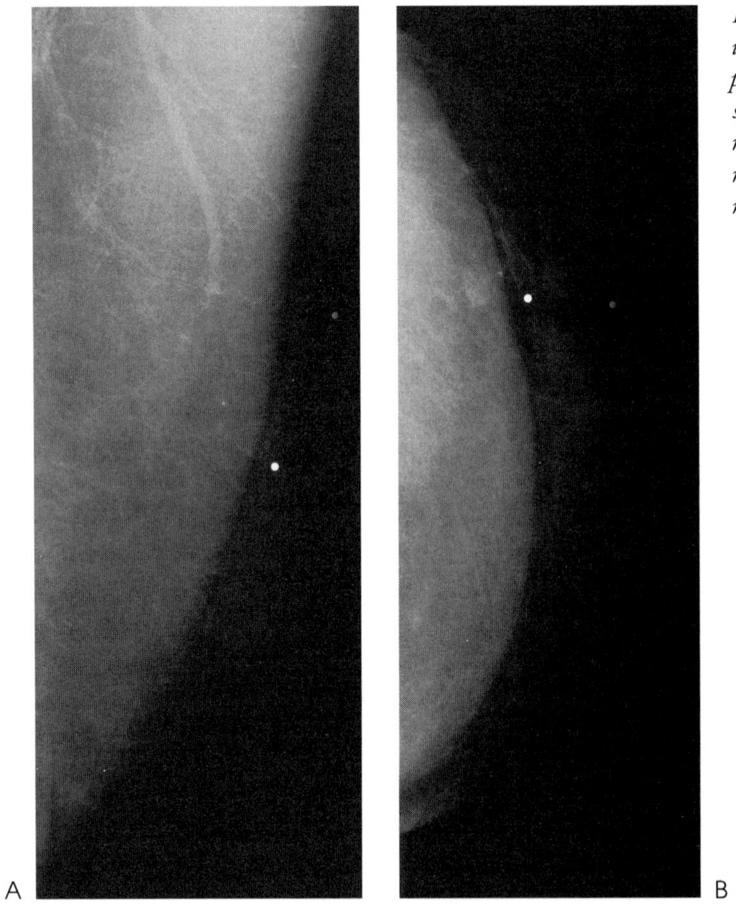

Figure 138–1. In the left upper breast, there are two palpable lumps that correspond to two ill-defined oval masses. (A). Left MLO mammogram. (B). Left CC mammogram.

Ultrasound

Frequency

- 13 MHz

Mass

- margin: ill defined
- echogenicity: isoechoic
- retrotumoral acoustic appearance: no shadowing
- shape: ellipsoid (Fig. 138-2)

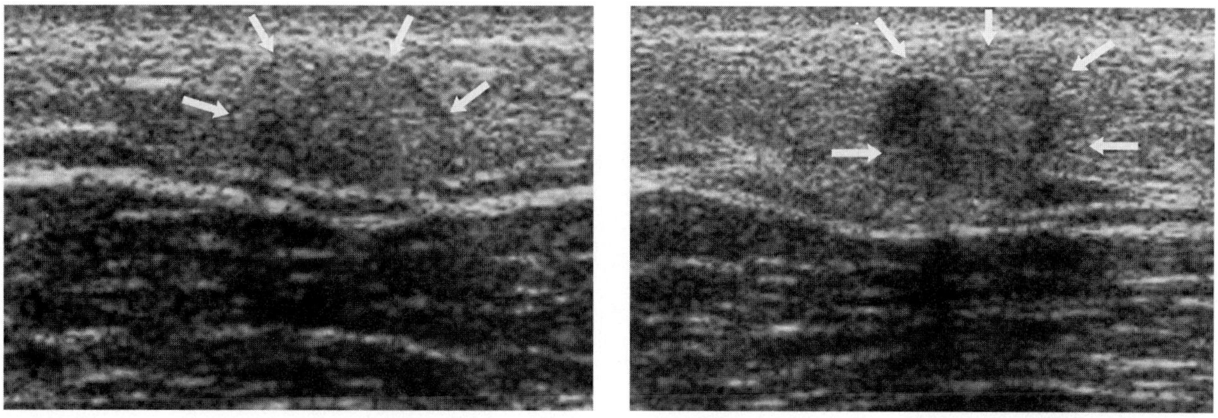

A B

Figure 138-2. The palpable lumps correspond to two solid masses. One mass (A) is an oval, ill-defined, isoechoic mass (arrows). The other mass (B) is an oval, ill-defined mass with heterogeneous echogenicity (arrows). (A). Left longitudinal breast sonogram. (B). Left longitudinal breast sonogram.

Pathology

- fat necrosis

Management

- BI-RADS Assessment Category 4, suspicious; biopsy should be considered

Pearls and Pitfalls

1. Fat necrosis in men is radiographically similar to women. Mammographically, fat necrosis produces either a well-defined fat density mass (oil cyst) or an ill-defined irregular mass. The latter abnormality generally cannot be differentiated from malignancy.
2. Sonographically, fat necrosis in the male breast is identical to the female breast. The mammographic irregular mass generally corresponds to an irregular hypoechoic mass. Occasionally, fat necrosis will have a more benign hyperechoic appearance.

Suggested Readings

1. Chantra PK, So GJ, Wollman JS, Bassett LW. Mammography of the male breast. *AJR* 1995;164:853-858.
2. Stewart RA, Howlett DC, Hearn FJ. Pictorial review: the imaging features of male breast disease. *Clin Radiol* 1997;52:739-744.

Case 139

Case History

A 72-year-old markedly obese male presents with left breast tenderness.

Physical Examination

- right breast: normal exam
- left breast: mildly tender, slight soft, fullness under the nipple without mass

Mammogram (Fig. 139–1)

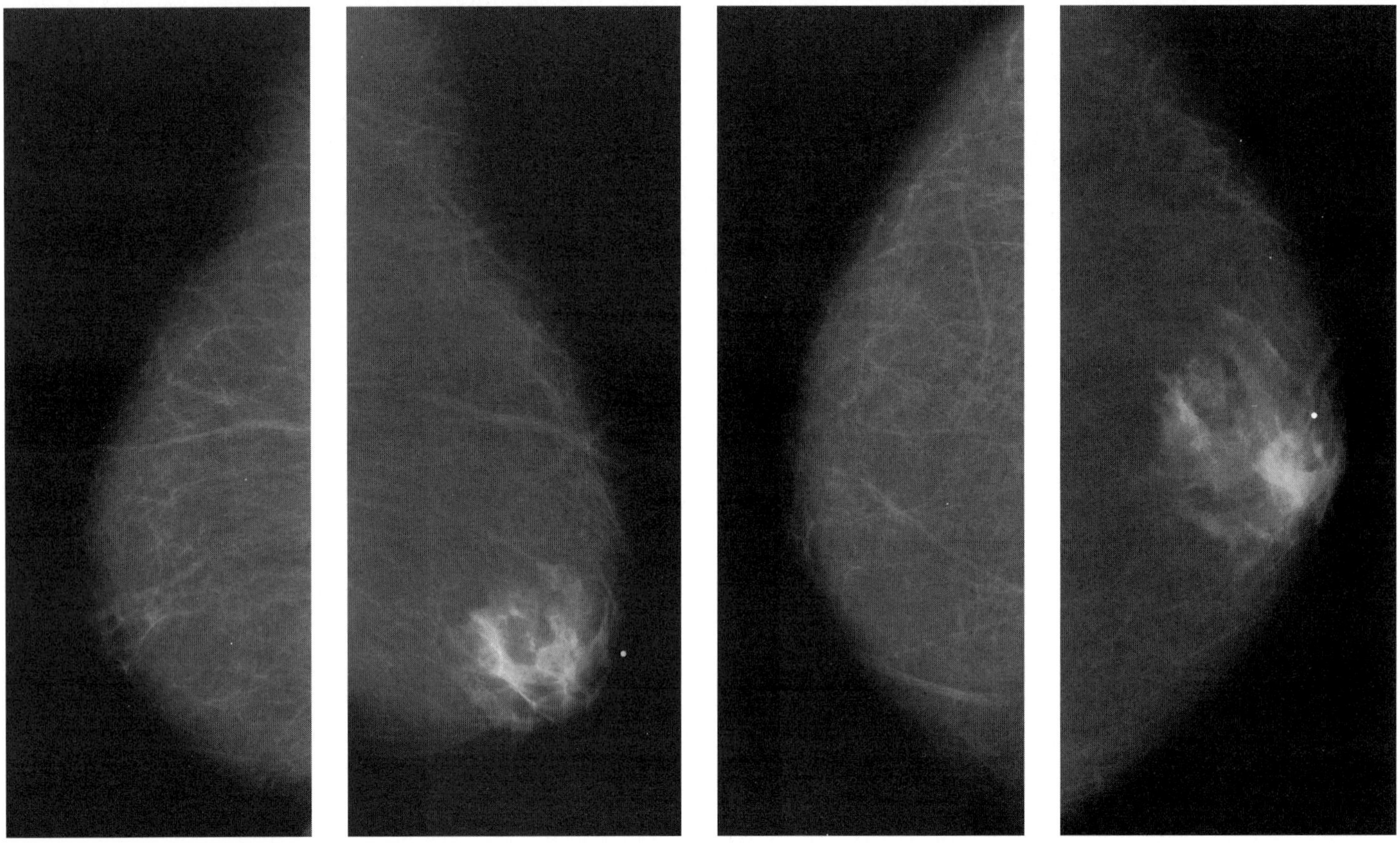

A B C D

Figure 139–1. The right breast is completely fatty. The left breast exhibits mild fan-shaped subareolar density. (A). Right MLO mammogram. (B). Left MLO mammogram. (C). Right CC mammogram. (D). Left CC mammogram.

Ultrasound (Fig. 139–2)

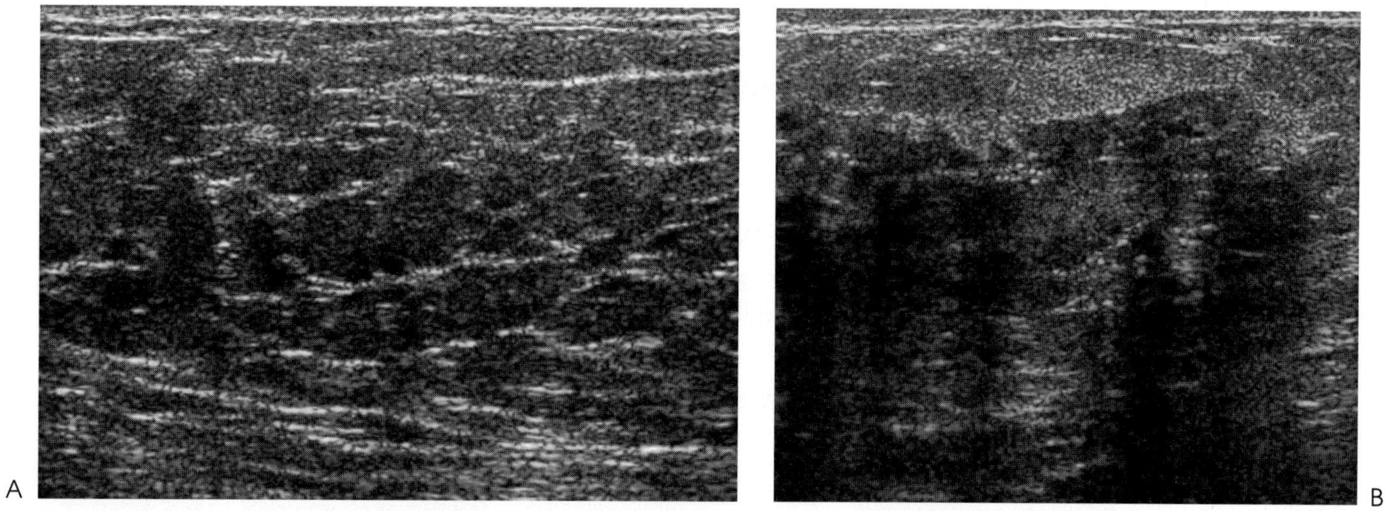

Figure 139–2. Right breast (A) exhibits normal predominantly fatty architecture. The tissue of the left breast is heterogeneous echogenicity with random intermittent shadowing. (A). Right radial breast sonogram. (B). Left radial breast sonogram.

Pathology

- gynecomastia

Management

- BI-RADS Assessment Category 2, benign finding

Pearls and Pitfalls

1. Gynecomastia is clinically defined as more than 2 cm of palpable subareolar tissue in the male breast. In one nonselective autopsy study of 100 men, 55% had gynecomastia. Clinically, most men present with unilateral symptoms. Only 20 to 30% of men note bilateral breast enlargement. The breast enlargement is due to benign ductal and stromal hyperplasia. In this case, the left breast exhibits nodular gynecomastia.
2. When males are overweight, breast enlargement is normal. Radiographically, the normal male breast will be predominantly fatty with very little linear or curvilinear density. This patient illustrates a normal right enlarged breast due to obesity.

Suggested Readings

1. Appelbaum AH, Evans GFF, Evans MB, Levy KR, Amirkhan RH, Schumpert TD. Mammographic appearances of male breast disease. *Radiographics* 1999;19:559–568.
2. Kapdi CC, Parekh NJ. The male breast. *Radiol Clin North Am* 1983;21:137–148.
3. Stewart RA, Howlett DC, Hearn FJ. Pictorial review: the imaging features of male breast disease. *Clin Radiol* 1997;52:739–744.
4. Tavassoli FA. *Pathology of the Breast.* 2nd ed. Stamford: Appleton and Lange; 1999:829–855.

Case 140

Case History

A 38-year-old man presents with new right breast soreness.

Physical Examination

- right breast: larger than left; no mass
- left breast: mildly prominent, otherwise normal

Mammogram (Fig. 140–1)

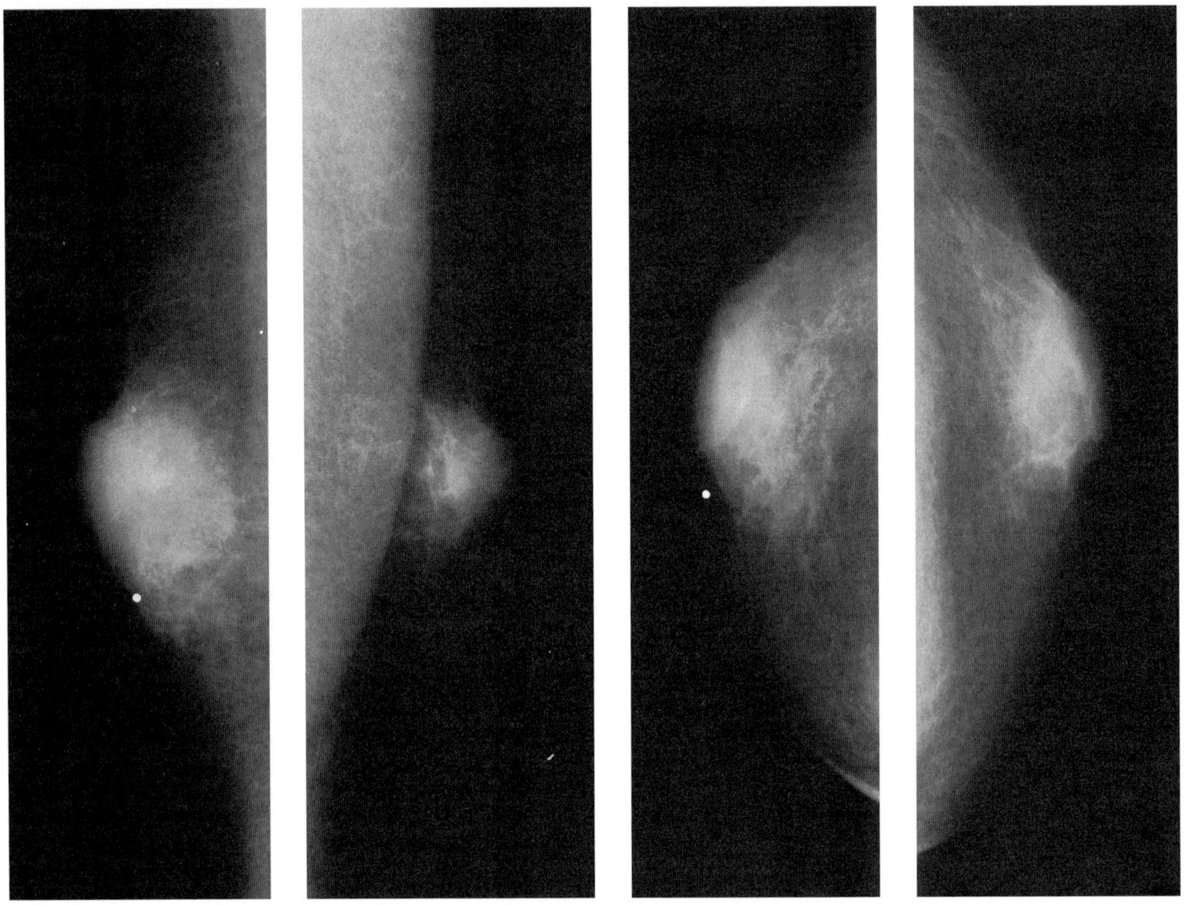

A B C D

Figure 140–1. Both breasts exhibit subareolar density. Left breast density is smaller than the right. (A). Right MLO mammogram. (B). Left MLO mammogram. (C). Right CC mammogram. (D). Left CC mammogram.

Ultrasound

Frequency

- 11.5 MHz

Mass

- margin: ill defined
- echogenicity: hypoechoic
- retrotumoral acoustic appearance: no shadowing
- shape: lobulated (Fig. 140–2)

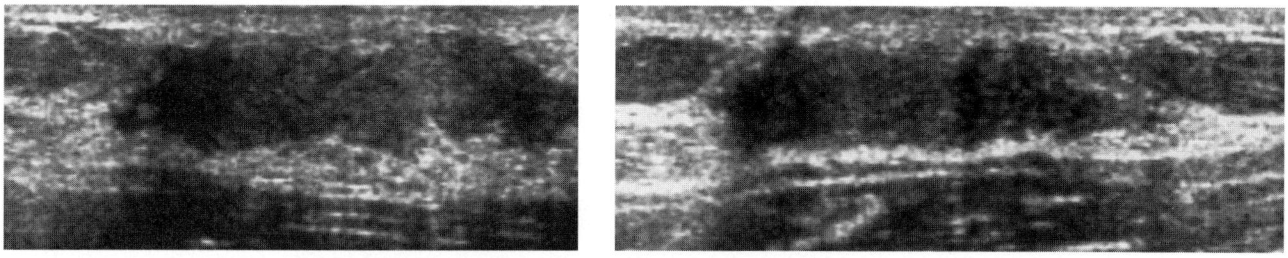

A B

Figure 140–2. The subareolar mammographic densities correspond to an ellipse of hypoechoic tissue. No separate focal mass is present in the right breast. (A). Right radial breast sonogram. (B). Left radial breast sonogram.

Pathology

- gynecomastia

Management

- BI-RADS Assessment Category 2, benign finding

Pearls and Pitfalls

1. Mammographically, there are three patterns of gynecomastia: nodular, dendritic, and diffuse. With the nodular pattern, the subareolar density is spherical with fan-shaped edges. The density is generally centered under the nipple, and the edges blend into the surrounding fat. Dendritic gynecomastia presents a flame-shaped subareolar density that radiates coarse linear or curvilinear densities into the surrounding breast tissue. The diffuse glandular pattern is similar to the heterogeneously dense female parenchymal pattern. This patient illustrates the nodular pattern of gynecomastia.
2. Sonographically, the nodular pattern may either present with a hypoechoic mass, enlarged ducts, or diffuse heterogeneous changes with no mass. Shadowing may be associated with the hypoechoic mass or heterogeneous echogencity. However, with the latter situation, the shadowing is random or intermittent. In this patient, since both breasts sonographically appeared similar, gynecomastia was easily confirmed even though a hypoechoic mass was present. Sonographically, the dendritic pattern demonstrates mild linear hyperechoic fibrous tissue without mass.

Suggested Readings

1. Jackson VP, Gilmore RL. Male breast carcinoma and gynecomastia: comparison of mammography and sonography. *Radiology* 1983;149:533–536.
2. So GJ, Chantra PK, Wollman JS, Bassett LW. The male breast. In: Bassett LW, Jackson VP, Jahan R, Fu YS, Gold RH, eds. *Diagnosis of Diseases of the Breast*. Philadelphia: WB Saunders; 1997:501–518.
3. Wigley KD, Thomas JL, Bernardino ME, Rosenbaum JL. Sonography of gynecomastia. *AJR* 1981;136:927–930.

Case 141

Case History

A 49-year-old man notes right breast lump. Eleven years ago, he saw a surgeon for a left breast lump.

Physical Examination

- right breast: soft, smooth, movable, subareolar lump
- left breast: normal exam

Mammogram (Figs. 141-1 and 141-2)

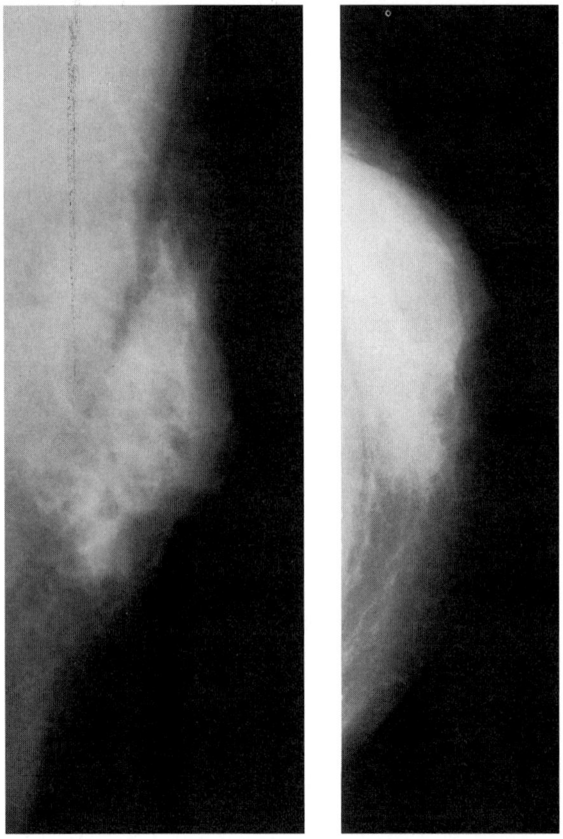

A B

Figure 141-1. Unilateral left breast mammogram was performed after patient noted a left breast lump for 2 months. His study demonstrates diffuse increased density of the left breast. (A). Left MLO mammogram. (B). Left CC mammogram.

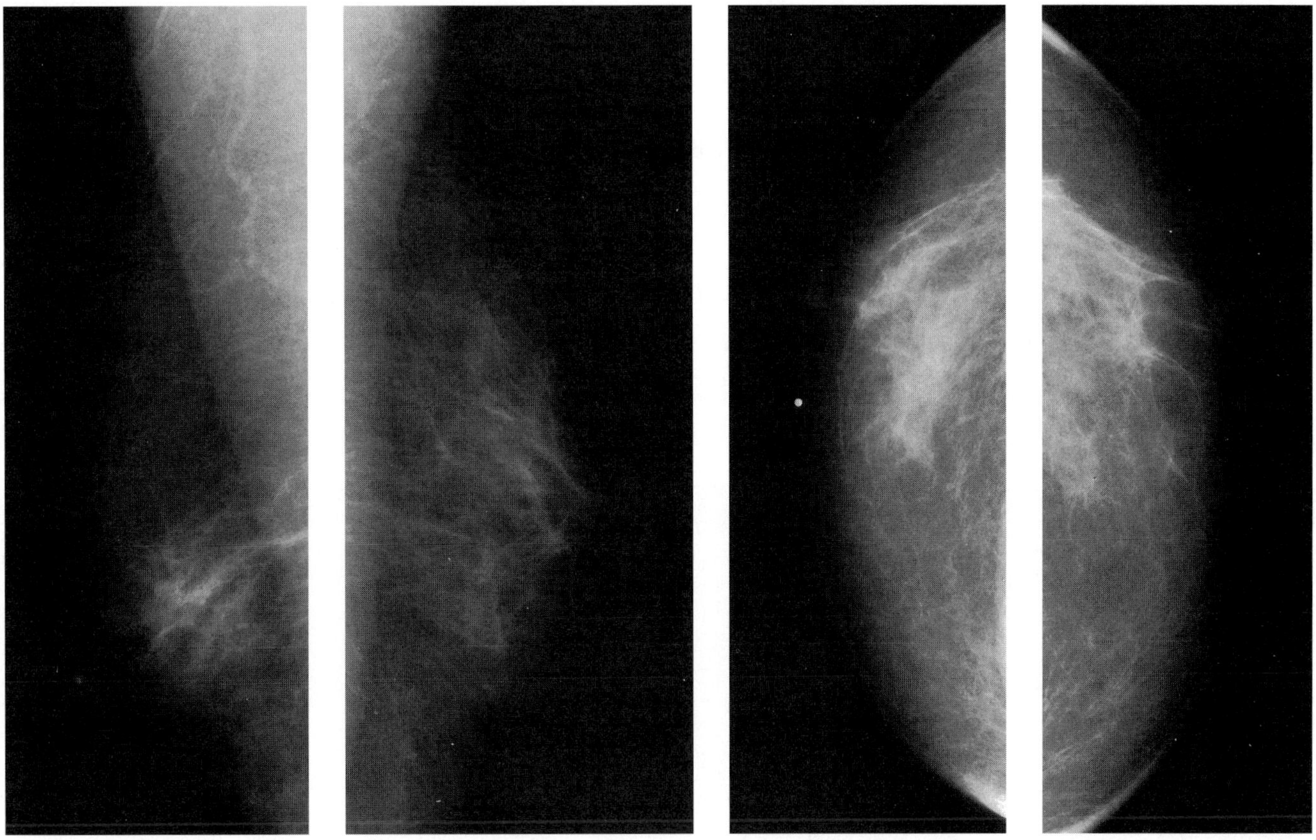

A B C D

Figure 141–2. This bilateral study was performed 11 years after Figure 141–1. Both breasts exhibit mild coarse subareolar linear densities. (A). Right MLO mammogram. (B). Left MLO mammogram. (C). Right CC mammogram. (D). Left CC mammogram.

Pathology

- gynecomastia

Management

- BI-RADS Assessment Category 2, benign finding

Pearls and Pitfalls

1. The radiographic appearance of gynecomastia is linked to the pathologic findings. Patients with acute symptoms less than 4 months have the florid histology that is associated with the radiographic nodular pattern.
2. Patients with gynecomastia longer than 1 year tend to have the fibrous histology that is associated with the dendritic mammographic pattern. This case demonstrates the evolution of nodular (Figures 141–1A,B) to the dendritic pattern (Figures 141–2A,B,C,D).

Suggested Readings

1. Michels LG, Gold RH, Arndt RD. Radiography of gynecomastia and other disorders of the male breast. *Radiology* 1977;122:117–122.
2. Tavassoli FA. *Pathology of the Breast.* 2nd ed. Stamford: Appleton and Lange; 1999:829–855.

Case 142

Case History

A 70-year-old man presents with cirrhosis. He is also taking spironolactone.

Physical Examination

- bilateral breasts: bilaterally enlarged with small subareolar firm nodules

Mammogram (Fig. 142–1)

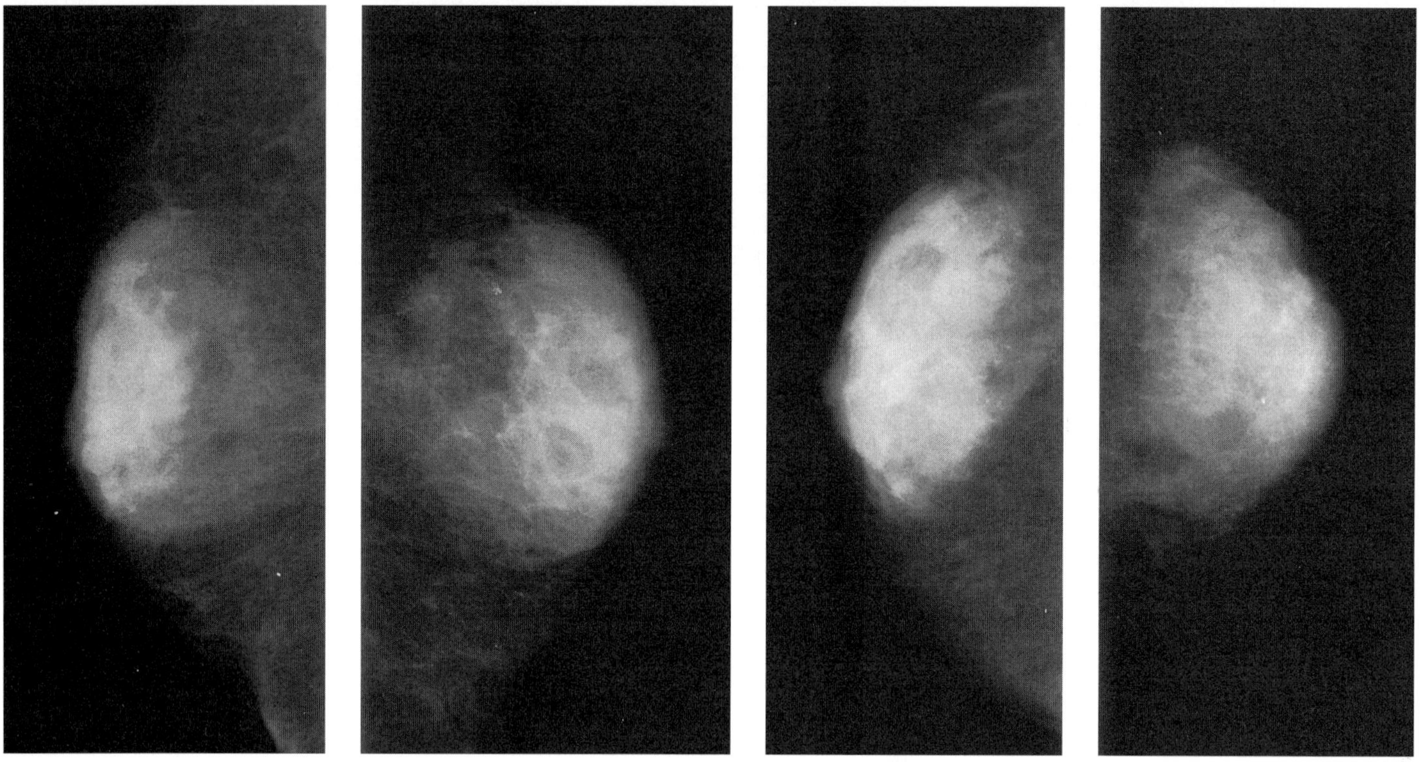

A B C D

Figure 142–1. Both breasts are enlarged and exhibit diffusely heterogeneous density. (A). Right MLO mammogram. (B). Left MLO mammogram. (C). Right CC mammogram. (D). Left CC mammogram.

Pathology

- gynecomastia

Management

- BI-RADS Assessment Category 2, benign finding

Pearls and Pitfalls

1. This patient exhibits the diffuse glandular pattern of gynecomastia.
2. Gynecomastia is due to increased estrogen, enhanced breast sensitivity to estrogen, decreased testosterone, or reduced breast sensitivity to testosterone. Causes for excess estrogen are the following: (1) puberty, (2) hermaphroditism, (3) testicular tumors, (4) nontesticular tumors skin (nevus, adrenal, lung, mesothelioma, hepatocellular), (5) endocrine abnormalities, (6) cirrhosis, (7) severe changes in nutrition, (8) drugs with estrogenic effect (steroid, digitalis estrogens, heroin, tamoxifen, marijuana). Abnormalities that create deficient androgen include: (1) senescence, (2) testicular failure (e.g., Klinefelter's syndrome, trauma, orchitis), (3) drugs that inhibit effect or synthesis of testosterone (antineoplastic agents, cimetidine, diazapam, phenytoin, spironolactone). Idiopathic causes for gynecomastia include: (1) drugs (furosemide, methyldopa, reserpine, theophylline, tricyclic antidepressants, verapamil), (2) renal failure, (3) nonneoplastic lung disease, (4) chest wall trauma, (5) pituitary adenoma, (6) acquired immunodeficiency syndrome (AIDS) and human immunodefiency virus (HIV) infection.

Suggested Readings

1. Bland KI, Graves TA, Page DL. Gynecomastia. In: Bland KI, Copeland EM. *The Breast.* 2nd ed. Philadelphia: WB Saunders; 1998:153–189.

Case 143

Case History

A 42-year-old man presents with a right breast lump.

Physical Examination

- right breast: soft lump in the outer inferior quadrant
- left breast: normal exam

Mammogram (Fig. 143–1)

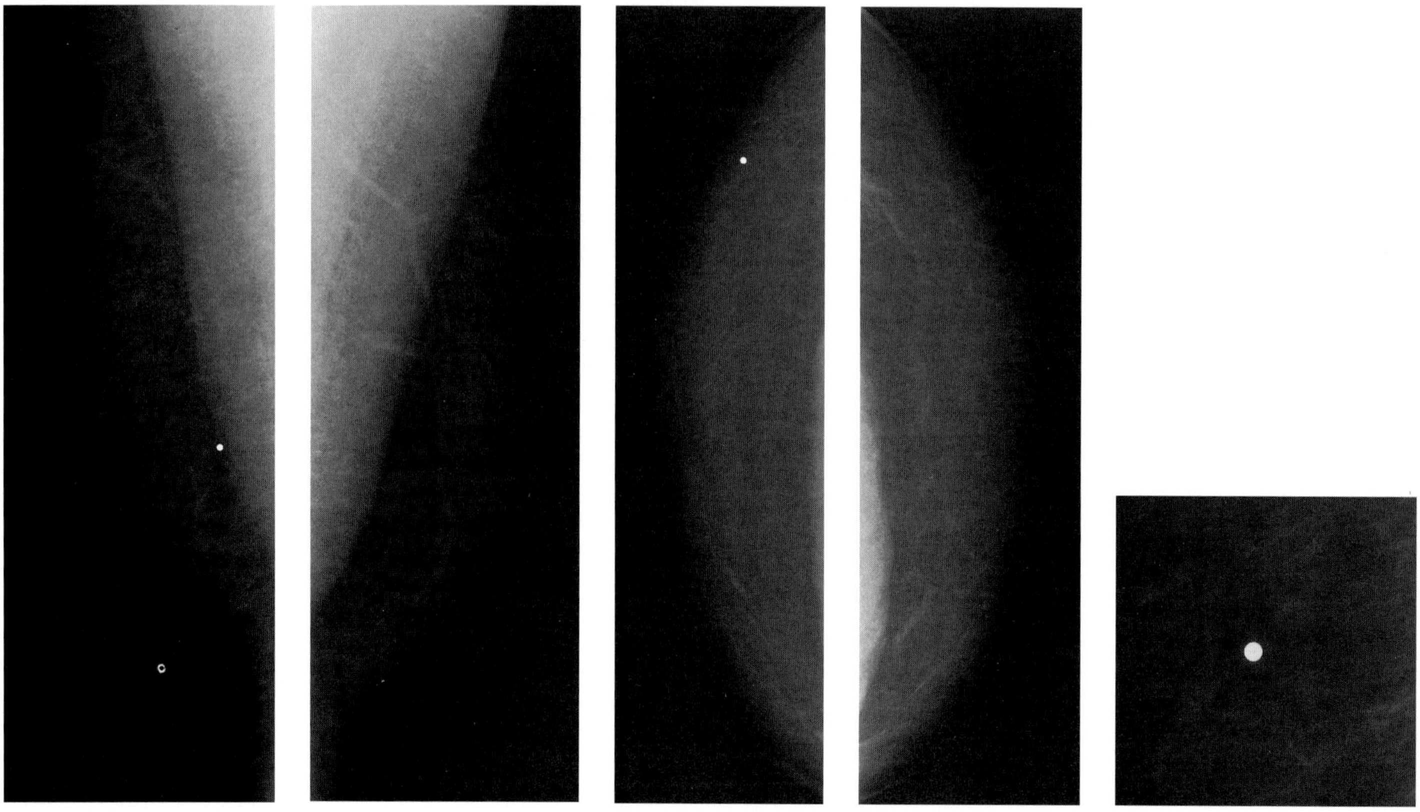

A B C D E

Figure 143–1. Bilateral normal male mammograms. No mass is identified in the area of the palpable mass. (A). Right MLO mammogram. (B). Left MLO mammogram. (C). Right CC mammogram. (D). Left CC mammogram. (E). Right MLO spot magnification mammogram.

Ultrasound

Frequency

- 11.5 MHz

Mass

- margin: well defined
- echogenicity: hyperechoic
- retrotumoral acoustic appearance: no shadowing
- shape: ellipsoid (Figs. 143–2 and 143–3)

Figure 143-2. Right radial breast sonogram: The palpable breast lump corresponds to a well-defined hyperechoic oval mass.

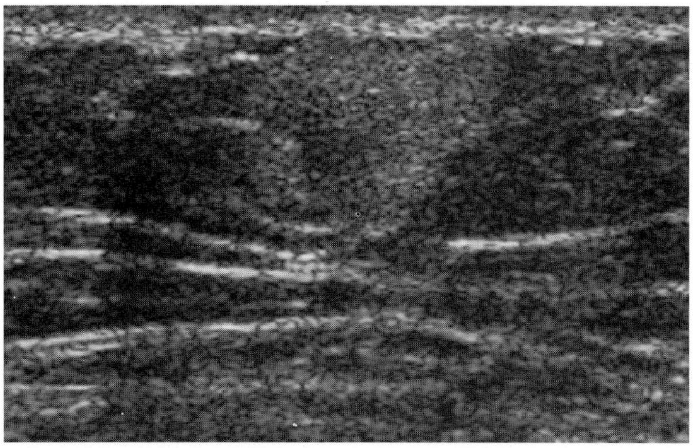

Figure 143-3. Longitudinal abdominal sonogram: On the anterior abdominal wall, a palpable lump corresponds to a well-defined hyperechoic mass that is similar to the breast mass.

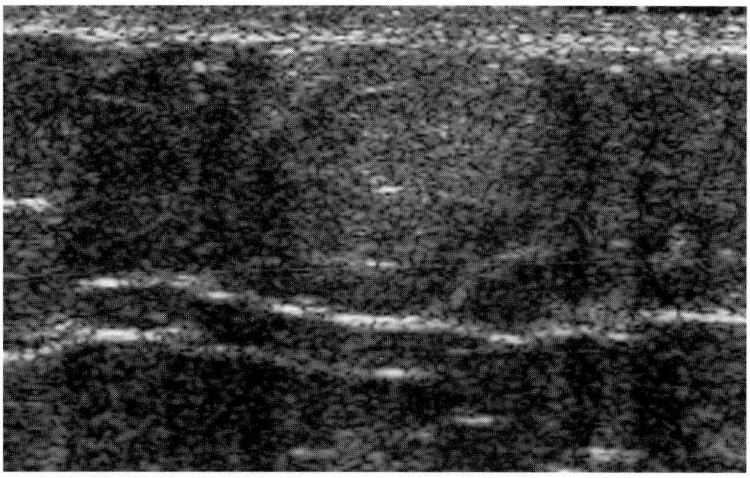

Pathology

- lipoma

Management

- BI-RADS Assessment Category 2, benign finding

Pearls and Pitfalls

1. Lipomas are composed of mature lipocytes that are surrounded by a fibrous capsule. Lipomas are present in any organ containing fat and are commonly multiple.
2. Mammographically, lipomas are well-circumscribed fat density masses. If the capsule is thin, the capsule may not be radiographically evident.
3. Sonographically, the lipoma is a well-defined mass that is isoechoic, hypoechoic, hyperechoic, or heterogeneous echogenicity compared to subcutaneous fat.

Suggested Readings

1. Stewart RA, Howlett DC, Hearn FJ. Pictorial review: the imaging features of male breast disease. *Clin Radiol* 1997;52:739–744.

Case 144

Case History

An 84-year-old obese man has a palpable lump in the right breast.

Physical Examination

- right breast: firm, movable nodule in the peripheral right upper outer quadrant
- left breast: normal exam

Mammogram

- mass: circumscribed
- shape: lobular
- density: equal

Associated Findings

- lymph node accounting for palpable lump in male patient with pseudogynecomastia (Fig. 144–1)

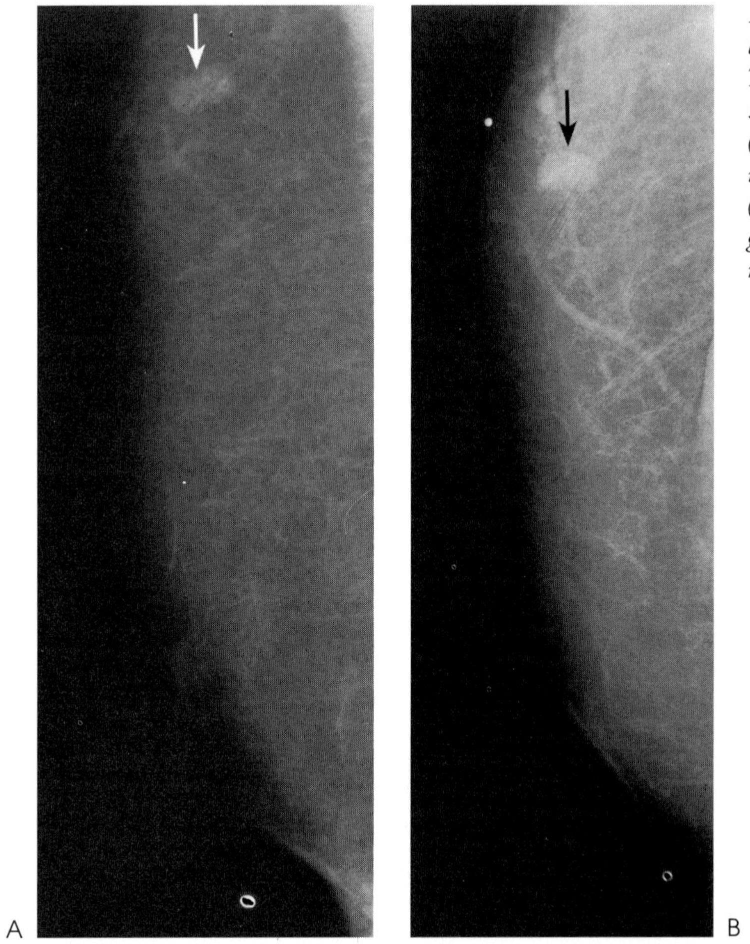

Figure 144–1. Right breast is primarily fatty. The palpable lump corresponds to a lobulated mass (arrow) in the extreme upper outer quadrant (B). (A). Right MLO mammogram. (B). Right XCCL mammogram.

Pathology

- intramammary lymph node/pseudogynecomastia

Management

- BI-RADS Assessment Category 2, benign finding

Pearls and Pitfalls

1. This patient demonstrates pseudogynecomastia or enlarged fatty breast associated with obesity. This condition is not true gynecomastia.
2. The palpable mammographic nodule has the characteristic central lucency consistent with a lymph node.

Suggested Readings

1. Michels LG, Gold RH, Arndt RD. Radiography of gynecomastia and other disorders of the male breast. *Radiology* 1977;122:117–122.

Case 145

Case History

A 61-year-old man presents with fullness of the right breast.

Physical Examination

- right breast: vague firm area in the 11:00 position
- left breast: normal exam

Mammogram

Mass

- margin: circumscribed
- shape: lobular
- density: high density (Fig. 145–1)

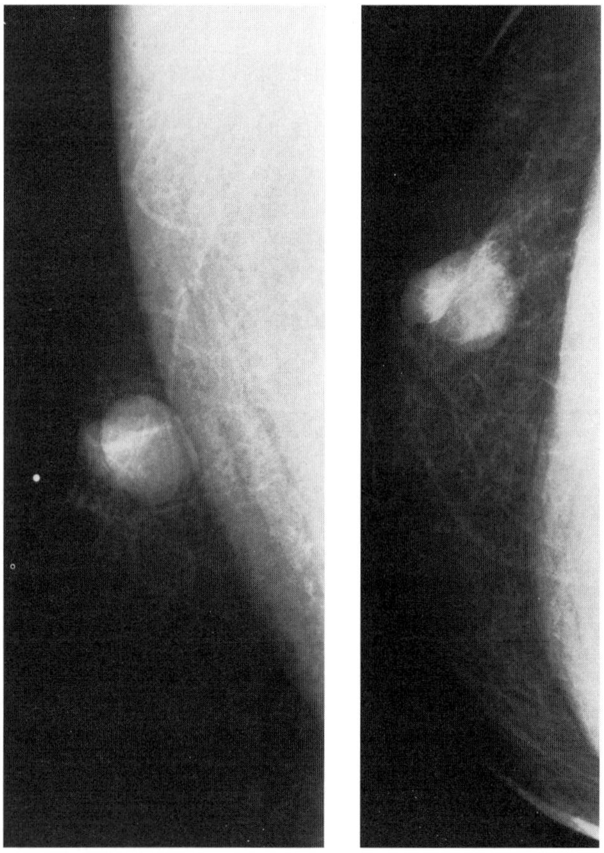

A B

Figure 145–1. A circumscribed lobulated mass is present in the right upper outer breast. (A). Right MLO mammogram. (B). Right CC mammogram.

Ultrasound

Frequency

- 14 MHz

Mass

- margin: well defined
- echogenicity: hypoechoic
- retrotumoral acoustic appearance: increased posterior acoustic enhancement
- shape: lobulated (Fig. 145–2)

A 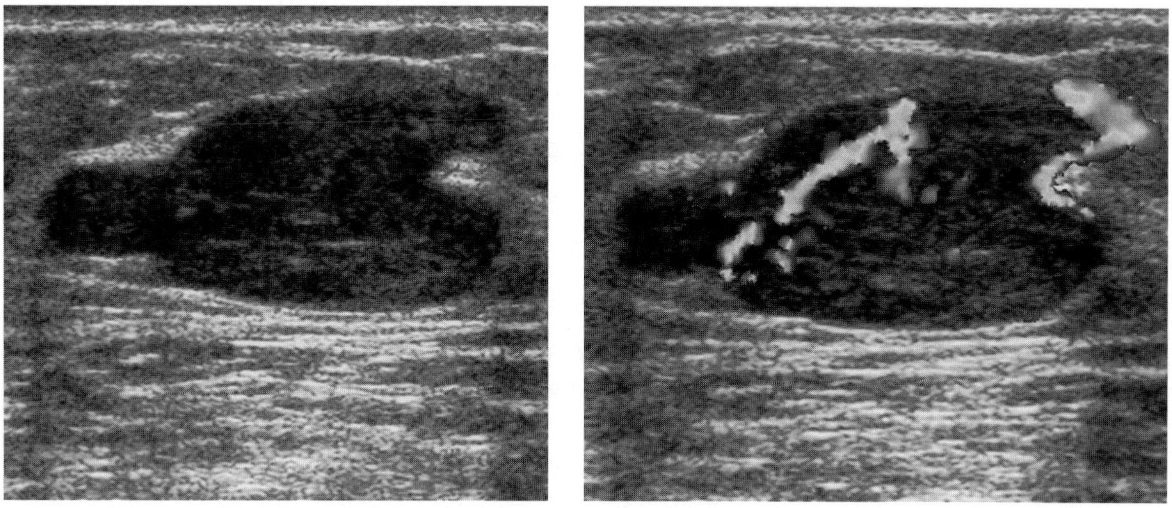 B

Figure 145–2. The palpable firmness in the right upper outer quadrant corresponded to a well-defined, lobulated, hypoechoic mass. (A) Right radial breast sonogram. (B). Right radial color Doppler breast sonogram (see Color Plate 145–2B).

Pathology

- myofibroblastoma

Management

- BI-RADS Assessment Category 4, suspicious; biopsy should be considered

Pearls and Pitfalls

1. Myofibroblastoma is a benign mass consisting of proliferating spindle-shaped cells. This tumor primarily affects men in the late 50s or early 60s. The lesion presents as a nontender, solitary, firm, movable mass.
2. Mammographically, myofibroblastomas are noncalcified well-defined, lobulated masses.
3. Sonographically, these tumors are well defined, lobulated, hypoechoic solid masses that may or may not shadow. Mammographically and sonographically, these tumors resemble fibroadenomas.

Suggested Readings

1. Greenberg JS, Kaplan SS, Grady C. Myofibroblastoma of the breast in women: imaging appearances. *AJR* 1998;171:71–72.
2. Miller JA, Levine C, Simmons MZ. Imaging characteristics of giant myofibroblastoma of the breast diagnosed by ultrasound-guided core biopsy. *J Clin Ultrasound* 1997;25:395–397.
3. Rebner M, Faju U. Myofibroblastoma of the male breast. *Breast Dis* 1993;6:157–160.
4. Tavassoli FA. *Pathology of the Breast.* 2nd ed. Stamford: Appleton and Lange; 1999:686–691.

Case 146

Case History

A 73-year-old male has a right breast mass, which has been present for many years.

Physical Examination

- right breast: mildly enlarged; small, firm area in outer breast
- left breast: normal exam

Mammogram

Mass

- margin: circumscribed
- shape: oval
- density: equal density (Fig. 146–1)

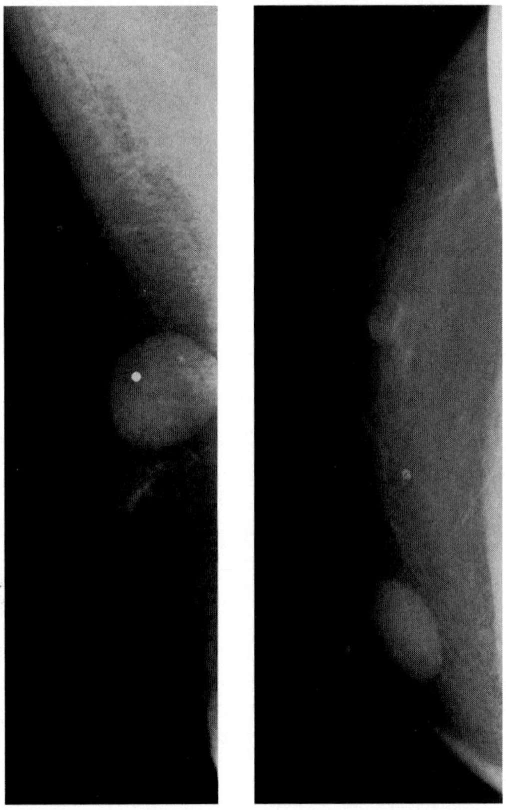

A B

Figure 146–1. In the right upper outer quadrant, there is a well-circumscribed oval subcutaneous mass. (A). Right MLO mammogram. (B). Right CC mammogram.

Ultrasound

Frequency

- 11.5 MHz

Mass

- margin: well defined
- echogenicity: hypoechoic
- retrotumoral acoustic appearance: increased posterior acoustic transmission
- shape: ellipsoid (Fig. 146–2)

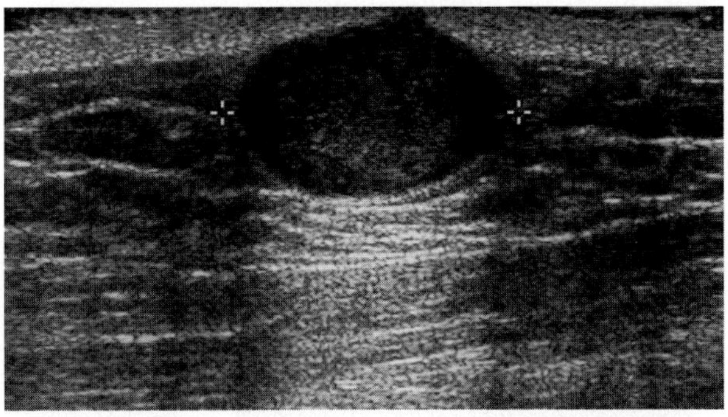

Figure 146–2. Right antiradial breast sonogram: The mammographic mass corresponds to a well-circumscribed hypoechoic oval mass with strong acoustic enhancement. The mass demonstrates continuity with the dermis through a small "beak" in its anterior margin.

Pathology

- sebaceous cyst

Management

- BI-RADS Assessment Category 2, benign finding

Pearls and Pitfalls

1. Epidermal inclusion and sebaceous cysts occur in cutaneous or subcutaneous tissues. Epidermal inclusion cysts usually arise from either hair follicles or squamous metaplasia of sweat ducts. Sebaceous cysts result from obstructed sebaceous glands.
2. Sebaceous cysts and epidermal inclusion cysts have similar mammographic findings. They are both circumscribed round masses. The appearance of these entities is the same as in females. Occasionally, the cyst may rupture and cause an inflammatory mass, which is indistinguishable from malignancy.
3. Sonographically, these cysts appear as well-defined, anechoic, or hypoechoic fluid collections with increased posterior acoustic transmission.

Suggested Readings

1. Appelbaum AH, Evans GFF, Levy KR, Amirkhan RH, Schumpert TD. Mammographic appearances of male breast disease. *Radiographics* 1999;19:559–568.
2. Jackson VP, Jahan R, Fu YS. Benign breast lesions. In: Bassett LW, Jackson VP, Jahan R, Fu YS, Gold RH, eds. *Diagnosis of the Diseases of the Breast*. Philadelphia: WB Saunders; 1997:357–443.
3. Wigley KD, Thomas JL, Bernardino ME, Rosenbaum JL. Sonography of gynecomastia. *AJR* 1981;136:927–930.

Case 147

Case History

A 77-year-old man presents with right bloody nipple discharge.

Physical Examination

- right breast: bloody discharge easily expressed from nipple at 2:00; normal nipple and areola
- left breast: normal exam

Mammogram (Fig. 147–1)

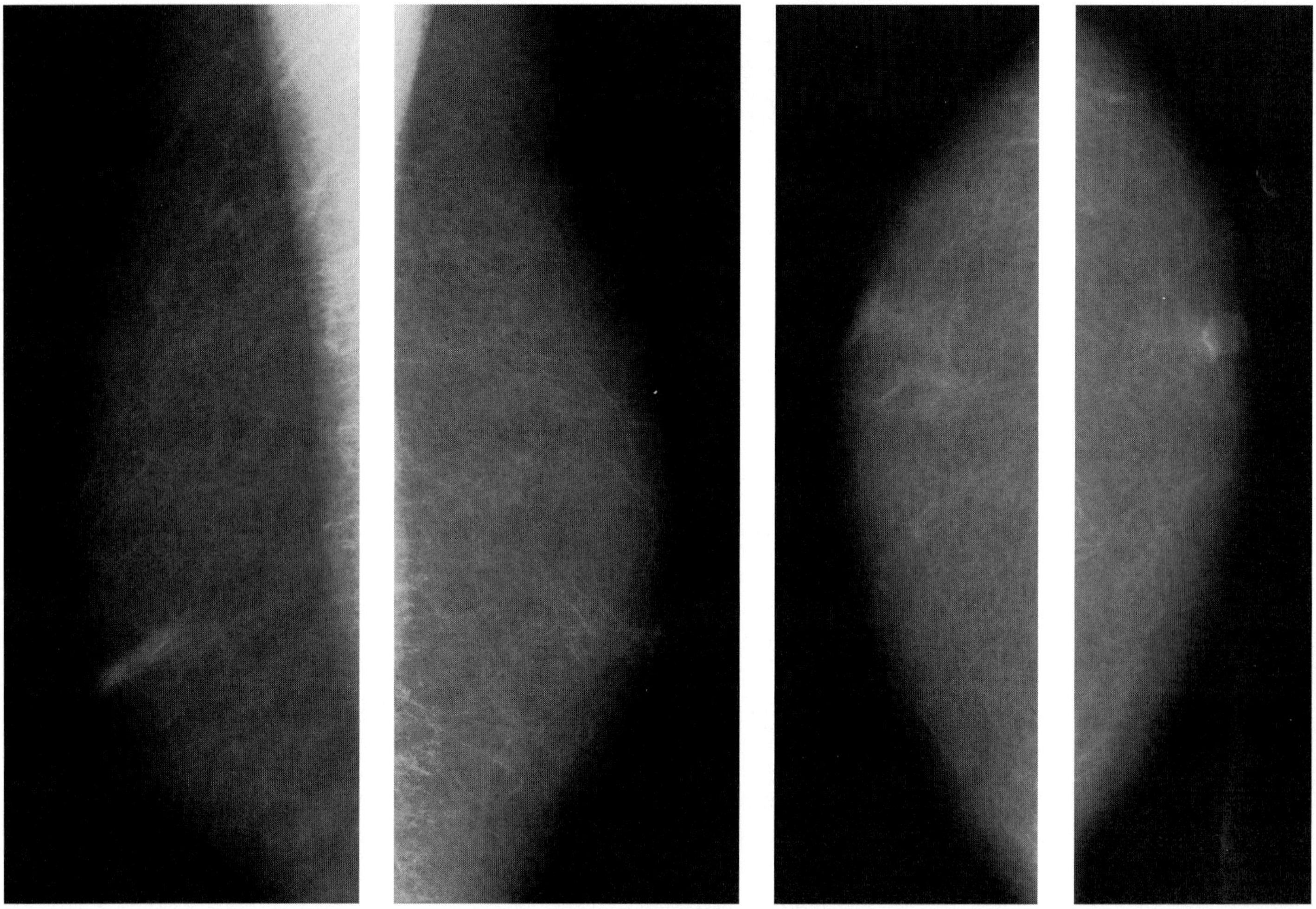

A B C D

Figure 147–1. There is mild prominence of a right subareolar duct. The left breast is normal. (A). Right MLO mammogram. (B). Left MLO mammogram. (C). Right CC mammogram. (D). Left CC mammogram.

Pathology

- ductal carcinoma in situ

Management

- BI-RADS Assessment Category 0, need additional imaging

Pearls and Pitfalls

1. Male breast cancer consists of less than 1% of all new breast cancer cases and only 0.2% of all newly discovered cancers in men. Infiltrating ductal carcinoma is the most common histology (about 85% of cases). Ductal carcinoma in situ comprises 5% of male breast cancers. Men develop ductal carcinoma in situ and invasive cancer later than women. Mean age at presentation is in the mid 60s. These tumors generally present with a nontender palpable mass. Nipple discharge is relatively common and is present in about 35% patients with ductal carcinoma in situ and in 10 to 20% of those with invasive tumors. Other associated findings include skin thickening, nipple retraction, and axillary adenopathy.
2. Mammographically, invasive malignancies have a wide variety of appearances. They may be either well or ill defined. Their shapes include round, oval, lobulated, or irregular. Microcalcifications are present in 25 to 30% of tumors. Commonly these calcifications are coarser than the ones found in female breast cancer.
3. Sonographically, male invasive malignancies have the same appearances as female tumors. However, male ductal carcinoma in situ differs from female ductal carcinoma in situ. The papillary subtype predominates in men so male ductal carcinoma in situ lesions sonographically commonly appear associated with fluid collections or ducts.
4. Bloody discharge, a prominent duct, and no palpable mass suggest that ductography may be useful to identify the intraductal abnormality. Sonography may also be used to identify a focally dilated ductal system and guide intraoperative excision. However, this patient had no further imaging. The patient's ducts were initially surgically excised. When ductal carcinoma in situ was identified, a mastectomy was performed.

Suggested Readings

1. American Cancer Society. *Cancer Facts and Figures—2001*. Atlanta: ACS; 2001.
2. Appelbaum AH, Evans GFF, Evans MB, Levy KR, Amirkhan RH, Schumpert TD. Mammographic appearances of male breast disease. *Radiographics* 1999;19:559–568.
3. Camus MG, Joshi MG, Mackarem G, et al. Ductal carcinoma in situ of the male breast. *Cancer* 1994;74:1289–1293.
4. Hittmair AP, Lininger RA, Tavassoli FA. Ductal carcinoma in situ (DCIS) in the male breast. *Cancer* 1998;83:2139–2149.
5. Ouimet-Oliva D, Hebert G, Ladouceur J. Radiographic characteristics of male breast cancer. *Radiology* 1978;129:37–40.
6. Scott-Conner CEH, Jochimsen PR, Menck HR, Winchester DJ. An analysis of male and female breast cancer treatment and survival among demographically identical pairs of patients. *Surgery* 1999;126:775–780.

Case 148

Case History

A 68-year-old patient presents with left breast swelling and shortness of breath.

Physical Examination

- left breast: entire breast is hard and lumpy; diffuse skin thickening and erythema present; palpable nodes present in the left axillary and supraclavicular areas
- right breast: normal exam
- chest: decreased breath sounds bilaterally at bases

Mammogram

Mass

- margin: indistinct
- shape: irregular
- density: high density
- skin thickening
- trabecular thickening (Fig. 148–1)

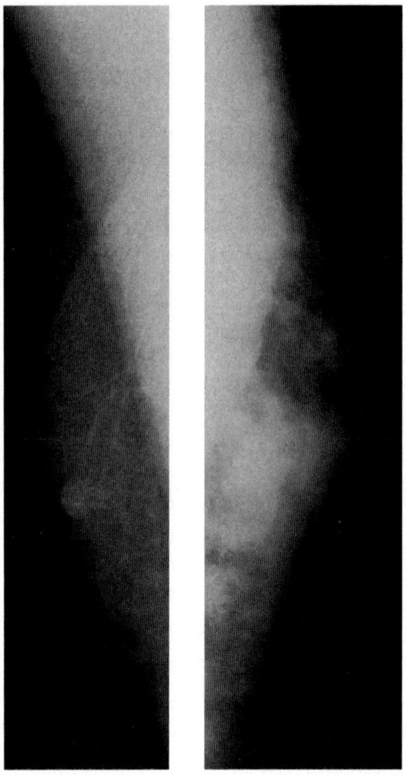

A B

Figure 148–1. The left breast shows marked, diffuse increase in density compared with the right breast. There is associated skin thickening and diffuse nodularity throughout the left breast. (A). Right MLO mammogram. (B). Left MLO mammogram.

Other Modalities (Figs. 148–2 and 148–3)

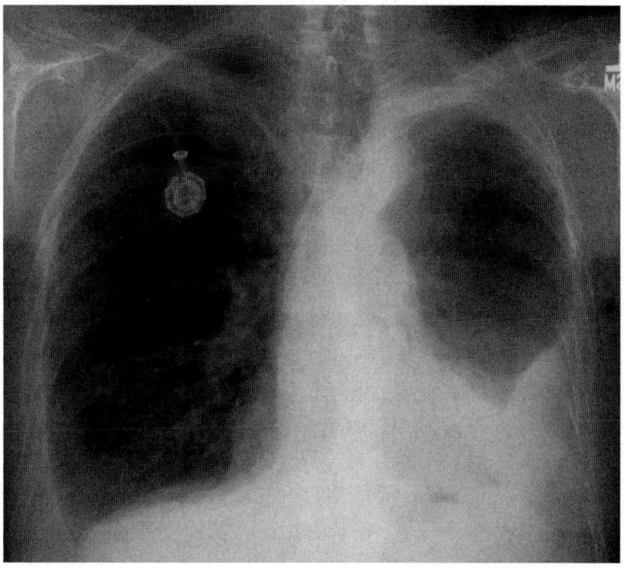

Figure 148–2. Posterior anterior (PA) chest radiograph: There are bilateral pleural effusions and mild right lower lobe increased interstitial densities.

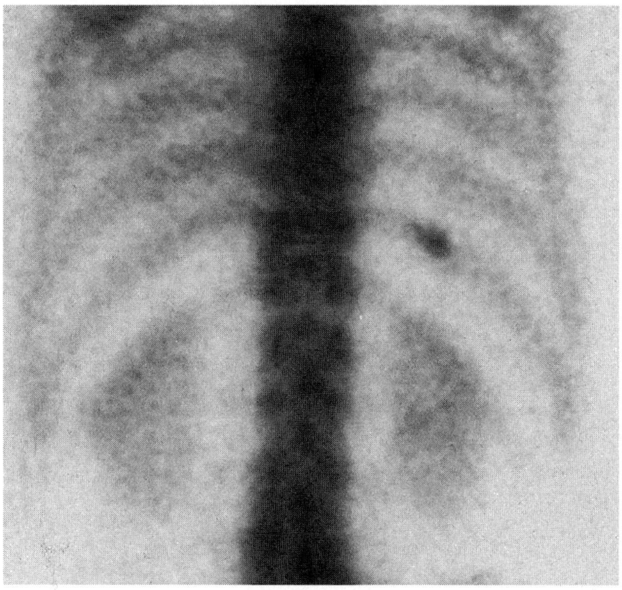

Figure 148–3. Bone scan, Tc-99m MDP (methylene diphophonate): There is a focal area of increased radionuclide uptake in the right 11th posterior rib.

Pathology

- inflammatory carcinoma

Management

- BI-RADS Assessment Category 5, highly suggestive of malignancy

Pearls and Pitfalls

1. Inflammatory breast cancer comprises 0.5 to 2% of male breast malignancies. The number of men presenting with inflammatory breast cancer is extremely small but they appear to have a poor prognosis.
2. Like female breast cancer, prognosis of male breast cancer is related to tumor, node, metastases (TNM) stage, as well as tumor histologic grade. Although there is conflicting data, it appears that male survival is comparable to female survival for similar stage disease. Five-year survival rates are the following: Stage I, 82 to 100%; Stage II, 63 to 83%; Stage III, 74%. Unfortunately, men commonly present later than women and have more advanced disease. Besides axillary and supraclavicular adenopathy, this patient had pulmonary and bony metastatic disease. He died about 3 years after initial presentation.

Suggested Readings

1. Donegan WL, Redlich PN, Lang PJ, Gall MT. Carcinoma of the breast in males: a multiinstitutional survey. *Cancer* 1998;83:498–509.
2. Joshi MG, Lee AK, Loda M, et al. Male breast carcinoma: an evaluation of prognostic factors contributing to a poorer outcome. 1996;77:490–498.
3. Tavassoli FA, Fattaneh A. *Pathology of the Breast.* 2nd ed. Stamford: Appleton and Lange; 1999:837–843.
4. Wilhelm MC, Langenburg SC, Wanebo HJ. Cancer of the male breast. In: Bland KI, Copeland EM, eds. *The Breast.* 2nd ed. Philadelphia: WB Saunders; 1998:1416–1420.

Case 149

Case History

A 55-year-old presents with right areolar ulcer and bloody nipple discharge. Patient was initially sent for breast sonogram because of areolar induration. He has had removal of two previous squamous cell carcinomas on his face.

Physical Examination

- right breast: the nipple areolar complex is replaced by a large ulceration; area also indurated and erythematous
- left breast: normal exam
- neck: large left supraclavicular mass

Mammogram

Mass

- margin: circumscribed
- shape: oval
- density: high density

Calcifications

- type: pleomorphic/heterogeneous
- distribution: grouped/clustered (Fig. 149–1)

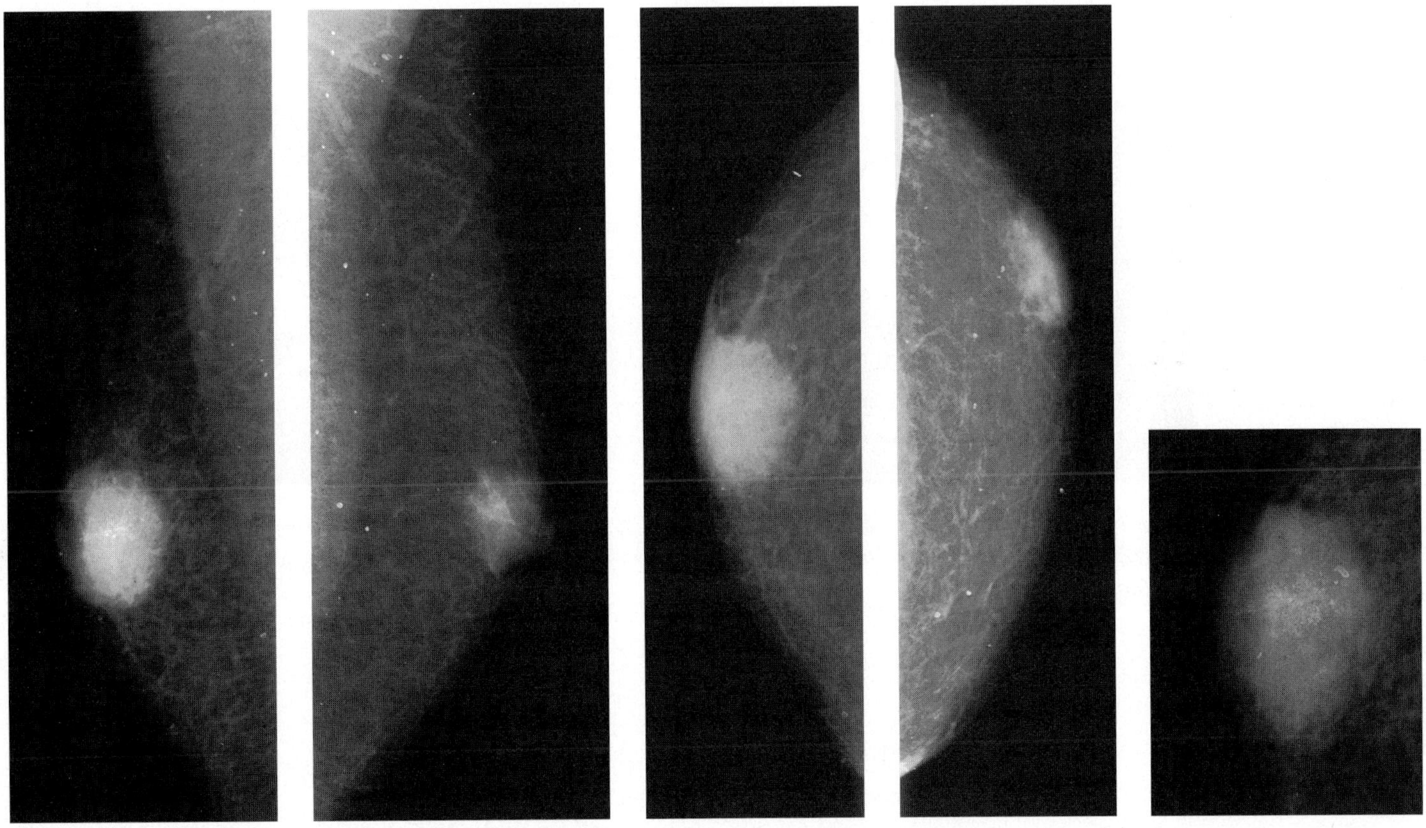

A B C D E

Figure 149–1. The sonographic mass corresponds to a right oval subareolar mammographic mass with heterogeneous calcifications. Although the mass appears circumscribed on the routine views (A,C), spot compression image (E) demonstrates that the mass has ill-defined margins. (A). Right MLO mammogram. (B). Left MLO mammogram. (C). Right CC mammogram. (D). Left CC mammogram. (E). Right CC spot compression mammogram.

Ultrasound

Frequency

- 10 MHz

Mass

- margin: well defined
- echogenicity: hypoechoic
- retrotumoral acoustic appearance: increased acoustic transmission
- shape: ellipsoid (Fig. 149-2)

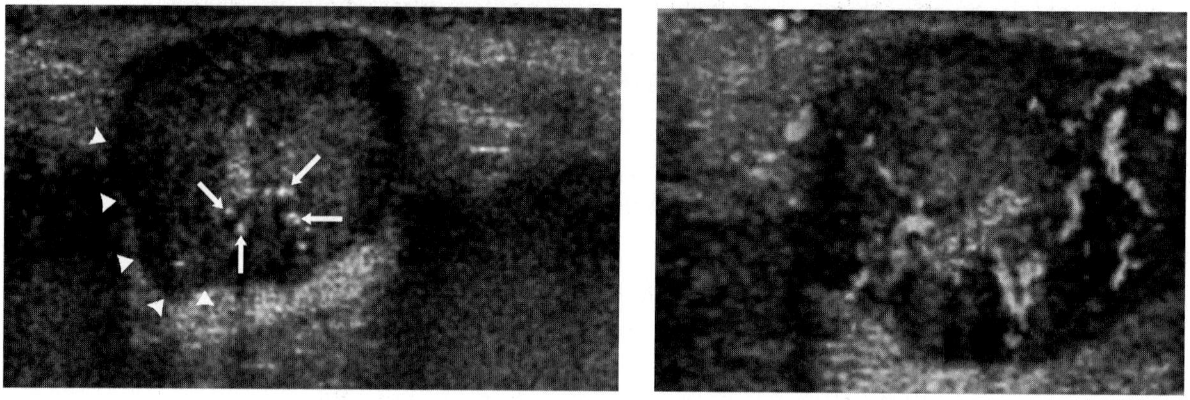

Figure 149-2. In the right subareolar area, there is an oval, hypoechoic solid mass with calcifications (arrows). Although the margins are generally well defined, there is mild irregularity of the contour of the mass (arrowheads). (A). Right radial breast sonogram. (B). Right radial color Doppler breast sonogram (see Color Plate 149–2 B).

Other Modalities (Figs. 149-3 and 149-4)

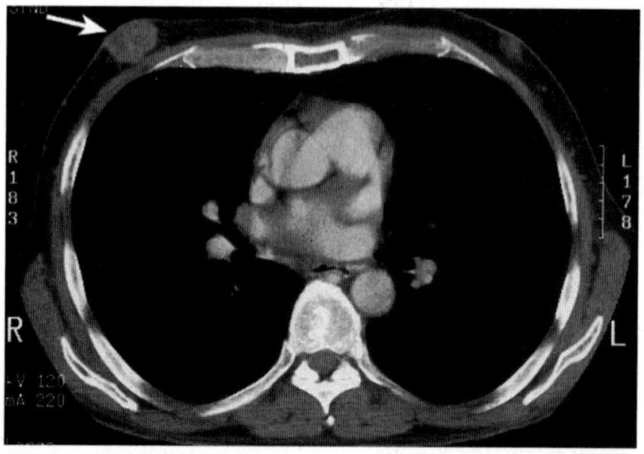

Figure 149-3. Transverse contrast-enhanced computed tomography: Right breast subareolar soft tissue mass is evident (arrow).

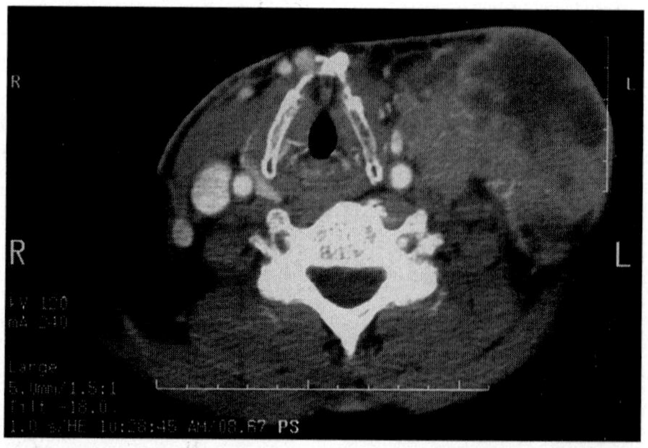

Figure 149-4. Transverse contrast-enhanced computed tomography: There is a large partially enhancing solid mass in the left neck, which extends to the clavicle.

Pathology

- metastases
- biopsy of right areola and neck mass: poorly differentiated squamous carcinoma

Management

- BI-RADS Assessment Category 4, suspicious; biopsy should be considered

Pearls and Pitfalls

1. This patient had metastatic squamous carcinoma to the breast. The most common metastatic tumor to the male breast is prostate carcinoma. Clinically, patients present with a palpable tumor. Nipple discharge or retraction is unusual.
2. The imaging appearance of metastatic tumors in men are the same as in women. Mammographically, these masses are superficial, circumscribed oval or lobulated masses. Sonographically, they are hypoechoic and generally do not shadow.

Suggested Readings

1. Cappabianca S, Grassi R, D'Alessandro P, Vecchio DA, Maioli A, Donogrio V. Metastasis to the male breast from carcinoma of the urinary bladder. *Br J Radiol* 2000;73:1326–1328.
2. Demirkazik FB, Baskan O, Aydingoz U, Tacal T, Firat P. Case report: squamous cell carcinoma of the skin metastasizing to the breast—imaging findings. *Br J Radiol* 1996;69:678-680.
3. Salyer WR, Salyer DC. Metastases of prostatic carcinoma to the breast. *J Urol* 1973;109:671-675.
4. Yang WT, Muttarak M, Ho LWC. Nonmammary malignancies of the breast: ultrasound, CT, and MRI. *Semin Ultrasound CT MR* 2000;21:375-394.

Case 150

Case History

A 57-year-old male presents with bloody nipple discharge. He has a long history of primary testicular failure and gynecomastia.

Physical Examination

- right breast: firm, small, subareolar nodule
- left breast: normal exam

Mammogram

Mass

- margin: circumscribed
- shape: oval
- density: equal density

Calcifications

- type: pleomorphic/heterogeneous
- distribution: grouped/clustered (Fig. 150–1)

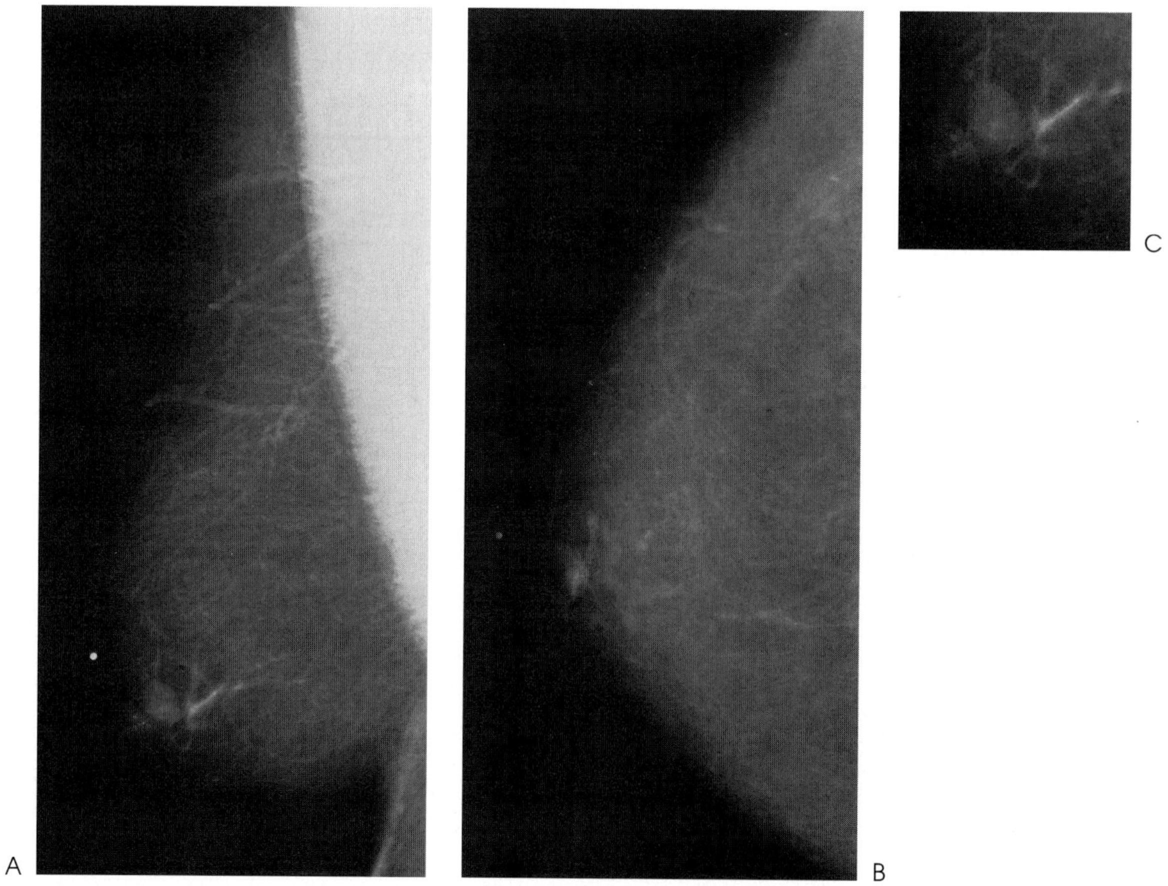

Figure 150–1. In the subareolar area, the palpable mass corresponds to an oval mass with heterogeneous calcifications. (A). Right MLO mammogram. (B). Right CC mammogram. (C). Right MLO mammogram (lesion enlarged).

Ultrasound

Frequency

- 11.5 MHz

Mass

- margin: well defined
- echogenicity: heterogeneous
- retrotumoral acoustic appearance: bilateral edge shadowing
- shape: ellipsoid (Fig. 150–2)

A 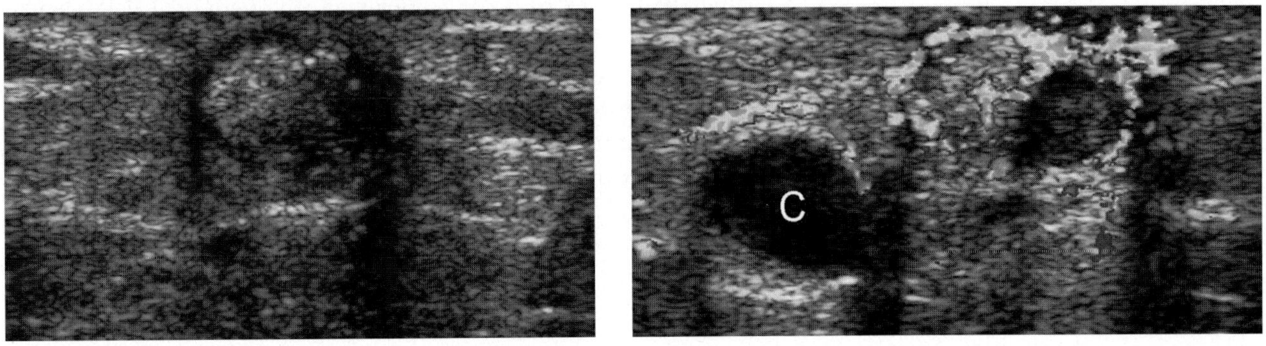 B

Figure 150–2. The mammographic mass corresponds to an oval mass with heterogeneous echogenicity. The mass has calcifications and is asymmetrically bordered by a cyst (C). (A). Right longitudinal breast sonogram. (B). Right transverse color Doppler sonogram (see Color Plate 150–2 B).

Pathology

- intracystic papillary carcinoma

Management

- BI-RADS Assessment Category 4, suspicious; biopsy should be considered

Pearls and Pitfalls

1. Male nipple discharge has been reported in 2% of benign lesions and about 4 to 20% of malignancies. Half of the benign masses presenting with nipple discharge were papillomas. Serosanguinous discharge is strongly associated with malignancy.
2. Complex cysts are more likely to be malignant in males than in females. Therefore, any cystic mass should be carefully sonographically examined. Any cyst with a thick wall or intracystic mass should be biopsied. Besides papillary carcinoma, the papillary subtype of ductal carcinoma in situ has also been reported to present as a complex cystic mass.

Suggested Readings

1. Fallentin E, Rothman L. Intracystic carcinoma of the male breast. *J Clin Ultrasound* 1994;22:118–120.
2. Goss PE, Reid C, Pintilie M, Lim RK, Miller N. Male breast carcinoma: a review of 229 patients who presented to the Princess Margaret Hospital during 40 years: 1955–1996. *Cancer* 1999;85:629–639.
3. Madden CM, Reynolds HE. Intracystic papillary carcinoma of the male breast. *AJR* 1995;165:1011–1012.
4. So GJ, Chantra PK, Wollman JS, Bassett LW. The male breast. In: Bassett LW, Jackson VP, Jahan R, Fu YS, Gold RH, eds. *Diagnosis of Diseases of the Breast*. Philadelphia: WB Saunders; 1997:501–518.
5. Stebbings W, George B, Boyle S, Plowman PN, Gilmore OJ. Malignant cysts of male breast. *Postgrad Med* J 1987;63:985–987.
6. Treves N, Robbins GF, Amoroso WL. Serous and serosanguinous discharge from the male nipple. *Arch Surg* 1956;73:319–329.
7. Yang WT, Whitman GJ, Yuen EHY, Tse GMK, Stelling CB. Sonographic features of primary breast cancer in men. *AJR* 2001;176:413–416.

Section IX

Postsurgical Findings

I. Solving imaging problems after augmentation mammoplasty

A. The following diagram illustrates the diagnostic approach to identifying implant rupture.

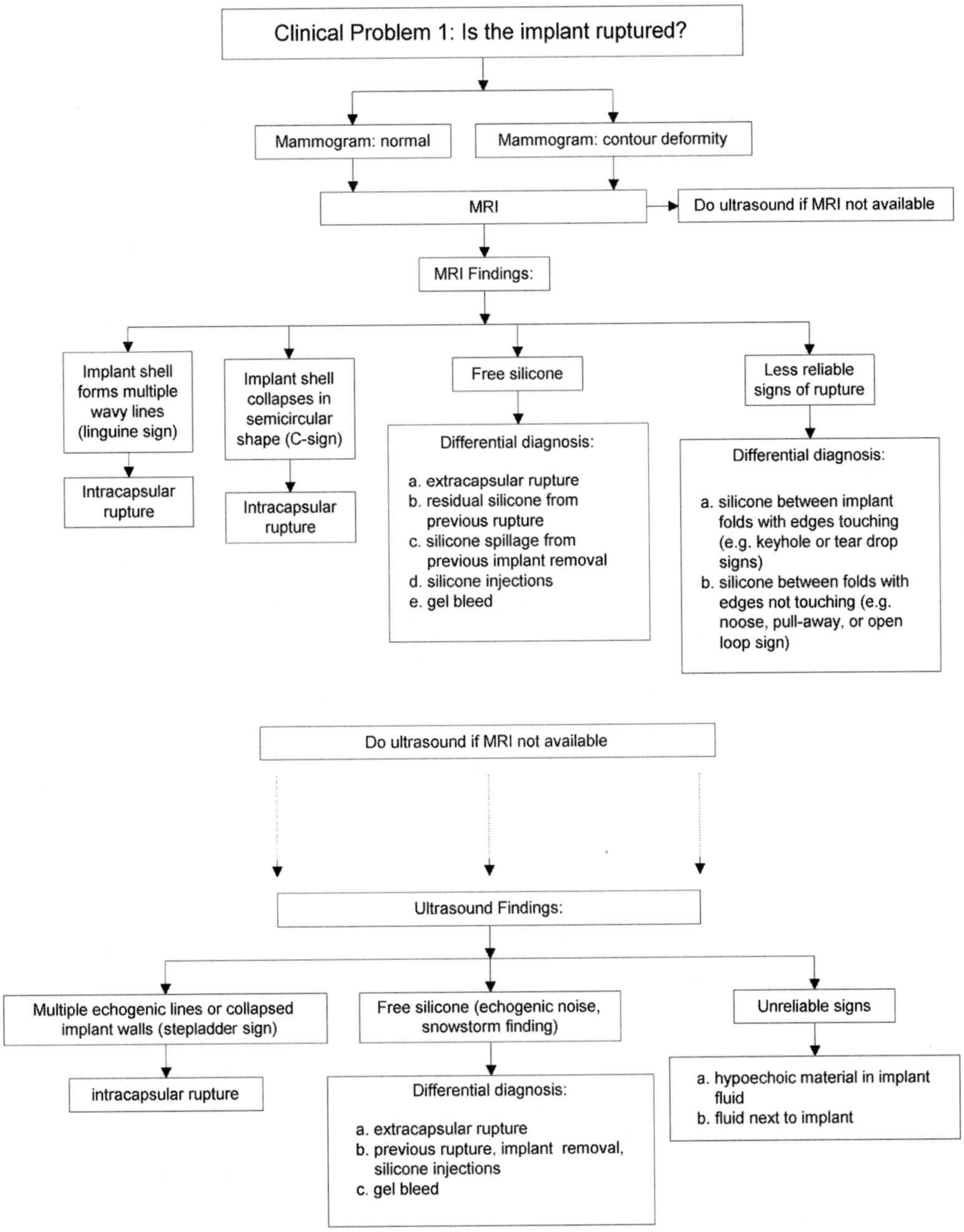

B. Patients with implants should be screened for breast cancer in a manner similar to patients who have not had surgery. The workup of malignancy in these patients is similar to those without implants.

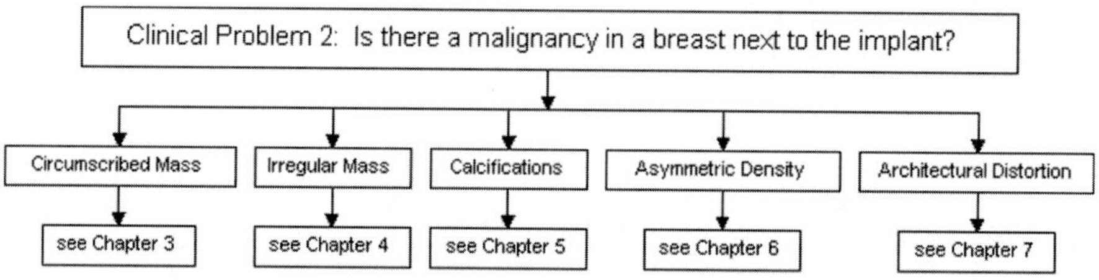

II. Solving problems after reduction mammoplasty

A. One should be aware of the common mammographic changes after reduction surgery.

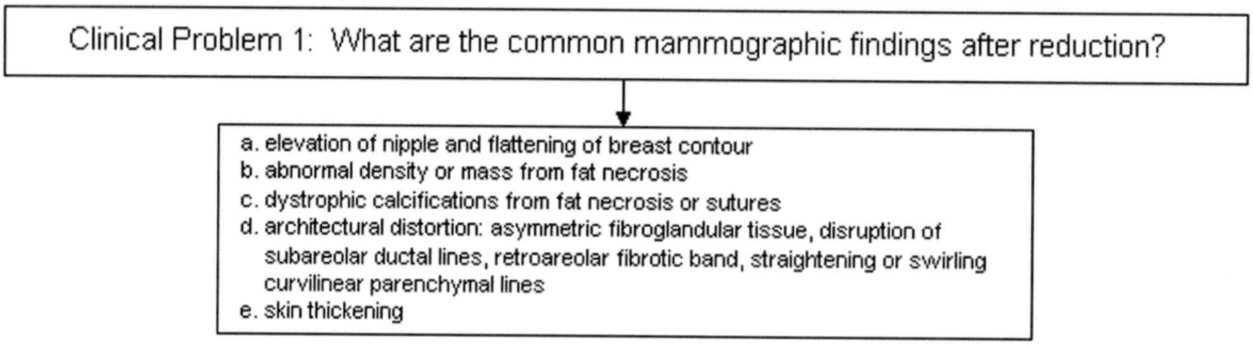

B. New or changing mammographic lesions in patients who have had reduction surgery should be treated similarly to those who have never had surgery.

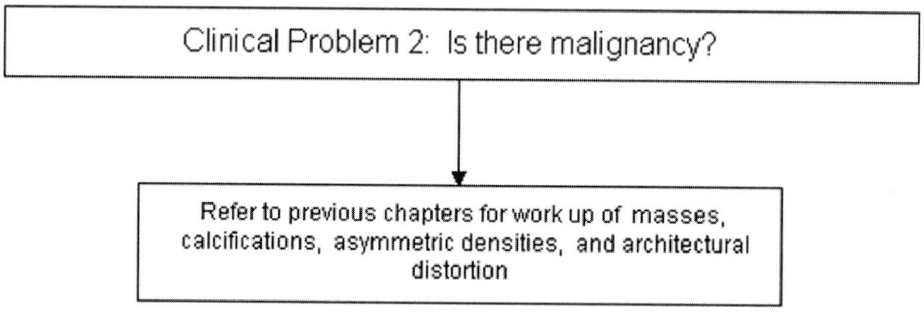

III. Solving problems after surgical treatment for breast malignancy

A. This diagram outlines the approach to the presence of an irregular mass in a patient who has had lumpectomy.

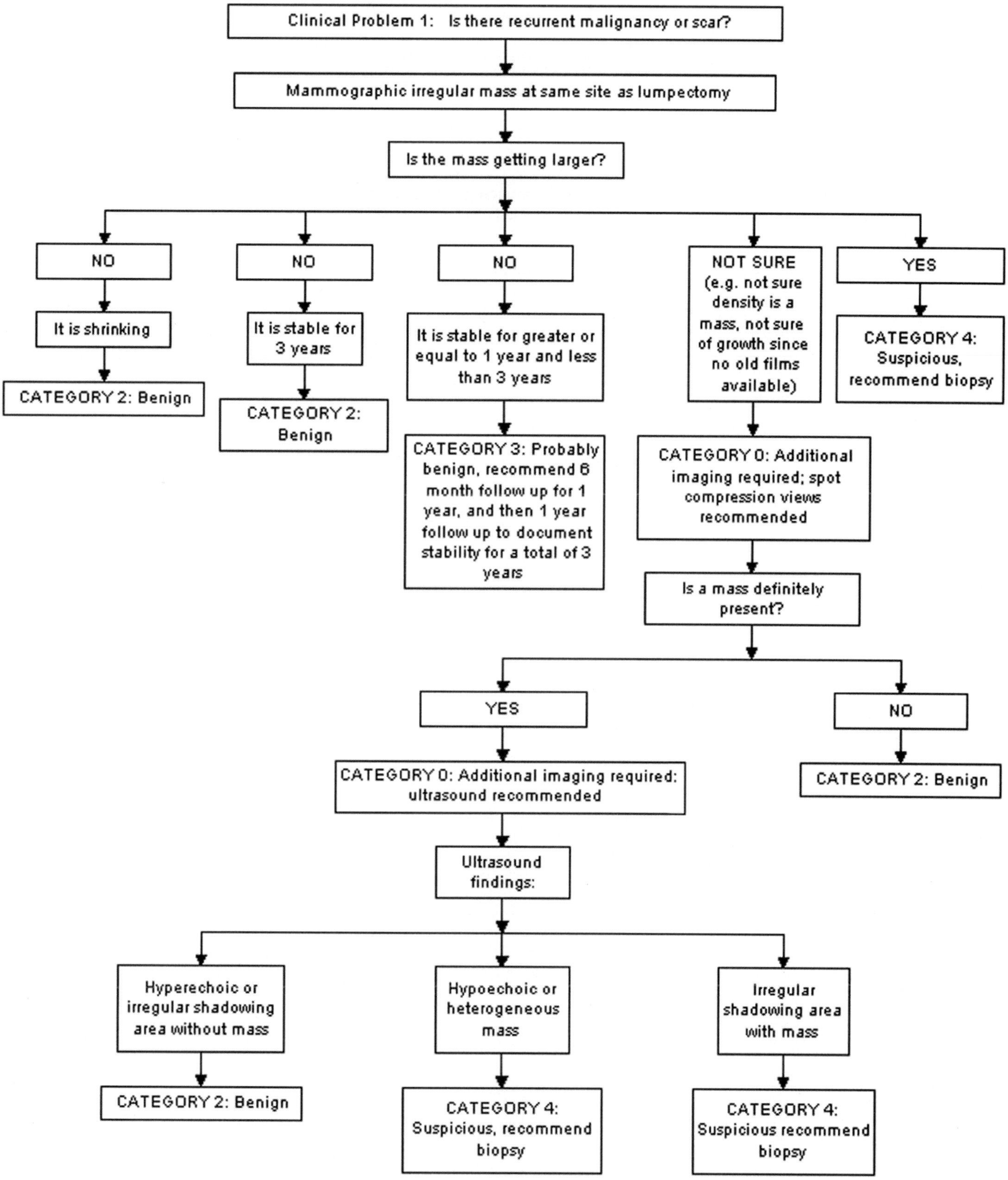

B. In the patient who has had lumpectomy, the workup of calcifications, architectural distortion, and asymmetric density is similar to the approach outlined in previous chapters.

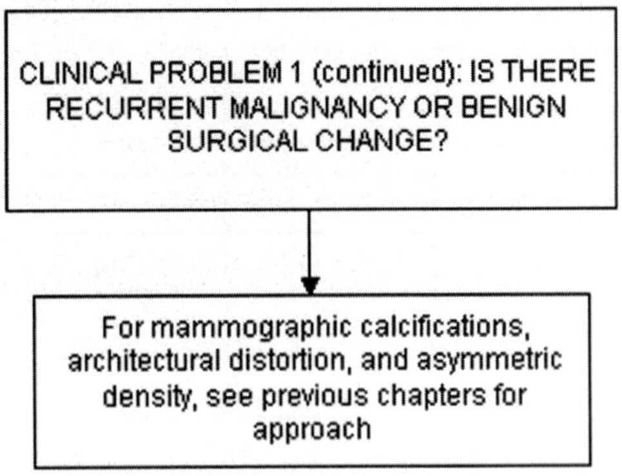

Case 151

Case History

A 47-year-old women presents with right breast pain. She had undergone bilateral breast augmentation 20 years prior to evaluation.

Physical Examination

- right breast: swollen and firm
- left breast: normal exam

Mammogram (Fig. 151–1)

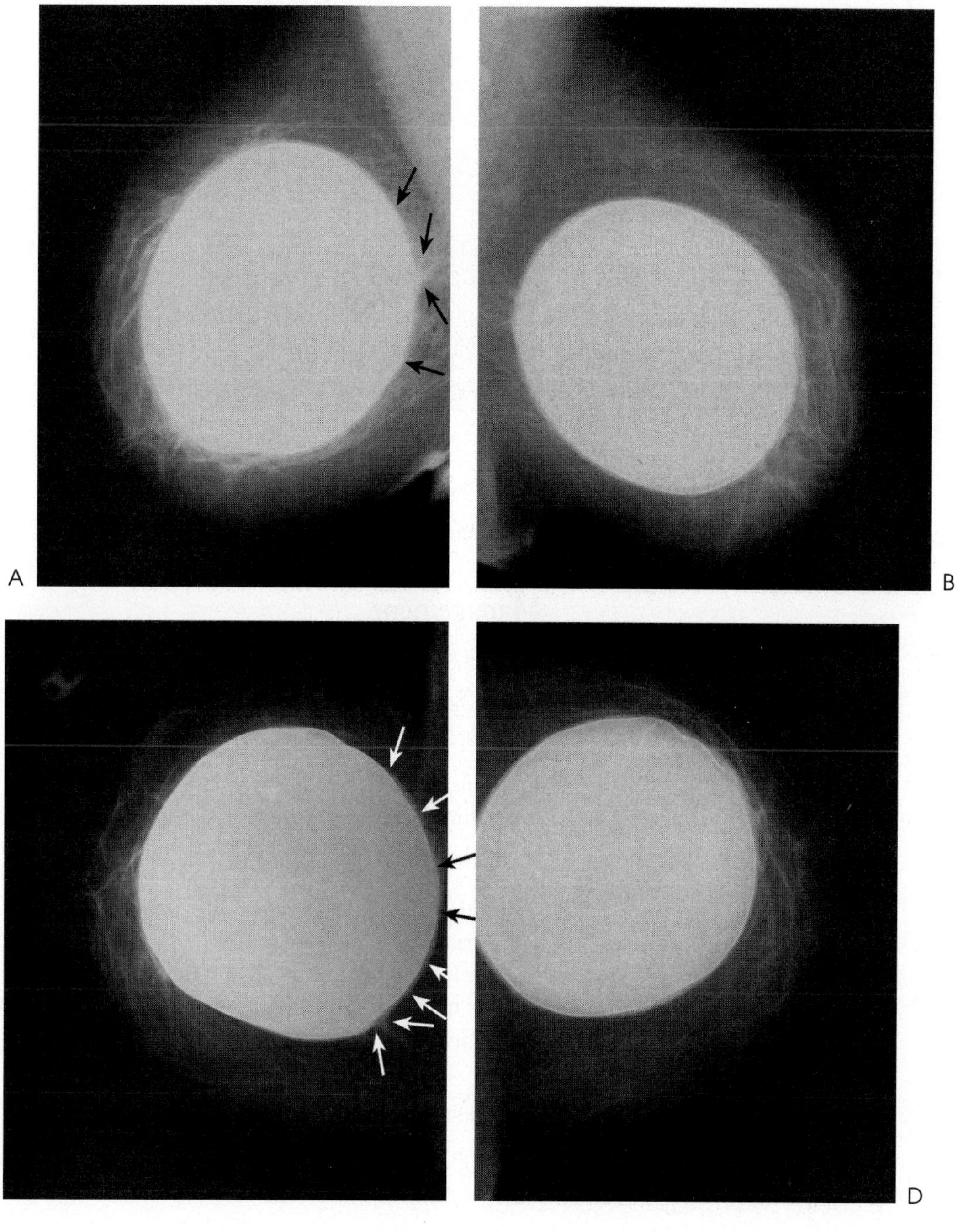

Figure 151–1. Bilateral subglandular implants are present. There is increased density associated with the posterior deep margin of the right implant (arrows). (A). Right MLO mammogram. (B). Left MLO mammogram. (C). Right CC mammogram. (D). Left CC mammogram.

Ultrasound

Frequency

- 7 MHz

Mass

- echogenicity: hypoechoic
- retrotumoral acoustic appearance: increased acoustic enhancement (Fig. 151–2)

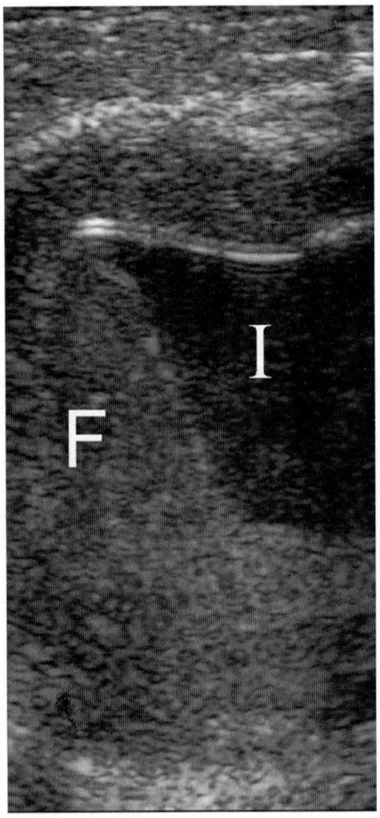

Figure 151–2. Right transverse breast sonogram 10:00 position: The density identified in Figure 151–1 corresponds to a complex hypoechoic fluid collection (F). The adjacent implant is anechoic (I).

Pathology

- infected fluid

Management

- BI-RADS Assessment Category 2, benign finding

Pearls and Pitfalls

1. Implants are generally located either deep to the pectoralis muscle (retropectoral) or within the breast glandular tissue anterior to the pectoralis (subglandular). Subglandular implants generally obscure more breast parenchyma than subpectoral implants. To improve visualization of the parenchyma, Eklund or implant-displaced views should be routinely done in patients with implants. Although we always perform implant-displaced views, these views are not shown in this book unless they have specific information for the case.
2. The main complications associated with implants include bleeding or hematoma, infection, capsule contracture, rupture, and silicone granulomas.

Suggested Readings

1. Steinbach BG, Hardt NS, Abbitt PL, Lanier L, Caffee HH. Breast implants, common complications, and concurrent breast disease. *Radiographics* 1993;13:95–118.

Case 152

Case History

A 47-year-old woman presents for screening mammogram.

Physical Examination

- normal exam

Mammogram (Fig. 152–1)

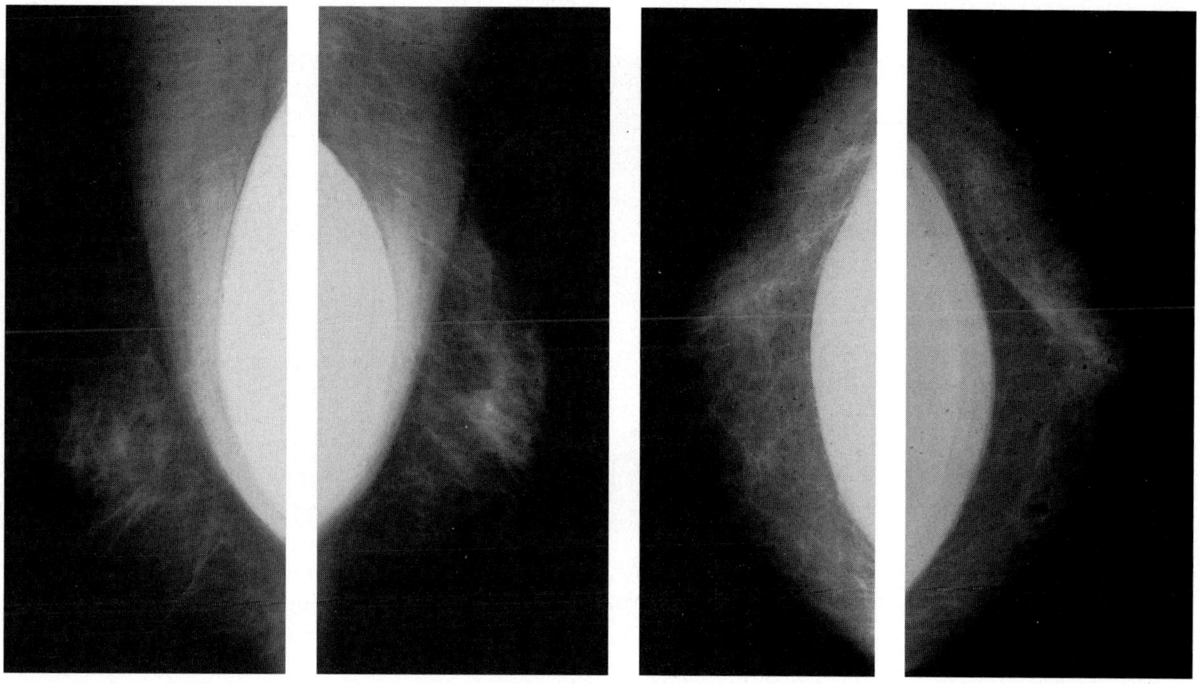

A B C D

Figure 152–1. Bilateral implant views: The subpectoral implants are normal. (A). Right MLO implant view. (B). Left MLO implant view. (C). Right CC implant view. (D). Left CC implant view.

Pathology

- normal implant

Management

- BI-RADS Assessment Category 1, negative

Pearls and Pitfalls

The advantage of subpectoral implants is that they interfere less with imaging the breast parenchyma and are associated with a lower rate of capsular contraction.

Suggested Readings

1. Biggs TM, Yarish RS. Augmentation mammoplasty: retropectoral versus retromammary implantation. *Clin Plast Surg* 1988;15:549–555.
2. Vazquez B, Given KS, Houston GC. Breast augmentation: a review of subglandular and submuscular implantation. *Anesthetic Plast Surg* 1987;11:101–105.

Case 153

Case History

A 49-year-old woman presents with chronic pain in her left breast. She received breast augmentation 10 years prior to evaluation.

Physical Examination

- normal exam

Other Modalities (Figs. 153-1 and 153-2)

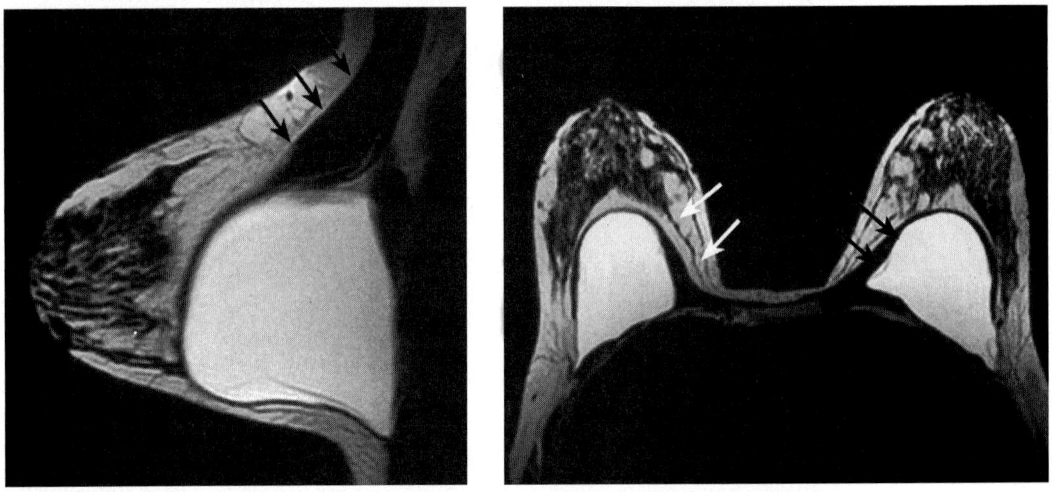

Figure 153-1. The implants are subpectoral in location and normal in appearance. Pectoralis muscle (arrows). (A) Right breast T2-weighted with water saturation longitudinal magnetic resonance imaging (MRI). (B). Bilateral breasts T2-weighted with water saturation transverse MRI.

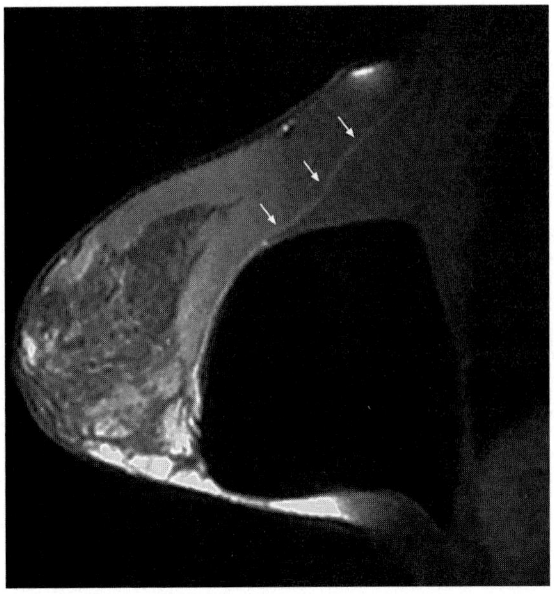

Figure 153-2. Right breast T1-weighted with fat saturation longitudinal MRI: Pectoralis (arrows) is not well identified on this sequence. This sequence is excellent for identifying free silicone due to extracapsular rupture.

Pathology

- normal implant

Management

- BI-RADS Assessment Category 1, negative

Pearls and Pitfalls

MRI is an excellent method to identify implant rupture. With an MRI T2-weighted series, the fibrous capsule and the implant shell are dark lines, which are normally inseparable except for normal folds of the shell. Silicone and water are bright on T2 series. If water saturation is added to the T2 sequence, then silicone will be brighter than water. This T2 method displays intracapsular rupture well. A T1 series with fat saturation will cause fat to be dark, but with this technique, fat is lighter than silicone. Therefore, a T1 series with fat saturation is a useful technique to identify extracapsular rupture by displaying free silicone.

Suggested Readings

1. Middleton MS. Breast implants and soft tissue silicone. In: Stark DD, Bradley WG, eds. *Magnetic Resonance Imaging.* 3rd ed. St. Louis: Mosby; 1999:335–353.

Case 154

Case History

A 66-year-old woman, who had silicone injections over 40 years ago, presents for annual mammogram.

Physical Examination

- bilateral breasts: lobulated pattern in both breasts, which is more prominent in the upper outer quadrants

Mammogram (Fig. 154–1)

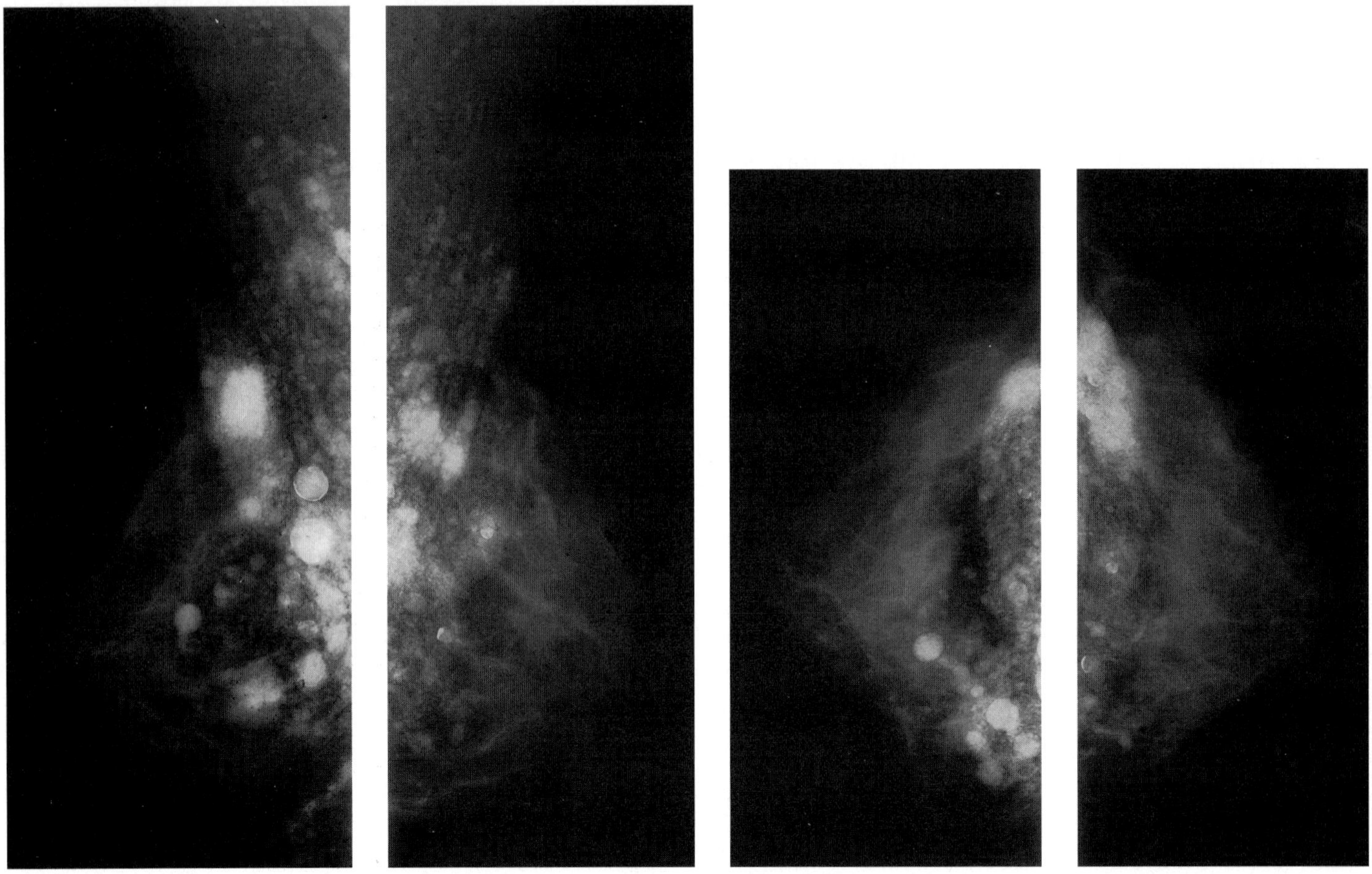

A B C D

Figure 154–1. Both breasts exhibit high-density material posteriorly in breast parenchyma, lymph nodes, and within the pectoralis muscles. (A). Right MLO mammogram. (B). Left MLO mammogram. (C). Right CC mammogram. (D). Left CC mammogram.

Pathology

- free silicone

Management

- BI-RADS Assessment Category 1, negative

Pearls and Pitfalls

1. Silicone was developed in the 1940s and injected into breasts for augmentation in the 1950s and 1960s. Unfortunately, silicone injections resulted in painful hardening of the breast, sloughing of skin, granulomatous hepatitis, and pulmonary embolism. The U.S. Food and Drug Administration banned these injections in 1965.
2. Mammographically, silicone injections result in high-density round or oval masses and architectural distortion. In the areas containing silicone, neoplasms may be hidden by the silicone masses.

Suggested Readings

1. Ganott MA, Harris KM, Ilkhanipour ZS, Costa-Greco MA. Augmentation mammoplasty: normal and abnormal findings with mammography and US. *Radiographics* 1992;12:281–295.
2. Liebman AJ, Sybers R. Mammographic and sonographic findings after silicone injection. *Ann Plast Surg* 1994;33:412–414.

Case 155

Case History

A 66-year-old woman presents with right breast pain and increasing "dimpling" at the edge of her augmentation scar.

Physical Examination

- right breast: tenderness and subtle nodularity in the upper outer quadrant
- left breast: normal exam

Mammogram (Fig. 155–1)

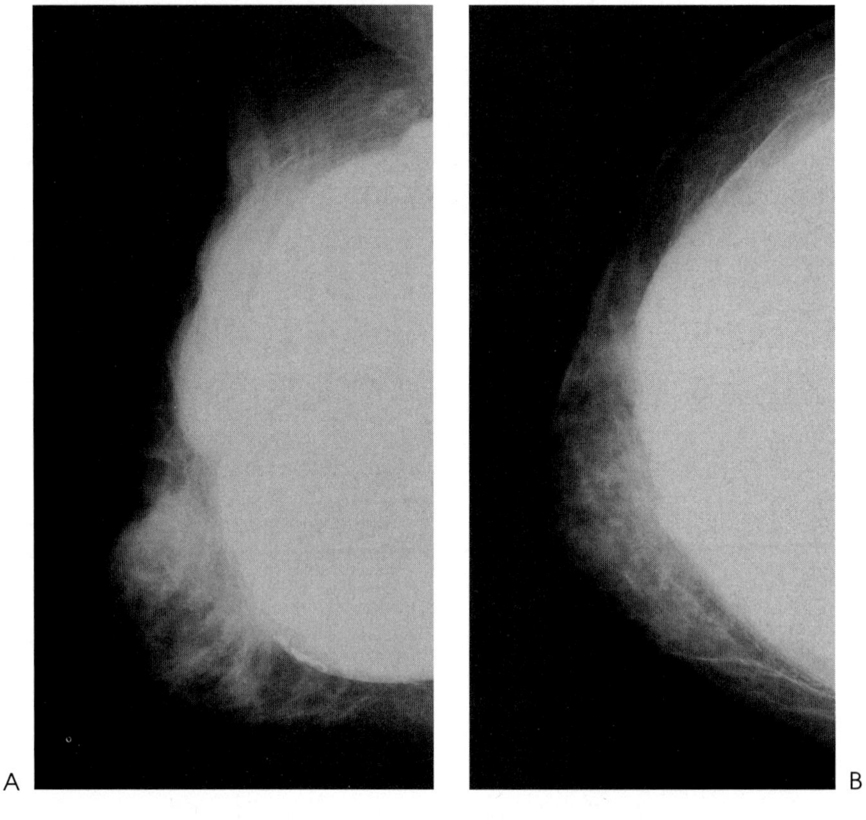

Figure 155–1. In the upper outer quadrant of the right breast, there is a contour bulge, which is only visible on the MLO view. (A). Right MLO implant mammogram. (B). Right CC implant mammogram.

Other Modalities (Figs. 155–2 and 155–3)

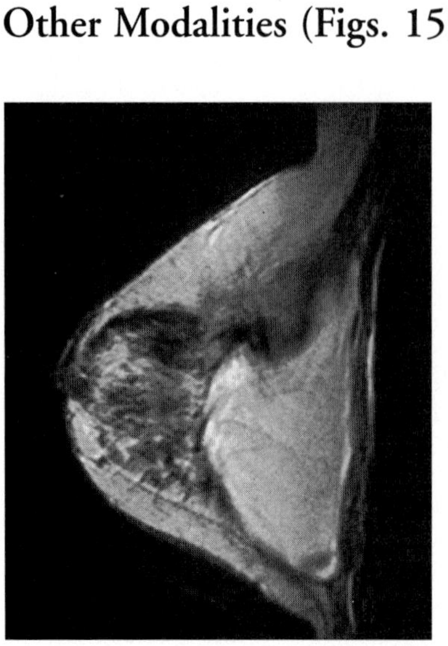

Figure 155–2. Right breast T2-weighted longitudinal MRI: The superior edge of the implant demonstrates a contour deformity that corresponds to the mammographic abnormality. There is no evidence of capsular rupture.

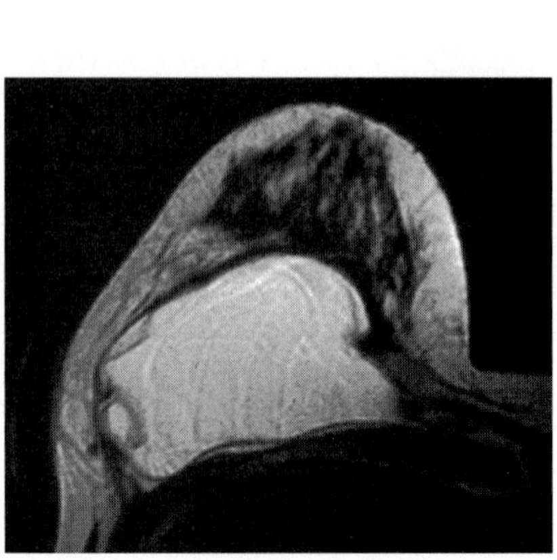

155-3

Figure 155–3. Right breast T2-weighted transverse MRI: Normal folds extend from the lateral aspect of the implant.

Pathology

- normal implant

Management

- BI-RADS Assessment Category 1, negative

Pearls and Pitfalls

1. About half of all implants demonstrate small focal contour deformities without rupture. Wrinkling is more common with saline implants compared with silicone prostheses. The most common location for contour deformities in silicone implants is the superior edge of the implant in the MLO view as illustrated in this case.
2. Contour deformities should be differentiated from implant herniation. Both contour deformities and implant folds are normal findings of an intact implant. Herniation is when an intact implant shell is extruded through the fibrous capsule. Capsular herniation is distinguished from a contour bulge by identifying bunching of the implant at the location of the ruptured capsule.

Suggested Readings

1. Destouet JM, Monsees BS, Oser RF, Nemecek JR, Young VL, Pilgram TK. Screening mammography in 350 women with breast implants: prevalence and findings of implant complications. *AJR* 1992;159:973–978.
2. Ganott MA, Harris KM, Ilkhanipour ZS, Costa-Greco MA. Augmentation mammoplasty: normal and abnormal findings with mammography and US. *Radiographics* 1992;12:281–295.
3. Middleton MS. Breast implants and soft tissue silicone. In: Stark DD, Bradley WG, eds. *Magnetic Resonance Imaging.* 3rd ed. St. Louis: Mosby; 1999:335–353.

Case 156

Case History

A 57-year-old woman, who had a right mastectomy 5 years ago with breast reconstruction using a subpectoral silicone implant, is worried about her implant.

Physical Examination

- right breast: implant smaller than left breast, otherwise normal
- left breast: normal exam

Ultrasound

Frequency

- 7 MHz (Fig. 156–1)

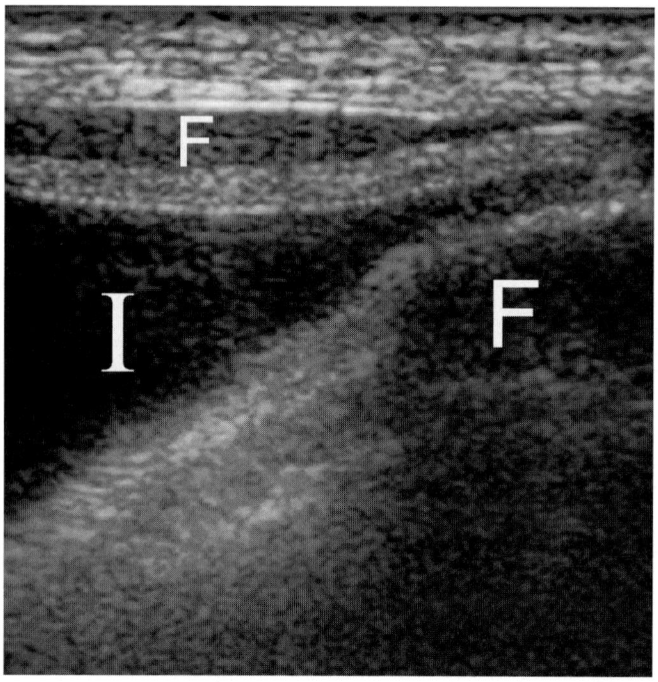

Figure 156–1. Right transverse breast sonogram: The implant (I) wall is intact but there is a thin fluid collection (F) outside the implant.

Pathology

- normal implant

Management

- BI-RADS Assessment Category 1, negative

Pearls and Pitfalls

Small fluid collections of water may form outside the nonruptured implant. These collections are identifiable by sonography or MRI and should not be mistaken for signs of extracapsular rupture.

Suggested Readings

1. Caskey CI, Hamper UM. Sonographic evaluation of breast implants. In: Sohn C, Blohmer JU, Hamper UM eds. *Breast Ultrasound.* New York: Thieme; 1999:143–165.
2. Middleton MS. Breast implants and soft tissue silicone. In: Stark DD, Bradley WG, eds. *Magnetic Resonance Imaging.* 3rd ed. St. Louis: Mosby; 1999:335–353.
3. Reynolds HE. Evaluation of the augmented breast. *Radiol Clin North Am* 1995;33:1131–1145.

Case 157

Case History

A 66-year-old woman presents with angina. She has had breast implants for over 20 years.

Physical Examination

- bilateral breasts: normal exam

Mammogram (Fig. 157–1)

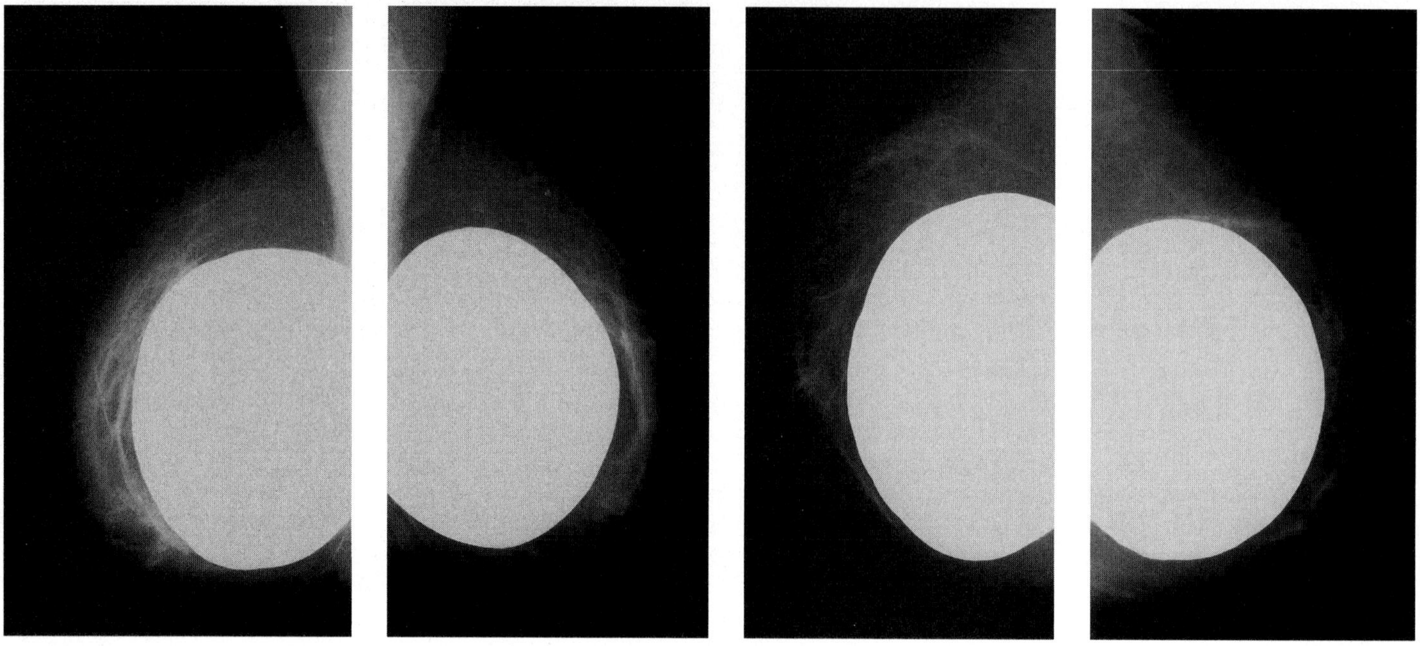

A B C D

Figure 157–1. Bilateral implants exhibit normal contours and shape. (A). Right MLO mammogram. (B). Left MLO mammogram. (C). Right CC mammogram. (D). Left CC mammogram.

Other Modalities (Fig. 157-2)

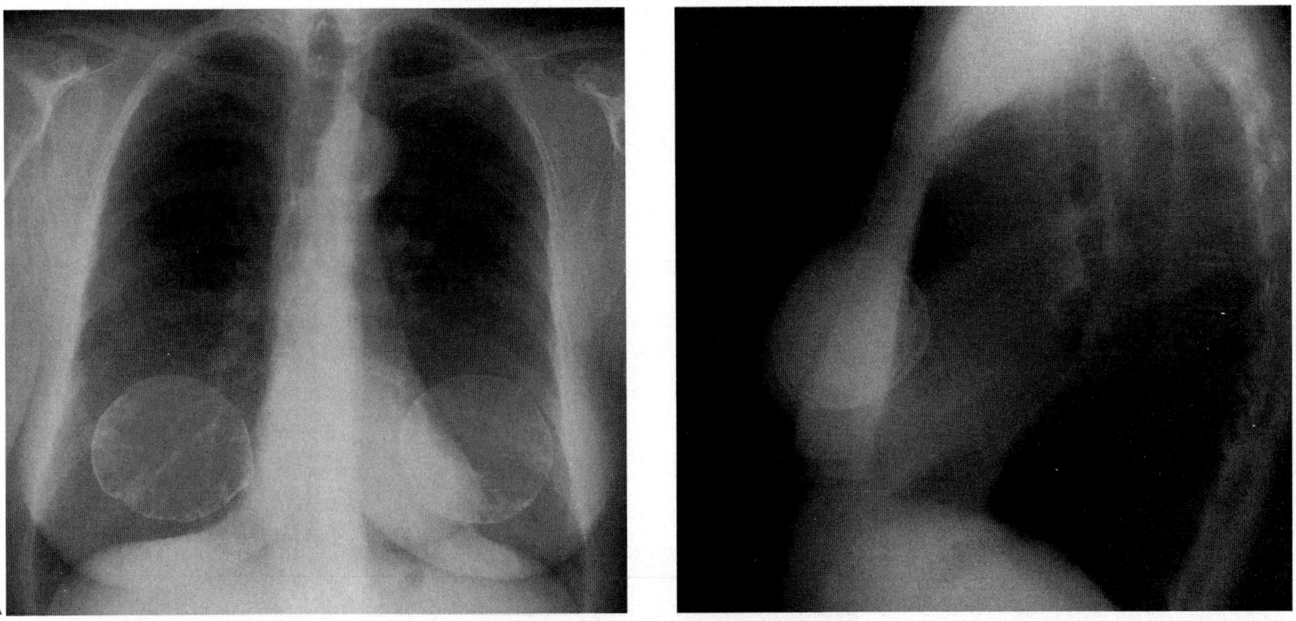

Figure 157-2. Chest radiograph demonstrates round densities within the breasts, which represent the patient's calcified implants. (A). Posterior anterior (PA) Chest radiograph. (B). Lateral chest radiograph.

Pathology

- calcified implants

Management

- BI-RADS Assessment Category 2, benign finding

Pearls and Pitfalls

Implant calcification is common and generally not associated with a significant clinical problem. About 20% of all types of implants demonstrate at least a small amount of calcification. In a few cases, heavy calcification has been associated with severe capsular contracture, which has been labeled the Krakatau syndrome. This syndrome is named after the famous volcano in Indonesia because when this abnormal implant is removed, the breast exhibits a craterlike depression.

Suggested Readings

1. Ganott MA, Harris KM, Ilkhanipour ZS, Costa-Greco MA. Augmentation mammoplasty: normal and abnormal findings with mammography and US. *Radiographics* 1992;12:281-291.
2. Koide T, Katayama H. Calcification in augmentation mammoplasty. *Radiology* 1979;130:337-340.
3. Steinbach BG, Hardt NS, Abbitt PL. Mammography: breast implants—types, complications, and adjacent breast pathology. *Curr Probl Diagn Radiol* 1993;22:39-86.
4. Vuursteen PJ. The Krakatau syndrome: a late complication of retroglandular mammary augmentation. *Br J Plast Surg* 1992;45:34-37.

Case 158

Case History

A 64-year-old woman has a history of implant rupture 28 years ago. She removed her implants 15 years ago.

Physical Examination

- bilateral breasts: multilobulated but stable

Mammogram (Fig. 158–1)

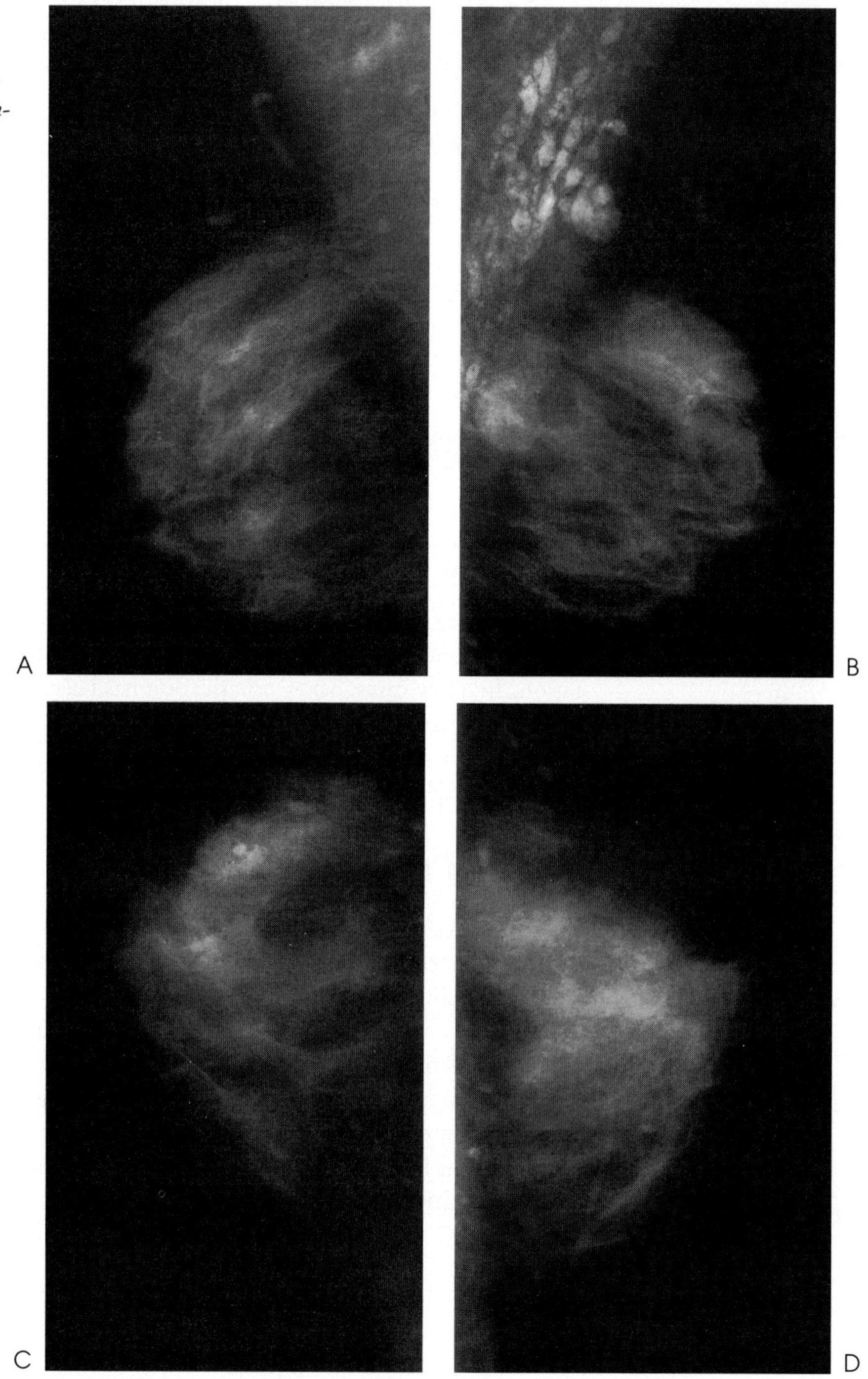

Figure 158–1. There are scattered small, oval, high-density masses in the breast parenchyma and numerous densities in the axilla. (A). Right MLO mammogram. (B). Left MLO mammogram. (C). Right CC mammogram. (D). Left CC mammogram.

Pathology

- free silicone

Management

- BI-RADS Assessment Category 2, benign finding

Pearls and Pitfalls

Reasons for free silicone in the breast include silicone injections, ruptured implant, or escape of silicone from an intact implant elastomer shell (gel bleed). The elastomer shell is a semiporous membrane that allows silicone to flow into the surrounding tissues without rupture of the shell. The most comon migration of free silicone is to the upper outer or upper medial soft tissues. Rarely silicone will migrate to the breast or axilla from a distal injection site such as the arm.

Suggested Readings

1. Hayes MD, Gold RH, Bassett LW. Mammographic findings after the removal of breast implants. *AJR* 1993;160:487–490.
2. Middleton MS. MR evaluation of breast implants and soft tissue silicone. *Top Magn Reson Imaging* 1998;9:92–137.
3. Roux SP, Bertucci GM, Ibarra JA, Blatt G, Ashworth CR. Unilateral axillary adenopathy secondary to a silicone wrist implant: report of a case detected at screening mammography. *Radiology* 1996;198:345–346.

Case 159

Case History

A 60-year-old woman, who has had removal of bilateral implants, presents for her annual mammogram.

Physical Examination

- normal exam

Mammogram

Calcifications

- type: dystrophic (Fig. 159–1)

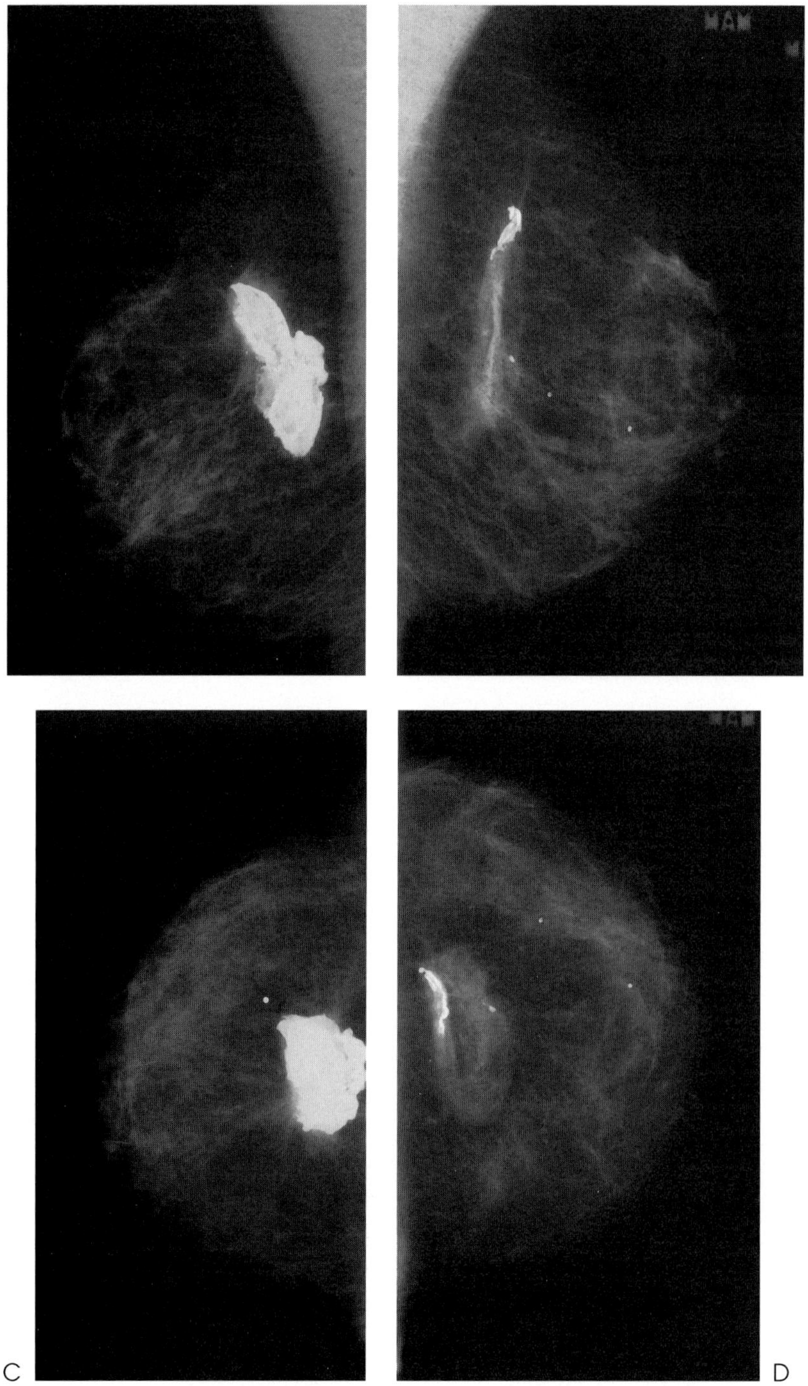

A B C D

Figure 159–1. There are large dystrophic calcifications and scarring in the areas of the patient's previous implants. (A). Right MLO mammogram. (B). Left MLO mammogram. (C). Right CC mammogram. (D). Left CC mammogram.

Pathology

- scar

Management

- BI-RADS Assessment Category 2, benign finding

Pearls and Pitfalls

The appearance and location of the large coarse calcifications, architectural distortion, and oval densities are characteristic of mammographic changes after implant removal. The abnormalities in this case may also be due to retained portions of the fibrous capsule that previously surrounded the patient's implants.

Suggested Readings

1. Hayes MD, Gold RH, Bassett LW. Mammographic findings after the removal of breast implants. *AJR* 1993;160:487–490.

Case 160

Case History

A 38-year-old woman removed her implants 1 year ago.

Physical Examination

- normal exam

Mammogram (Figs. 160–1 and 160–2)

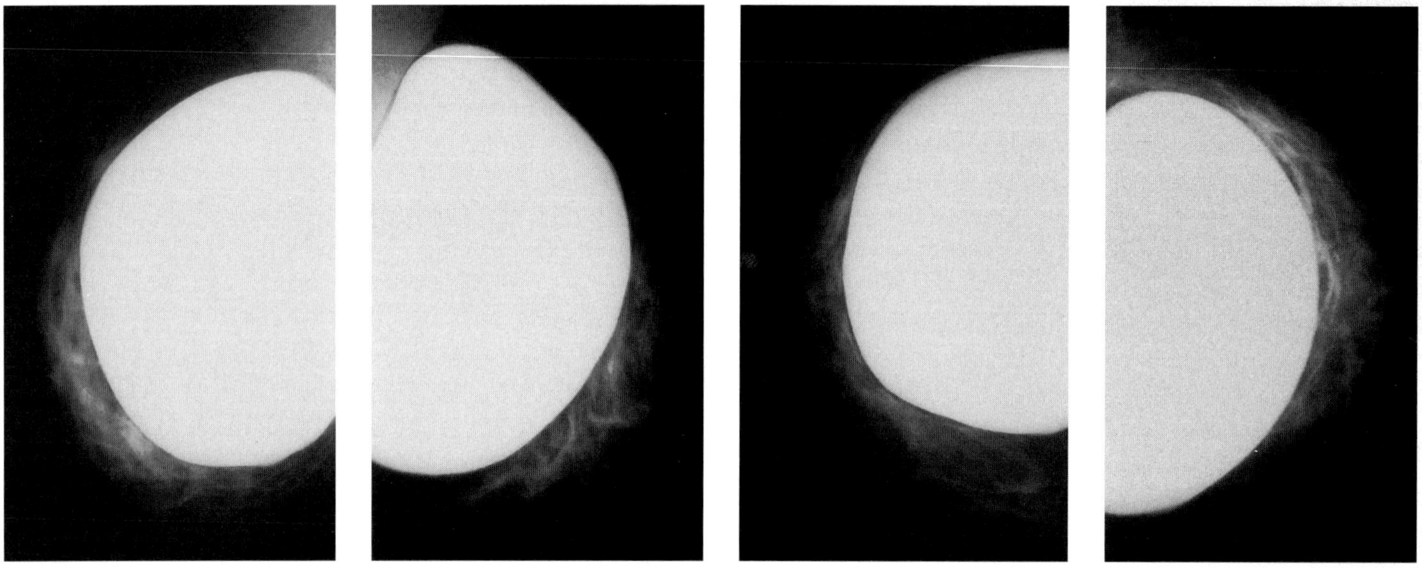

A B C D

Figure 160–1. Normal bilateral breast implant views. (A). Right MLO implant mammogram. (B). Left MLO implant mammogram. (C). Right CC implant mammogram. (D). Left CC implant mammogram.

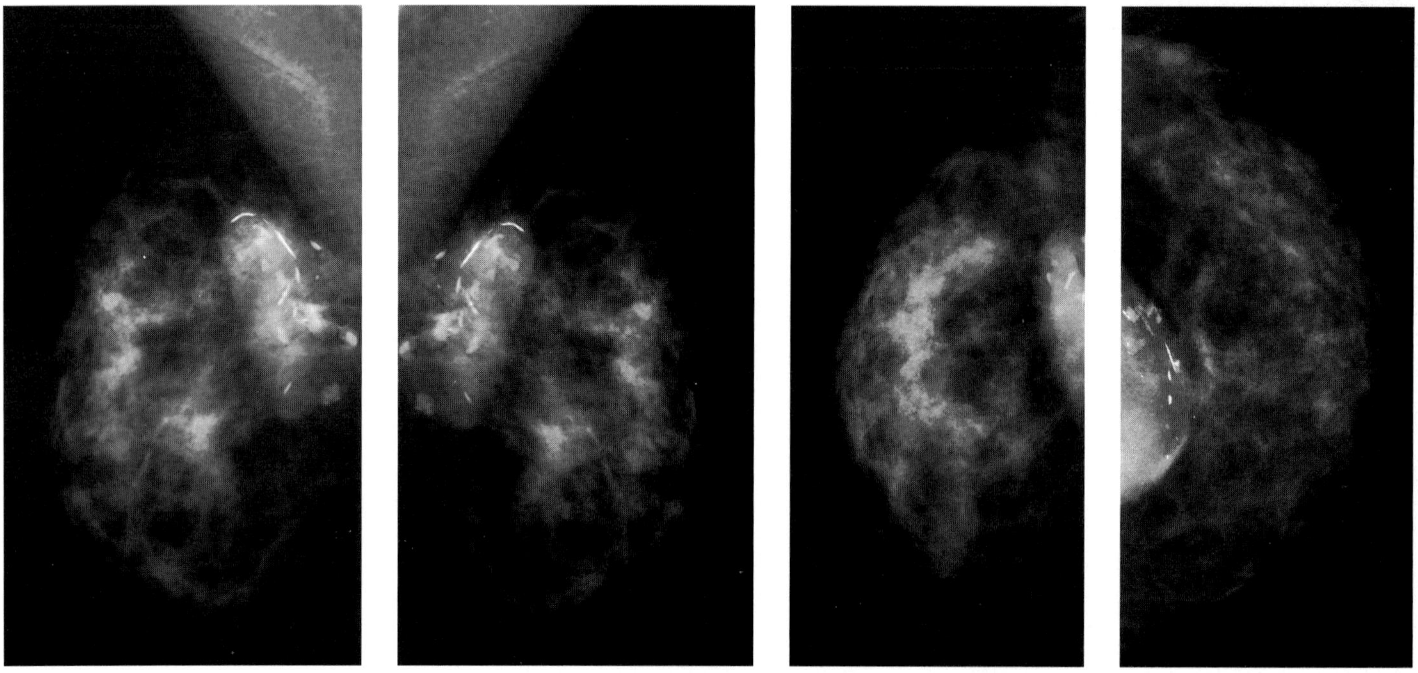

A B C D

Figure 160–2. This mammographic exam was performed 4 years after the mammograms in Figure 160–1 and 1 year after removal of implants. There are oval densities with calcifications in the areas of the previous implants. (A). Right MLO mammogram. (B). Left MLO mammogram. (C). Right CC mammogram. (D). Left CC mammogram.

Pathology

- scar

Management

- BI-RADS Assessment Category 2, benign finding

Pearls and Pitfalls

Mammographic findings after removal of breast implants include fat necrosis, scarring, architectural distortion, skin thickening, silicone in the breast parenchyma and axilla, and calcifications. Usually the fibrous capsule surrounding the implants is removed with the implants. In this case, some or all of the fibrous capsule was left within the breast. These fibrous capsules were subsequently removed.

Suggested Readings

1. Hayes MD, Gold RH, Bassett LW. Mammographic findings after the removal of breast implants. *AJR* 1993;160:487–490.

Case 161

Case History

A 52-year-old woman has had the same saline implants for over 25 years. After partial mastectomy for breast cancer, the woman noticed that her left breast is larger than her right and there is a new thickening in the lumpectomy site.

Physical Examination

- right breast: mild nodularity of healing scar in the inner inferior breast; right breast smaller than left breast
- left breast: normal exam

Mammogram (Fig. 161–1)

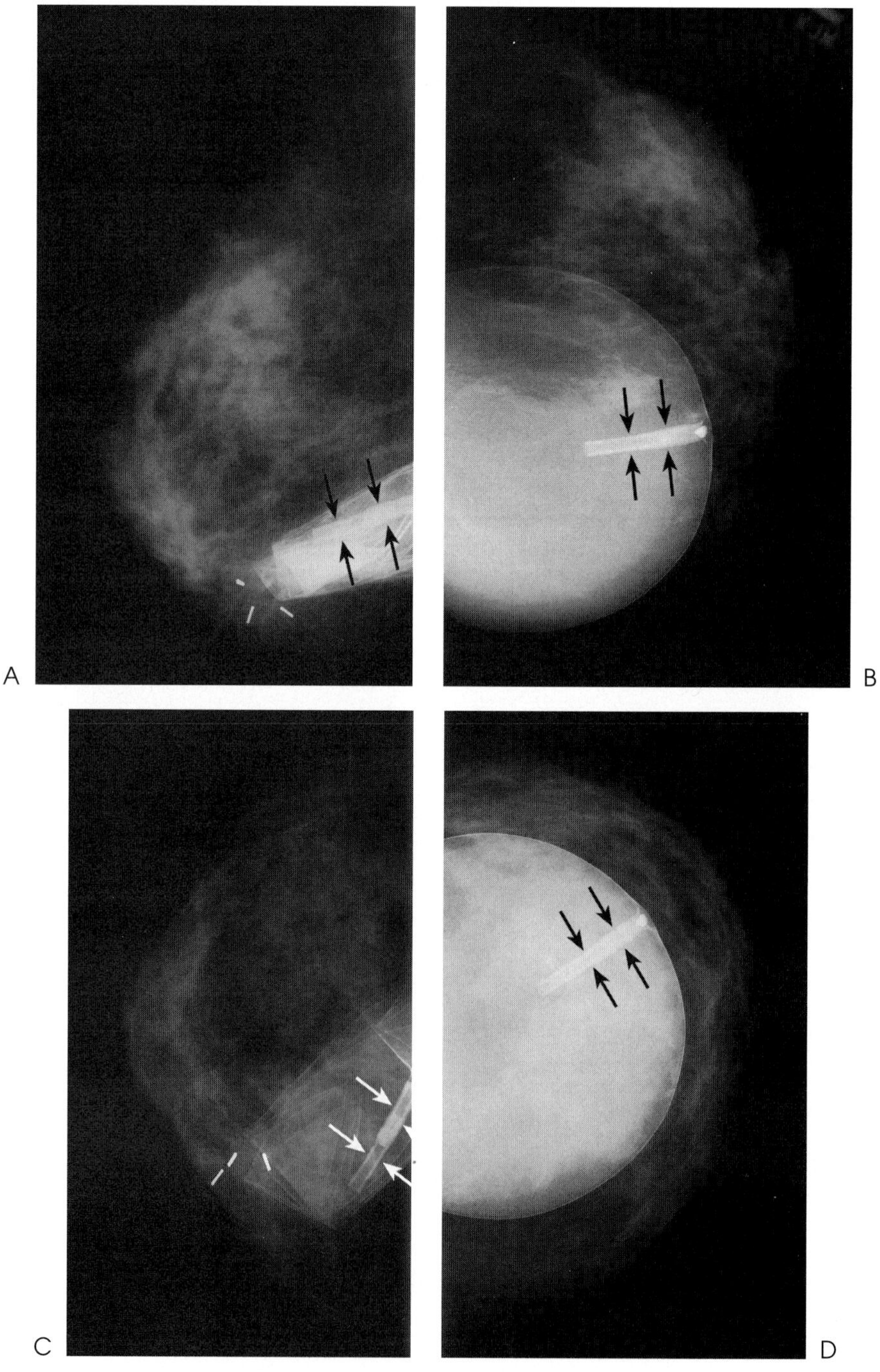

Figure 161–1. Patient has bilateral saline implants. The tubular structure (arrows) is the valve that was used to fill the implant. The right implant has ruptured and completely collapsed. The clips mark the location of the recent lumpectomy. (A). Right MLO mammogram. (B). Left MLO mammogram. (C). Right CC mammogram. (D). Left CC mammogram.

Ultrasound (Figs. 161-2 and 161-3)

Figure 161-2. Right breast sonogram: The breast sonogram was performed before the mammograms to investigate the palpable abnormality in the lumpectomy scar. The palpable thickening corresponds sonographically to a deformed, collapsed implant.

Figure 161-3. Left breast sonogram: The left implant is normal without evidence of rupture. The linear lines within the implant correspond to the valve identified in Figure 161-1.

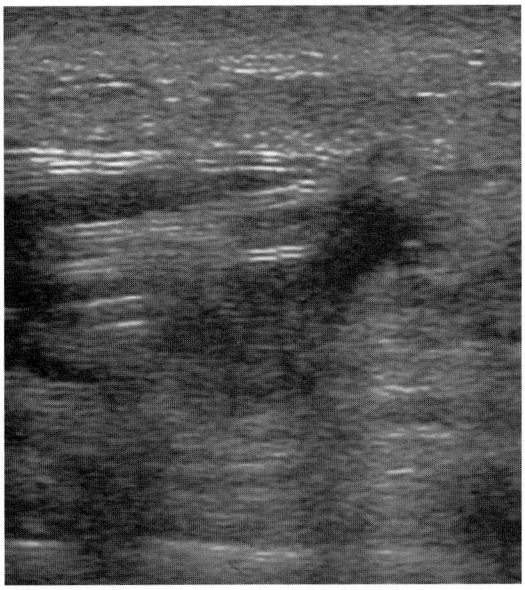

161-2

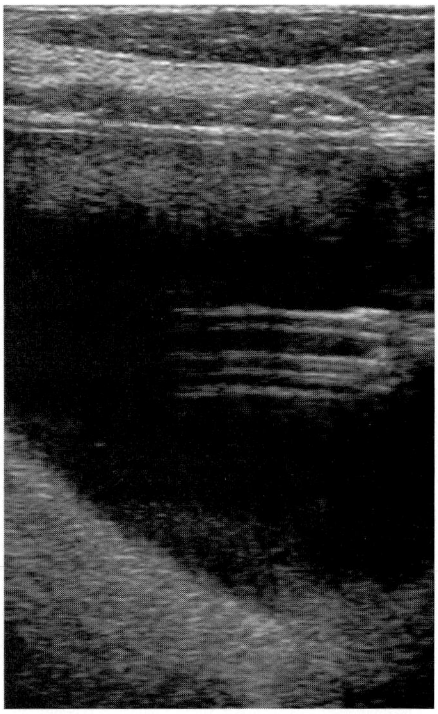

161-3

Pathology

- ruptured implant

Management

- BI-RADS Assessment Category 2, benign finding

Pearls and Pitfalls

1. When an implant is inserted, a fibrous capsule develops around the implant elastomer shell. There are two types of implant failure: intracapsular and extracapsular. Intracapsular failure involves rupture of the implant elastomer shell without rupture of the surrounding fibrous capsule. With intracapsular rupture, the liquid contents of the implant are contained within the fibrous capsule. Extracapsular failure is when both the implant elastomer shell and the fibrous capsule have been ruptured. As a result of this type of rupture, the internal contents of the implant (silicone or water) are extruded outside the capsule into the surrounding tissues.
2. Saline implants have a higher rate of leakage and a less natural feel than silicone implants. The advantages of saline are that they have a lower reported incidence of contracture and that leakage from the implant is undesirable but harmless.

Suggested Readings

1. Ganott MA, Harris KM, Ilkhanipour ZS, Costa-Greco MA. Augmentation mammoplasty: normal and abnormal findings with mammography and US. *Radiographics* 1992;12:281–291.
2. Lavine DM. Saline inflatable prostheses: 14 years' experience. *Aesthetic Plast Surg* 1993;17:325–330.
3. Newman J. Mammographic evaluation of the augmented breast. *Radiol Technol* 1998;69:319–338.
4. Steinbach BG, Hardt NS, Abbitt PL. Mammography: breast implants—types, complications, and adjacent breast pathology. *Curr Probl Diagn Radiol* 1993;22:39–86.

Case 162

Case History

A 39-year-old woman who has had breast augmentation with saline implants notes a new palpable abnormality in her left breast.

Physical Examination

- left breast: deformed and small implant
- right breast: normal exam

Mammogram (Fig. 162–1)

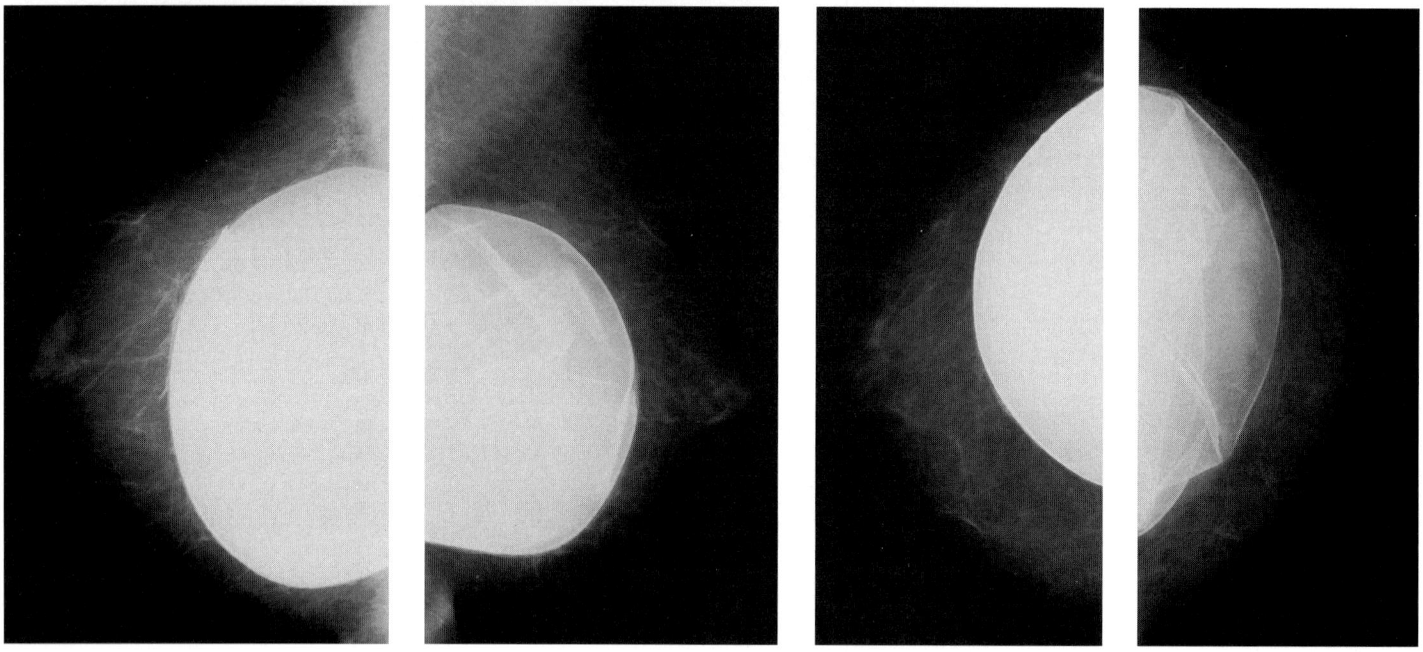

A B C D

Figure 162–1. The left implant is deformed and smaller than the right. (A). Right MLO mammogram. (B). Left MLO mammogram. (C). Right CC mammogram. (D). Left CC mammogram.

Ultrasound

Frequency

- 11.5 MHz (Figs. 162–2 and 162–3)

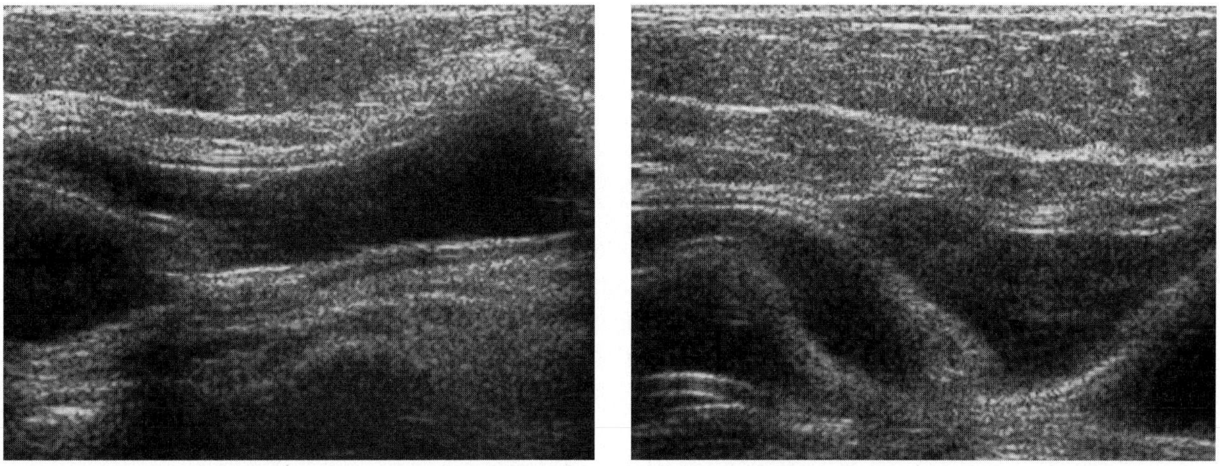

A B

Figure 162–2. *Sonography of the left implant demonstrates a distorted, small implant with multiple linear invaginations, suggesting implant rupture. (A). Left radial breast implant sonogram. (B). Left antiradial implant sonogram.*

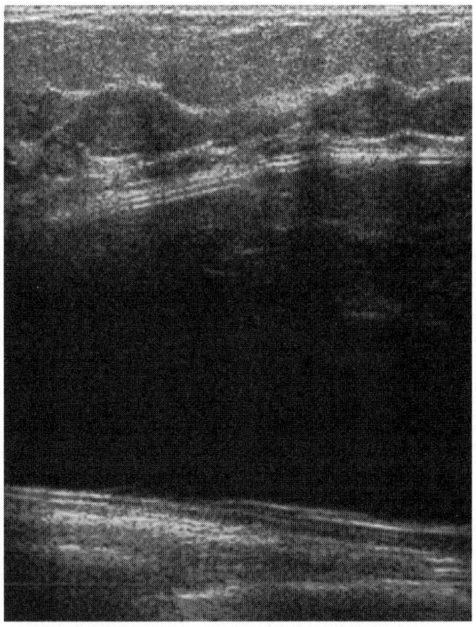

Figure 162–3. *Right radial implant sonogram: Right implant is normal.*

Pathology

- deflation of saline implant

Management

- BI-RADS Assessment Category 2, benign finding

Pearls and Pitfalls

1. Sonography is better than mammography but not as accurate as MRI in identifying implant rupture. One article reviewing the literature found that mammography has a sensitivity of 28.4% and specificity of 92.9%. Ultrasound's sensitivity and specificity are 59.0% and 76.8%. MRI's sensitivity and specificity are 78.1% and 80.0%.
2. The main pitfalls of sonographically identifying implant rupture include mistaking normal implant folds for collapsed walls, confusing normal perimplant fluid for abnormal leakage, and identifying silicone collections or nodes that are due to normal seepage of silicone through an intact implant shell or due to a previously ruptured implant.

Suggested Readings

1. Goodman CM, Cohen V, Thornby J, Netscher D. The life span of silicone gel breast implants and a comparison of mammography, ultrasonography, and magnetic resonance imaging in detecting implant rupture: a meta-analysis. *Ann Plast Surg* 1998;41:577–586.
2. Samuels JB, Rohrich RJ, Weatherall PT, Angelena MWH, Goldberg KL. Radiographic diagnosis of breast implant rupture: current status and comparison of techniques. *Plast Reconstr Surg* 1995;96:865–877.

Case 163

Case History

A 46-year-old woman has had subglandular silicone gel implants for 13 years.

Physical Examination

- bilateral breasts: both implants feel irregular in shape

Mammogram (Fig. 163–1)

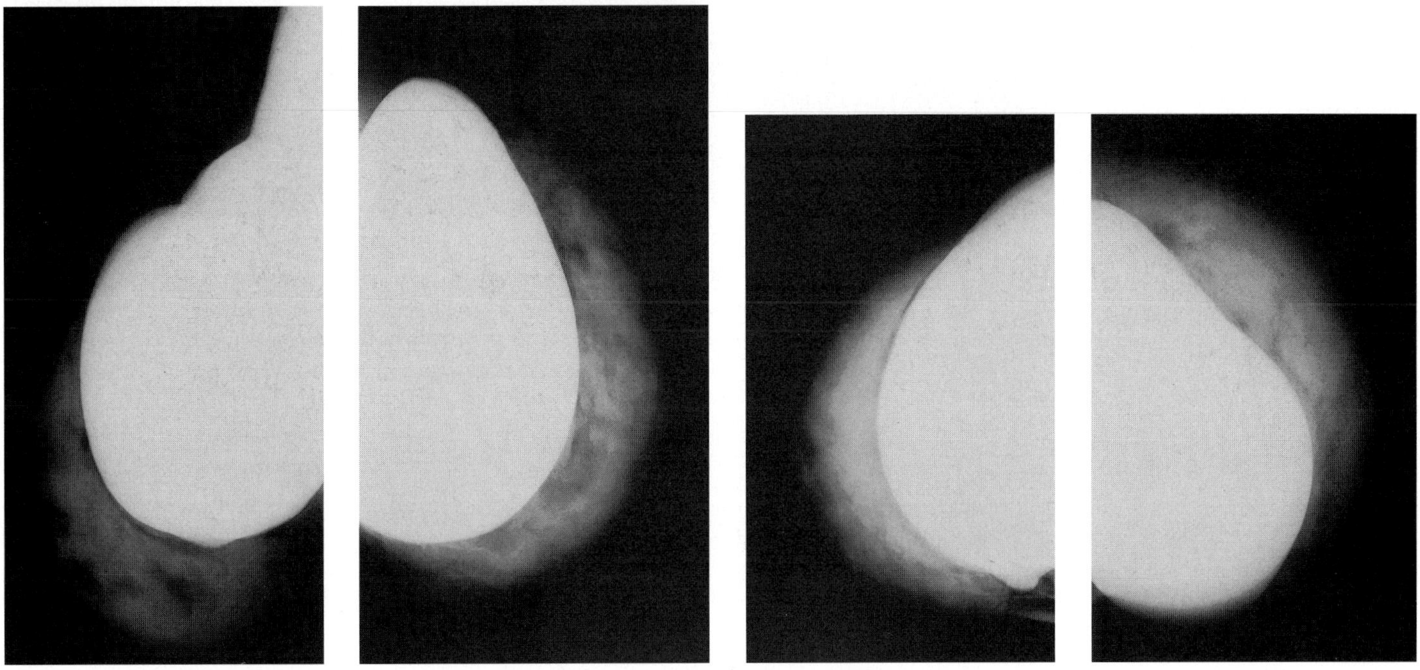

A B C D

Figure 163–1. There is asymmetric extension of the right implant in the right upper outer quadrant. There is also a focal contour bulge in the medial aspect of the implant on the CC view. (A). Right MLO mammogram. (B). Left MLO mammogram. (C). Right CC mammogram. (D). Left CC mammogram.

Ultrasound (Figs. 163-2 and 163-3)

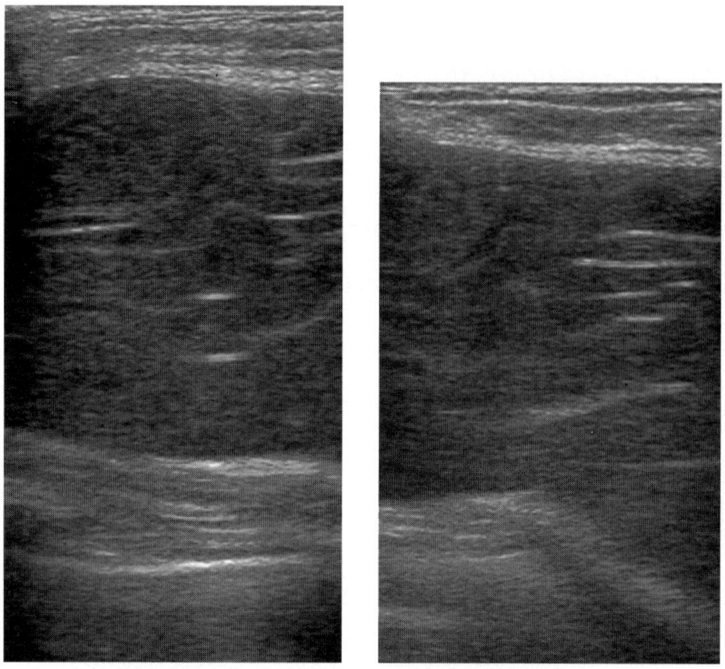

Figure 163-2. (A) Transverse right breast implant sonogram: The right implant is filled with hypoechoic fluid and exhibits multiple echogenic lines within it. (B) Transverse right breast implant sonogram: This is a different position from Figure 163-2A. This figure illustrates the stepladder sign created by the echogenic lines.

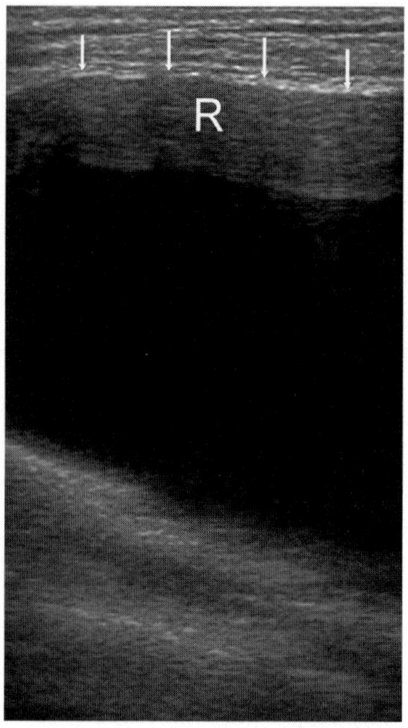

Figure 163-3. Transverse left breast sonogram: Left implant appears normal. The fluid is anechoic and there are no echogenic lines. The hypoechoic band (R) next to the implant shell (arrows) is acoustic reverberation artifact.

Pathology

- ruptured right implant

Management

- BI-RADS Assessment Category 2, benign finding

Pearls and Pitfalls

1. Implant rupture increases with increasing prosthesis age. A review of over 1000 silicone gel implants found that the median life span for those implants was 16.4 years. About 79% of silicone implants were intact at 10 years. Only 49% were unruptured by 15 years.
2. With experienced operators, sonography is a useful method to identify implant rupture. The most reliable sign of rupture is identification of multiple horizontal, straight, or curvilinear lines (stepladder sign) within the silicone gel. This sonographic finding corresponds to the MRI "linguini" sign. The lines represent the collapsed walls of the implant. Another important sonographic sign of rupture is the presence of "echodense noise" (snowstorm appearance), which indicates free silicone. Hypoehoic debris within the implant is a less reliable finding of rupture.

Suggested Readings

1. DeBruhl ND, Gorczyca DP, Ahn CY, Shaw WW, Bassett LW. Silicone breast implants: US evaluation. *Radiology* 1993;189:95–98.
2. Goodman CM, Cohen V, Thornby J, Netscher D. The life span of silicone gel breast implants and a comparison of mammography, ultrasonography, and magnetic resonance imaging in detecting implant rupture: a meta-analysis. *Ann Plast Surg* 1998;41:577–586.

Case 164

Case History

A 31-year-old woman is concerned that her implants feel asymmetric.

Physical Examination

- right breast: implant is irregular in shape
- left breast: normal exam

Other Modalities (Figs. 164–1 and 164–2)

Figure 164–1. Right breast T2-weighted transverse MRI: This image illustrates mild collapse of the implant shell with silicone on both sides of the collapsing walls. Two mild or indirect signs of intracapsular rupture are the keyhole sign (arrow) and the noose sign (arrowhead).

Figure 164–2. Right breast T2-weighted longitudinal MRI: This image demonstrates more small areas (arrows) where the implant shell has separated from the fibrous capsule.

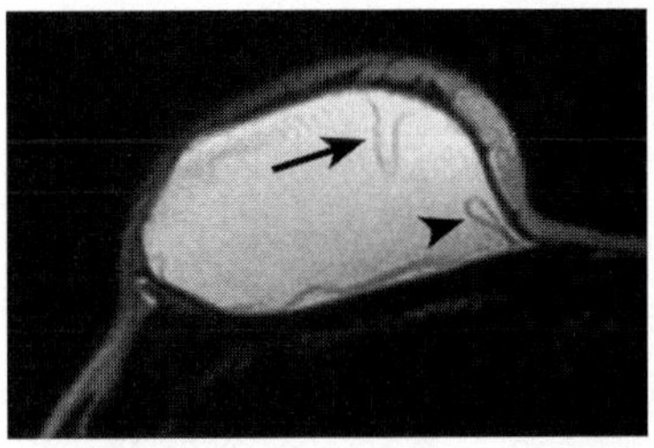

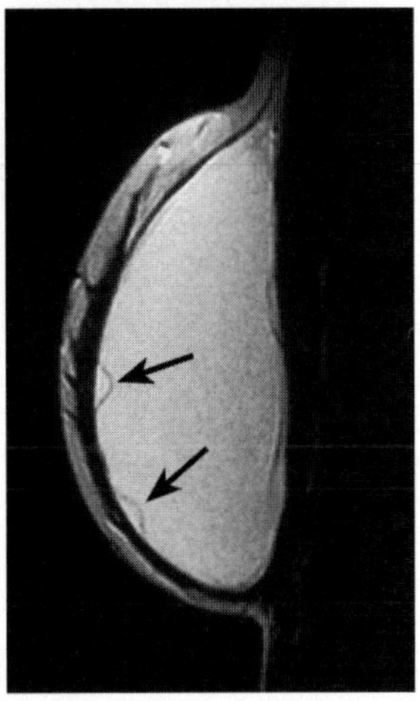

164-2

Pathology

- intracapsular implant rupture

Management

- BI-RADS Assessment Category 2, benign finding

Pearls and Pitfalls

MRI findings of intracapsular rupture include multiple wavy lines (linguine sign) and curvilinear lines that form a semicircular shape with the fibrous capsule (C-sign). The least reliable signs of rupture are the group that demonstrates silicone on both sides of the folded implant wall. When the edges of the fold are touching, the sign is called the keyhole or teardrop sign. When the walls are not touching, the abnormality has a variety of names including noose, pull-away, or open loop sign.The reason that these signs may be misleading is that these findings are also present when nonruptured silicone is against the wall. Furthermore, complex normal implant folds may also be misinterpreted as representing one of these findings.

Suggested Readings

1. Soo MS, Kornguth PJ, Walsh R, Elenberger CD, Georgiade GS. Complex radial folds versus subtle signs of intracapsular rupture of breast implants: MR findings with surgical correlation. *AJR* 1996;166:1421–1427.

Case 165

Case History

A 57-year-old woman presents for screening mammogram. She has no breast symptoms.

Physical Examination

- breast exam: normal exam

Mammogram (Fig. 165–1)

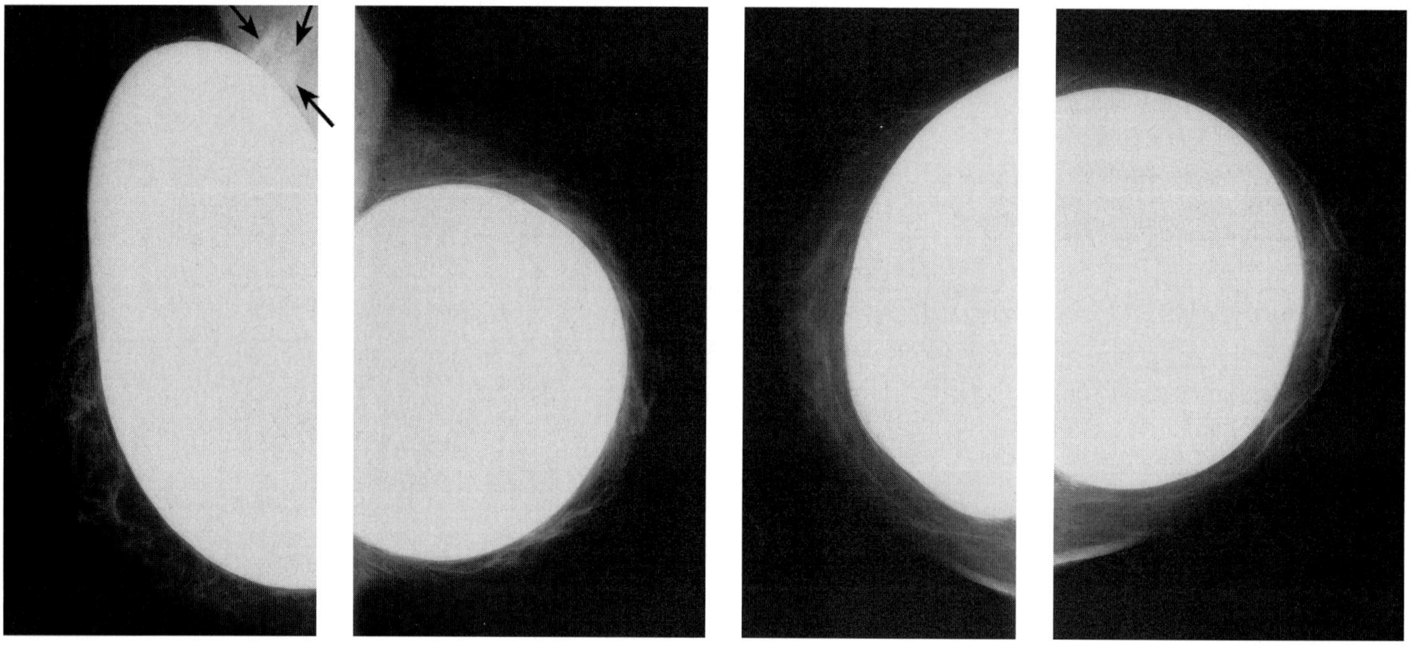

A B C D

Figure 165–1. In the right axilla, there are some oval high-density collections (arrows) consistent with silicone. These collections have been present for at least 7 years. (A). Right MLO mammogram. (B). Left MLO mammogram. (C). Right CC mammogram. (D). Left CC mammogram.

Other Modalities (Fig. 165–2)

Figure 165–2. There are multiple curvilinear lines consistent with implant shell rupture. (A). Right breast T2 transverse MRI. (B). Right breast T2 longitudinal MRI.

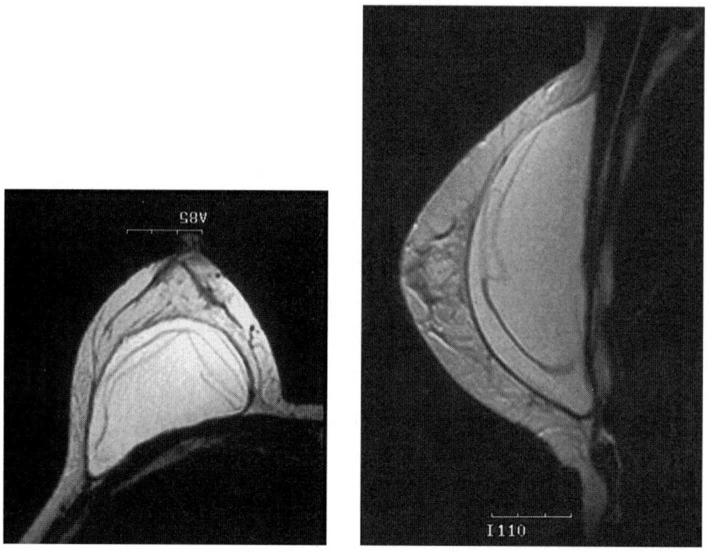

A B

Pathology

- implant rupture

Management

- BI-RADS Assessment Category 2, benign finding

Pearls and Pitfalls

Only an intracapsular rupture was identified by MRI. The right axillary silicone identified mammographically may either be the result of an occult capsular rupture or due to passage of silicone through the fibrous capsule without a rupture in the capsule. This patient elected not to remove the implants.

Suggested Readings

1. Middleton MS. MR evaluation of breast implants and soft tissue silicone. *Top Magn Reson Imaging* 1998;9:92–137.

Case 166

Case History

A 40-year-old woman had implants for 20 years. She notes an enlarging bulge in the lateral side of her right implant.

Physical Examination

- right breast: implant is contracted and irregular in contour
- left breast: normal exam

Mammogram (Fig. 166–1)

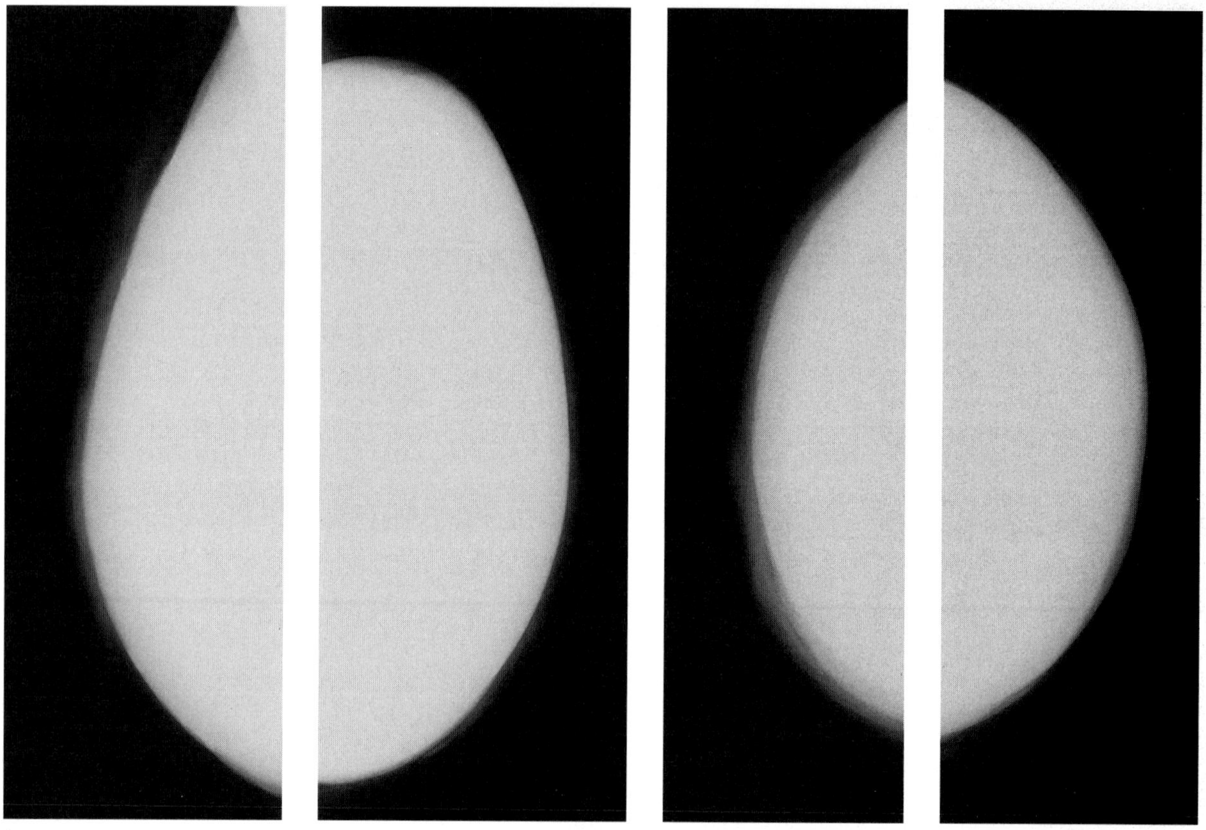

A B C D

Figure 166–1. There is mild asymmetry in the shape of the implants. Otherwise the exam is normal. (A). Right MLO implant mammogram. (B). Left MLO implant mammogram. (C). Right CC implant mammogram. (D). Left CC implant mammogram.

Other Modalities (Figs. 166–2 through 166–4)

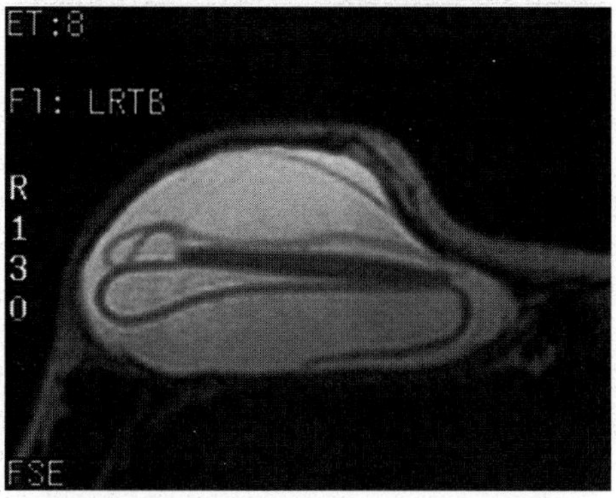

Figure 166–2. Right breast T2-weighted transverse MRI: Right breast implant demonstrates multiple wavy lines (linguine sign), which represent the collapse of the implant shell.

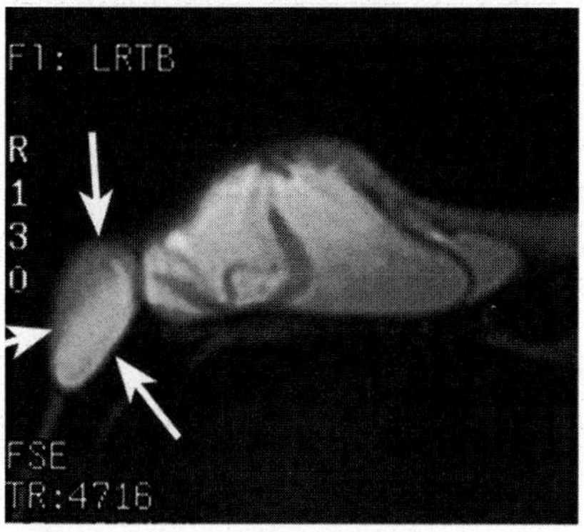

Figure 166–3. Right breast T2-weighted transverse MRI: An oval collection of silicone is present lateral to the edge of the implant (arrows).

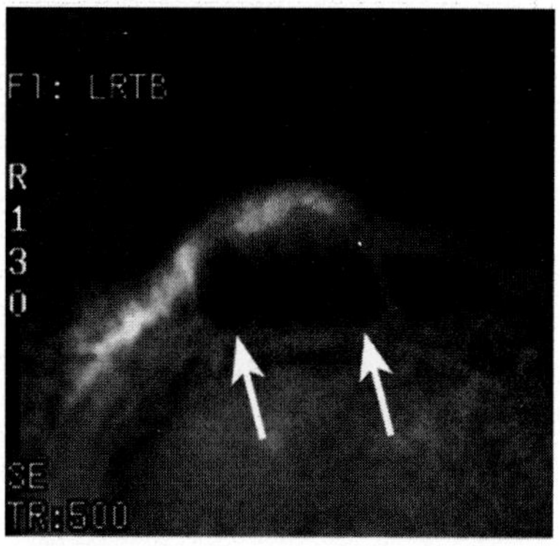

Figure 166–4. Right breast T1-weighted transverse MRI: Oval collections of extracapsular silicone (which is dark with this technique) are present superior to the fibrous capsule (arrows).

Pathology

- extracapsular rupture

Management

- BI-RADS Assessment Category 2, benign finding

Pearls and Pitfalls

The most dramatic and reliable MRI sign of capsular rupture is the demonstration of multiple curvilinear low signal lines that correspond to the collapsed elastomer shell (linguine sign). The collapsed ruptured shell and the free silicone are stronge evidence for extracapsular rupture.

Suggested Readings

1. Orel SG. MR Imaging of the Breast. *Radiol Clin North Am* 2000;38:899–913.

Case 167

Case History

A 56-year-old woman presents with a new right breast lump. She has bilateral breast implants.

Physical Examination

- right breast: implant irregular; palpable lump at 6:00 position adjacent to implant
- left breast: normal exam

Mammogram (Fig. 167–1)

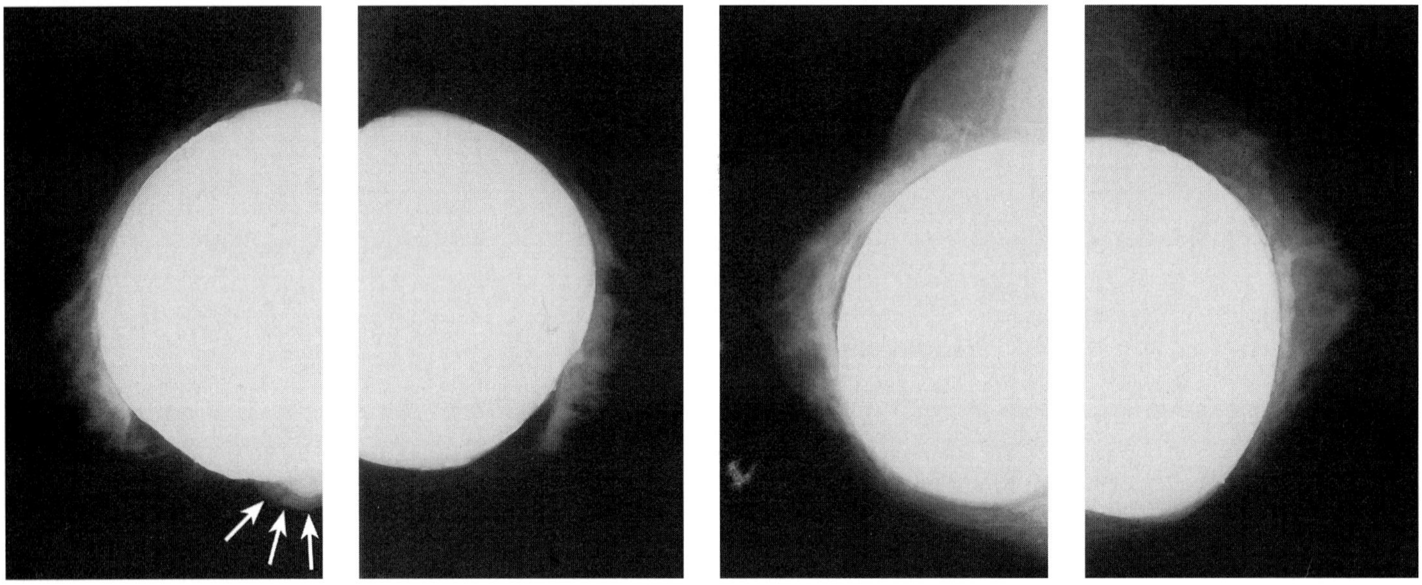

A B C D

Figure 167–1. An oval density is present in the right inferior breast adjacent to the implant (arrows). It corresponds to the palpable lump. (A). Right MLO mammogram. (B). Left MLO mammogram. (C). Right CC mammogram. (D). Left CC mammogram.

Ultrasound

Frequency

- 13 MHz (Fig. 167–2)

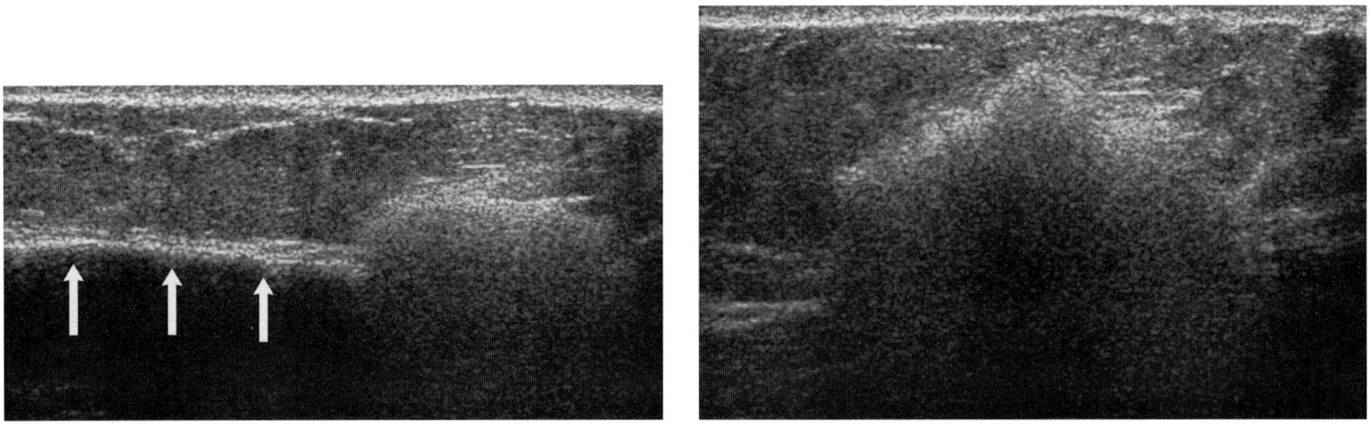

A B

Figure 167–2. The right palpable lump at 6:00 corresponds to a focal area of echogenic noise. The wall of the implant and the fibrous capsule form a well-defined hyperechoic line (arrows) adjacent to this mass. (A). Right longitudinal breast sonogram. (B). Right transverse breast sonogram.

Other Modalities (Figs. 167-3 and 167-4)

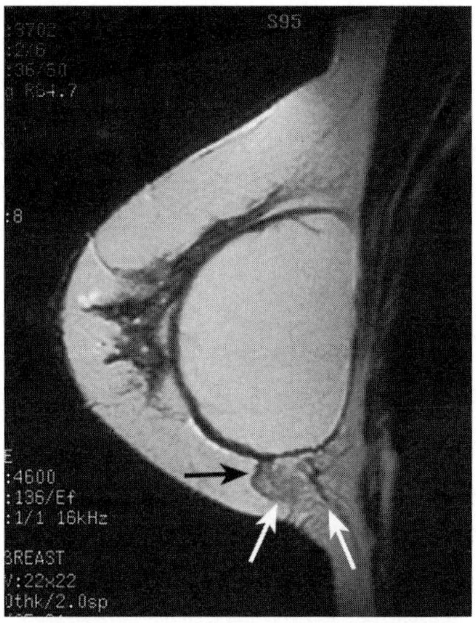

Figure 167-3. Right breast T2-weighted longitudinal MRI: Inferior to the breast (in the areas of the palpable mass) there is a faint mass (arrows). It does not appear as bright as the intracapsular silicone.

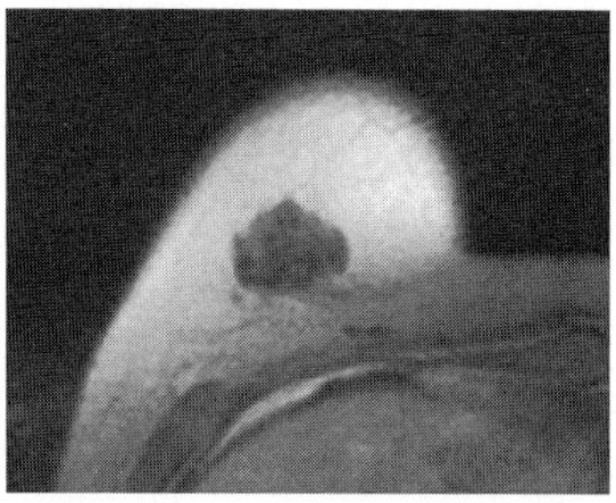

Figure 167-4. Right breast T1-weighted with fat saturation transverse MRI: The extracapsular silicone identified sonographically corresponds to the low signal intensity (dark) focus in the breast.

Pathology

- extracapsular ruptured implant
- grossly ruptured right implant when removed
- palpable lump corresponded microscopically to a silicone granuloma

Management

- BI-RADS Assessment Category 2, benign finding

Pearls and Pitfalls

Five appearances of extracapsular silicone have been described with MR: (1) cyst, (2) granuloma, (3) infiltration of fatty breast parenchyma, (4) infiltration of muscle, (5) globules in muscle. If the silicone forms a fluid collection, it will appear as a cystic mass that has the same high intensity on T2-weighted sequences as intracapsular silicone. If the silicone becomes infiltrated with scar (granuloma formation), then the intensity will vary depending upon the concentration of silicone within the granuloma. Less than 5 to 15% silicone concentration is probably not detectable with current MRI techniques. Irregular, lacy silicone infiltration of both breast tissue and muscle will be bright on T2-weighted sequences. Usually this pattern is due to previous silicone injection. Silicone muscle globules are similar in appearance to silicone cysts in the breast. Globules are a rarer presentation of silicone migration to muscle.

Suggested Readings

1. Castkey CI, Berg WA, Hamper UM, Sheth S, Chang BW, Anderson ND. Imaging spectrum of extracapsular silicone: correlation of us, MR imaging, mammographic and histopathologic findings. *Radiographics* 1999;19:S39–S51.
2. Middleton MS. Breast implants and soft tissue silicone. In: Stark DD, Bradley WG, eds. *Magnetic Resonance Imaging.* 3rd ed. St. Louis: Mosby; 1999:335–353.

Case 168

Case History

A 47-year-old woman with left axillary lumps and a breast lump. She had bilateral augmentation mammoplasties with silicone implants 25 years ago. Seven years ago, they became contractured and the right implant ruptured, so both were replaced at that time.

Physical Examination

- left breast: palpable mass at 3:00. Three palpable lymph nodes are identified.
- right breast: normal exam

Mammogram (Fig. 168–1)

Figure 168–1. There is a mass in the left outer breast, which corresponds to the palpable lump. A high-density lymph node is present in the left axilla. (A). Right MLO mammogram. (B). Left MLO mammogram. (C). Right CC mammogram. (D). Left CC mammogram.

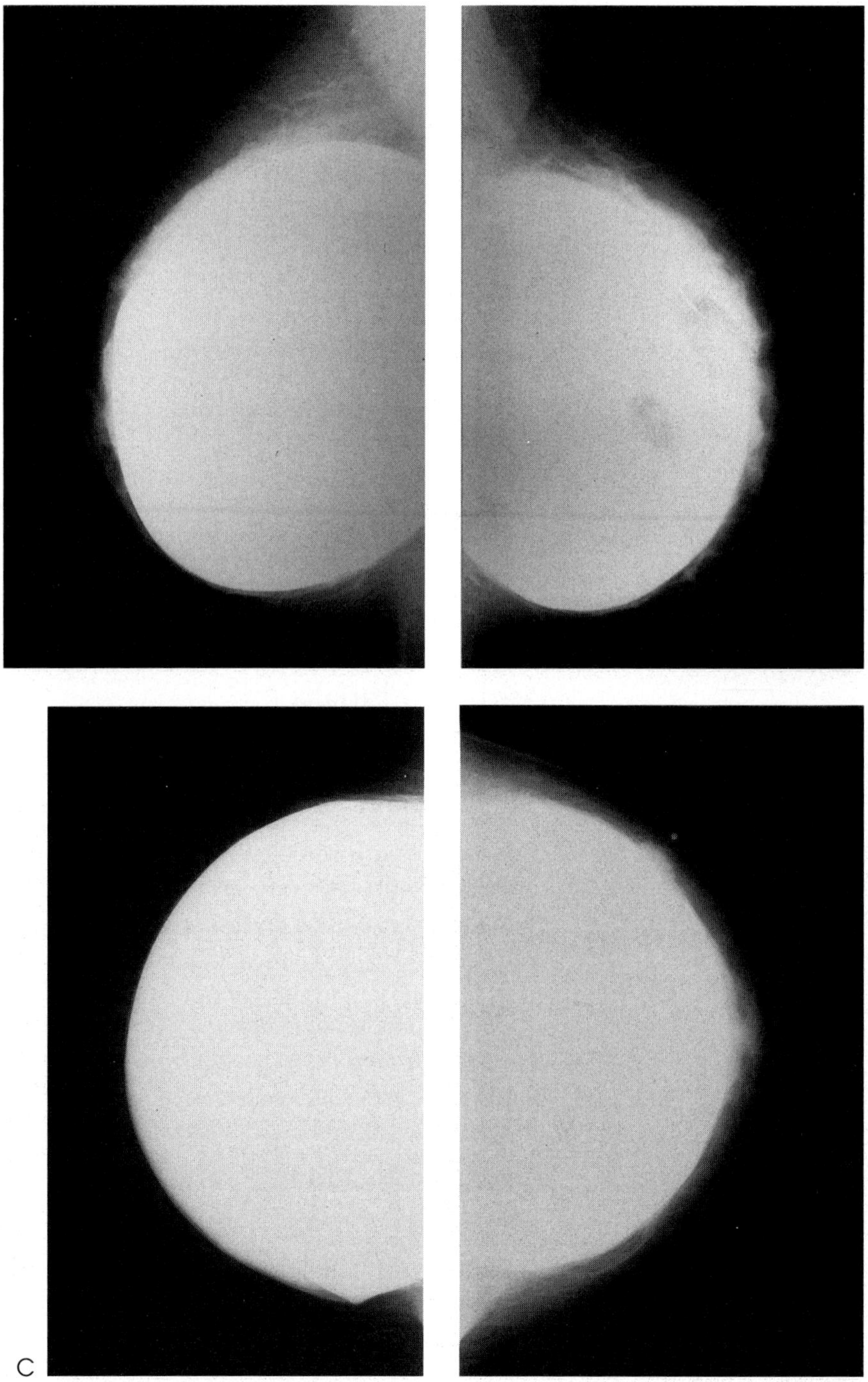

A B C D

Ultrasound

Frequency

- 13 MHz (Figs. 168–2 through 168–3)

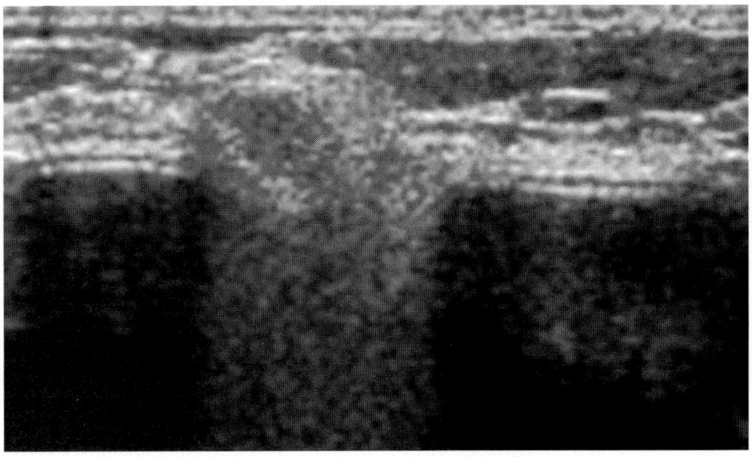

Figure 168–2. Left transverse breast sonogram: The palpable lump corresponds to a hyperechoic mass with echogenic noise characteristic of silicone.

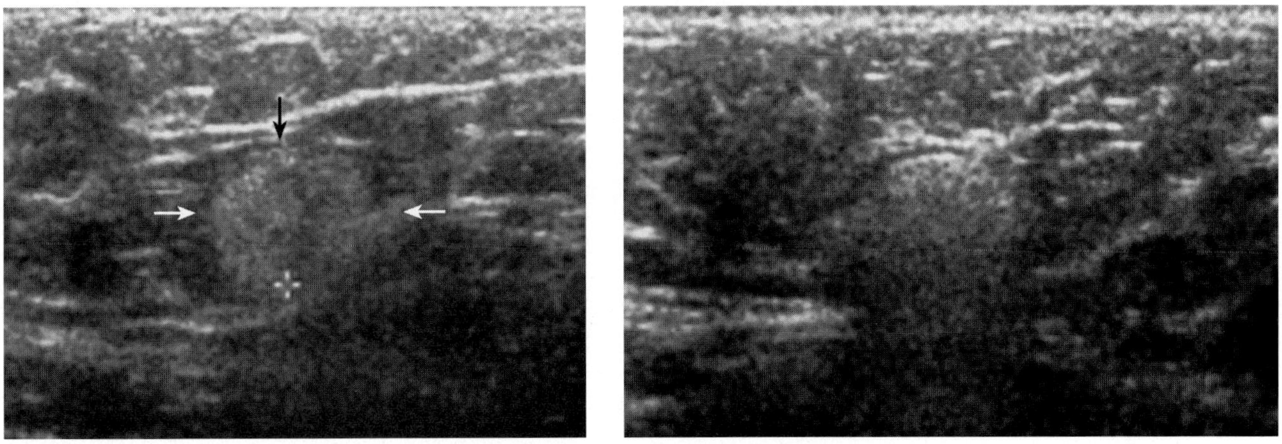

Figure 168–3. Within the axilla, two abnormal hyperechoic masses were identified. The internal architecture of the mass (A: arrows) is suggestive of silicone within a lymph node. The mass (B) could either be a silicone-laden node or a granuloma. (A). Longitudinal left axillary sonogram of mass #1. (B). Longitudinal left axillary sonogram of mass #2.

Other Modalities (Fig. 168-4)

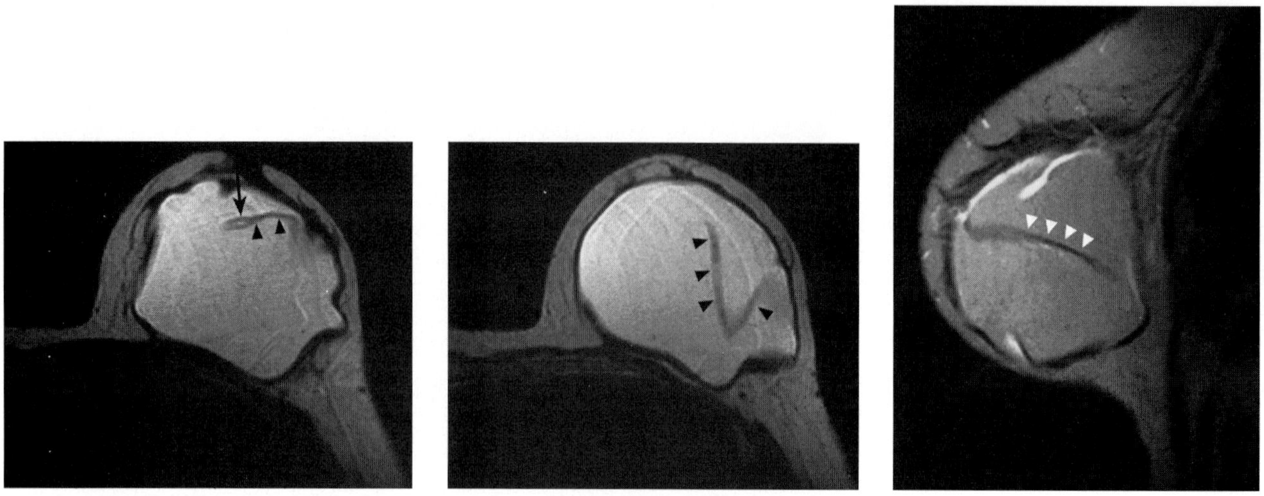

A B C

Figure 168-4. These T2-weighted images demonstrate a pseudokeyhole sign (arrow) that is created by a complex normal fold of the implant. In the transverse plane (A, B), the fold (arrowheads) forms an S-shaped line that ends with the pseudokeyhole (arrow). In the longitudinal plane (C), the sheetlike configuration of this fold (arrowheads) is confirmed. This fold meets the surface of the implant close to the region of the palpable lump. (A). Left breast T2-weighted transverse MRI. (B). Left breast T2-weighted transverse MRI: This image is inferior to A. (C). Left breast T2-weighted longitudinal MRI.

Pathology

- intact implant, extracapsular silicone

Management

- BI-RADS Assessment Category 2, benign finding

Pearls and Pitfalls

The left breast implant was removed and no rupture was identified. The palpable breast lump was histologically found to be a silicone granuloma. The patient also had silicone axillary adenopathy. This case demonstrates some pitfalls in the identification of implant rupture. In this case, complex implant folds (radial folds) simulated collapse of the ruptured implant shell. Furthermore, silicone outside of the capsule was not a result of extracapsular rupture. In this patient, the free silicone may either be due to silicone that leaked during the previous replacement surgery or due to silicone that has seeped through an intact implant shell (gel bleed).

Suggested Readings

1. Castkey CI, Berg WA, Hamper UM, Sheth S, Chang BW, Anderson ND. Imaging spectrum of extracapsular silicone: correlation of US, MR imaging, mammographic and histopathologic findings. *Radiographics* 1999;19:S39–S51.

Case 169

Case History

A 55-year-old woman presents with a left breast lump. She has had bilateral augmentation mammoplasty. This is her baseline examination.

Physical Examination

- left breast: mass on medial breast
- right breast: normal exam

Mammogram

Mass

- margin: spiculated
- shape: irregular
- density: equal density

Calcifications (Fig. 169–1)

- type: pleomorphic/heterogeneous
- distribution: grouped/clustered

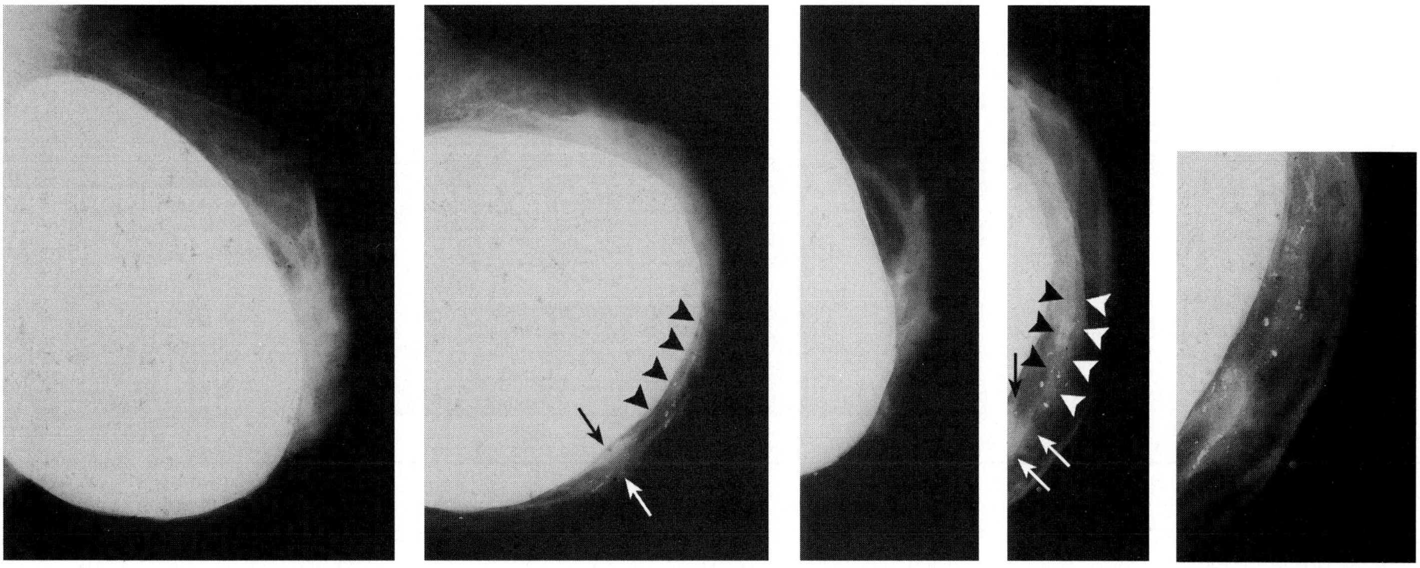

A B C D E

Figure 169–1. In the left medial breast there is an irregular density (arrows) containing heterogeneous calcifications. Adjacent to the mass are more heterogeneous calcifications (arrowheads). (A). Left MLO implant mammogram. (B). Left CC implant mammogram. (C). Left MLO implant displaced mammogram. (D). Left CC implant displaced mammogram. (E). Close-up of left medial breast.

Ultrasound

Low Frequency

Frequency

- 7.5 MHz

Mass

- margin: ill defined
- echogenicity: hypoechoic
- retrotumoral acoustic appearance: no shadowing
- shape: irregular (Fig. 169–2)

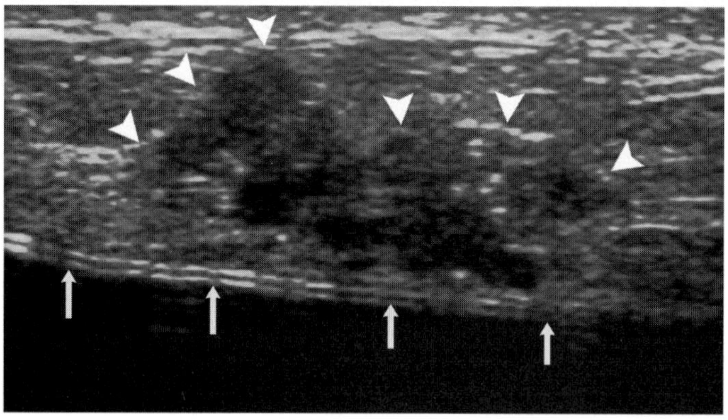

Figure 169–2. Left radial breast sonogram: The mammographic spiculated density and palpable mass correspond to an irregular hypoechoic mass with calcifications. With the lower frequency the mass does not shadow. No second mass is identified. Implant shell (arrows) (see Color Plate 169–2).

High Frequency

Frequency

- 13 MHz (Fig. 169–3)

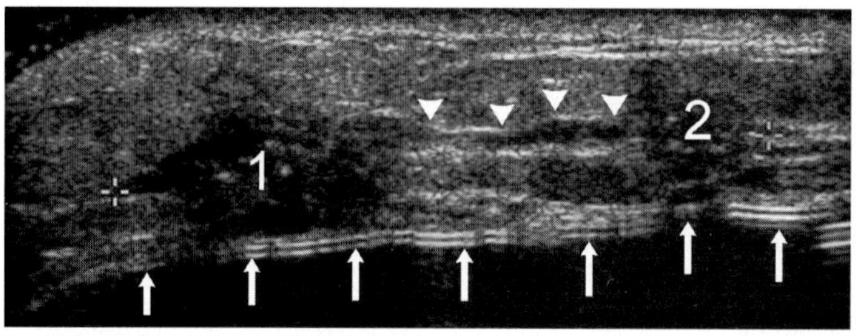

Figure 169–3. Left radial breast sonogram: With higher frequency, two masses are identified. One mass (labeled 1) corresponds to the mass previously identified with the lower-frequency exam. The second mass (labeled 2) is closer to the nipple and connected to the first mass with a dilated duct (arrowheads). Implant shell (arrows).

Other Modalities (Fig. 169–4 and 169–5)

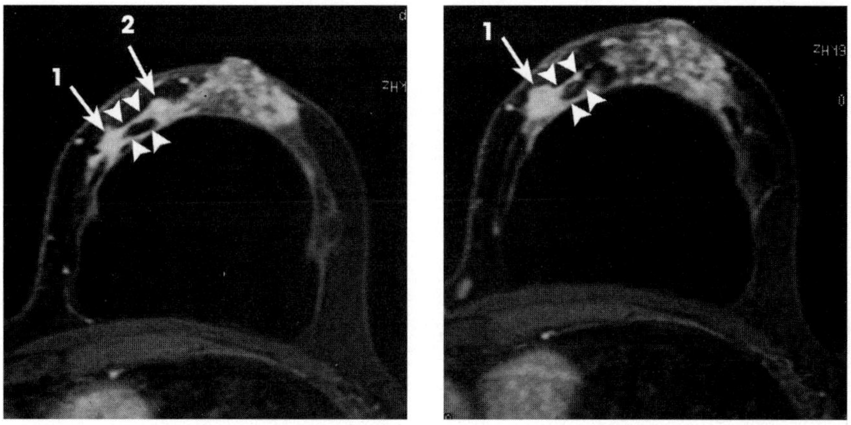

A B

Figure 169–4. *Both the masses identified sonographically are evident. The larger mass (labeled 1) is the mass identified on the mammogram and the lower-frequency sonogram. The smaller mass closer to the nipple (labeled 2) is the second mass identified on the high-frequency sonogram. Abnormal contrast enhancement connects the two masses (arrowheads). (A). Left transverse dynamic bolus three-dimensional (3-D) volume gradient series breast MRI. (B). Left transverse dynamic bolus 3-D volume gradient series breast MRI: This image is slightly cranial to Figure 169–4A.*

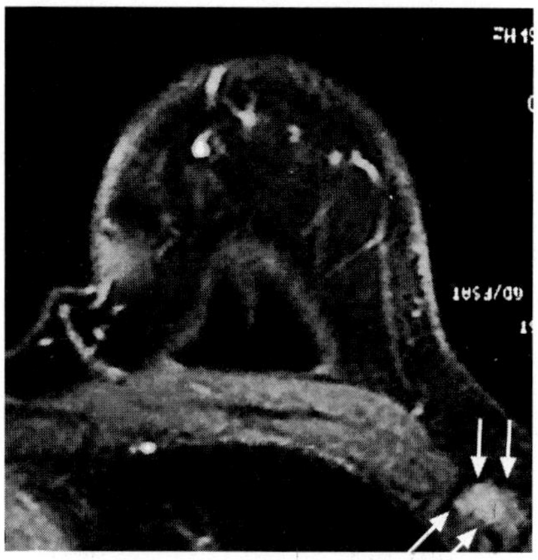

Figure 169–5. *Left transverse dynamic bolus 3-D volume gradient series breast MRI: Besides the abnormal breast masses, enhancing axillary lymphadenopathy is evident (arrows).*

Pathology

Infiltrating ductal carcinoma. Microscopically, the two sonographic masses corresponded to two separate masses of infiltrating ductal carcinoma. These masses were connected with an area of ductal carcinoma in situ. Sixteen of 21 axillary nodes were postive for metastatic disease.

Management

- BI-RADS Assessment Category 4, suspicious; biopsy should be considered

Pearls and Pitfalls

1. Because implants commonly obscure breast parenchyma, it is a challenge to optimize imaging of the surrounding tissues. An important routine technique for implant examination is performing the Eklund or implant-displaced views. By displacing the implant posteriorly, one can enhance imaging the breast tissue. However, even with Eklund views, visualization may be difficult. In this patient, the abnormality could only be identified in one orientation.
2. This case illustrates that higher-frequency sonography provides more information than lower-frequency sonography by demonstrating the presence of multifocal disease. One should be suspicious of multifocal disease from the mammographic calcifications. However, because these calcifications could not be optimally imaged mammographically, sonographic confirmation of multifocal disease was useful. Both masses were biopsied sonographically.

Suggested Readings

1. Barloon TJ, Young DC, Bergus G. The role of diagnostic imaging in women with breast implants. *Am Fam Physician* 1996;54:2029–2036.
2. Eklund GW, Busby RC, Miller SH, Job JS. Improved imaging of the augmented breast. *AJR* 1988;151:469–473.

Case 170

Case History

A 51-year-old woman notes two lumps on the lateral aspect of her right breast. She has had implants for more than 20 years.

Physical Examination

- right breast: two masses; one at 7:00 and the other subareaolar at 10:00
- left breast: normal exam

Mammogram (Fig. 170–1)

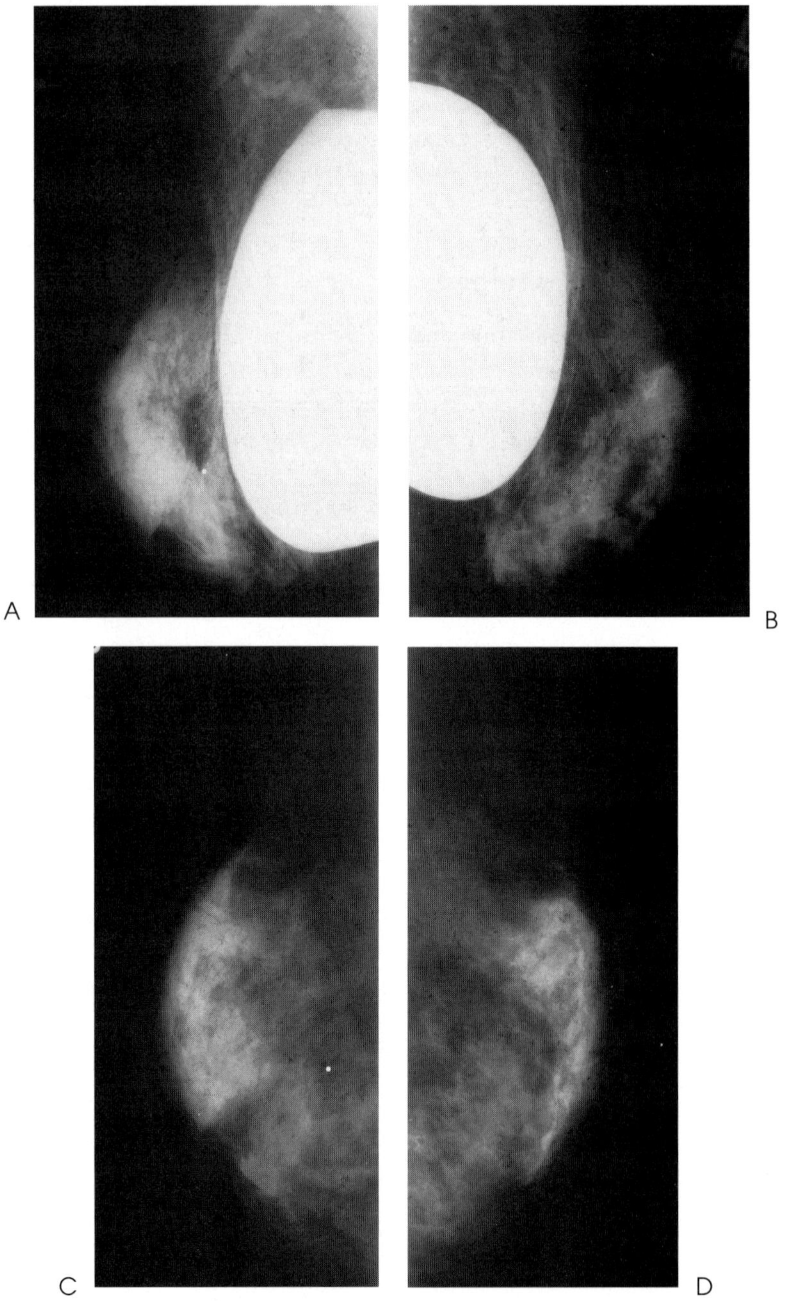

Figure 170–1. The mammograms are normal. No mammographic masses are associated with the palpable masses. (A). Right MLO implant mammogram. (B). Left MLO implant mammogram. (C). Right MLO implant-displaced mammogram. (D). Left MLO implant-displaced mammogram.

Figure 170–1 continued on next page ▷

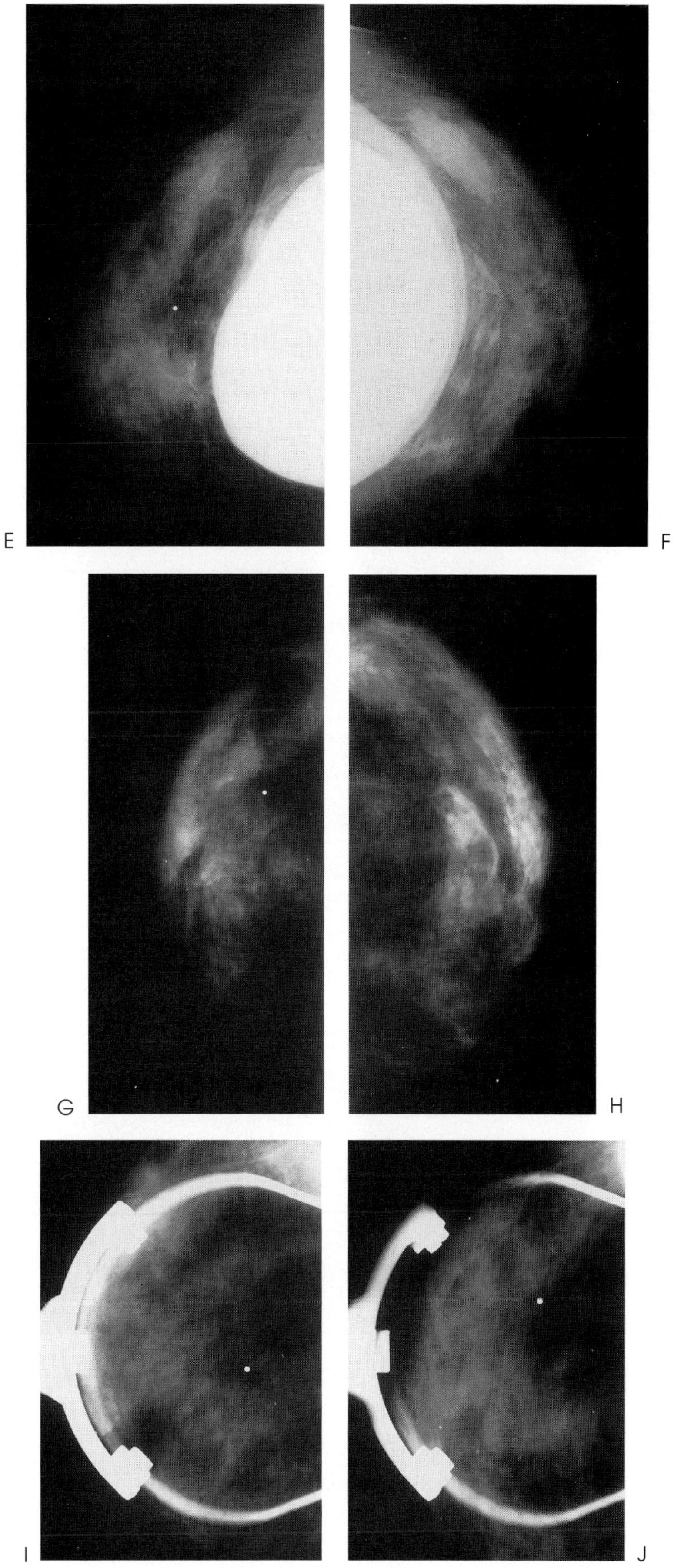

Figure 170–1. (continued from previous page) *(E). Right CC implant mammogram. (F). Left CC implant mammogram. (G). Right CC implant-displaced mammogram. (H). Left CC implant-displaced mammogram. (I). Right MLO spot compression mammogram. (J). Right CC spot compression mammogram.*

Ultrasound

Frequency

- 10 MHz

Mass (Figs. 170-2 and 170-3)

- margin: irregular
- echogenicity: hypoechoic
- retrotumoral acoustic appearance: no shadowing
- shape: lobulated

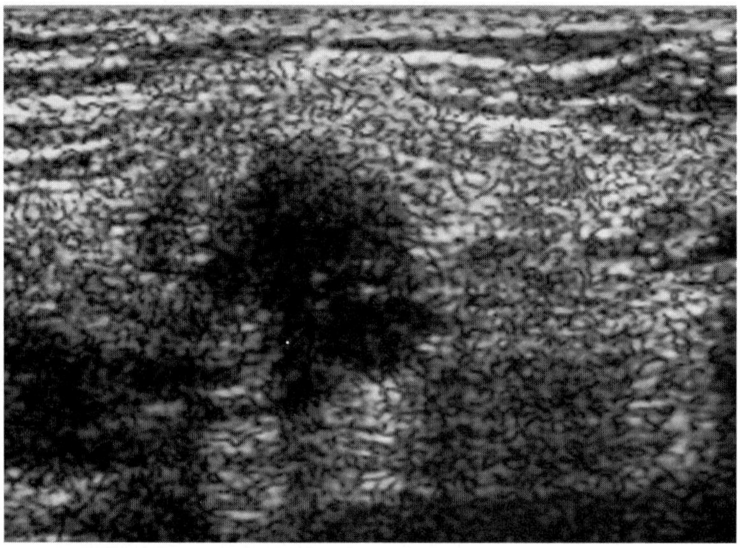

Figure 170-2. Right antiradial breast sonogram: At the 7:00 position, a palpable lump corresponds to an irregular, hypoechoic mass with calcifications.

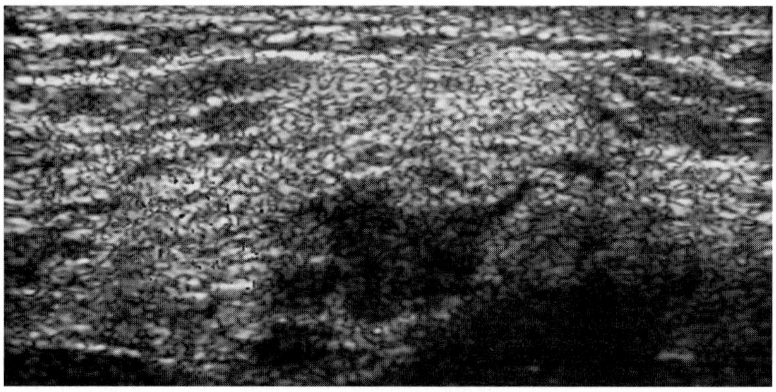

Figure 170-3. Right antiradial breast sonogram: At the 10:00 position, the second palpable mass corresponds to another irregular, hypoechoic mass.

Pathology

- infiltrating ductal carcinoma
- two separate but histologically similar nodules of infiltrating ductal carcinoma. Mass at 7:00 has <25% ductal carcinoma in situ and mass at 10:00 has no ductal carcinoma in situ.

Management

- BI-RADS Assessment Category 4, suspicious; biopsy should be considered

Pearls and Pitfalls

The risk of breast cancer is not increased in patients with breast augmentation. Palpable lumps should be examined in a manner similar to patients without augmentation. In this case, sonography was useful to identify multicentric disease.

Suggested Readings

1. Berkel H, Birdsell DC, Jenkins H. Breast augmentation: a risk factor for breast cancer? *N Engl J Med* 1992;326:1649–1653.
2. Leibman AJ, Kruse B. Breast cancer: mammographic and sonographic findings after augmentation mammoplasty. *Radiology* 1990;174:195–198.
3. Leibman AJ, Kruse BD. Imaging of breast cancer after augmentation mammoplasty. *Ann Plast Surg* 1993;30:111–115.

Case 171

Case History

A 61-year-old woman had reduction mammoplasty 2 years ago.

Physical Examination

- bilateral breasts: bilateral reduction scars, otherwise normal

Mammogram (Figs. 171–1 and 171–2)

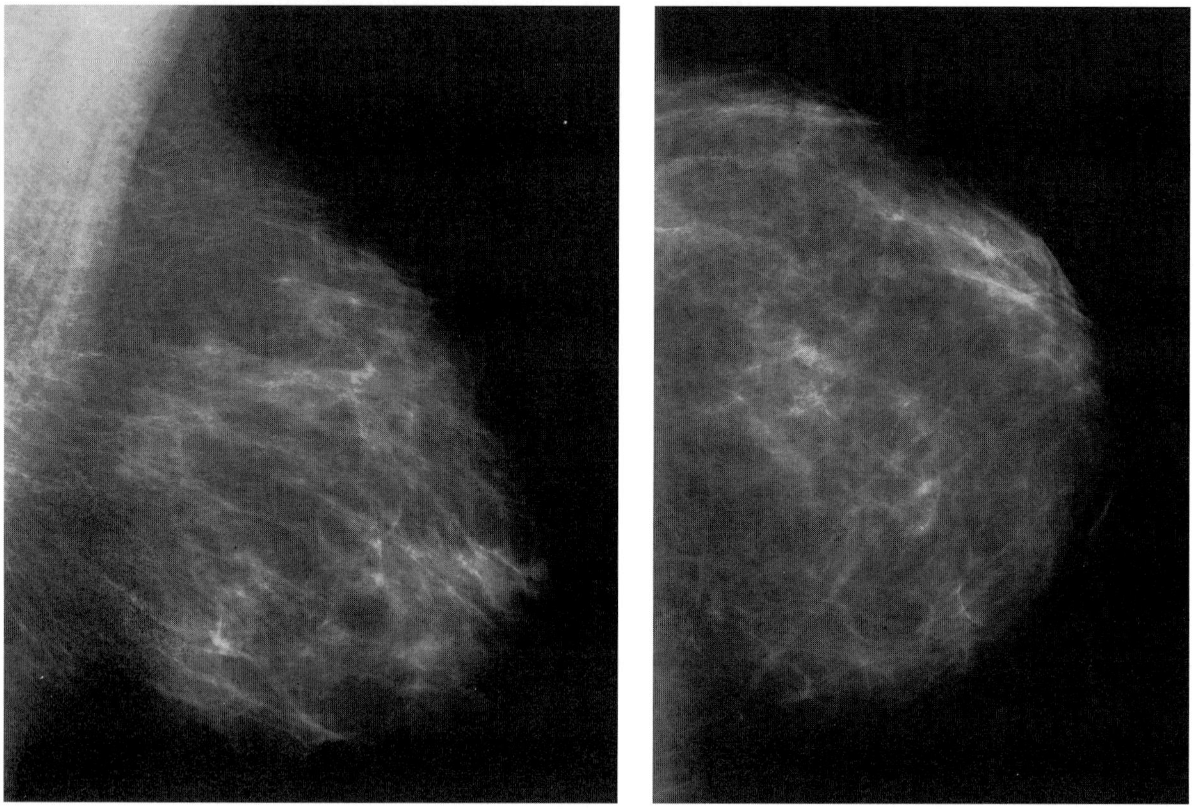

A B

Figure 171–1. Normal mammogram prior to reduction mammoplasty. (A). Left MLO mammogram. (B). Left CC mammogram.

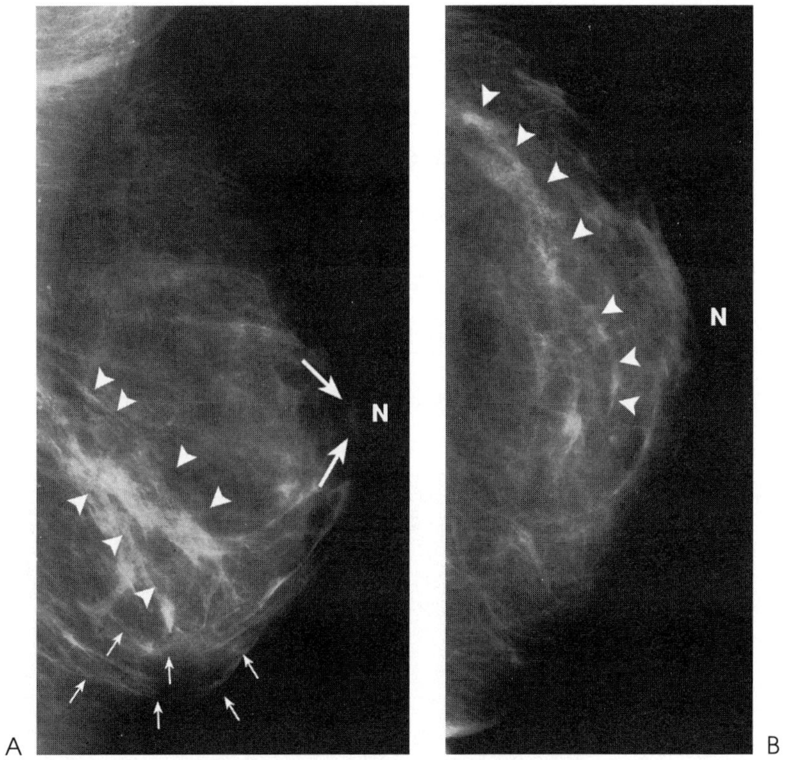

Figure 171–2. Normal mammogram 2 years after reduction mammoplasty. The nipple (N) is higher in position and the contour of the breast is flatter. Architectural distortion has resulted in (1) swirled lines (small arrows), (2) disruption of the normal subareolar ductal lines (large arrows), (3) increase in the density of the inferior breast, which in this patient is associated with straight parenchymal bands (arrowheads). (A). Left MLO mammogram. (B). Left CC mammogram.

Pathology

- changes from reduction mammoplasty

Management

- BI-RADS Assessment Category 2, benign finding

Pearls and Pitfalls

The various reduction mammoplasty procedures involve removing tissue from the inferior breast. The residual upper breast tissue is brought together in the midline to reform a smaller breast, and the nipple areolar complex is transposed superiorly. After these procedures, mammograms exhibit the following findings: (1) elevation of the nipple with flattening of the breast contour, (2) architectural distortion, (3) fat necrosis, (4) dystrophic calcifications, and (5) skin thickening.

Suggested Readings

1. Jackson VP. Reduction mammoplasty. In: Bassett LW, Jackson VP, Jahan R, Fu YS, Gold RH, eds. *Diagnosis of Diseases of the Breast.* Philadelphia: WB Saunders; 1997:581–587.

Case 172

Case History

An 85-year-old woman presents for screening mammogram.

Physical Examination

- bilateral breasts: reduction mammoplasty scars, otherwise normal

Mammogram (Fig. 172–1)

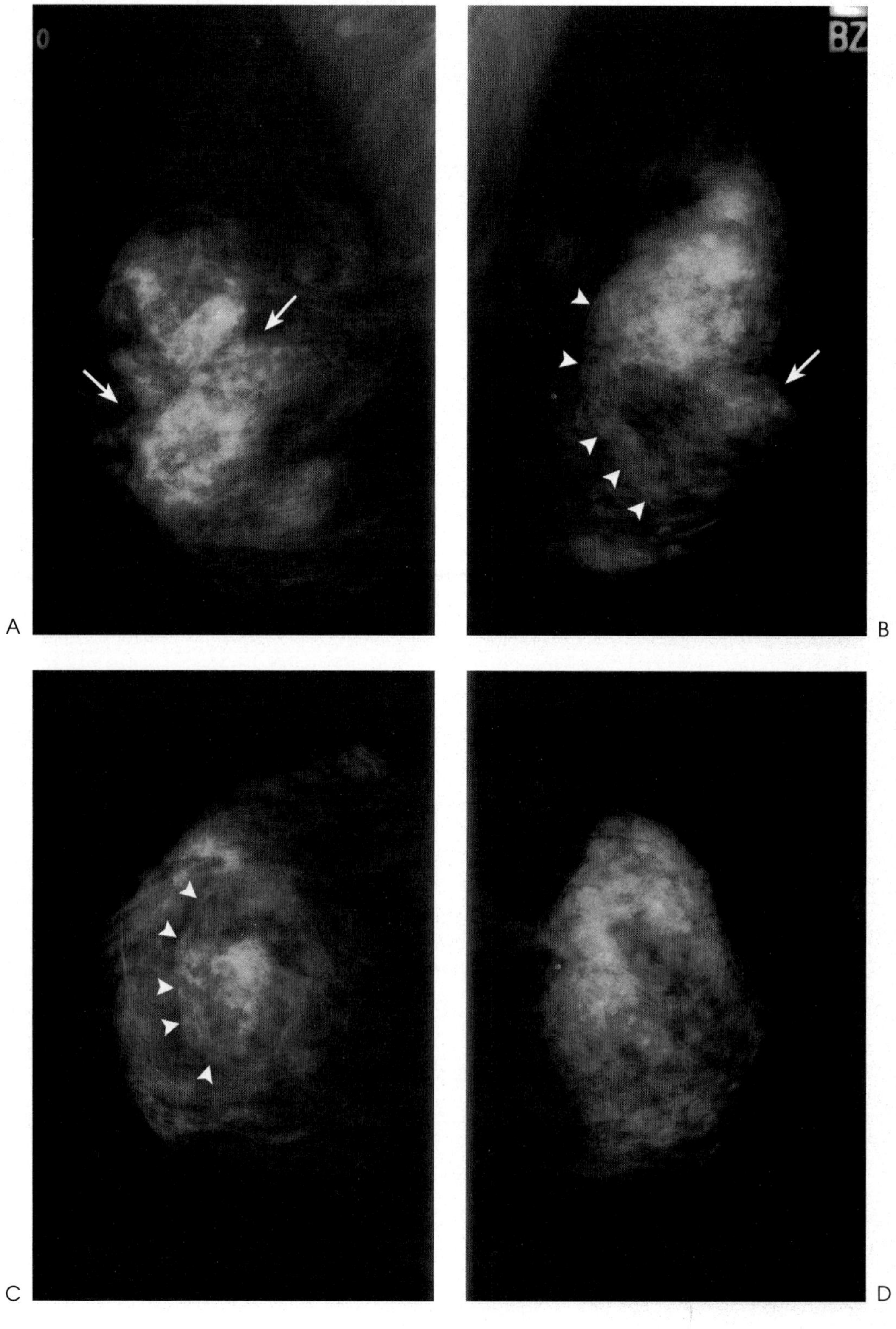

Figure 172–1. *Bilateral normal mammograms after reduction: Architectural distortion from reduction has resulted in asymmetry in both the anterior and posterior contours of the breasts. There are unusual indentations in the parenchymal outline (arrows). There are also linear and curvilinear parenchymal bands (arrowheads). (A). Right MLO mammogram. (B). Left MLO mammogram. (C). Right CC mammogram. (D). Left CC mammogram.*

Pathology

- changes from reduction mammoplasty

Management

- BI-RADS Assessment Category 2, benign finding

Pearls and Pitfalls

Architectural distortion from reduction includes unusual straight linear or swirling curvilinear parenchymal lines, loss of the normal subareolar ductal pattern, retroareolar fibrotic band, asymmetric parenchymal contours, and asymmetric parenchymal density.

Suggested Readings

1. Miller CL, Feig SA, Fox JW. Mammographic changes after reduction mammoplasty. *AJR* 1987;149:35–38.

Case 173

Case History

A 65-year-old woman presents with a palpable lump or thickening at the right 12:00 periareolar position. One year ago, she had reduction mammoplasty.

Physical Examination

- right breast: ill-defined subareolar thickening at 12:00
- left breast: less prominent but similar subareolar thickening

Mammogram (Fig. 173–1 and 173–2)

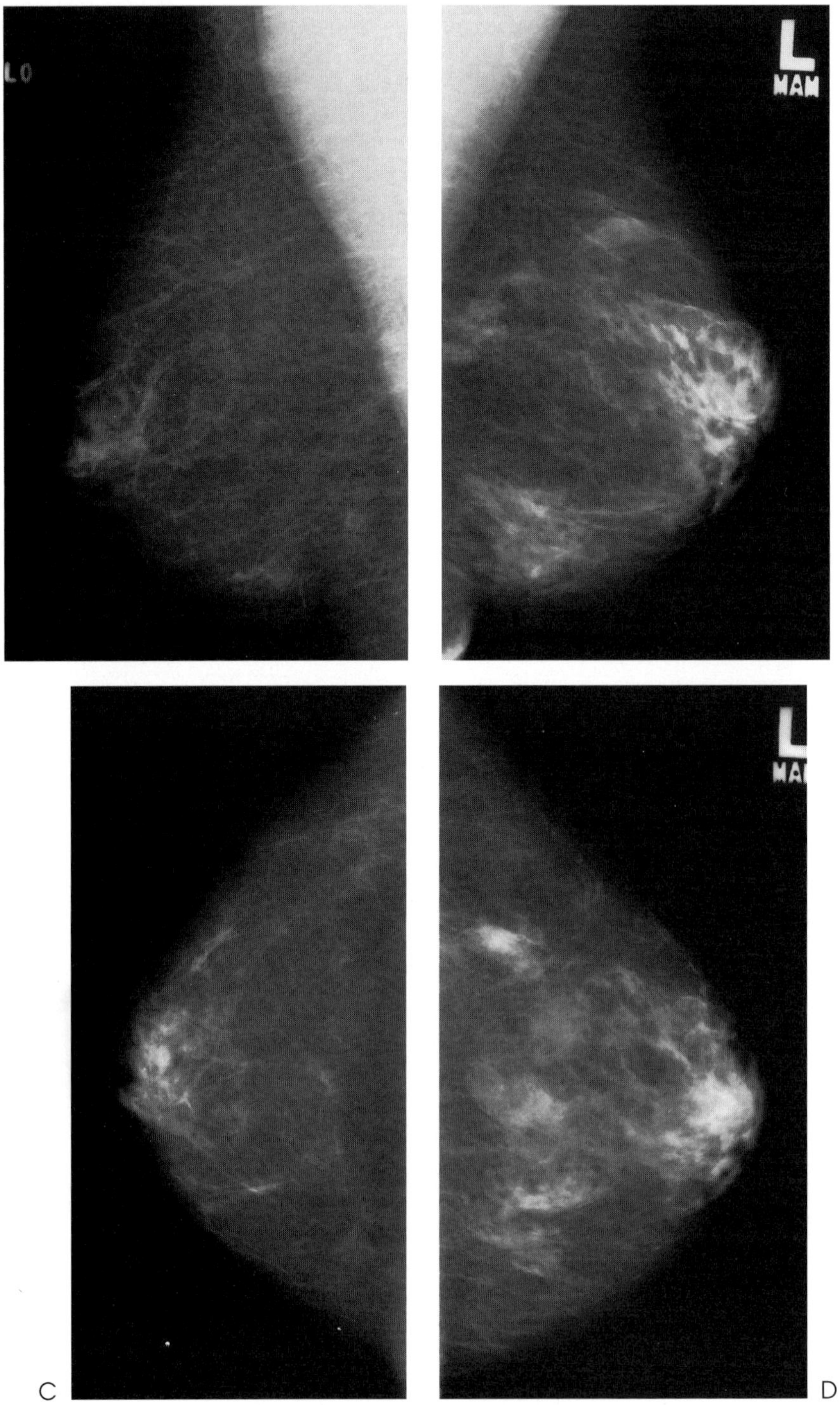

A B C D

Figure 173–1. The mammograms demonstrate changes due to previous reduction. The left breast exhibits asymmetric parenchymal densities, particularly in the inferior breast. This breast also demonstrates parenchymal swirls. Right breast does not exhibit any abnormal mass. (A). Right MLO mammogram. (B). Left MLO mammogram. (C). Right CC mammogram. (D). Left CC mammogram.

Ultrasound (Fig. 173-2)

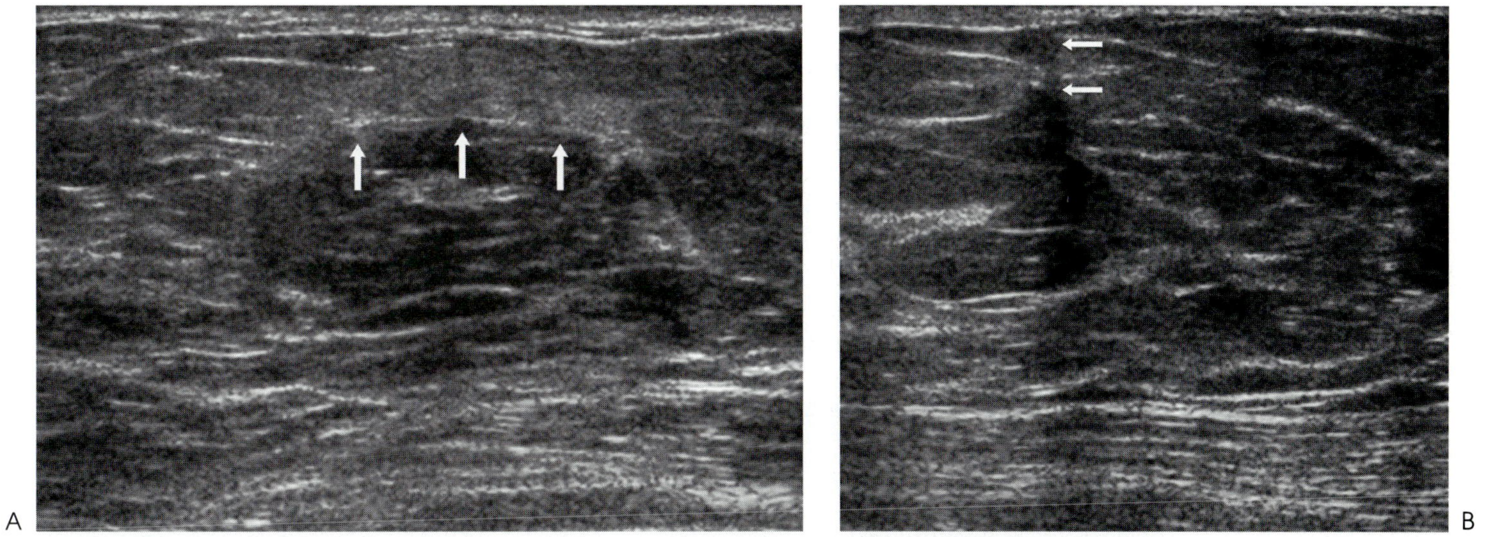

Figure 173-2. Sonographic examination of the right breast demonstrates that the periareolar thickening corresponds to an irregular hyperechoic line. This line represents a scar (arrows), which is wider in the antiradial view (A) compared to the radial view (B). In the radial view, the scar (arrows) appears as a thin straight line associated with shadowing. (A). Right antiradial breast sonogram. (B). Right radial breast sonogram.

Pathology

- scar

Management

- BI-RADS Assessment Category 2, benign finding

Pearls and Pitfalls

After the acute postsurgical changes have resolved, the most common palpable masses that develop after breast reduction are scar, fat necrosis, and carcinoma. The mammographic and sonographic identification of palpable masses in these women is similar to women who have not had reduction. Sonographically, scars may be differentiated from carcinoma if there is no mass associated with the architectural distortion (such as in this case).

Suggested Readings

1. Beer GM, Kompatscher P, Hergan K. Diagnosis of breast tumors after breast reduction. *Aesthetic Plast Surg* 1996;20:391-397.

Case 174

Case History

A 50-year-old woman presents for screening mammogram.

Physical Examination

- bilateral breasts: bilateral reduction mammoplasty scars, otherwise normal

Mammogram (Figs. 174–1 and 174–2)

Figure 174–1. These normal bilateral mammograms were performed prior to reduction mammoplasty. (A). Right MLO mammogram. (B). Left MLO mammogram. (C). Right CC mammogram. (D). Left CC mammogram.

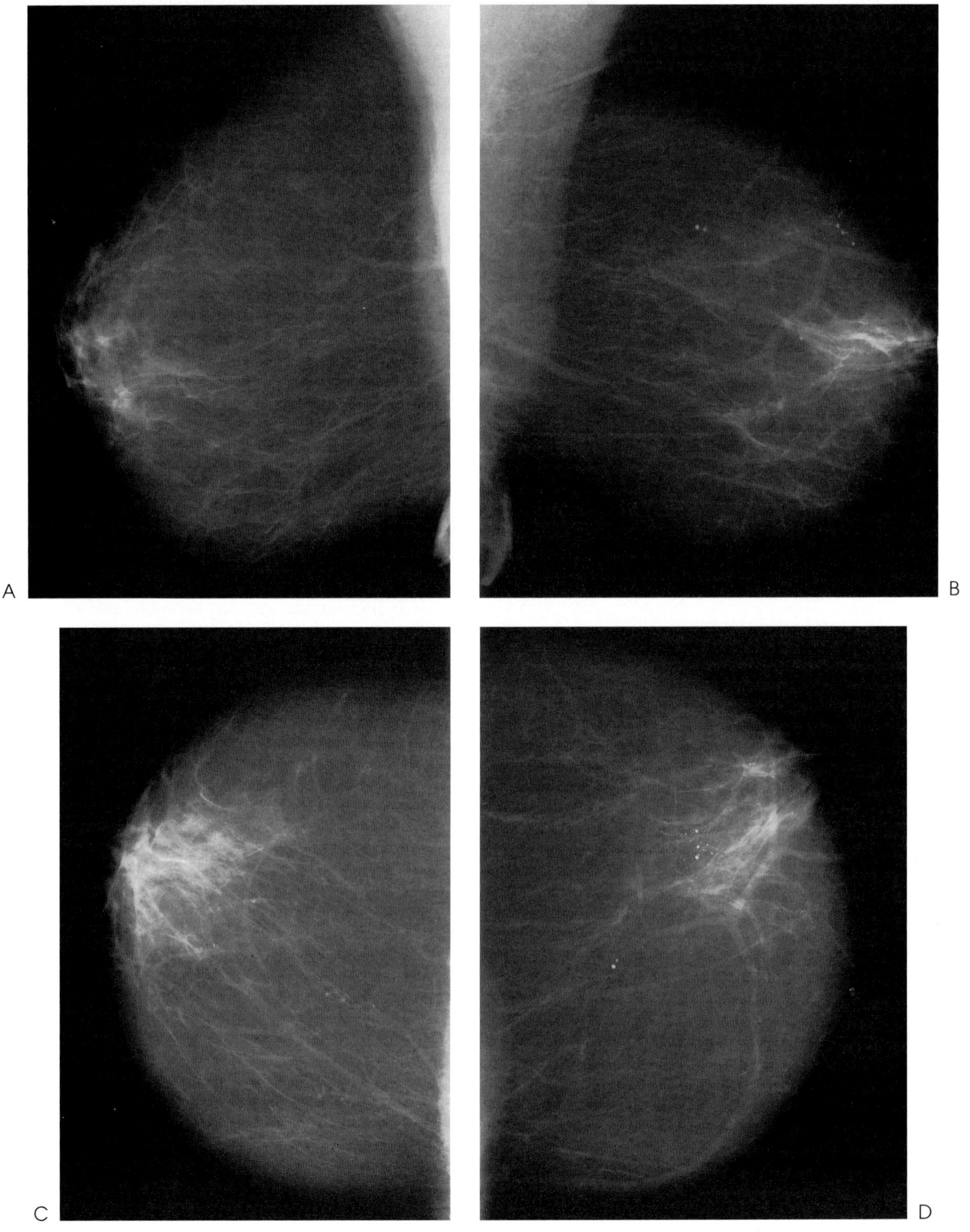

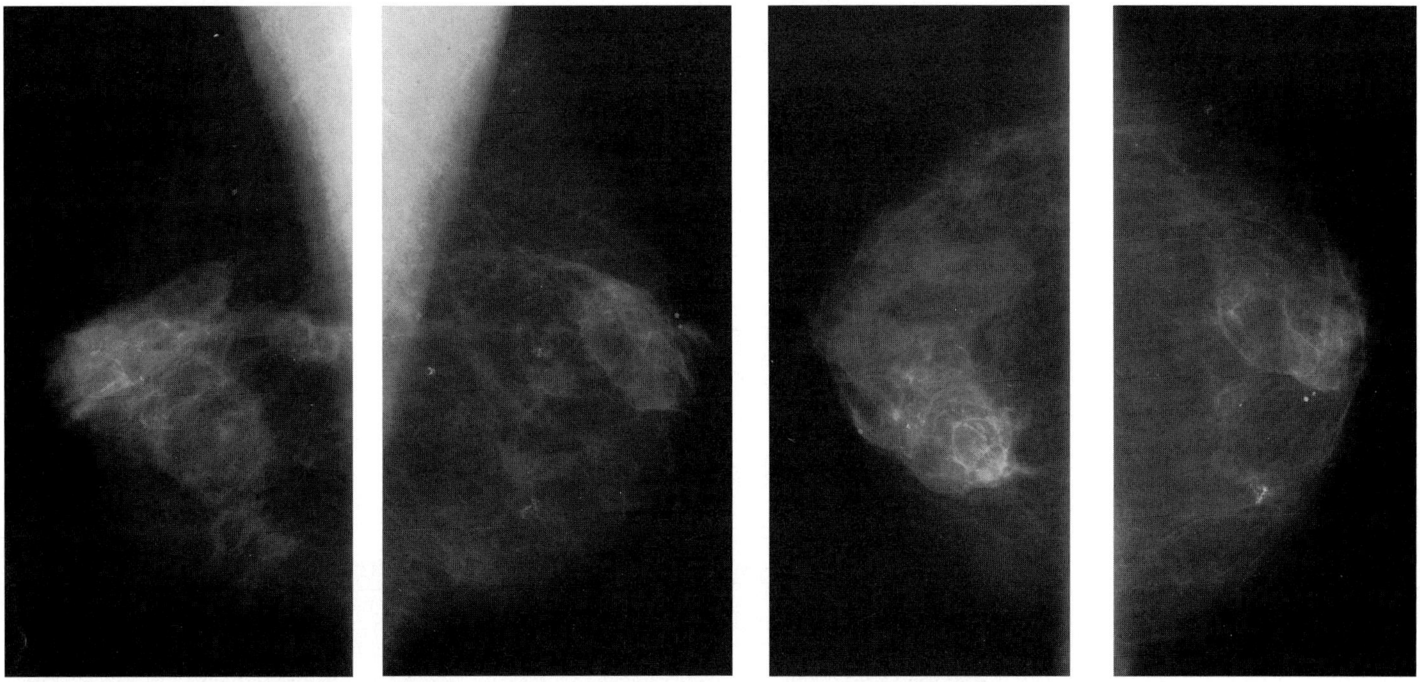

A B C D

Figure 174–2. Bilateral mammograms after reduction mammoplasty: Both breasts exhibit new dystrophic calcifications. There are also multiple rounded lucencies indicating fat necrosis. (A). Right MLO mammogram. (B). Left MLO mammogram. (C). Right CC mammogram. (D). Left CC mammogram.

Pathology

- fat necrosis

Management

- BI-RADS Assessment Category 2, benign finding

Pearls and Pitfalls

1. Benign calcifications are a common finding after breast reduction: 20 to 50% of patients develop new calcifications, and most of these calcifications develop 2 years after the patient's reduction mammoplasty. The most common benign calcifications are either characteristic of oil cysts or are large, coarse, and dystrophic in appearance. Less commonly, suture calcifications may appear. Calcifications are commonly located in the periareolar or inferior aspect of the breast.
2. Fat necrosis is mammographically evident in about 10% of patients after breast reduction. Although fat necrosis is generally easily identifiable mammographically, occasionally fat necrosis will produce an irregular mass and/or heterogeneous calcifications that simulate malignancy.

Suggested Readings

1. Brown FE, Sargent SK, Cohen SR, Morain WD. Mammographic changes following reduction mammoplasty. *Plast Reconst Surg* 80;1987:691–698.
2. Miller JA, Festa S, Golstein M. Benign fat necrosis simulating bilateral breast malignancy after reduction mammoplasty. *South Med J* 1998;91:765–767.
3. Mitnick JS, Roses DF, Harris MN, Colen SR. Calcifications of the breast after reduction mammoplasty. *Surg Gynecol Obstet* 1990;171;409–412.

Case 175

Case History

A 77-year-old woman presents for screening right breast mammogram. She had a left mastectomy for neoplasm and a benign right excisional biopsy several years ago.

Physical Examination

- normal exam

Mammogram (Fig. 175–1)

A 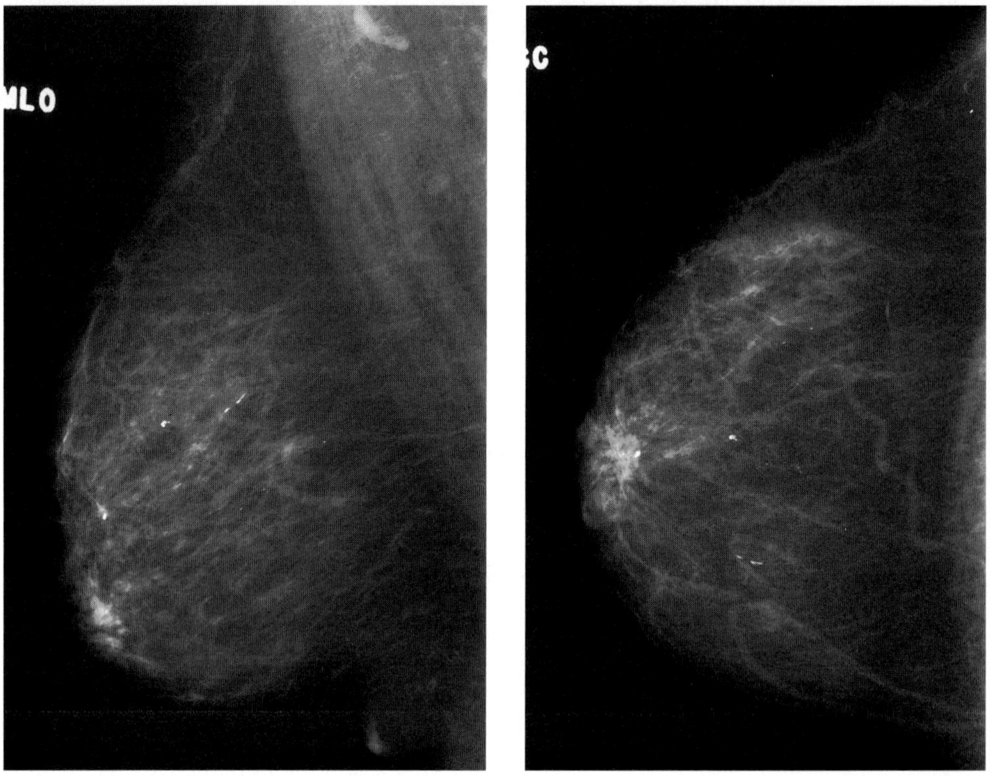 B

Figure 175–1. *In the right subareolar area, there is disruption and distortion of the ductal system. This architectural distortion resulted from the patient's benign excisional biopsy and has been stable for at least 10 years. (A). Right MLO mammogram. (B). Right CC mammogram.*

Pathology

- scar

Management

- BI-RADS Assessment Category 2, benign finding

Pearls and Pitfalls

Mammographically, scar presents as architectural distortion or irregular density. Patients treated for malignancy demonstrate scarring more often than those treated for benign lesions. One year after surgery, more than 90% of patients treated with lumpectomy and radiation therapy have mammographically detectable scars compared with less than 50% for those experiencing benign excisional biopsies. Five years after surgery, architectural distortion is mammographically evident in 70 and 20%, respectively.

Suggested Readings

1. Brenner RJ, Pfaff JM. Mammographic features after conservation therapy for malignant breast disease: serial findings standardized by regression analysis. *AJR* 1996;167:171–178.
2. Mendelson EB. Evaluation of the postoperative breast. *Radiol Clin North Am* 1992;30:107–138.
3. Sickles EA, Herzog KA. Mammography of the postsurgical breast. *AJR* 1981;136:585–588.

Case 176

Case History

A 66-year-old woman had a left breast lumpectomy and radiation therapy 6 months ago.

Physical Examination

- left breast: large scar; otherwise normal exam
- right breast: normal exam

Mammogram

Mass (Fig. 176–1)

- margin: spiculated
- shape: irregular
- density: high

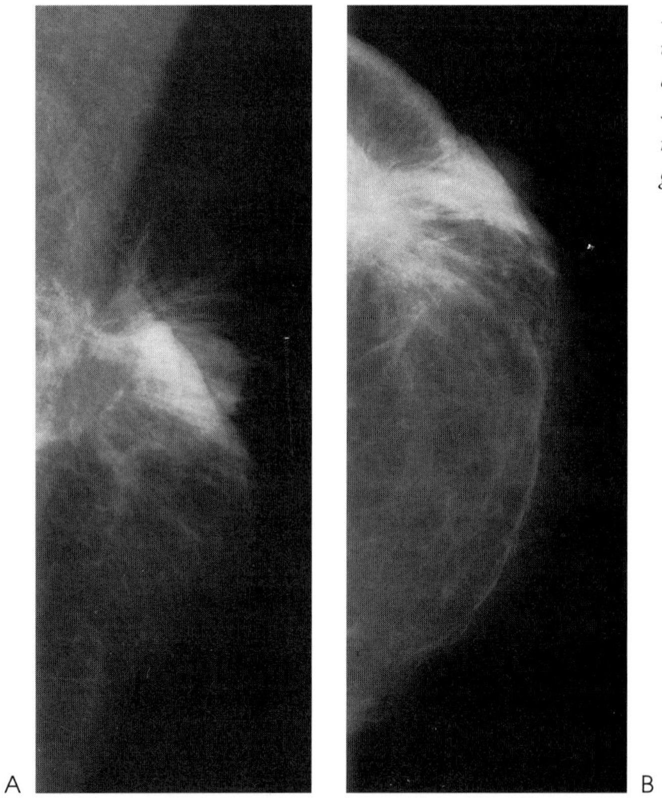

Figure 176–1. *In the site of previous lumpectomy, there is irregular density, architectural distortion, spiculation, skin thickening, and retraction. (A). Left MLO mammogram. (B). Left CC mammogram.*

Pathology

- scar

Management

- BI-RADS Assessment Category 2, benign finding

Pearls and Pitfalls

Within the first year, the density associated with breast excision is a combination of hematoma, fat necrosis, and scar. The combination of these abnormalities will produce either an ill-defined regional density or a focal irregular mass. When the postoperative lesion is a regional density, the density may decrease in size but it tends to persist even after 5 years. However, when the postsurgical abnormality is a mass, it tends to completely resolve.

Suggested Readings

1. Brenner RJ, Pfaff JM. Mammographic features after conservation therapy for malignant breast disease: serial findings standardized by regression analysis. *AJR* 1996;167:171–178.

Case 177

Case History

A 77-year-old woman had right lumpectomy and radiation 2 years ago.

Physical Examination

- right breast: lumpectomy scar; otherwise normal exam
- left breast: normal exam

Mammogram

Mass (Figs. 177–1 and 177–2)

- margin: spiculated
- shape: irregular
- density: equal density

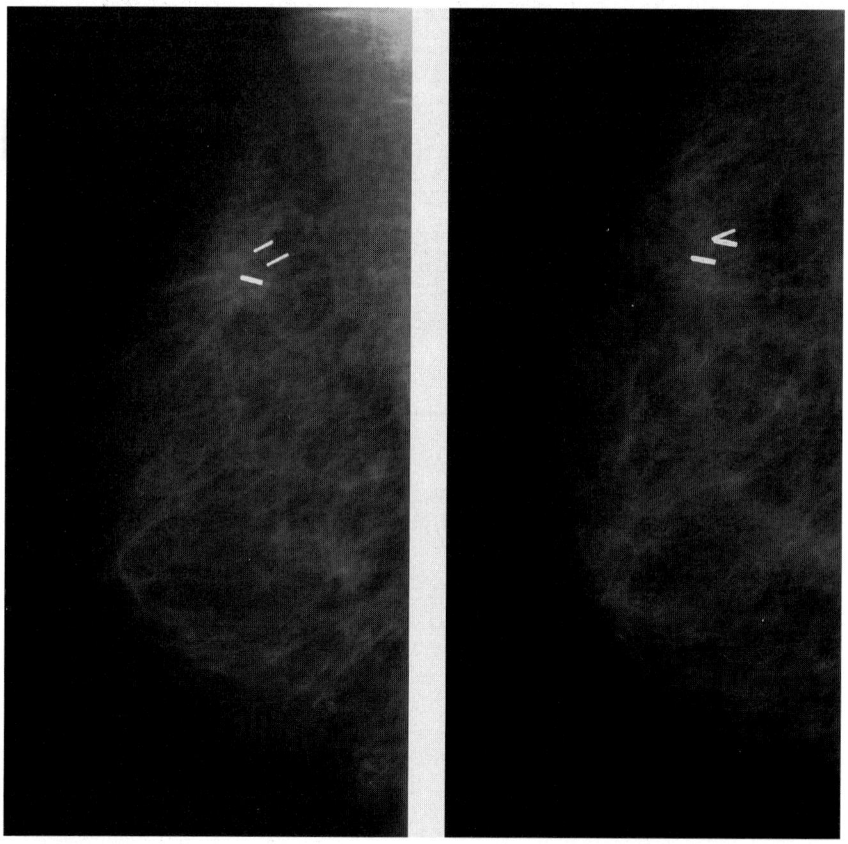
A B

Figure 177–1. These mammograms were performed 1 year after lumpectomy and radiation therapy. There is an ill-defined density associated with the clips from the previous lumpectomy. (A). Right MLO mammogram. (B). Right exaggerated CC mammogram.

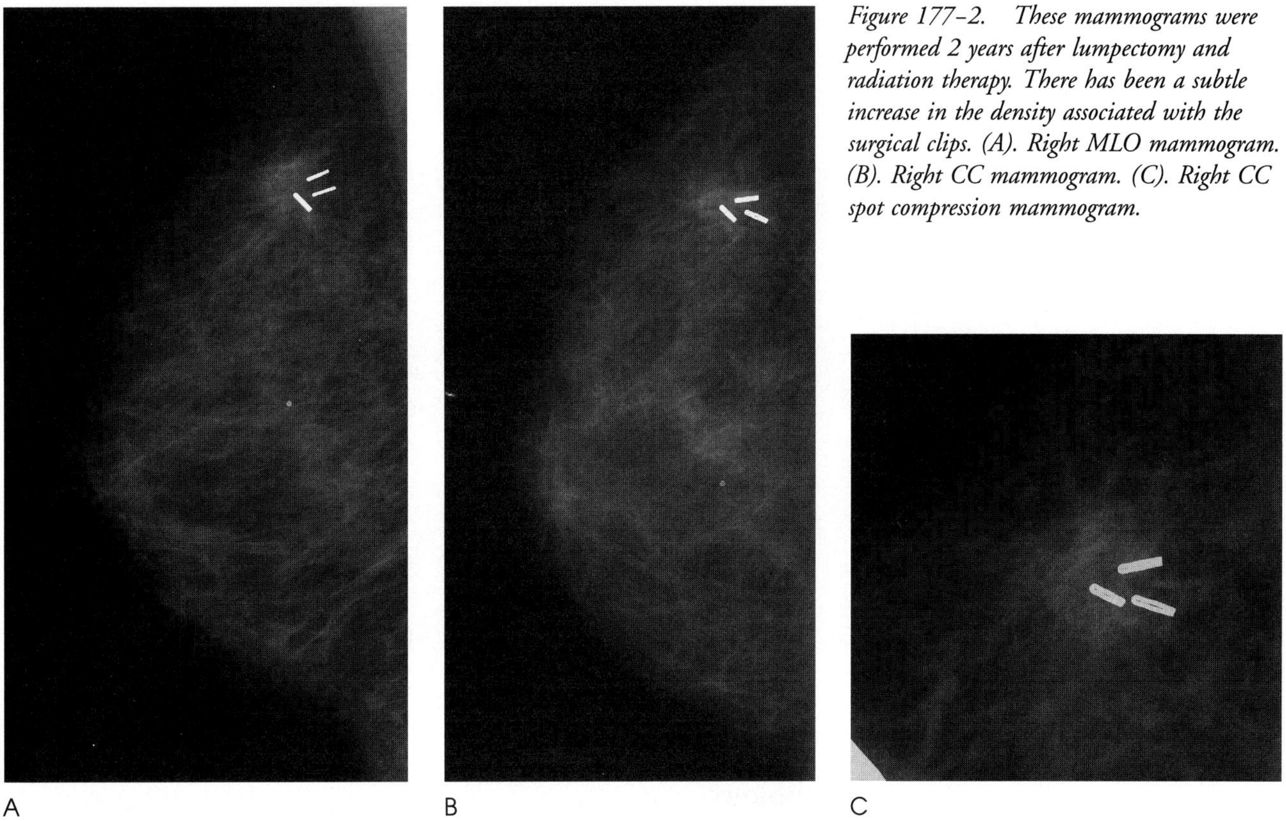

Figure 177–2. These mammograms were performed 2 years after lumpectomy and radiation therapy. There has been a subtle increase in the density associated with the surgical clips. (A). Right MLO mammogram. (B). Right CC mammogram. (C). Right CC spot compression mammogram.

Ultrasound

Low Frequency

Frequency

- 7 MHz

Mass

- margin: spiculation/architectural distortion
- echogenicity: hypoechoic
- retrotumoral acoustic appearance: severe shadowing, mass completely obscured
- shape: irregular (Fig. 177–3)

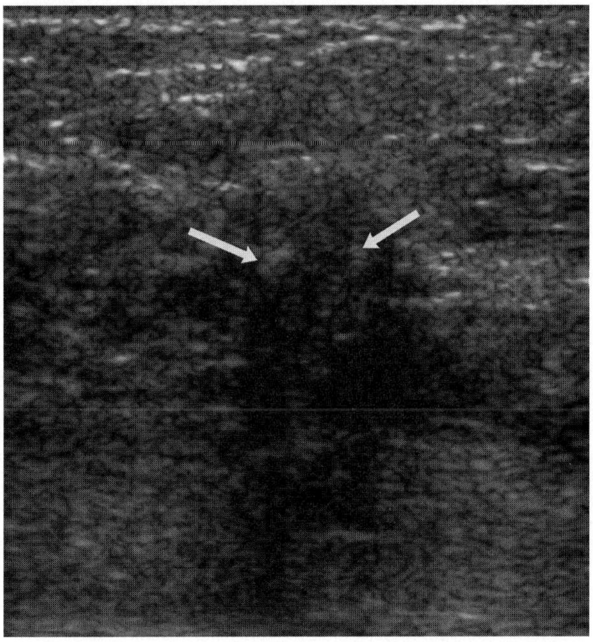

Figure 177–3. Right breast radial sonogram: With lower-frequency sonography, the lumpectomy site still exhibits an irregular, hypoechoic solid mass. Surgical clips (arrows) (see Color Plate 177–3).

High Frequency

Frequency

- 11.5 MHz (Fig. 177–4)

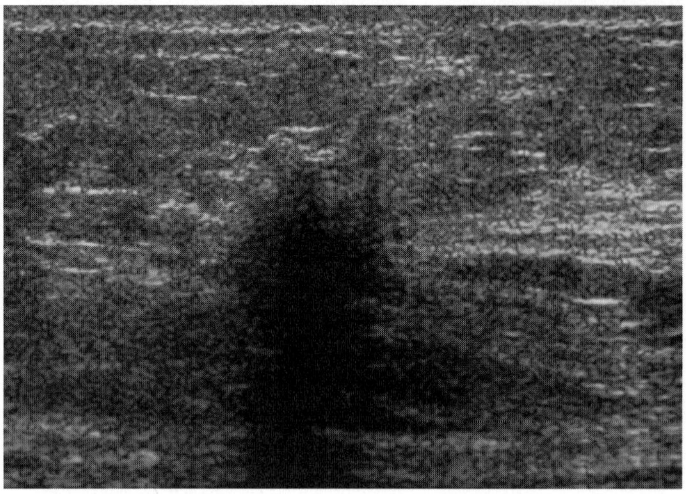

Figure 177–4. Right breast radial sonogram: With high-frequency sonography, the lumpectomy site is an irregular hypoechoic, heavily shadowing mass.

Pathology

- scar

Management

- BI-RADS Assessment Category 4, suspicious; biopsy should be considered

Pearls and Pitfalls

1. Usually, scars remain unchanged or diminish in mammographic density and size. However, if the mammographic density of an excisional site increases and the site exhibits a sonographic mass, then biopsy is indicated.
2. Sonographically, scars commonly cause severe posterior acoustic shadowing. If this shadowing is present when using a high frequency, then one should switch to low frequency. A benign scar produces a hyperechoic irregularity without a mass. However, this case illustrates that some scars appear identical to malignancies.

Suggested Readings

1. Mendelson EB. Imaging the post-surgical breast. *Semin Ultrasound CT MR* 1989;10:154–170.

Case 178

Case History

A 61-year-old woman has had 6 months of left breast pain. She had a benign left breast biopsy 20 years ago.

Physical Examination

- left breast: scar in left upper outer quadrant; also extremely tender to palpation in the upper outer quadrant
- right breast: diffusely mildly tender, otherwise normal exam

Mammogram (Fig. 178–1)

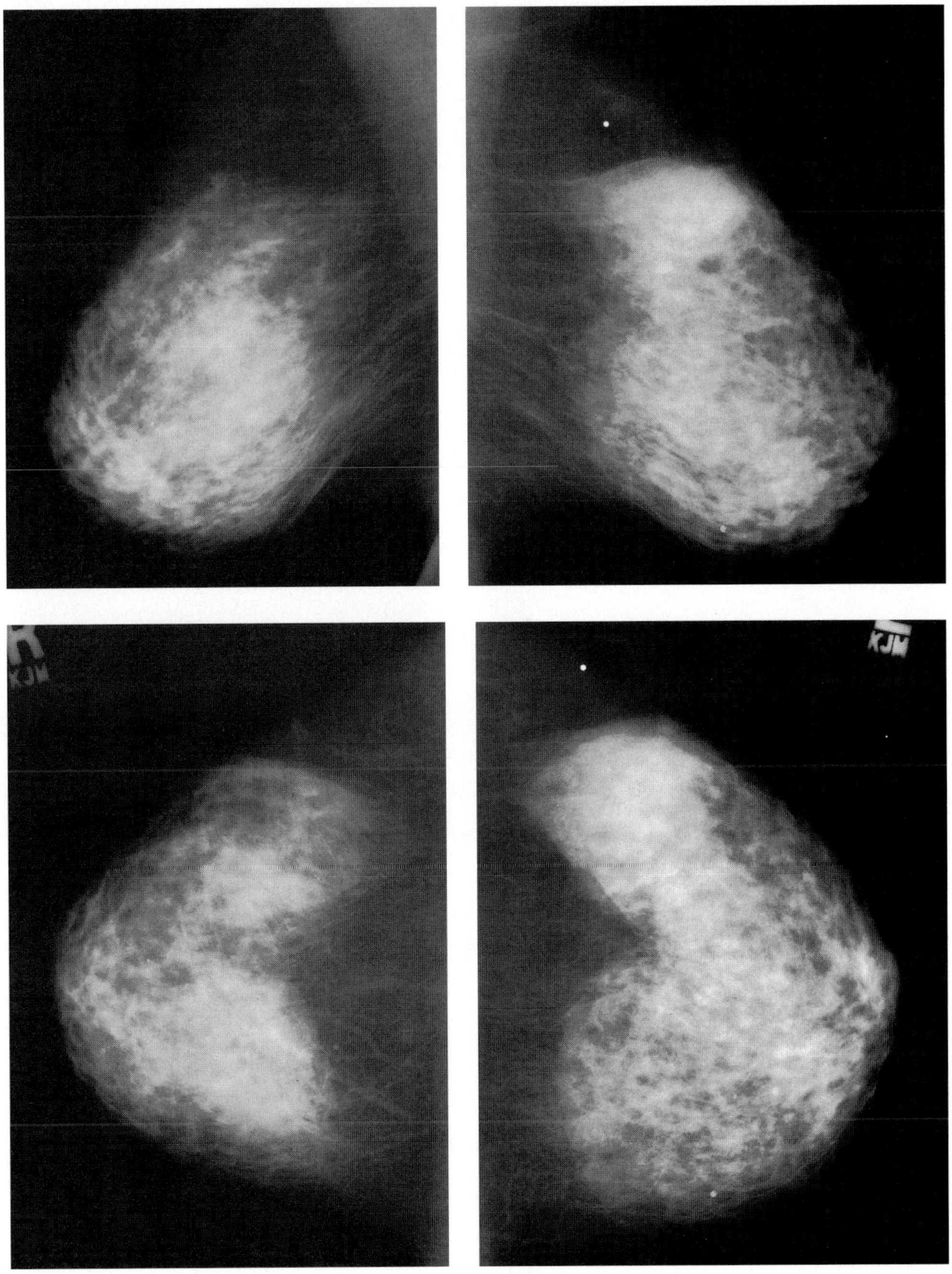
A B C D

Figure 178–1. *Bilateral normal mammograms. (A). Right MLO mammogram. (B). Left MLO mammogram. (C). Right CC mammogram. (D). Left CC mammogram.*

Ultrasound

Low Frequency

Frequency

- 10 MHz (Fig. 178-2)

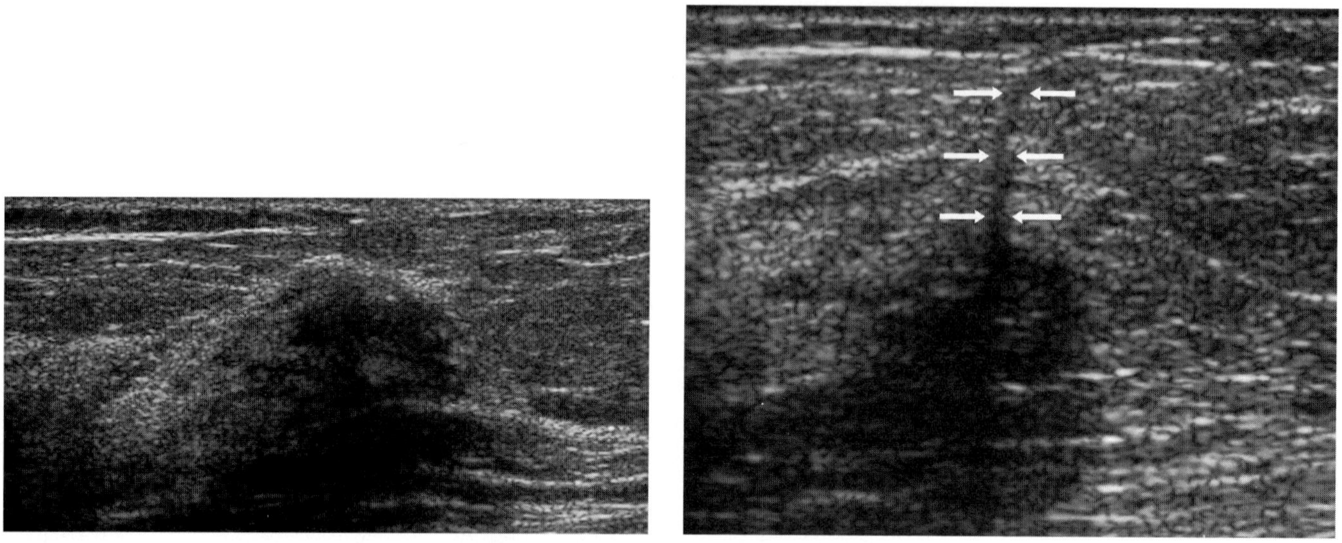

Figure 178-2. With lower frequency in the radial view (A) the scar appears to be a hypoechoic area, but the antiradial view (B) demonstrates that the lesion corresponds to a thin line of architectural distortion associated with shadowing (arrows). (A). Left radial breast sonogram. (B). Left antiradial breast sonogram.

High Frequency

Frequency

- 13 MHz (Fig. 178-3)

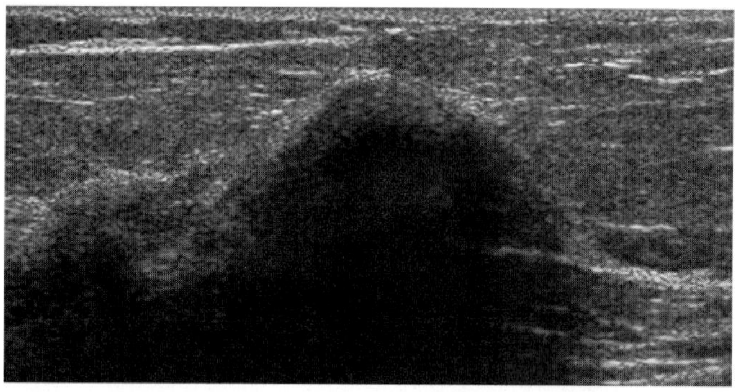

Figure 178-3. Left radial breast sonogram: The patient's scar was in the middle of the area of tenderness. With high frequency, the scar creates severe shadowing so the benign nature of this lesion is not visible.

Pathology

- scar

Management

- BI-RADS Assessment Category 2, benign finding

Pearls and Pitfalls

1. In an area of surgical excision, one may mammographically differentiate scar from neoplasm in the following ways: (1) identify lucencies within the center of the scar; (2) observe that the scar changes in appearance with different views; and (3) note decreases in size or density of the lesion on sequential exams.
2. Sonographically, scars have the following characteristics: (1) scars are hyperechoic; (2) they exhibit different appearances with different angles; and (3) benign scars have no associated hypoechoic mass (which is visible on two views). Because scars strongly attenuate sound, lower-frequency sonography is generally better than higher-frequency sonography in characterizing scars.

Suggested Readings

1. Mendelson EB. Evaluation of the postoperative breast. *Radiol Clin North Am* 1992;30:107–138.

Case 179

Case History

A 63-year-old woman presents 3 months after right lumpectomy for breast cancer. She now has a lump in her surgical site.

Physical Examination

- right breast: tender palpable lump in the lumpectomy site
- left breast: normal exam

Mammogram

Mass (Figs. 179–1 and 179–2)

- margin: circumscribed
- shape: oval
- density: equal density

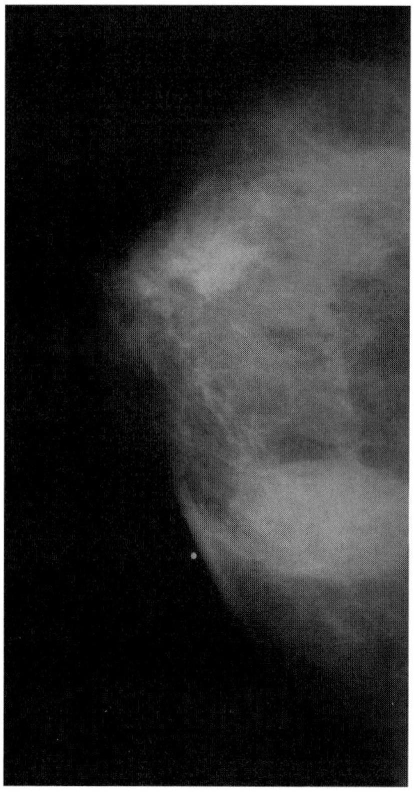

A

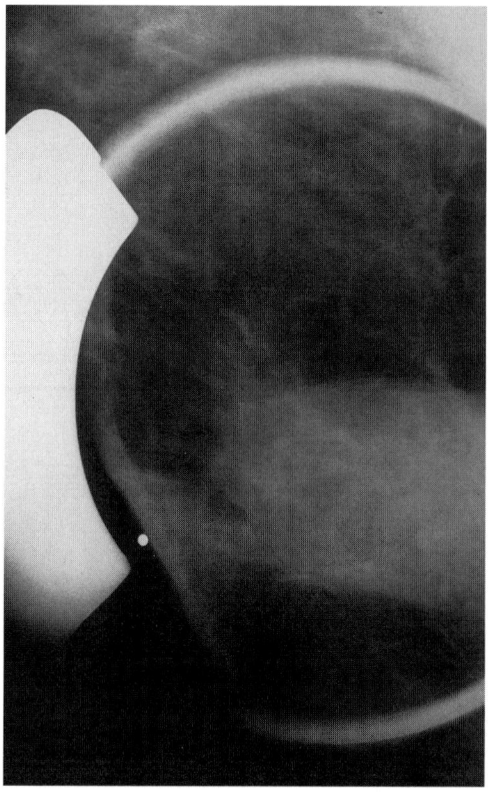

B

Figure 179–1. Three months after patient's right lumpectomy, there is an ill-defined oval mass associated with the lumpectomy site. The palpable lump corresponds to this mass. (A). Right CC mammmogram. (B). Right CC spot compression mammogram.

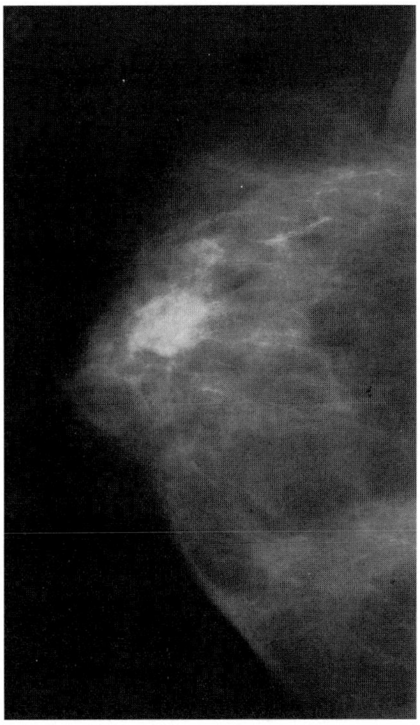

Figure 179–2. *Right CC mammogram: Ten months after the patient's surgery, the oval mass has decreased in size and density.*

Ultrasound

Frequency

- 7 MHz

Mass

- margin: well defined
- echogenicity: heterogeneous (mixed)
- retrotumoral acoustic appearance: increased acoustic transmission
- shape: ellipsoid (Figs. 179–3 and 179–4)

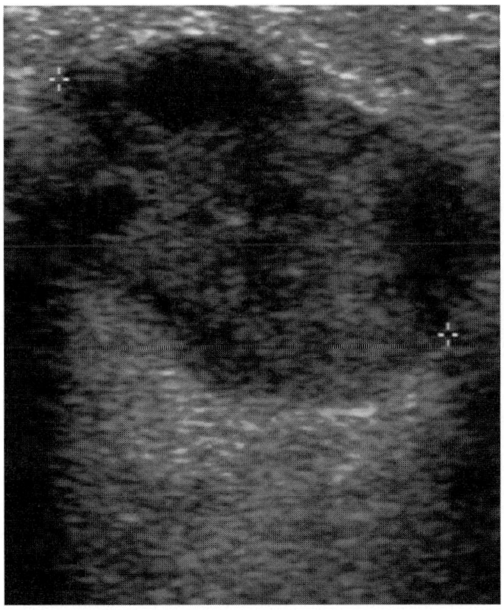

Figure 179–3. *Right transverse breast sonogram: Three months after surgery, the palpable lump is a sonographically complex, well-defined fluid collection with heterogeneous echogenicity and increased acoustic transmission.*

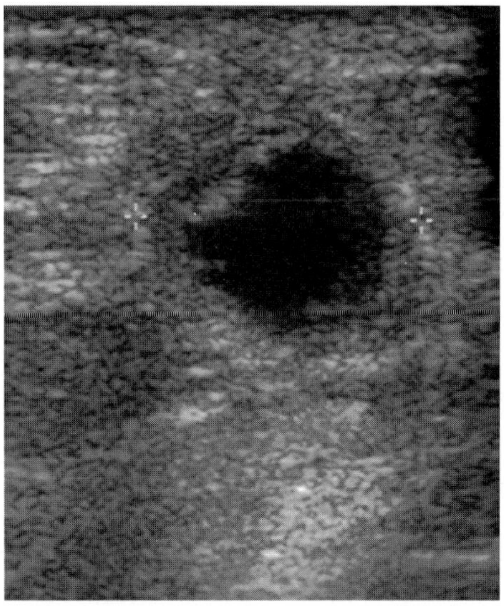

Figure 179–4. *Right transverse breast sonogram: Sonographic examination 10 months after surgery demonstrates that the fluid collection has greatly decreased in size. The fluid is anechoic and surrounded by thick walls. Anterior to the fluid, there is architectural distortion with skin thickening.*

Pathology

- hematoma

Management

- BI-RADS Assessment Category 2, benign finding

Pearls and Pitfalls

1. Hematomas or seromas have been observed in 50% of patients 1 month after surgery. These lesions tend to resolve so only 25% of patients exhibit fluid collections 6 months after excision. However, rarely patients will have persistent seromas years later.
2. Mammographically, the hematoma/seroma typically appears as an oval mass of water density. Sometimes, the mass may demonstrate fat-fluid layering on 90 degree lateral views. The margins may be well defined, ill defined, or spiculated.
3. Sonographically, the hematoma/seroma is a hypoechoic, anechoic, or heterogeneous fluid collection. Internal septations and dependent solid material may be present.

Suggested Readings

1. Soo MS, Williford ME. Seromas in the breast: imaging findings. *Crit Rev Diagn Imaging* 1995;36:385–440.

Case 180

Case History

A 59-year-old woman had excision of ductal carcinoma in situ and radiation therapy 4 months ago. She now notes a ridge next to her lumpectomy site.

Physical Examination

- left breast: vague ridge of tissue in the axilla near healing scar
- right breast: normal exam

Mammogram

- asymmetric density (Fig. 180–1)

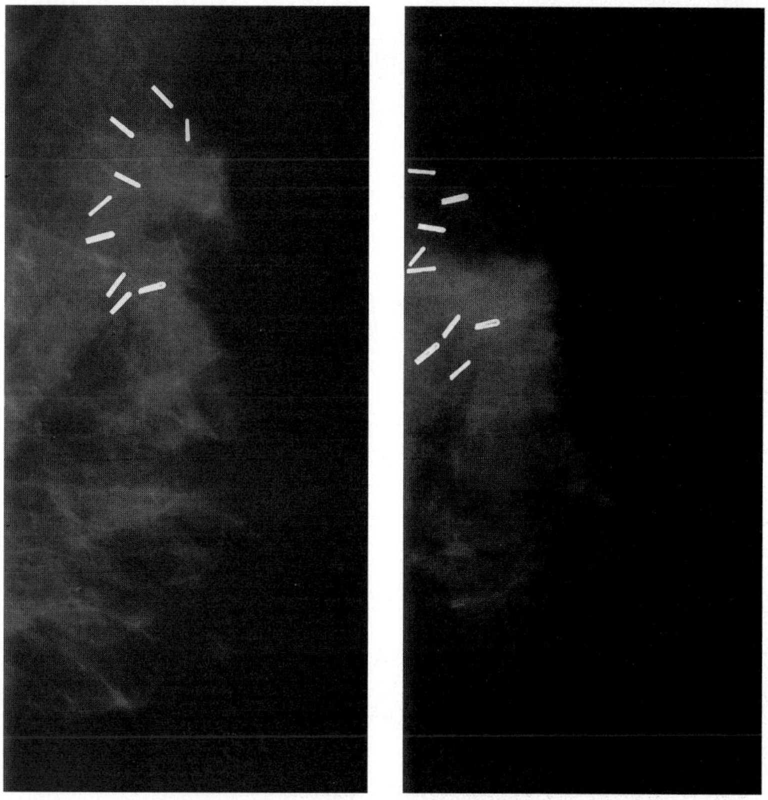

A B

Figure 180–1. In the left upper outer breast there are clips and ill-defined density in the lumpectomy site. (A). Left MLO mammogram. (B). Left exaggerated CC mammogram.

Ultrasound

Frequency

- 14 MHz

Mass

- margin: ill defined
- echogenicity: hypoechoic
- retrotumoral acoustic appearance: single edge shadowing
- shape: irregular (Figs. 180–2 and 180–3)

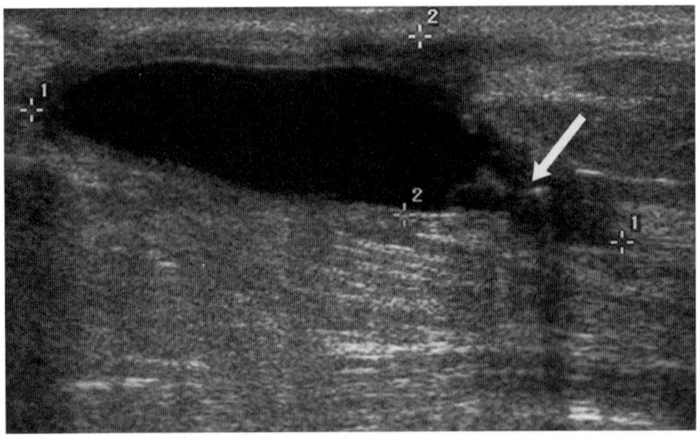

Figure 180–2. Left radial breast sonogram: Within the lumpectomy site there is a well-defined anechoic fluid collection that is characteristic of a hematoma or seroma. Anteriorly there is architectural distortion and skin thickening. At the edge of the fluid is a hyperechoic, shadowing focus (arrow), which is one of the clips.

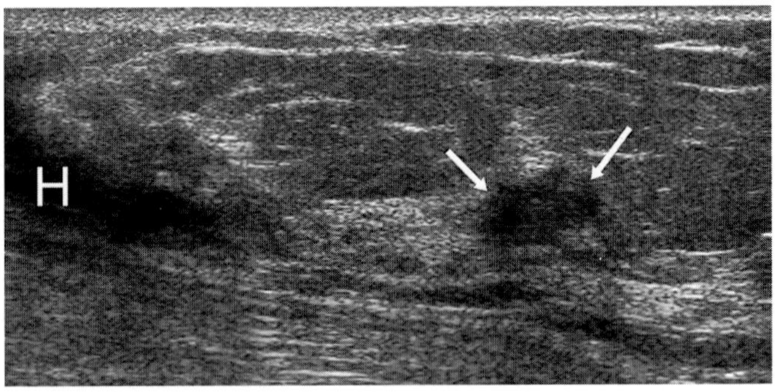

Figure 180–3. Left radial breast sonogram: Next to the hematoma (H), there is a small irregular hypoechoic mass (arrows).

Pathology

- fat necrosis

Management

- BI-RADS Assessment Category 4, suspicious; biopsy should be considered

Pearls and Pitfalls

When surgical trauma ruptures adipocytes, the released fat may incite a fibrotic response, which produces an ill-defined, irregular mass. This type of fat necrosis cannot be differentiated mammographically or sonographically from neoplasm.

Suggested Readings

1. Bassett LW, Gold RH, Cove HC. Mammographic spectrum of traumatic fat necrosis: the fallibility of "pathognomonic" signs of carcinoma. *AJR* 1978;130:119–122.
2. Tohno D, Cosgrove DO, Sloane JP, eds. *Ultrasound Diagnosis of Breast Diseases*. New York: Churchill Livingston; 1994:140–143.

Case 181

Case History

A 52-year-old woman presents for diagnostic postoperative mammogram. She had lumpectomy and radiation therapy 2 years prior for primary breast lymphoma. She currently has no symptoms.

Physical Examination

- left breast: well-healed scar; otherwise normal
- right breast: normal exam

Mammogram

Mass (Figs. 181-1 and 181-2)

- margin: circumscribed
- shape: oval
- density: fat-containing

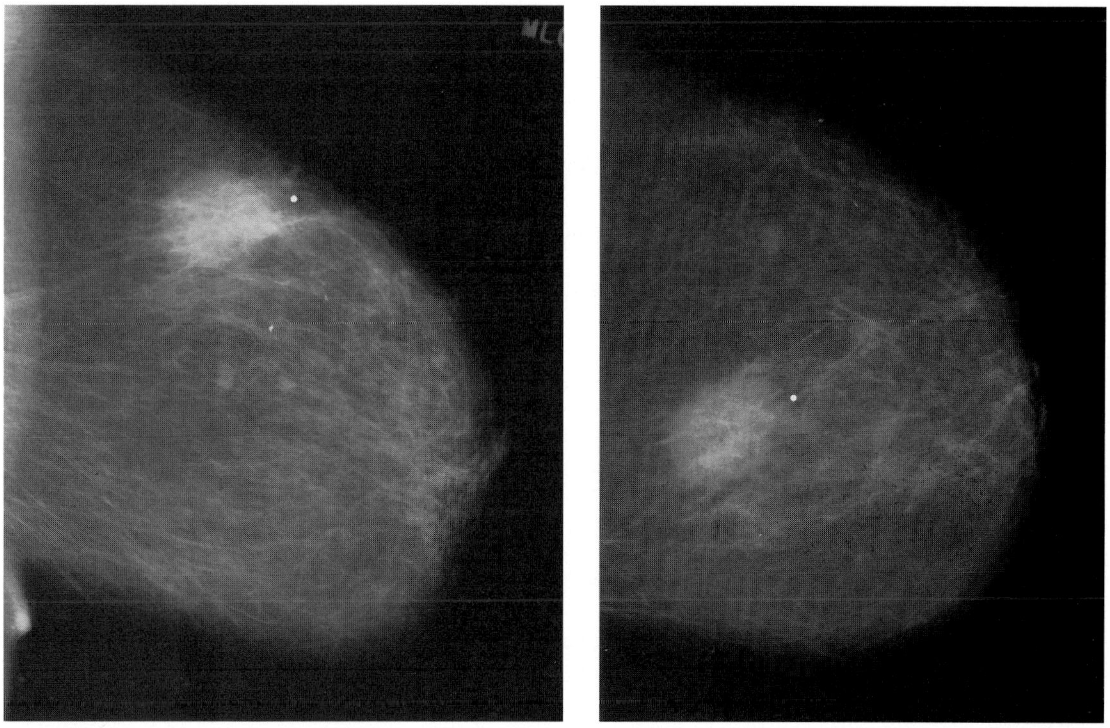

A B

Figure 181-1. This mammogram was performed 6 months after the lumpectomy. Ill-defined increased density, multiple lucencies, and skin retraction are within the area of the excision. (A). Left MLO mammogram. (B). Left CC mammogram.

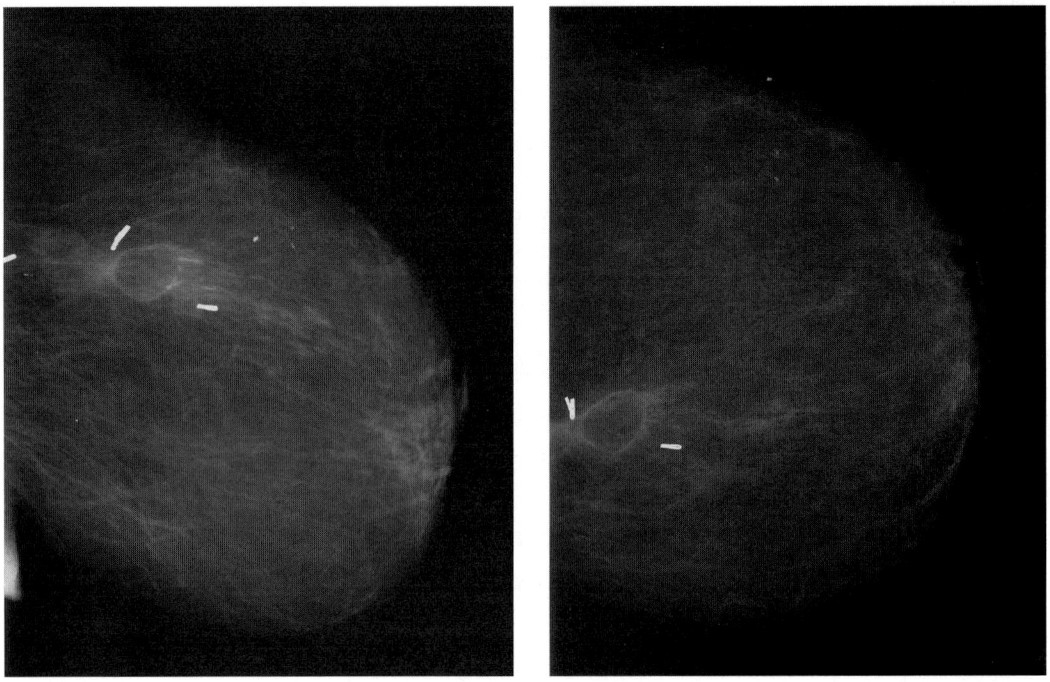

A B

Figure 181–2. This study was done 2 years after the lumpectomy. In the area of the excision, the density has decreased and an oil cyst has formed. (A). Left MLO mammogram. (B). Left CC mammogram.

Pathology

- fat necrosis

Management

- BI-RADS Assessment Category 2, benign finding

Pearls and Pitfalls

When fat necrosis results, a release of lipid occurs, which does not cause a fibrotic reaction. The material forms an oil cyst. The mammographic appearance of this round or oval, circumscribed, fat density mass is characteristic of this lesion.

Suggested Readings

1. Morgan CL, Trought, Peete W. Xeromammographic and ultrasonic diagnosis of a traumatic oil cyst. *AJR* 1978;130:1189–1190.

Case 182

Case History

A 45-year-old woman presents for preoperative evaluation for sentinel node biopsy. Her left breast tumor was biopsied with sonographic guidance 3 weeks ago.

Physical Examination

- left breast: healed biopsy incision in upper outer quadrant; otherwise normal exam
- right breast: normal exam

Mammogram (Fig. 182–1)

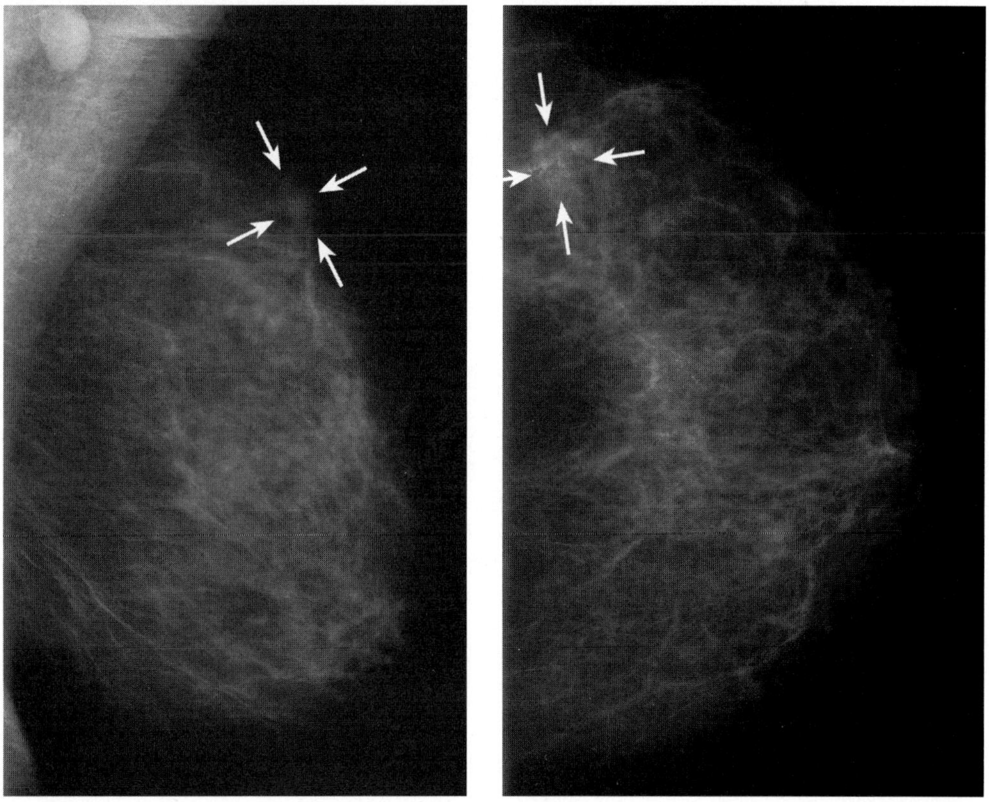

A B

Figure 182–1. In the upper outer quadrant there is an ill-defined mass (arrows). After this mammogram was performed, the mass was biopsied and found to be infiltrating ductal carcinoma. (A). Left MLO mammogram. (B). Left CC mammogram.

Ultrasound

Frequency

- 10 MHz

Mass

- margin: well defined
- echogenicity: heterogeneous
- retrotumoral acoustic appearance: increased acoustic enhancement
- shape: ellipsoid (Fig. 182–2)

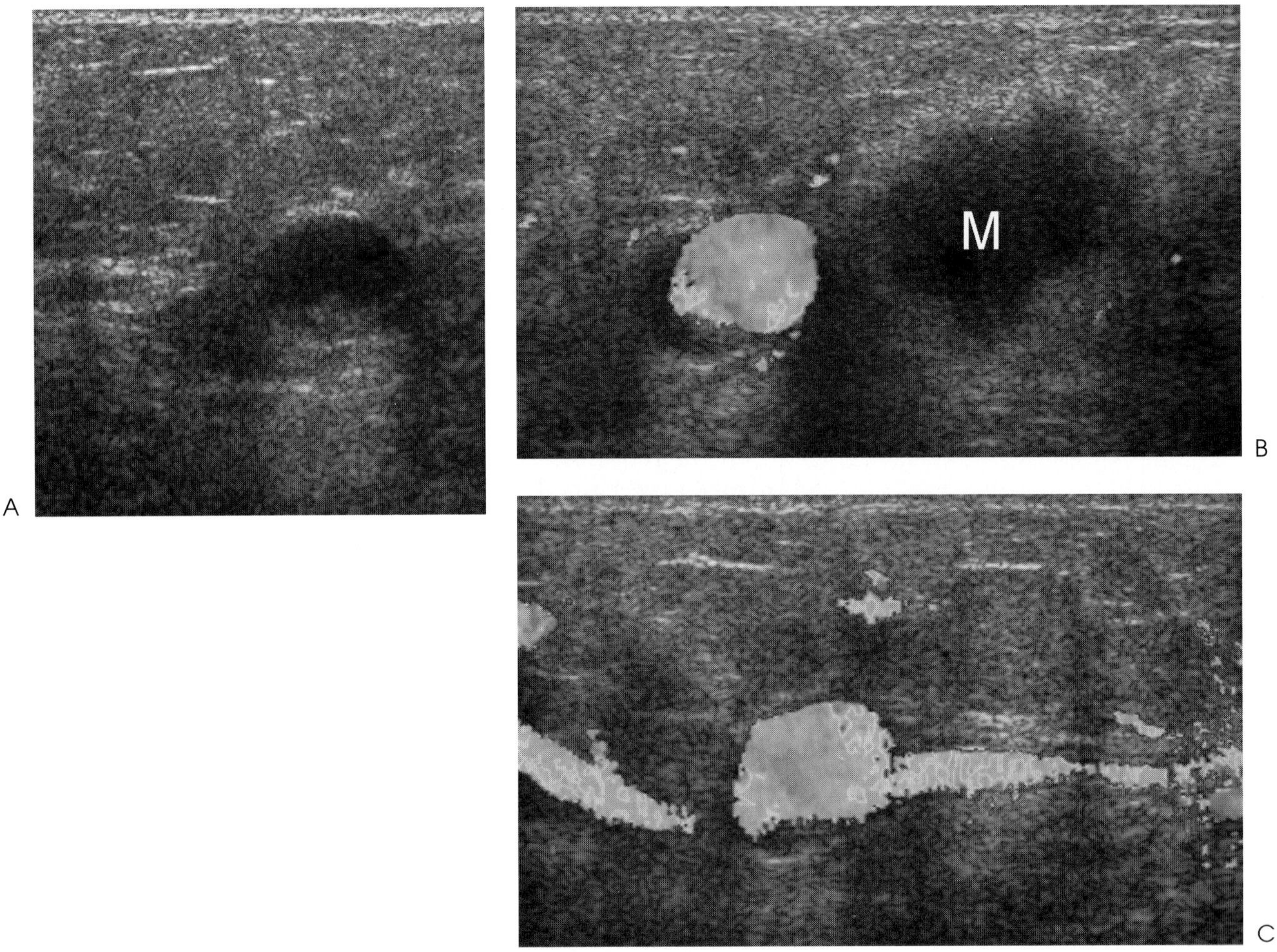

Figure 182–2. *In the left upper outer quadrant, there was an ill-defined hypoechoic mass (M) that corresponded to the tumor (B). Adjacent to the tumor was an oval fluid collection, which was predominantly anechoic except for its hypoechoic inferior rim (A). Color Doppler demonstrates that the hypoechoic lesion is filled with high-velocity swirling bloodflow characteristic of a pseudoaneurysm. (A). Left antiradial breast sonogram: Pseudoaneurysm without color Doppler. (B). Left antiradial color Doppler breast sonogram: Pseudoaneurysm next to mass (M). (C). Left antiradial color Doppler breast sonogram: Pseudoaneurysm with feeding and draining vessels (see Color Plate 182–2B and C).*

Pathology

- pseudoaneurysm

Management

- BI-RADS Assessment Category 2, benign finding

Pearls and Pitfalls

As a result of core needle biopsies, breast imagers have reported breast pseudoaneurysms. Researchers have described treatments including manual compression and placement of coils. Because this pseudoaneurysm was adjacent to a malignancy, it was removed with the tumor.

Suggested Readings

1. Beres RA, Harington DG, Wenzel MS. Percutaneous repair of breast pseudoaneurysm: sonographically guided embolization. *AJR* 1997;169:425–427.
2. Smith SM. Breast pseudoaneurysm after core biopsy. *AJR* 1996;167:817.

Case 183

Case History

A 74-year-old woman with left breast swelling. She had lumpectomy and axillary dissection 3 years ago. She had no symptoms until after she had coronary artery revascularization 3 months ago. During that procedure, her left internal mammary artery was harvested.

Physical Examination

- left breast: healed upper outer scar; entire breast is rock hard with diffuse skin thickening; no warmth or erythema; no arm edema
- right breast: normal exam

Mammogram (Fig. 183-1)

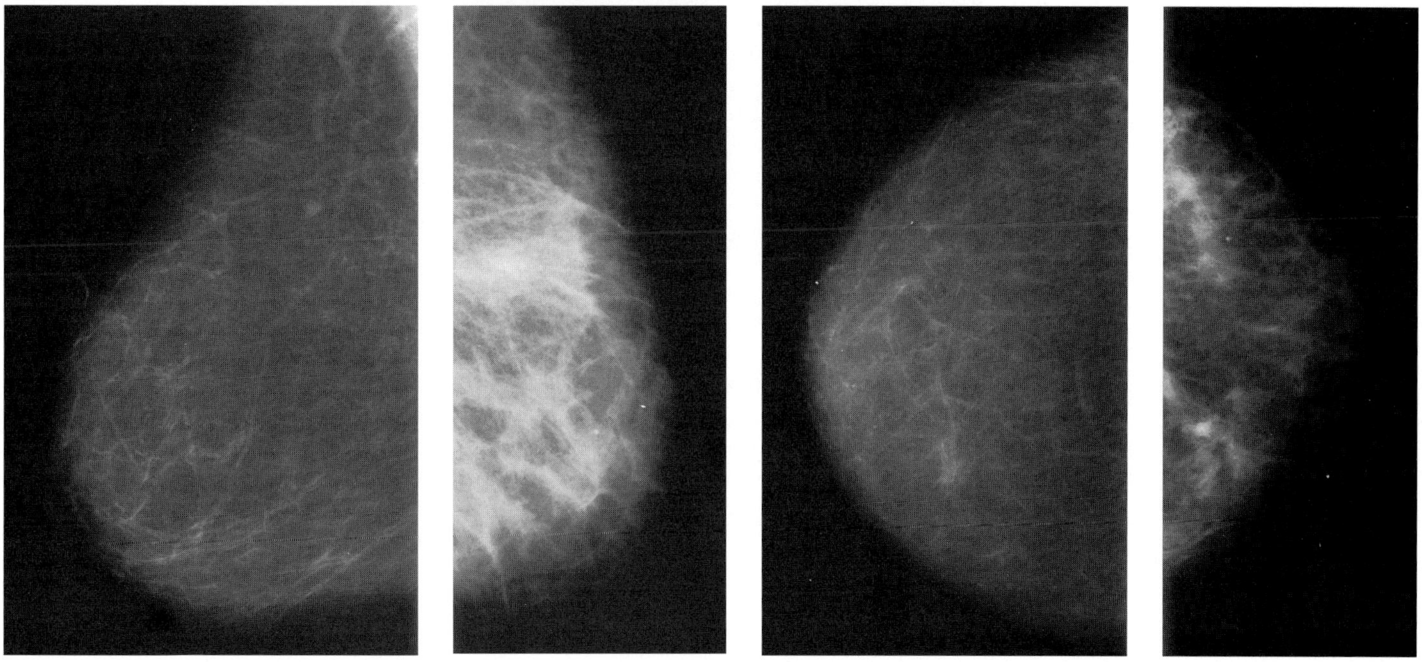

A B C D

Figure 183-1. The right breast is normal. The left breast is small and exhibits diffuse increased density. Lumpectomy site is in upper outer quadrant and is only partially evident on the left MLO view. (A). Right MLO mammogram. (B). Left MLO mammogram. (C). Right CC mammogram. (D). Left CC mammogram.

Ultrasound

Low Frequency

Frequency

- 8 MHz (Fig. 183-2)

Figure 183-2. Left radial breast sonogram: There is diffuse thickening of the parenchymal tissues with loss of normal architecture. The edematous tissue produces indistinct, random shadowing.

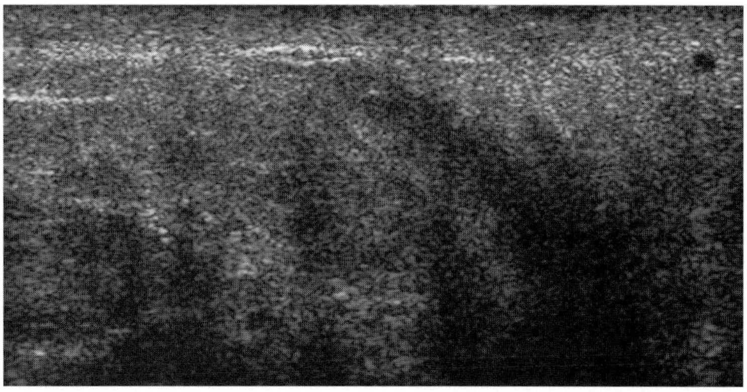

High Frequency

Frequency

- 13 MHz (Fig. 183–3)

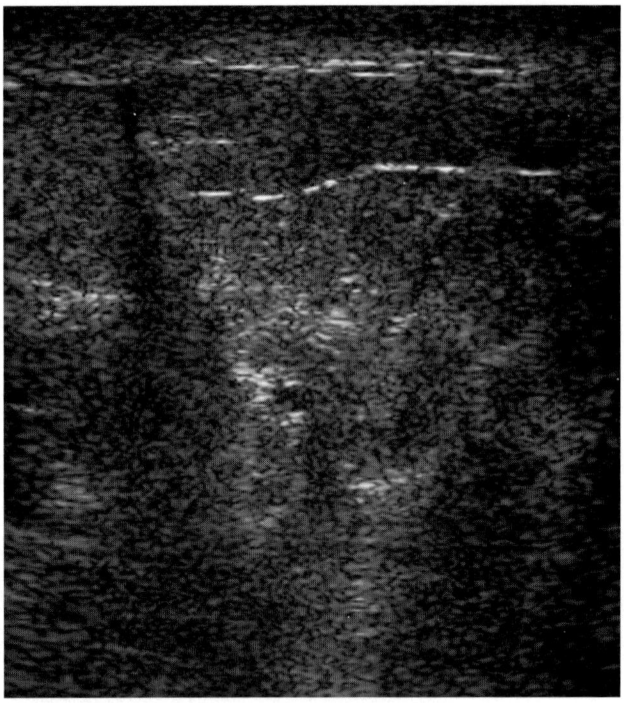

Figure 183–3. Left radial breast sonogram: Sonographic examination of the breast demonstrates irregular skin thickening. There is also intermittant loss of the border between the skin and the hyperechoic subcutaneous fat.

Pathology

- lymphedema

Management

- BI-RADS Assessment Category 3, probably benign; short-interval follow-up

Pearls and Pitfalls

Lymphedema is due to lymphatic obstruction (see Section 6). In this case, the patient's axillary lymphatic drainage had been damaged after the axillary dissection, and the internal mammary drainage was compromised by a combination of the median sternotomy and trauma from dissecting the internal mammary artery.

Suggested Readings

1. Tabar L, Dean PB. *Teaching Atlas of Mammography.* 3rd ed. New York: Thieme; 2001:239–246.

Case 184

Case History

A 47-year-old woman presents for first post-lumpectomy mammogram 6 months after the procedure.

Physical Examination

- right breast: healing excision site
- left breast: normal exam

Mammogram

Mass (Figs. 184–1 and 184–2)

- margin: spiculated

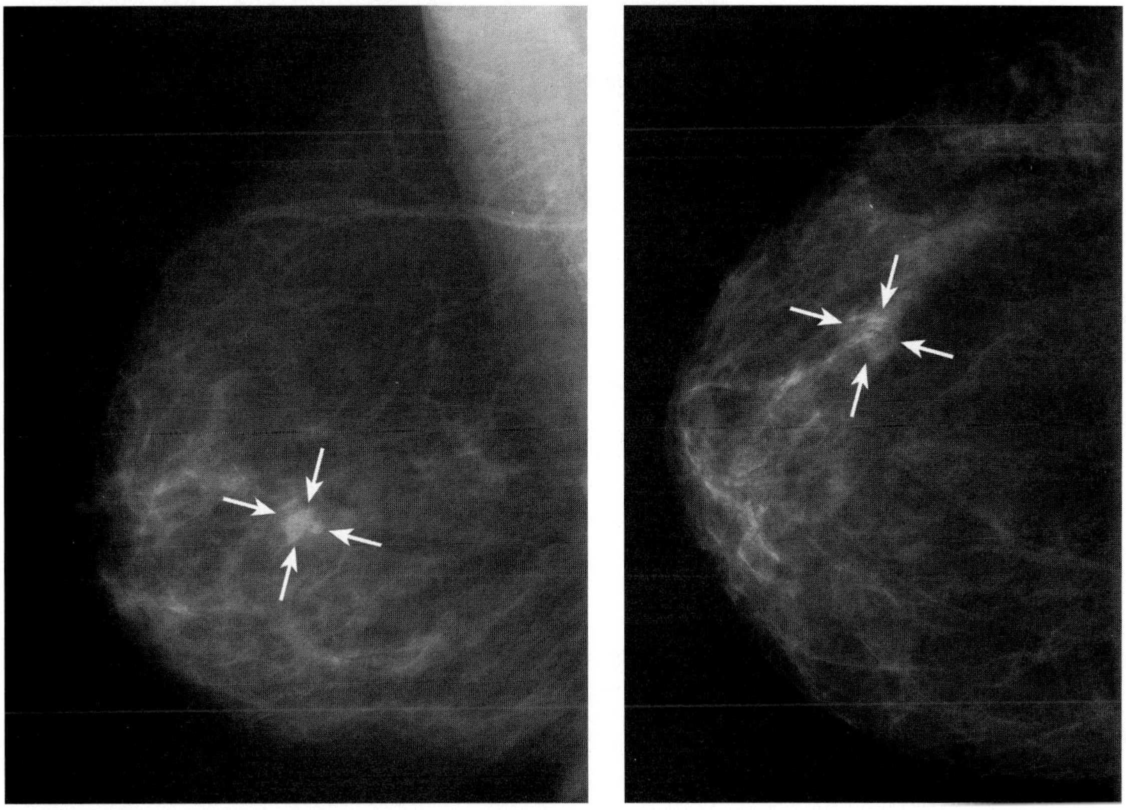

A B

Figure 184–1. This is the patient's screening mammogram prior to surgery. An ill-defined mass is present in the right outer breast (arrows). (A). Right MLO mammogram. (B). Right CC mammogram.

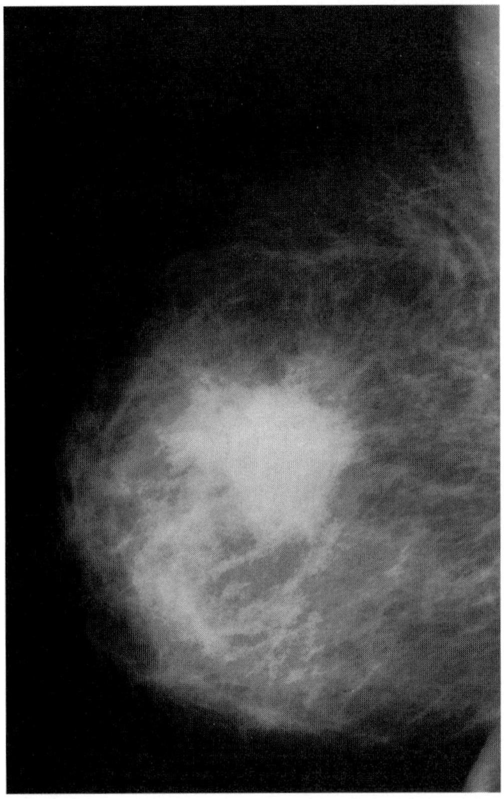

A

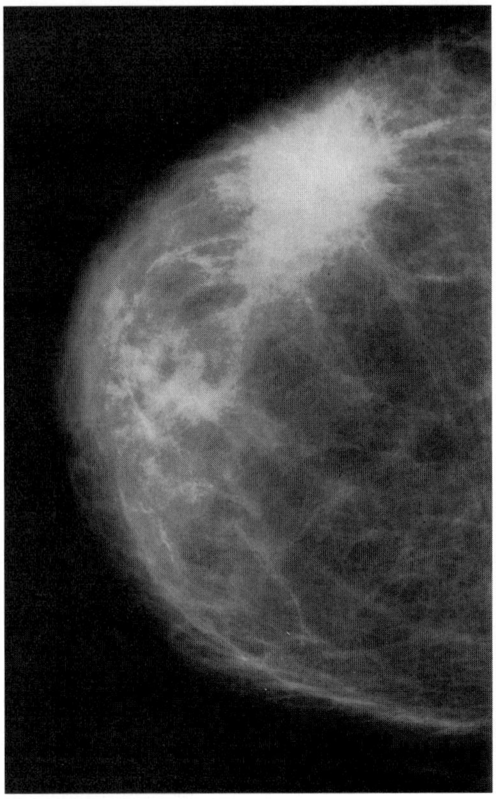

B

Figure 184–2. This study was performed 6 months after lumpectomy and radiation therapy. The right breast exhibits diffuse increased density. A large spiculated mass is present in the lumpectomy site. (A). Right MLO mammogram. (B). Right CC mammogram.

Pathology

- scar, lymphedema, seroma

Management

- BI-RADS Assessment Category 2, benign finding

Pearls and Pitfalls

Skin thickening and tissue edema are mammographically evident in 50 to 95% of patients 1 year after lumpectomy and radiation therapy. These abnormalities gradually diminish and stabilize between 2 and 3 years after treatment. After 5 years, 40 to 50% of patients still demonstrate either thickened skin or increased glandular density.

Suggested Readings

1. Brenner RJ, Pfaff JM. Mammographic features after conservation therapy for malignant breast disease: serial findings standardized by regression analysis. *AJR* 1996;167:171–178.
2. Dershaw DD, Shank B, Reisinger S. Mammographic findings after breast cancer treatment with local excision and definitive irradiation. *Radiology* 1987;164:455–461.
3. Destouet JM. Mammography of the altered breast. *Curr Opin Radiol* 1990;2:734–740.

Case 185

Case History

A 57-year-old woman presents with left nipple inversion. She had a left lumpectomy for infiltrating ductal carcinoma 3 years ago. She refused posterative radiation and chemotherapy after surgery.

Physical Examination

- left breast: healed incision in upper outer quadrant; no masses; inverted nipple; mild periareolar erythema and and peau d'orange.
- right breast: normal exam

Mammogram

Mass (Figs. 185–1 through 185–3)

- margin: spiculated

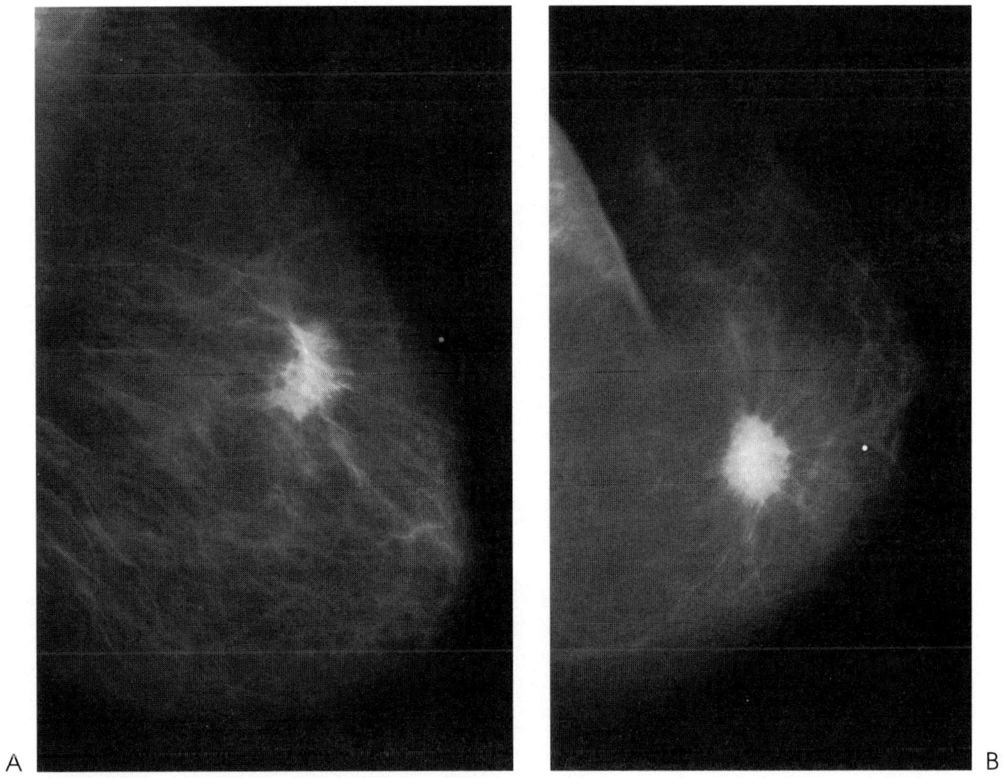

Figure 185–1. Screening mammogram prior to lumpectomy demonstrated a dense spiculated mass in the upper inner left breast. (A). Left MLO mammogram. (B). Left CC mammogram.

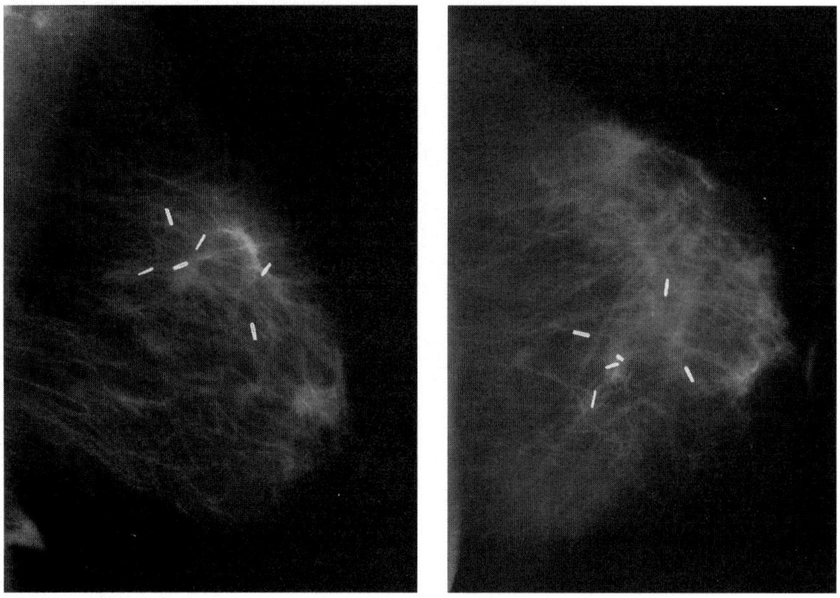

A B

Figure 185-2. *Two years after lumpectomy, there is mild ill-defined increased density and skin thickening and retraction associated with the lumpectomy site. This appearance had been stable for 1 year. (A). Left MLO mammogram. (B). Left CC mammogram.*

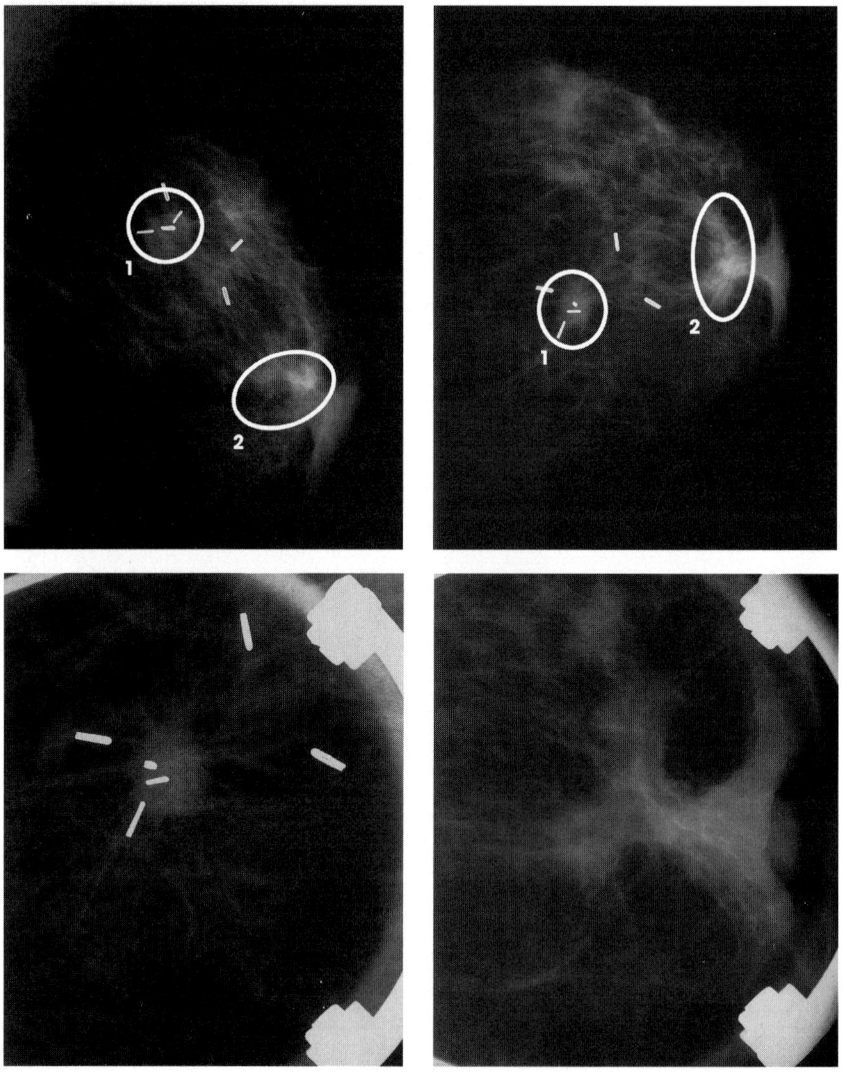

A B C D

Figure 185-3. *Three years after lumpectomy, there has been development of a spiculated mass in the lumpectomy site (lesion 1). There is also a subareolar lobular mass (lesion 2) associated with architectural distortion and skin thickening. (A). Left MLO mammogram. (B). Left CC mammogram. (C). Left CC spot compression of lesion 1. (D). Left CC spot compression of lesion 2.*

Ultrasound

Frequency

- 7 MHz

Mass

- margin: spiculation/architectural distortion
- echogenicity: hypoechoic
- retrotumoral acoustic appearance: posterior shadowing distal to mass
- shape: irregular (Figs. 185–4 and 185–5)

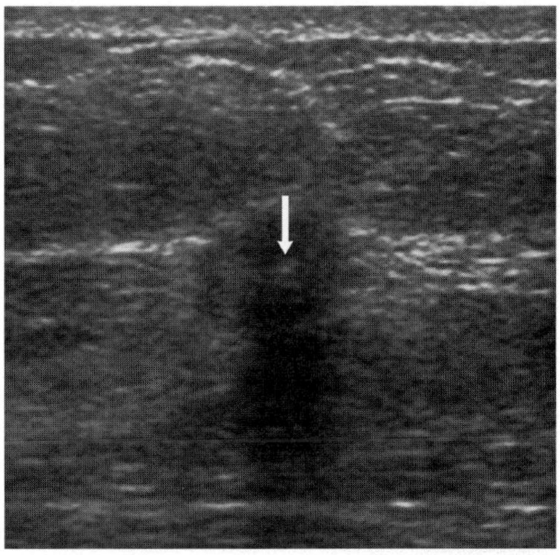

Figure 185–4. Left transverse breast sonogram: At the 11:00 position, there is a hypoechoic ill-defined mass that corresponds to the mammographic lesion 1. In the center of the mass is a hyperechoic focus, which is a clip (arrow) (see Color Plate 185–4).

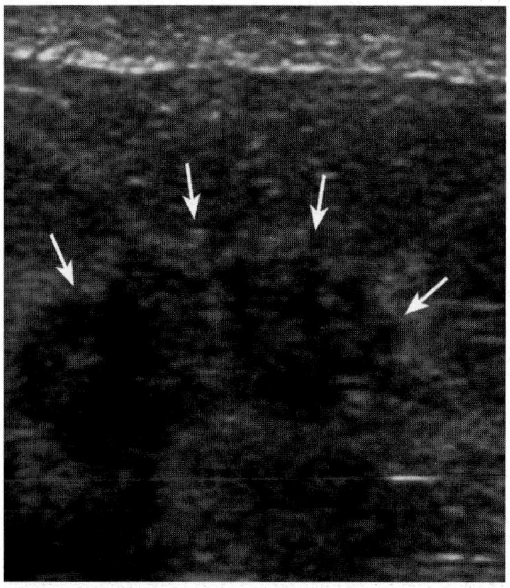

Figure 185–5. Left transverse breast sonogram: In the subareolar area there is a hypoechoic, ill-defined lobular mass that corresponds to the mammographic lesion 2 (see Color Plate 185–5).

Pathology

- infiltrating ductal carcinoma

Management

- BI-RADS Assessment Category 5, highly suggestive of malignancy

Pearls and Pitfalls

1. Although lumpectomy and radiation therapy for small tumors has the same clinical result as mastectomy, multiple studies have shown that lumpectomy alone has a higher recurrence rate compared to lumpectomy with radiation therapy. After 5 years, the local recurrence rate for lumpectomy and radiation therapy is about 3 to 5% but for lumpectomy alone the rate is between 12 and 19%.
2. Mammographically, the findings of recurrence include new calcifications, mass or enlarging density, architectural distortion, and inflammatory changes.

Suggested Readings

1. Orel SG, Troupin RH, Patterson EA, Fowble BL. Breast cancer recurrence after lumpectomy and irradiation: role of mammography in detection. *Radiology* 1992;183:201–206.
2. Stomper PC, Recht A, Berenberg AL, Jochelson MS, Harris JR. Mammographic detection of recurrent cancer in the irradiated breast. *AJR* 1987;148:39–43.
3. Veronesi U. Conservation surgery and irradiation in stages I and II disease: the European experience. In: Bland KI, Copeland EM, eds. *The Breast.* 2nd ed. Philadelphia: WB Saunders; 1998:1191–1196.

Case 186

Case History

A 67-year-old woman is referred for new left breast lump. She was treated for left breast cancer 15 years ago with left lumpectomy, axillary node dissection, and radiation therapy.

Physical Examination

- left breast: diffusely erythematous, thickened skin; no dominant masses; slightly inverted nipple
- right breast: single enlarged axillary node; otherwise normal exam

Mammogram (Fig. 186–1)

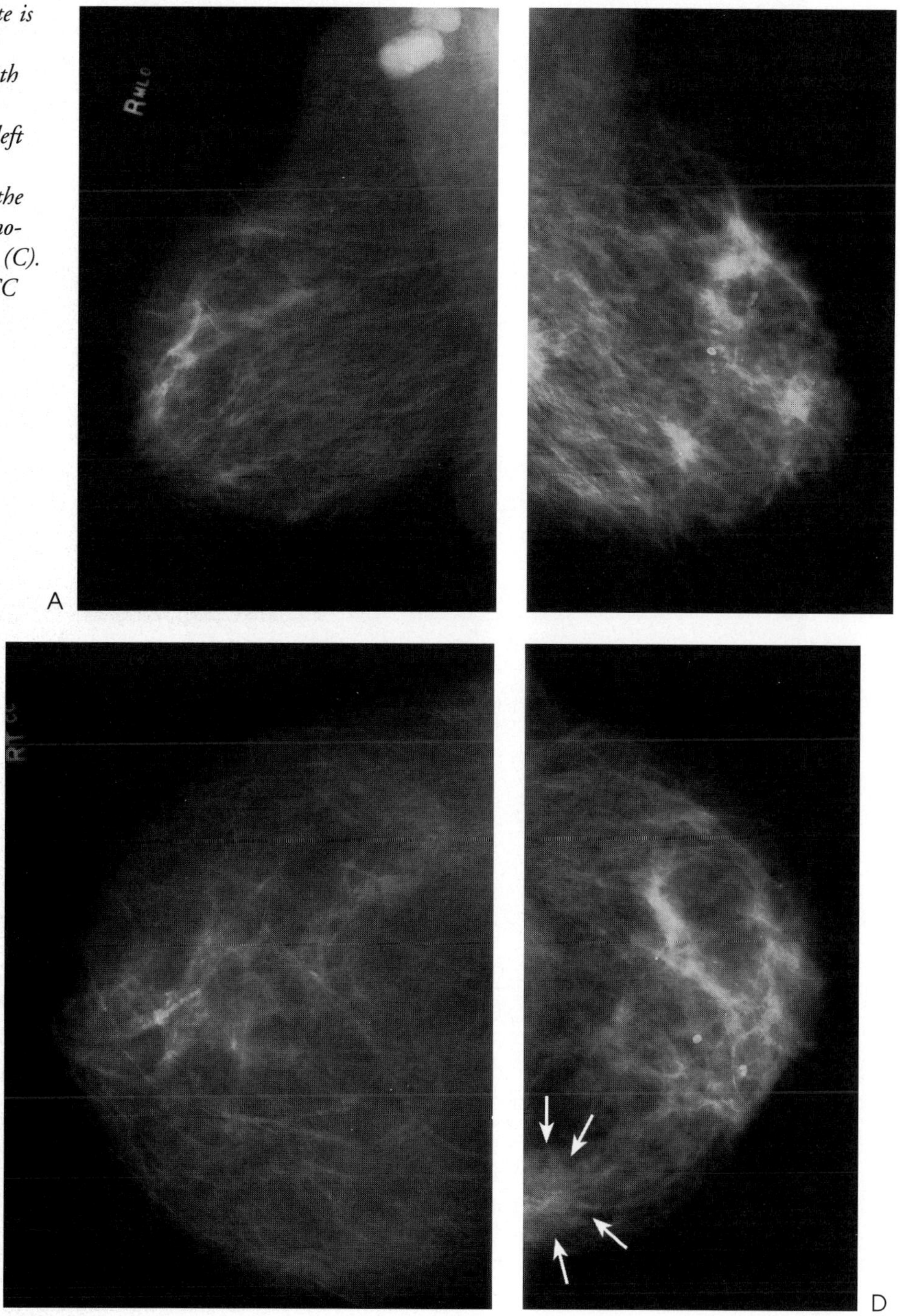

Figure 186–1. *Old lumpectomy site is in the left axilla. There is diffuse increased density of the left breast with skin and trabecular thickening. An asymmetric density is present in the left medial breast (arrows). Multiple enlarged, dense nodes are present in the right axilla. (A). Right MLO mammogram. (B). Left MLO mammogram. (C). Right CC mammogram. (D). Left CC mammogram.*

Ultrasound

Frequency

- 14 MHz (Figs. 186-2 and 186-3)

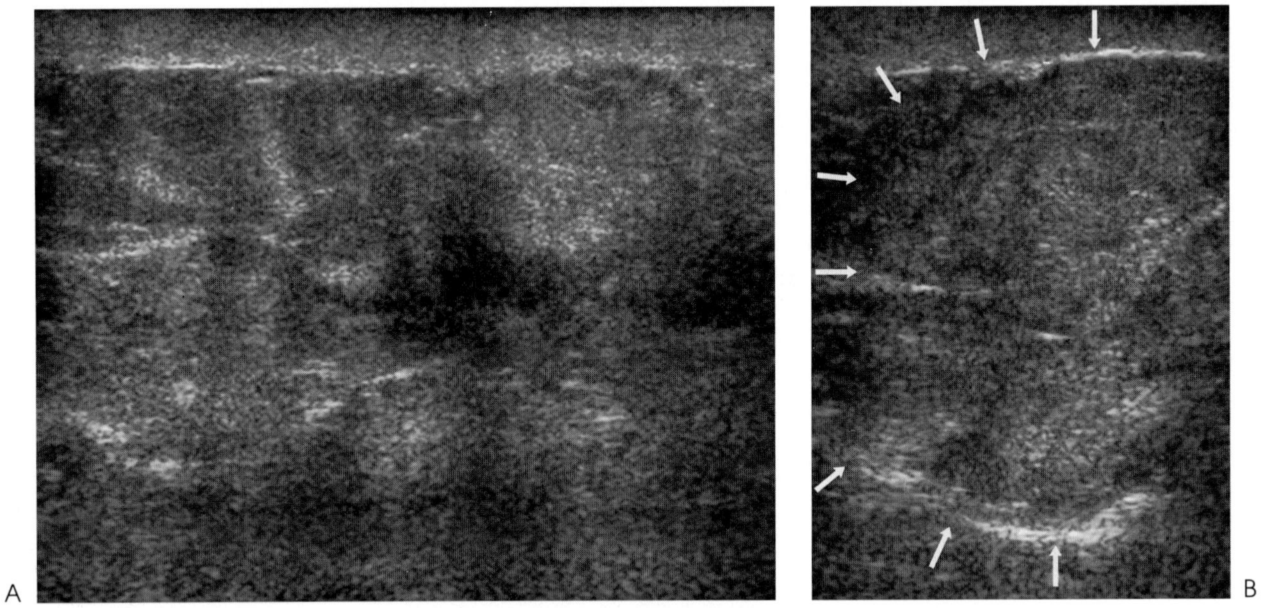

Figure 186-2. The left breast exhibits diffuse skin thickening (A). There is loss of the normal parenchymal architecture. No normal lobular lines or density are present. Ill-defined shadowing from random interfaces are evident. At the 9:00 position (B) there was a suggestion of a large, ill-defined lobular mass (arrows). This mass was difficult to separate from the rest of the abnormal parenchyma. (A). Left radial breast sonogram: Parenchyma at 3:00. (B). Left radial breast sonogram: Mass at 9:00.

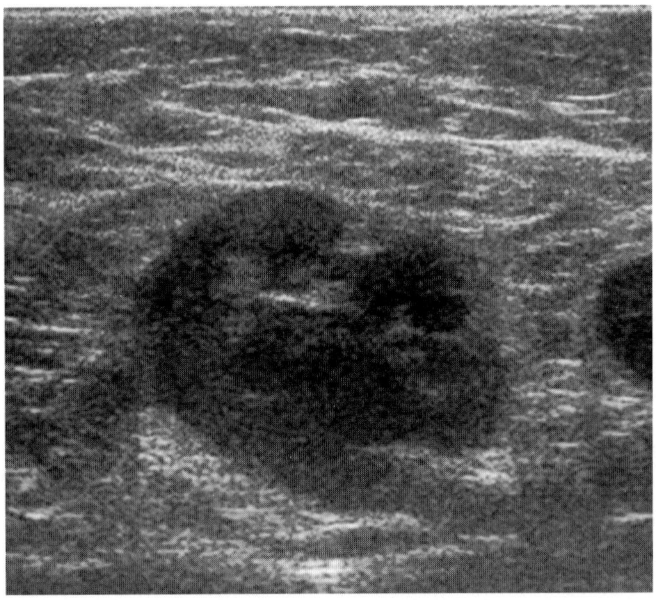

Figure 186-3. Right transverse breast sonogram: In the right axilla, there were multiple enlarged lymph nodes. This suspicious node is hypoechoic and has lost the normal internal hyperechoic hilus.

Other Modalities (Fig. 186–4)

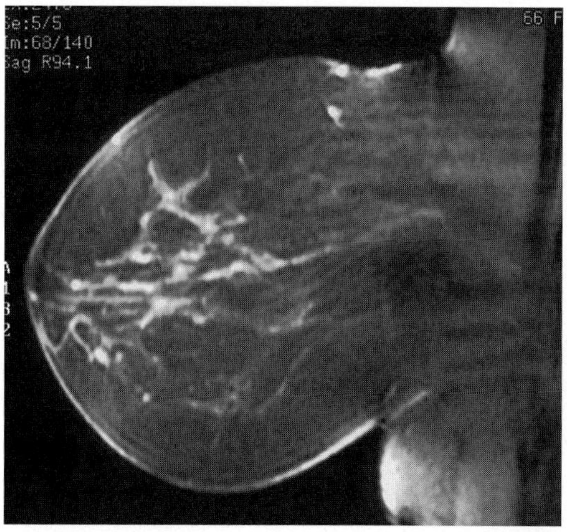

Figure 186–4. Right longitudinal dynamic bolus 3-D volume gradient series breast MRI: No abnormal enhancing masses are present in the right breast.

Pathology

Mixed lobular and infiltrating ductal carcinoma. Biopsies from the left 3:00 and 9:00 position produced similar histologies. Both were mixed lobular and infiltrating ductal carcinoma. The right lymph node biopsy demonstrated metastatic breast carcinoma.

Management

- BI-RADS Assessment Category 5, highly suggestive of malignancy

Pearls and Pitfalls

1. After lumpectomy, tumor recurrence within the same breast occurs at a rate of about 1% per year. Therefore, after 10 years, it is about 10%. There are three clinical and pathologic presentations for tumor recurrence within the breast. The most common recurrence (86%) is a focal mass. The second presentation (14%) is when the tumor is multifocal or highly infiltrative. This type is commonly associated with diffuse lymphatic extension and often involves the skin. The third type (<1%) is limited to the lymphatics and has no parenchymal component. This case illustrates the second presentation. The second presentation is clinically and radiographically similar to inflammatory breast cancer.
2. MRI was useful to clarify the origin of the right axillary nodal metastases. In this case, the lack of right breast tumor indicates that the nodal metastases are from the left malignancy. The origin of the nodal metastases determines the patient's clinical stage, and therefore, affects her treatment options.

Suggested Readings

1. Fisher B. Lumpectomy (segmental mastectomy) and axillary dissection. In: Bland KI, Copeland EM, eds. *The Breast.* Philadelphia: WB Saunders; 1998:917–939.

Case 187

Case History

A 54-year-old woman presents with new right breast lump. Twelve years ago, she had a right modified radical mastectomy for extensive ductal carcinoma in situ. She subsequently had breast reconstruction with placement of a permanent implant.

Physical Examination

- right breast: a hard mass at the 5:00 position; 3 cm palpable node in the right axilla
- left breast: normal exam

Mammogram

Mass (Fig. 187–1)

- margin: circumscribed
- shape: lobular
- density: high density

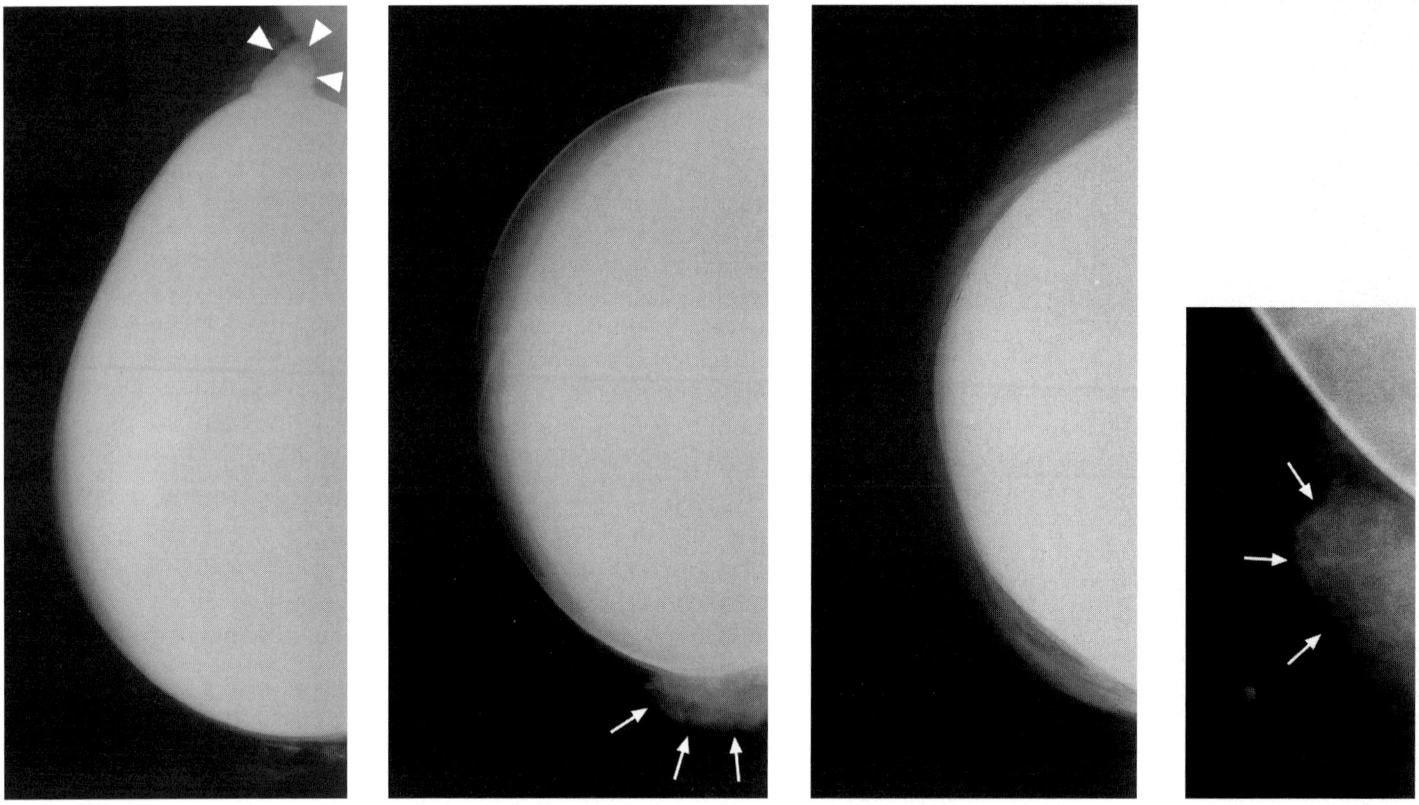

A B C D

Figure 187–1. In the inferior breast, there is an oval mass (arrows) with indistinct margins. There is also a circumscribed lobular mass in the axillary area (arrowheads). (A). Right MLO mammogram. (B). Repositioned right MLO mammogram. (C). Right CC mammogram. (D). Right MLO spot magnification mammogram.

Ultrasound

Frequency

- 11.5 MHz

Mass

- margin: ill defined
- echogenicity: hypoechoic
- shape: ellipsoid (Figs. 187-2 and 187-3)

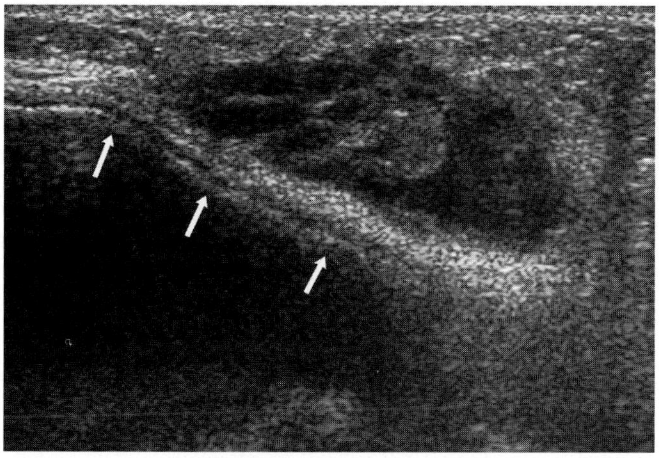

Figure 187-2. Right longitudinal breast sonogram: At the 5:00 position, there is an ellipsoid, hypoechoic, ill-defined mass that corresponds to the mammographic mass and the palpable lump. The mass is next to the implant wall (arrows).

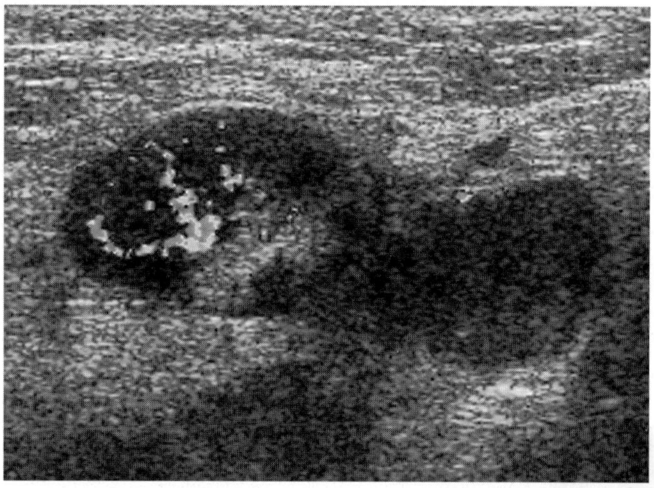

Figure 187-3. Right longitudinal color Doppler breast sonogram: The palpable right axillary node exhibits abnormal architecture. The hilum is located in an asymmetric position compared to the nodal mass (see Color Plate 187-3).

Pathology

Infiltrating ductal carcinoma. Both the palpable mass and the right axillary node had similar histologies.

Management

- BI-RADS Assessment Category 4, suspicious; biopsy should be considered

Pearls and Pitfalls

1. Risk of recurrence depends upon the patient's initial stage of disease. In patients with Stage I disease (tumor < 2 cm, no spread to axillary nodes or other areas), the disease-free survival after 10 years is 82% and after 20 years is 78%. The rate of recurrence peaks between the second to fifth year after diagnosis.
2. In Stages I to II disease, the first sites of recurrence after mastectomy are (in order of decreasing frequency): local/regional (chest wall, axilla, supraclavicular region), bone, lung, liver.

Suggested Readings

1. Moore MP, Kinne DW. Patterns of recurrence in breast cancer. In: Bland KI, Copeland EM, ed. *The Breast.* 2nd ed. Philadelphia: WB Saunders; 1998:395-399.

Section X

Masses Poorly Identified Mammographically

Any benign or malignant mass may be poorly identified mammographically. Visualization depends upon mammographic technique, breast radiographic density, and lesion location. The cases presented in this chapter are presented because of the following reasons: (1) The mass commonly presents as a palpable mass. (2) The case has a teaching point about the disease process that has not been illustrated in the rest of the book.
(3) The mass is an unusual histology that is not illustrated in the rest of the book.

Case 188

Case History

A 35-year-old woman is admitted for severe disseminated encephalomyelitis of unknown origin. She is comatose.

Physical Examination

- unresponsive patient
- right breast: palpable lump in upper outer quadrant
- left breast: normal exam

Ultrasound

Frequency

- 10 MHz

Mass

- margin: ill defined
- echogenicity: hypoechoic
- retrotumoral acoustic appearance: bilateral edge shadowing
- shape: lobulated (Fig. 188–1)

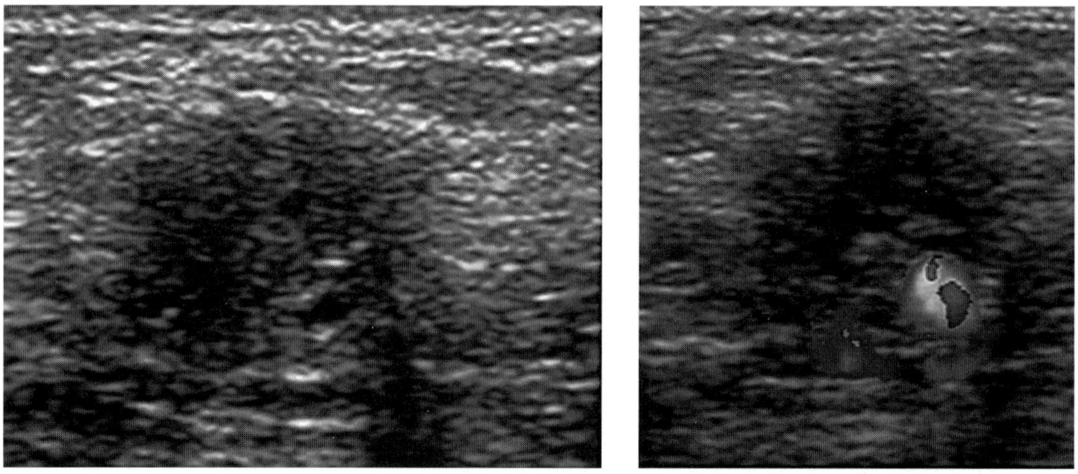

A B

Figure 188–1. The palpable lump corresponds to a lobulated hypoechoic mass. (A). Right radial breast sonogram. (B). Right radial color Doppler breast sonogram (see Color Plate 188–1B).

Other Modalities (Fig. 188–2)

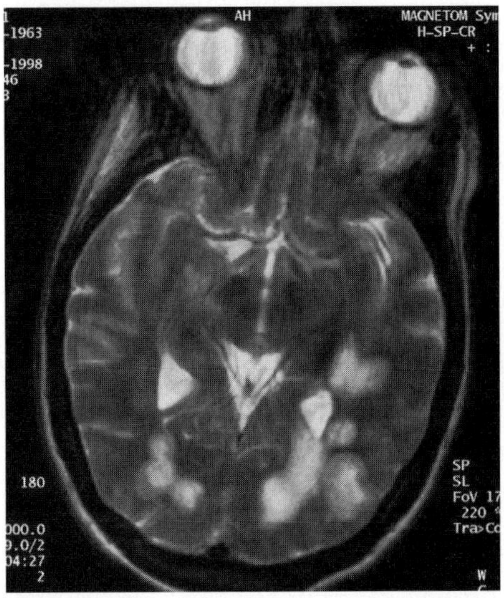

Figure 188–2. T2-weighted transverse image of the brain: There are numerous high-intensity white matter abnormalities.

Pathology

- infiltrating ductal carcinoma

Management

- BI-RADS Assessment Category 4, suspicious; biopsy should be considered

Pearls and Pitfalls

1. In this patient, the encephalomyelitis was a paraneoplastic syndrome caused by the breast cancer. The patient was treated with mastectomy and the patient's symptoms improved, but she retained chronic left-sided paralysis and contractures.
2. When tumors produce symptoms at anatomic locations that are distant from the primary tumor or its metastases, these symptoms are described as paraneoplastic syndromes. Paraneoplastic syndromes may be classified as: (1) endocrine (e.g., ectopic adrenocorticotropic hormone, inappropriate antidiuretic hormone); (2) hematologic (e.g., anemia, erythrocytosis, thrombophlebitis); (3) gastrointestinal (e.g., protein-losing enteropathy, anorexia-cachexia); (4) renal (e.g., membranous nephropathy, hemolytic uremic syndrome); (5) cutaneous (e.g., pigmented lesions, keratoses, erythemas, bullae, urticaria); (6) neurologic (e.g., encephalomyelitis, cerebellar degeneration, Lambert-Eaton myasthenic syndrome, dermatomyositis). Neurologic paraneoplastic syndromes occur in less than 1% of cancer patients. The etiology of encephalomyelitis is unknown. There is no specific treatment and patients generally suffer chronic severe debilitation.
3. In rare situations, patients cannot tolerate or cooperate adequately to produce a mammogram. In a clinically suspicious situation, if a palpable lump is present, sonography is useful for clarifying a specific problem. If no lump is present, then magnetic resonance imaging (MRI) is useful to evaluate the breasts.

Suggested Readings

1. Arnold SM, Patchell R, Lowy AM, Foon KA. Paraneoplastic syndromes. In: DeVita VT, Hellman S, Rosenberg SA, eds. *Cancer Principles and Practice of Oncology*. 6th ed. Philadelphia: Lippincott Williams and Wilkins; 2001:2511–2536.
2. Cosmacini P, Veronesi P, Galimberti V, Ferranti C, Viganotti G, Coopmans de Yoldi G. Ultrasonographic evaluation of palpable breast masses: analysis of 134 cases. *Tumori* 1990;76:495–498.
3. Dalmau JO, Posner JB. Paraneoplastic syndromes affecting the nervous system. *Semin Oncol* 1997;24:318–328.

Case 189

Case History

A 74-year-old woman presents with a left breast lump. She was identified with Type 1 diabetes 40 years ago and is on an insulin pump.

Physical Examination

- left breast: firm 2 cm palpable mass at the 6:00 position
- right breast: normal exam

Mammogram (Fig. 189–1)

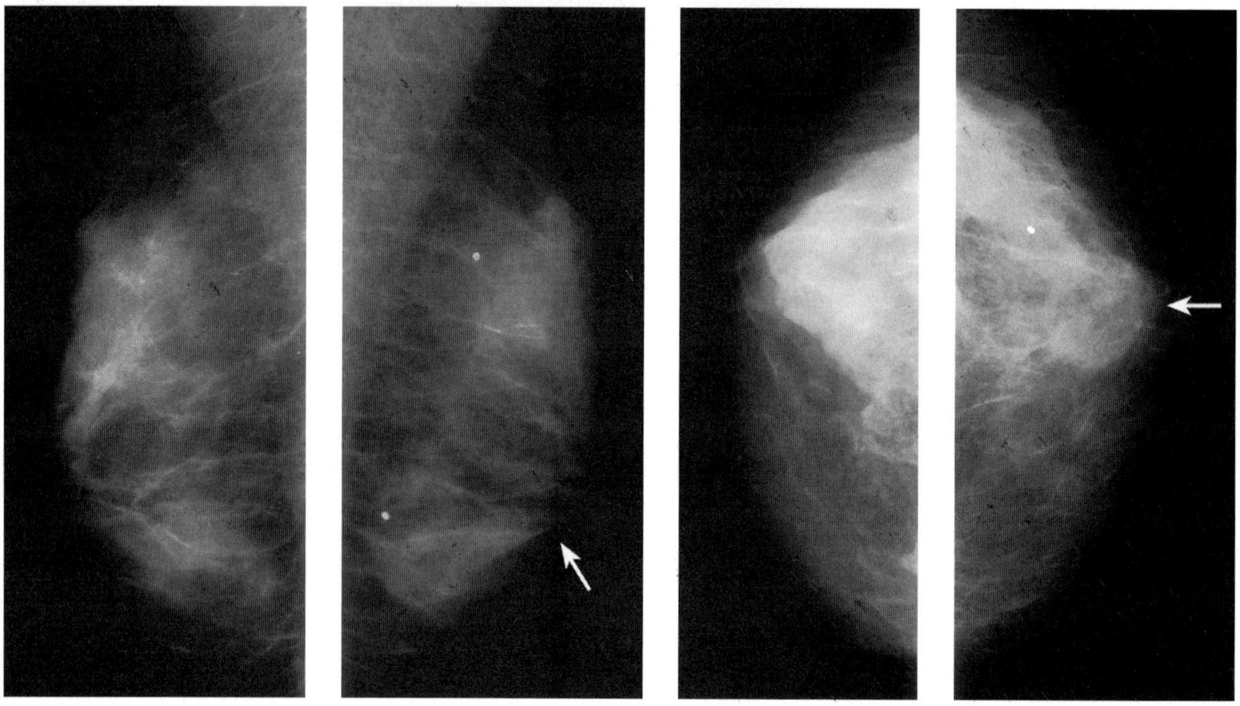

A B C D

Figure 189–1. The left palpable mass is marked with an arrow. No focal mass is identified. Bilateral mammograms are normal. (A). Right MLO mammogram. (B). Left MLO mammogram. (C). Right CC mammogram. (D). Left CC mammogram.

Ultrasound

Low Frequency

Frequency

- 6 MHz

Mass

- margin: ill defined
- echogenicity: hypoechoic
- retrotumoral acoustic appearance: severe shadowing, mass completely obscured
- shape: irregular (Fig. 189–2)

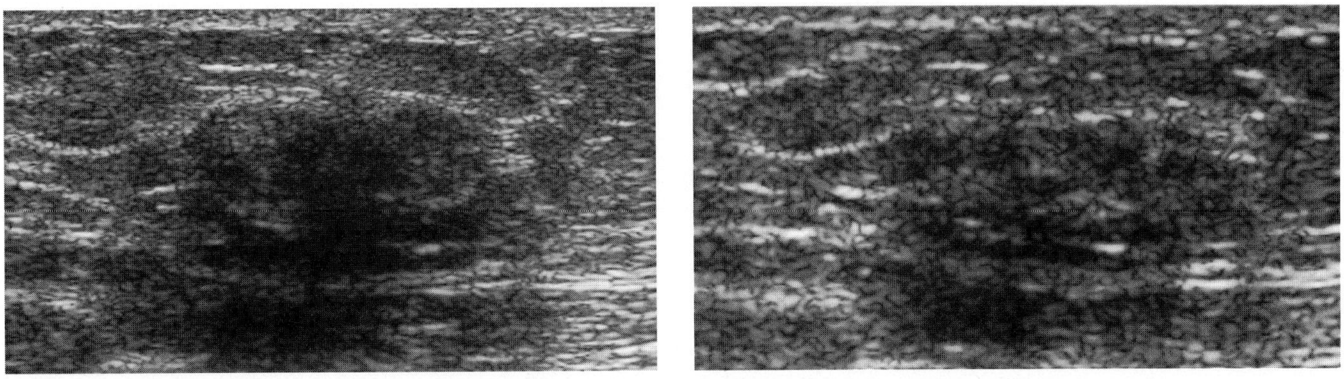

Figure 189-2. *Because the mass is obscured with the high-frequency examination (see Fig. 189-3), lower frequencies were applied. With 8 MHz (A), the mass is mildly hypoechoic. However, normal parenchymal lines are identified running through the "mass." With 6 MHz (B), the hypoechogenicity and mass almost disappear. (A). Left antiradial breast sonogram (8 MHz). (B). Left antiradial breast sonogram (6 MHz).*

High Frequency

Frequency

- 11.5 MHz

Associated Findings (Fig. 189-3)

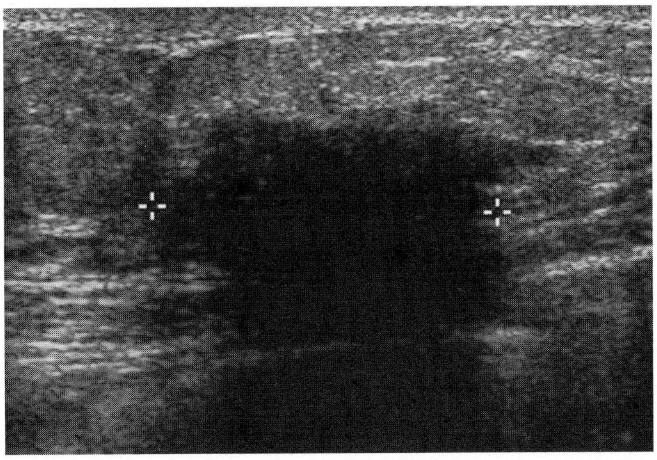

Figure 189-3. *Left antiradial breast sonogram: The palpable mass corresponds to a hypoechoic mass with severe shadowing.*

Pathology

- diabetic mastopathy

Management

- BI-RADS Assessment Category 4, suspicious; biopsy should be considered

Pearls and Pitfalls

1. Diabetic mastopathy is identified in less than 1% of benign breast biopsies, but represents about 13% of benign biopsies in women with Type 1 diabetes. Clinically, this abnormality affects young women between the ages of 25 and 40 years who have had a long history of diabetes (usually greater than 10 years). This patient is much older than most patients who present with this problem.The mastopathy presents as a painless, hard, irregular mass. About 50% of patients will have multiple masses.
2. Mammographically, these masses are commonly not identifiable. Sometimes there is an asymmetric focal density or ill-defined mass.
3. Sonographically, these masses highly attenuate sound. Therefore, if one uses a high-frequency transducer, the mass will appear as a focal area of heavy shadowing (Fig. 189–3). With lower frequencies, the shadowing and hypoechogenicity will decrease (Figs. 189–2A and B) and no definite masss is evident. Sonographically, these findings do not prevent a biopsy. However, if the biopsy result is diabetic mastopathy, then one may be confident that there is good sonographic and pathologic correlation.

Suggested Readings

1. Boullu S, Andrac L, Piana L, Darmon P, Dutour A, Oliver C. Diabetic mastopathy, complication of type 1 diabetes mellitus: report of two cases and a review of the literature. *Diabete Metab* 1998;24:448–454.
2. Hunfeld KP, Bassler R. Lymphocytic mastitis and fibrosis of the breast in long-standing insulin-dependent diabetics. *Gen Diagn Pathol* 1997;143:49–58.
3. Logan WW, Hoffman NY. Diabetic fibrous breast disease. *Radiology* 1989;172:667–670.

Case 190

Case History

A 14-year-old girl presents with new left breast lump.

Physical Examination

- left breast: 3 cm smooth mass extending from 10:00 to 2:00 along the areolar margin
- right breast: normal exam

Ultrasound

Frequency

- 7 MHz

Mass

- margin: well defined
- echogenicity: hypoechoic
- retrotumoral acoustic appearance: no shadowing
- shape: ellipsoid (Fig. 190–1)

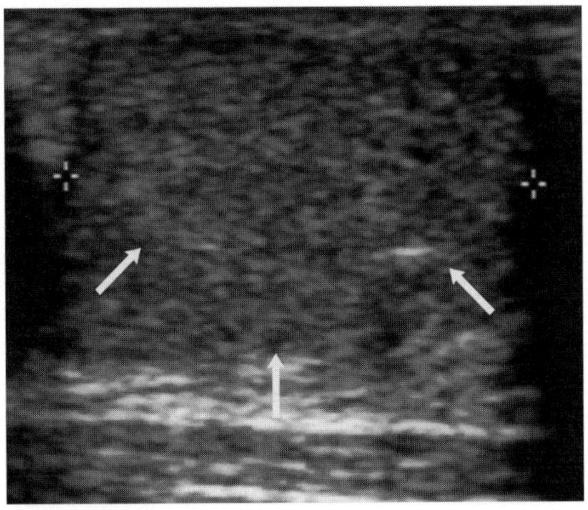

Figure 190–1. Left radial breast sonogram: The palpable mass corresponds to a well-defined hypoechoic mass with a thin lucent rim (arrows).

Pathology

- juvenile fibroadenoma

Management

- BI-RADS Assessment Category 3, probably benign; short-interval follow-up

Pearls and Pitfalls

1. Fibroadenoma is the most common mass in adolescent girls. Most of these fibroadenomas are the adult type of histology. However, some adolescents have juvenile fibroadenomas, which are variants of the adult type. These patients commonly present with a rapidly growing mass. Microscopically, the tumor demonstrates a pericanalicular growth pattern, as opposed to the usual intracanalicular pattern of adult fibroadenomas. Furthermore, the stroma is more cellular than the adult type.
2. Because these masses are palpable and occur in young women, they are generally initially identified sonographically. Their appearance is identical to adult fibroadenomas. They are generally well-defined oval or lobulated hypoechoic masses. Because these lesions tend to be large and growing, they are commonly biopsied even though their appearance is sonographically relatively benign (as in this case).

Suggested Readings

1. Ashikari R, Farrow JH, O'Hara J. Fibroadenomas in the breast of juveniles. *Surg Gynecol Obstet* 1971;132:259–262.
2. Devitt JE. Juvenile giant fibroadenoma of the breast. *Can J Surg* 1974;17:205–207.
3. Tavassoli FA, Fattaneh A. *Pathology of the Breast.* 2nd ed. Stamford: Appleton and Lange; 1999:583–586.

Case 191

Case History

A 37-year-old woman who is 9 months postpartum presents with a new right breast lump. She recently had symptoms of right breast mastitis, which have improved on antibiotics. She is still nursing her baby.

Physical Examination

- right breast: smooth, soft, mobile mass at 6:00
- left breast: normal exam

Ultrasound

Frequency

- 10 MHz

Mass

- margin: well defined
- echogenicity: heterogeneous
- retrotumoral acoustic appearance: no shadowing
- shape: ellipsoid (Fig. 191-1)

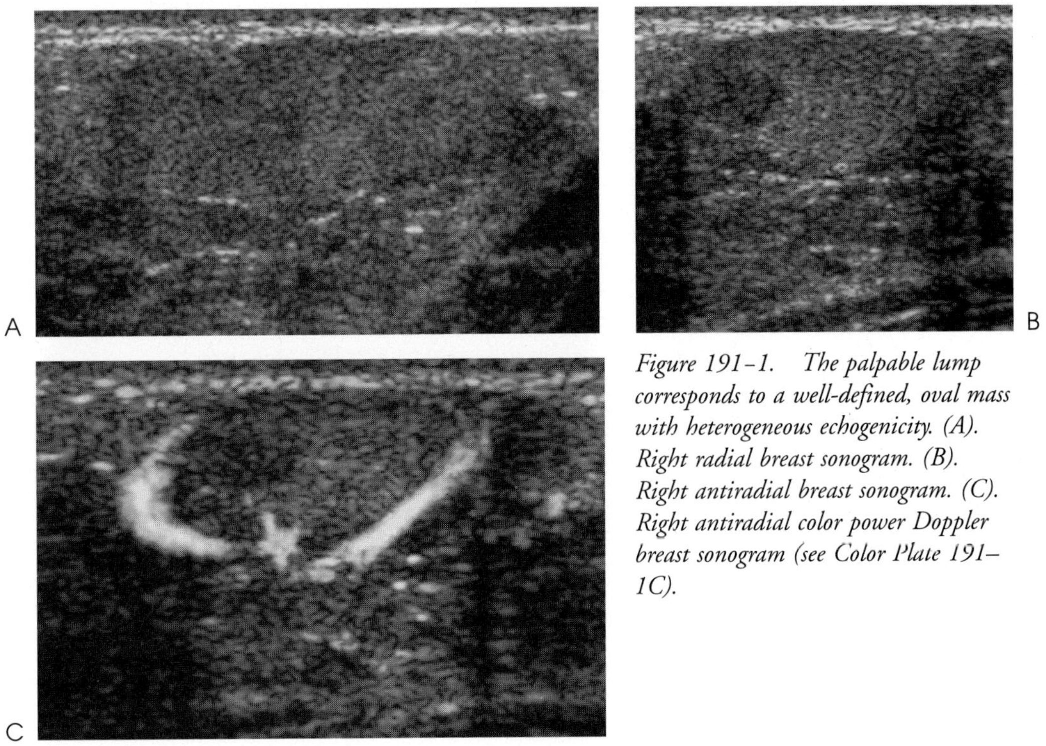

Figure 191-1. The palpable lump corresponds to a well-defined, oval mass with heterogeneous echogenicity. (A). Right radial breast sonogram. (B). Right antiradial breast sonogram. (C). Right antiradial color power Doppler breast sonogram (see Color Plate 191-1C).

Pathology

- lactating adenoma

Management

- BI-RADS Assessment Category 4, suspicious; biopsy should be considered

Pearls and Pitfalls

1. Adenomas are benign tumors consisting of epithelial and myoepithelial lined tubules. Adenomas differ from fibroadenomas because adenomas have little stroma. In fibroadenomas, stromal cells are the dominate feature.
2. Lactating adenomas occur in young women who are either pregnant or nursing. Of an Armed Forces Institute of Pathology (AFIP) series of 88 lactating adenomas, the oldest woman was 38 years.
3. Because lactating adenomas present as palpable masses in young pregnant or nursing women, these masses are commonly imaged only with sonography. They are generally well-defined, oval or lobulated masses that are hypoechoic or heterogeneous in echogenicity. They are sonographically similar to fibroadenomas.

Suggested Readings

1. Bassett LW, Ysrael M, Gold RH, Ysrael C. Usefulness of mammography and sonography in women less than 35 years of age. *Radiology* 1991;180:831–835.
2. Hertel BF, Zaloudek C, Kempson RI. Breast adenomas. *Cancer* 1976;37:2891–2905.
3. Tavassoli FA, Fattaneh A. *Pathology of the Breast.* 2nd ed. Stamford: Appleton and Lange; 1999:157–165.

Case 192

Case History

A 49-year-old woman presents with a red spot on her right breast.

Physical Examination

- right breast: tender mass present at the 1:30 position; diffuse erythema of the upper inner quadrant
- left breast: normal exam

Mammogram (Fig. 192–1)

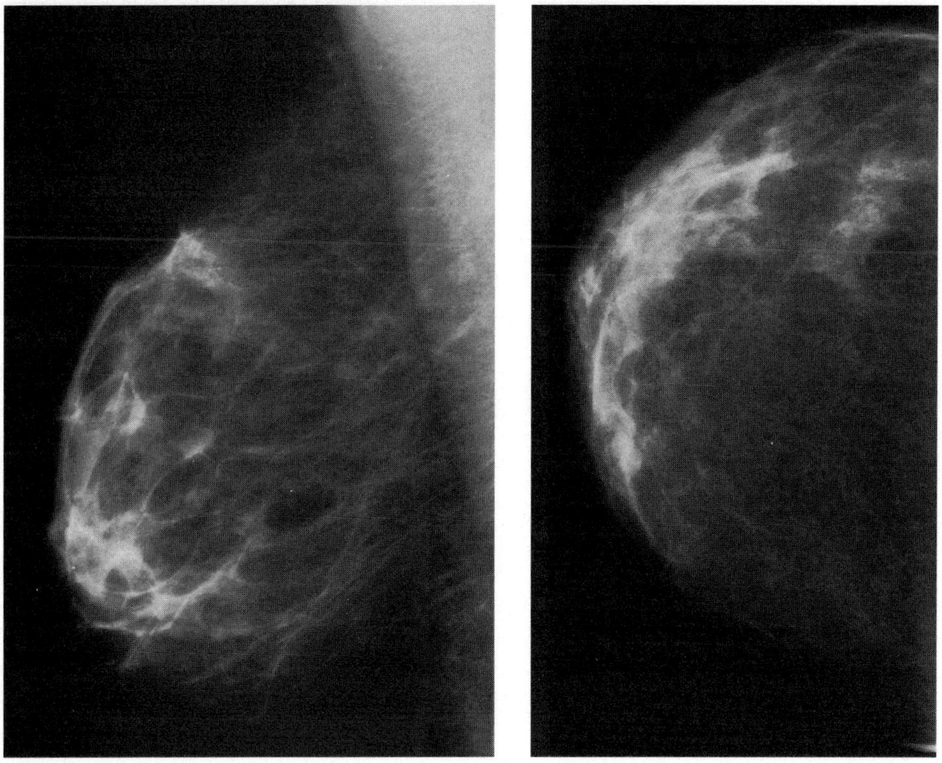

A B

Figure 192–1. Right breast mammogram is normal. (A). Right MLO mammogram. (B). Right CC mammogram.

Ultrasound

Frequency

- 7 MHz

Mass

- margin: ill defined
- echogenicity: heterogeneous
- retrotumoral acoustic appearance: no shadowing
- shape: ellipsoid (Fig. 192–2)

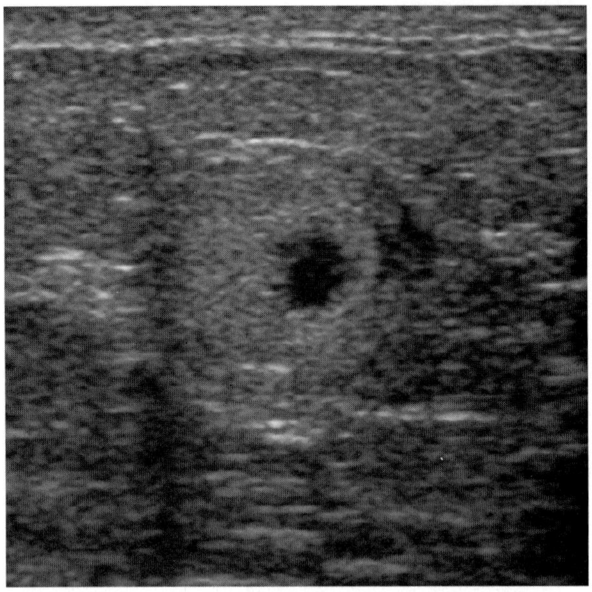

Figure 192–2. *Right radial breast sonogram: The palpable mass corresponds to a complex thick-walled mass that has fluid and solid components.*

Pathology

- abscess

Management

- BI-RADS Assessment Category 4, suspicious; biopsy should be considered

Pearls and Pitfalls

1. About 0.2 cc of yellow purulent material was aspirated and the patient's symptoms resolved with antibiotics.
2. Abscesses are most commonly the result of mastitis from either *Staphylococcus aureus* or streptococcal bacteria. These infections result from disruption of the skin with retrograde inflammatory progression.
3. Mammographically, an abscess may produce an ill-defined noncalcified mass. Rarely air may be identified. Commonly, abscesses may not be visible. The lack of findings may partially be due to inadequate compression due to severe breast tenderness.
4. Sonographically, abscesses commonly have thick walls and are oval or irregular in shape. The abscess cavity is comprised of cystic and solid components. The abscess fluid produces posterior acoustic enhancement. Sonography is an excellent method to identify and drain abscesses.

Suggested Readings

1. Bland KI. Inflammatory, infectious and metabolic disorders of the breast. In: Bland KI, Copeland EM, eds. *The Breast.* 2nd ed. Philadelphia: WB Saunders; 1998:75–108.
2. Hayes R, Michell M, Nunnerley HB. Acute inflammation of the breast—the role of breast ultrasound in diagnosis and management. *Clin Radiol* 1991;44:253–256.
3. Karstrup S, Solvig J, Nolsoe CP, et al. Acute puerperal breast abscesses: US-guided drainage. *Radiology* 1993;188:807–809.
4. Tohno D, Cosgrove DO, Sloane JP, eds. *Ultrasound Diagnosis of Breast Diseases.* New York: Churchill Livingston; 1994:136–138.

Case 193

Case History

A 68-year-old woman had right lumpectomy and radiation therapy 7 years ago for breast cancer. She now presents with new red skin lesions on the incision site.

Physical Examination

- right breast: three red quarter-sized lesions around the healed lumpectomy scar
- left breast: normal exam

Mammogram (Fig. 193–1)

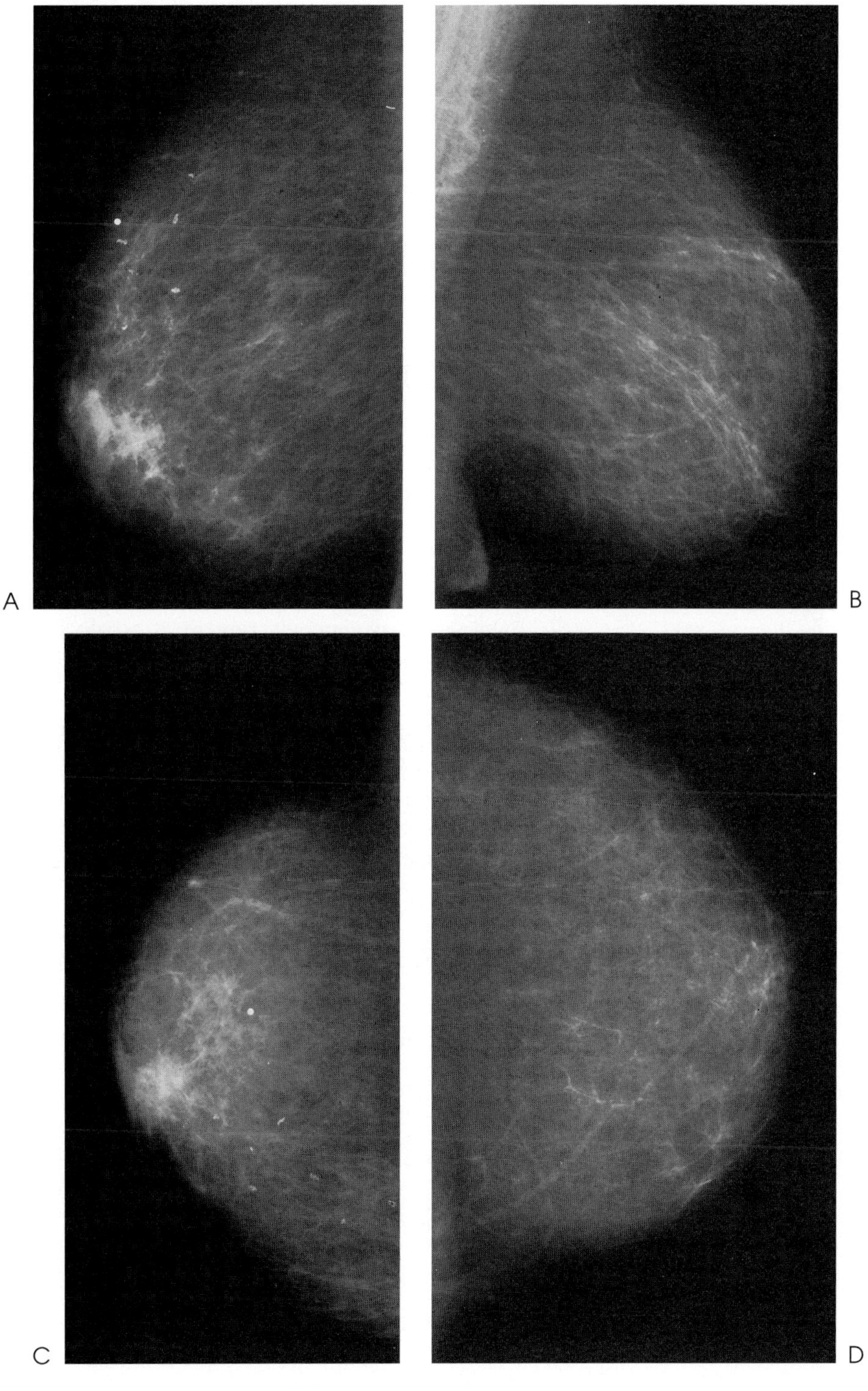

Figure 193–1. There is ill-defined increased density and coarsening of the trabecular pattern of the right breast consistent with previous radiation therapy. No mass corresponding to the skin abnormalities is identified. Left breast is normal. (A). Right MLO mammogram. (B). Left MLO mammogram. (C). Right CC mammogram. (D). Left CC mammogram.

Other Modalities (Fig. 193–2)

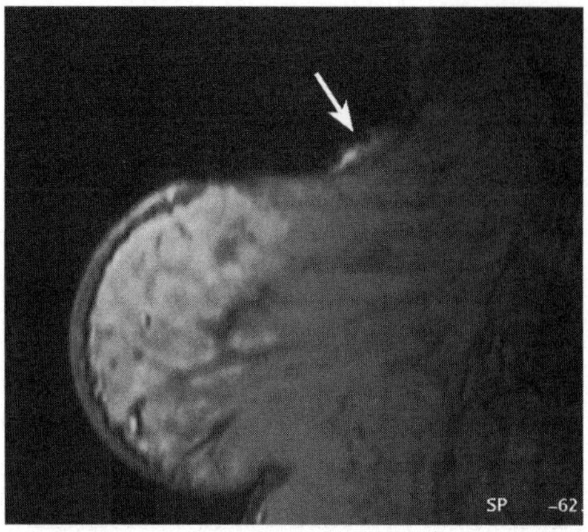

Figure 193–2. Right longitudinal dynamic bolus three-dimensional (3-D) volume gradient series breast MRI: There is abnormal enhancement of an irregular superficial mass (arrow) in the upper outer quadrant.

Pathology

- angiosarcoma

Management

- BI-RADS Assessment Category 4, suspicious; biopsy should be considered

Pearls and Pitfalls

1. The breast is a relatively common site for angiosarcoma. In a series of 33 patients from Sloan-Kettering, breast was fourth (9%) behind head (27%), thigh (18%), and arm (12%). However, compared with other breast malignancies, this tumor is rare. It accounts for less than 0.05% of primary breast cancers. Women who have had breast cancer have an increased risk for developing this tumor. The reason for this association is not clear.
2. Angiosarcomas generally present as a palpable mass. A blue-red skin discoloration is commonly present. Generally, nipple discharge, retraction, and axillary adenopathy are absent even with large masses.
3. Mammographically, these tumors are lobulated or irregular in shape and have ill-defined margins. Calcifications have been described in 10% of masses and skin thickening in 5% of cases. Many (35%) of these tumors are not visible mammographically.
4. Sonographically, these masses appear ellipsoid, lobulated, or irregular with either well-defined or ill-defined margins. The masses are hypoechoic, heterogeneous, or hyperechoic in echogenicity.
5. With MRI, these tumors have a low to intermediate signal intensity on T1-weighted studies and a high signal intensity on T2-weighted sequences.

Suggested Readings

1. Cozen W, Berstein L, Wang F, Press MF, Mack TM. The risk of angiosarcoma following primary breast cancer. *Br J Cancer* 1999;81:532–536.
2. Grant EG, Holt RW, Chun B, Richardson JD, Orson LW, Cigtay OS. Angiosarcoma of the breast: sonographic, xeromammographic, and pathologic appearance. *AJR Am J Roentgenol* 1983;141:691–692.
3. Lieberman L, Dershaw DD, Kaufman RJ, Rosen PP. Angiosarcoma of the breast. *Radiology* 1992;183:649–654.
4. Tavassoli FA, Fattaneh A. *Pathology of the Breast.* 2nd ed. Stamford: Appleton and Lange; 1999:633–673.

Case 194

Case History

A 42-year-old woman presents with new left breast lump.

Physical Examination

- left breast: ill-defined 5 cm area of thickening in the upper outer quadrant
- right breast: normal exam

Mammogram (Fig. 194-1)

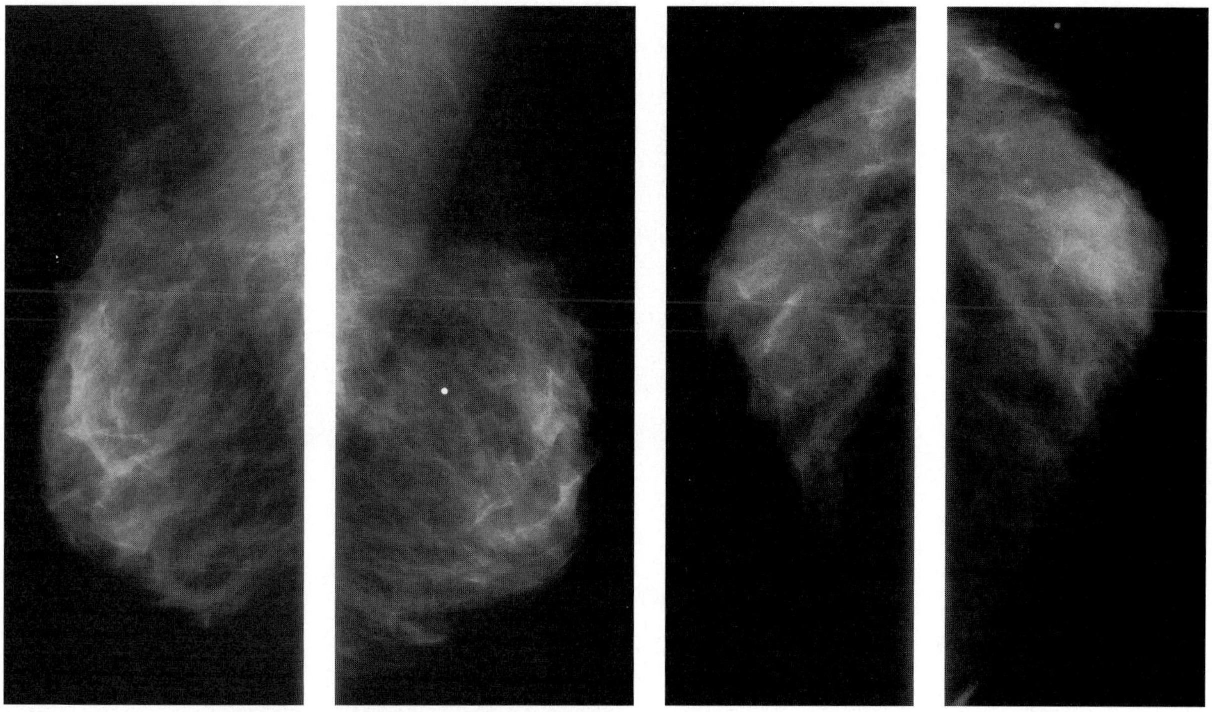

A B C D

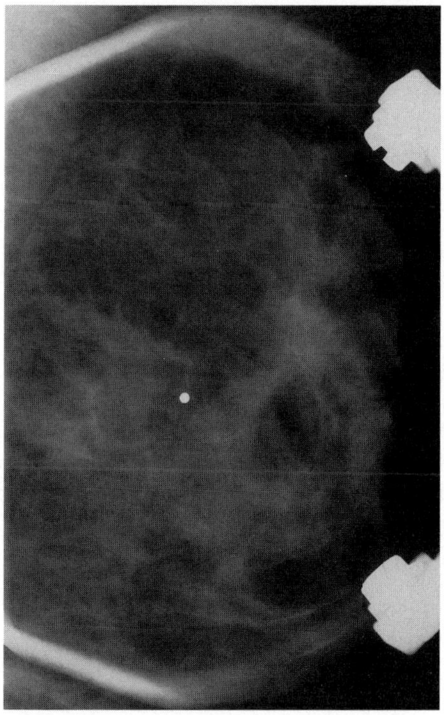

E

Figure 194-1. Bilateral mammograms demonstrate scattered fibroglandular densities. The palpable mass (labeled with a radiographic marker) is associated with an area of focal increased density in the left breast visible only on the MLO view (B,E). (A). Right MLO mammogram. (B). Left MLO mammogram. (C). Right CC mammogram. (D). Left CC mammogram. (E). Left MLO spot magnification mammogram of region of palpable mass.

Ultrasound

Frequency

- 11.5 MHz

Mass

- margin: ill defined
- echogenicity: hypoechoic
- retrotumoral acoustic appearance: no shadowing
- shape: ellipsoid (Fig. 194–2)

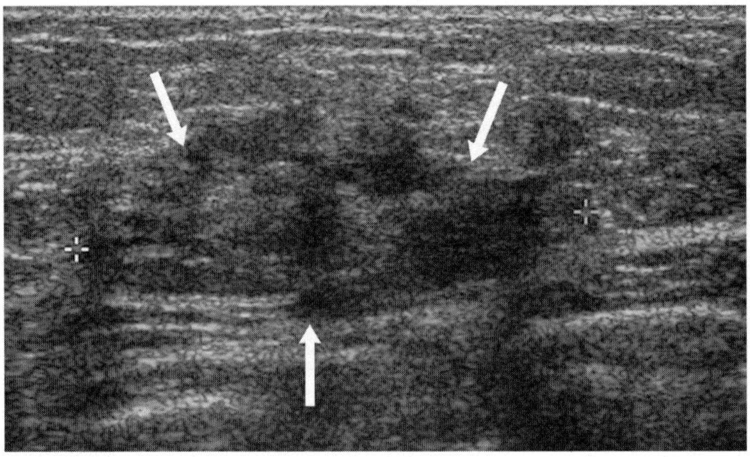

Figure 194–2. Left radial breast sonogram: The palpable thickening corresponded to an area of ill-defined hypoechogenicity (arrows) (see Color Plate 194–2).

Pathology

- ductal carcinoma in situ
- 4 cm of low-grade ductal carcinoma in situ

Management

- BI-RADS Assessment Category 4, suspicious; biopsy should be considered

Pearls and Pitfalls

Occasionally, ductal carcinoma in situ presents as a palpable mass. Sonographically, this malignancy is relatively difficult to identify. Sonographic findings include calcifications, irregular hypoechoic mass, focally dilated ducts, and ill-defined hypoechoic area. This case illustrates the last type of appearance.

Suggested Readings

1. Rickard MT. Ultrasound of malignant breast microcalcifications: role in evaluation and guided procedures. *Australas Radiol* 1996;40:26–31.
2. Schoonjans JM, Brem RF. Sonographic appearance of ductal carcinoma in situ diagnosed with ultrasonographically guided large core needle biopsy: correlation with mammographic and pathologic findings. *J Ultrasound Med* 2000;19:427–440.

Case 195

Case History

A 35-year-old woman found a right breast lump on breast self-examination.

Physical Examination

- right breast: irregular movable mass at the 10:00 position
- left breast: normal exam

Mammogram (Fig. 195–1)

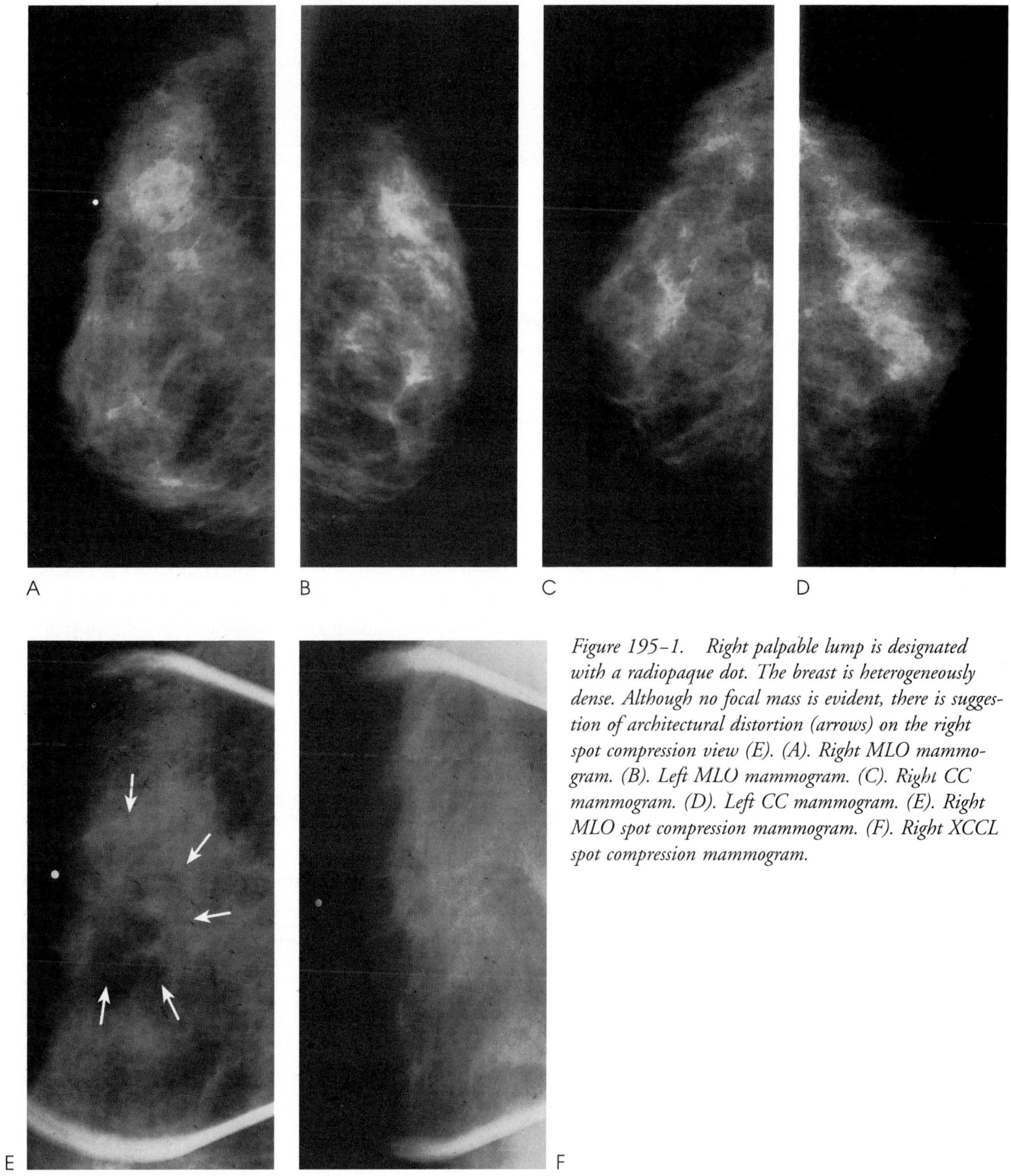

Figure 195–1. *Right palpable lump is designated with a radiopaque dot. The breast is heterogeneously dense. Although no focal mass is evident, there is suggestion of architectural distortion (arrows) on the right spot compression view (E). (A). Right MLO mammogram. (B). Left MLO mammogram. (C). Right CC mammogram. (D). Left CC mammogram. (E). Right MLO spot compression mammogram. (F). Right XCCL spot compression mammogram.*

Ultrasound

Frequency

- 11.5 MHz

Mass

- margin: ill defined
- echogenicity: hypoechoic
- retrotumoral acoustic appearance: posterior shadowing distal to mass
- shape: irregular (Fig. 195–2)

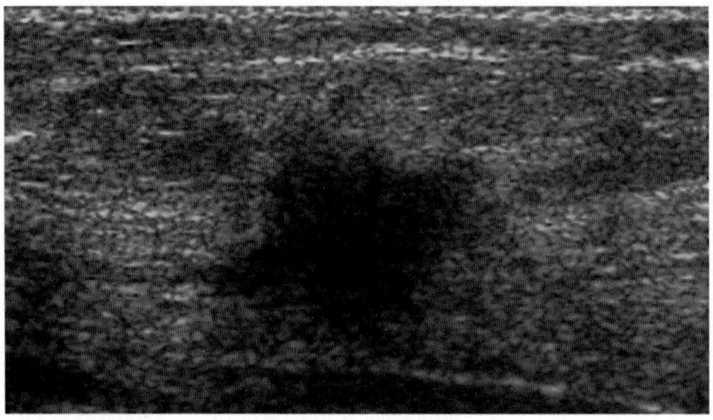

Figure 195–2. Right radial breast sonogram: An ill-defined irregular mass of heterogeneous echogenicity corresponds to the palpable mass.

Pathology

- invasive ductal carcinoma
- 1.6 cm primary tumor; one of eight axillary nodes positive for metastatic tumor

Management

- BI-RADS Assessment Category 4, suspicious; biopsy should be considered

Pearls and Pitfalls

One of the well-established reasons for breast sonography is examination of a palpable mass that is not mammographically identified. Lack of mammographic identification may be due to a variety of factors including suboptimal technique, unusual position of mass, or overlap of tumor with fibroglandular tissue.

Suggested Readings

1. Cosmacini P, Veronesi P, Galimberti V, Ferranti C, Viganotti G, Coopmans de Yoldi G. Ultrasonographic evaluation of palpable breast masses: analysis of 134 cases. *Tumori* 1990;76:495–498.
2. Dennis MA, Parker SH, Klaus AJ, Stavros AT, Kaske TI, Clark SB. Breast biopsy avoidance: the value of normal mammograms and normal sonograms in the setting of a palpable lump. *Radiology* 2001;219:186–291.
3. Zonderland HM. The role of ultrasound in the diagnosis of breast cancer. *Semin Ultrasound CT MR* 2000;21:317–324.

Case 196

Case History

- A 45-year-old woman presents with a palpable lump.

Physical Examination

- right breast: small palpable lump at 4:30 position associated with skin thickening and mild redness
- left breast: normal exam

Mammogram (Fig. 196–1)

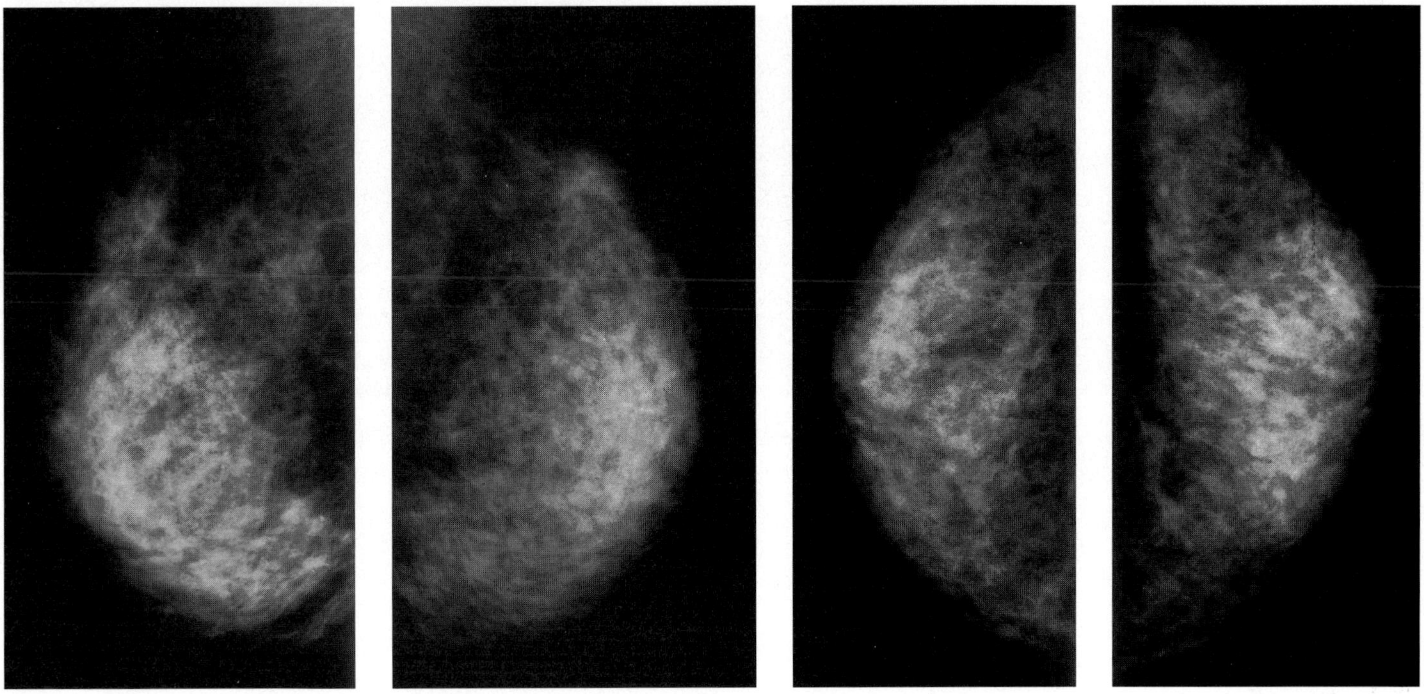

A B C D

Figure 196–1. The palpable mass is not evident on the heterogeneously dense mammograms. (A). Right MLO mammogram. (B). Left MLO mammogram. (C). Right CC mammogram. (D). Left CC mammogram.

Ultrasound

Frequency

- 13 MHz

Mass

- margin: ill defined
- echogenicity: hypoechoic
- retrotumoral acoustic appearance: bilateral edge shadowing
- shape: irregular (Fig. 196–2)

A 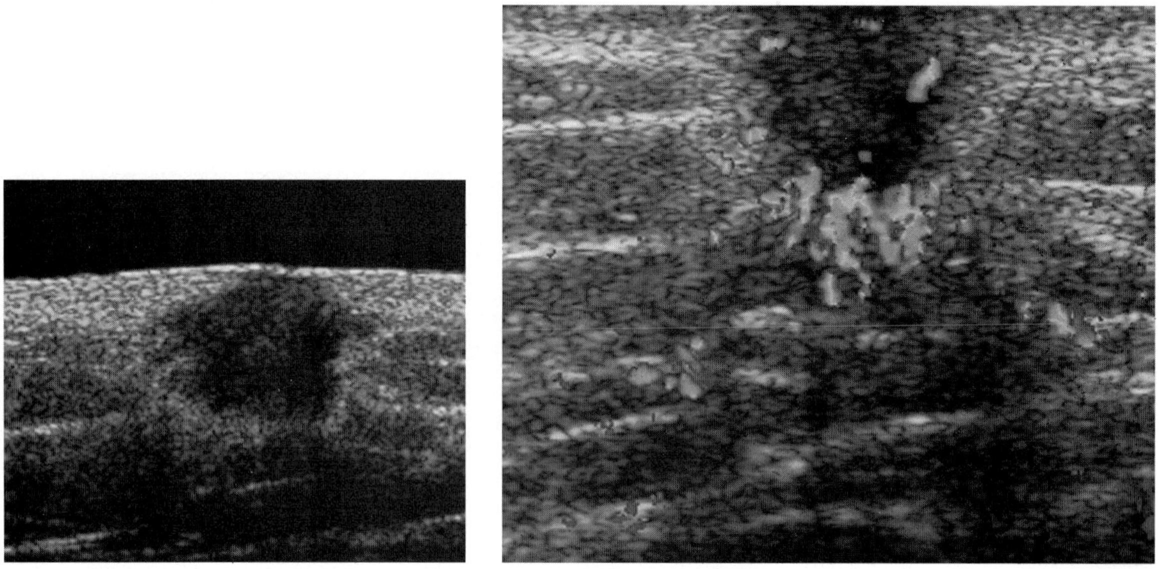 B

Figure 196–2. The palpable mass corresponds to an irregular, hypoechoic mass. The mass extends into the hyperechoic skin. (A). Right radial breast sonogram. (B). Right radial color Doppler breast sonogram (see Color Plate 196–2 B).

Pathology

- malignant fibrous histiocytoma

Management

- BI-RADS Assessment Category 4, suspicious; biopsy should be considered

Pearls and Pitfalls

1. Malignant fibrous histiocytomas are an unusual breast sarcoma. Most reported cases are idiopathic, but this lesion has been related to previous radiation therapy. In an AFIP series of 24 tumors, 5 tumors were in men. The mean patient age was 58 years.
2. We are unaware of radiographic descriptions of this entity. In this case, the tumor is an irregular, ill-defined, hypoechoic solid mass that is indistinguishable from other tumors.

Suggested Readings

1. Hori R, Fukuuchi A, Nishi T, Takanashi R. A case of malignant fibrous histiocytoma after breast conserving therapy for breast cancer. *Breast Cancer* 2000;7:75–77.
2. Tavassoli FA, Fattaneh A. *Pathology of the Breast.* 2nd ed. Stamford: Appleton and Lange; 1999:718–729.

Case 197

Case History

A 39-year-old woman presents with a palpable left breast lump.

Physical Examination

- left breast: 5 mm lump in the upper outer quadrant
- right breast: normal exam

Mammogram (Fig. 197–1)

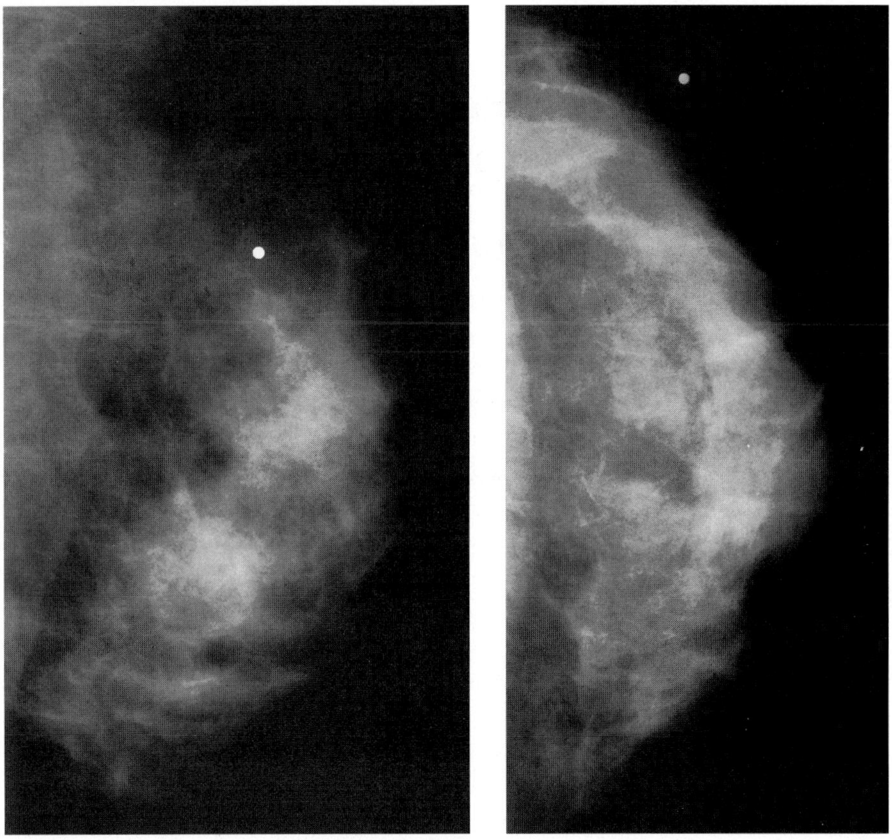

A B

Figure 197–1. *Normal left mammogram. Breast is extremely dense. No mass is associated with the palpable lump, which is marked with a radiopaque dot. (A). Left MLO mammogram. (B). Left CC mammogram.*

Ultrasound

Frequency

- 13 MHz (Fig. 197–2) .

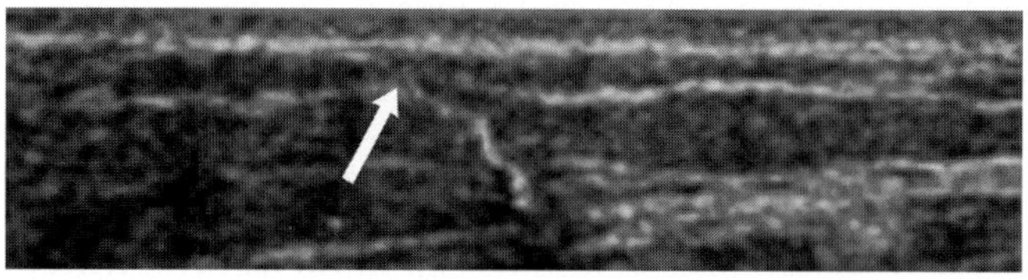

Figure 197–2. Left oblique breast color Doppler sonogram: The palpable lump corresponds to a Cooper's ligament attachment (arrow) (see Color Plate 197–2).

Pathology

- Cooper's ligament attachment

Management

- BI-RADS Assessment Category 2, benign finding

Pearls and Pitfalls

1. With higher-frequency sonography, the normal breast structures are better visualized. Many palpable lumps are due to normal breast structures. Cooper's ligament attachments are commonly palpable, particularly in the upright position. Sometimes one attachment is more prominent as illustrated in this case. After one identifies the attachment as the etiology of the lump, one can generally confirm the presence of similar (but less obvious) lumps throughout the breast that also correspond to these ligaments sonographically. Other common palpable lumps include lobular fibroglandular tissue, fat lobules, and blood vessels. To assign a BI-RADS Category 2 (benign) or 3 (probably benign) to a palpable lump, it is critical that the mammogram also be normal.
2. The main reasons for missing a neoplasm when one sonographically identifies "normal structures" include (1) not using high-resolution sonography; (2) not palpating the correct abnormality; (3) not correlating the sonogram to the mammogram; (4) not linking the palpable lump to a specific normal structure; (5) suboptimal sonographic technique (e.g., inadequate contrast). Some lesions such as ductal carcinoma in situ will be present with minimal disruption of breast architecture. Therefore, I would not assign a Category 2 to a "negative breast sonogram" for the following situations: (1) The patient is unusually high risk for cancer (e.g., previous history of cancer, high-risk gene pool). (2) The patient has any other symptoms besides a palpable lump (e.g., nipple discharge). (3) The lump size is discordant with the size of the normal structure. (4) The mammogram has any abnormality or asymmetry. (5) High-frequency sonography is not available.

Suggested Readings

1. Dennis MA, Parker SH, Klaus AJ, Stavros AT, Kaske TI, Clark SB. Breast biopsy avoidance: the value of normal mammograms and normal sonograms in the setting of a palpable lump. *Radiology* 2001;219:186–191.

Case 198

Case History

A 76-year-old woman presents with a new right palpable lump.

Physical Examination

- right breast: firm lump associated with a bruise in the 12:00 position
- left breast: normal exam

Mammogram (Fig. 198–1)

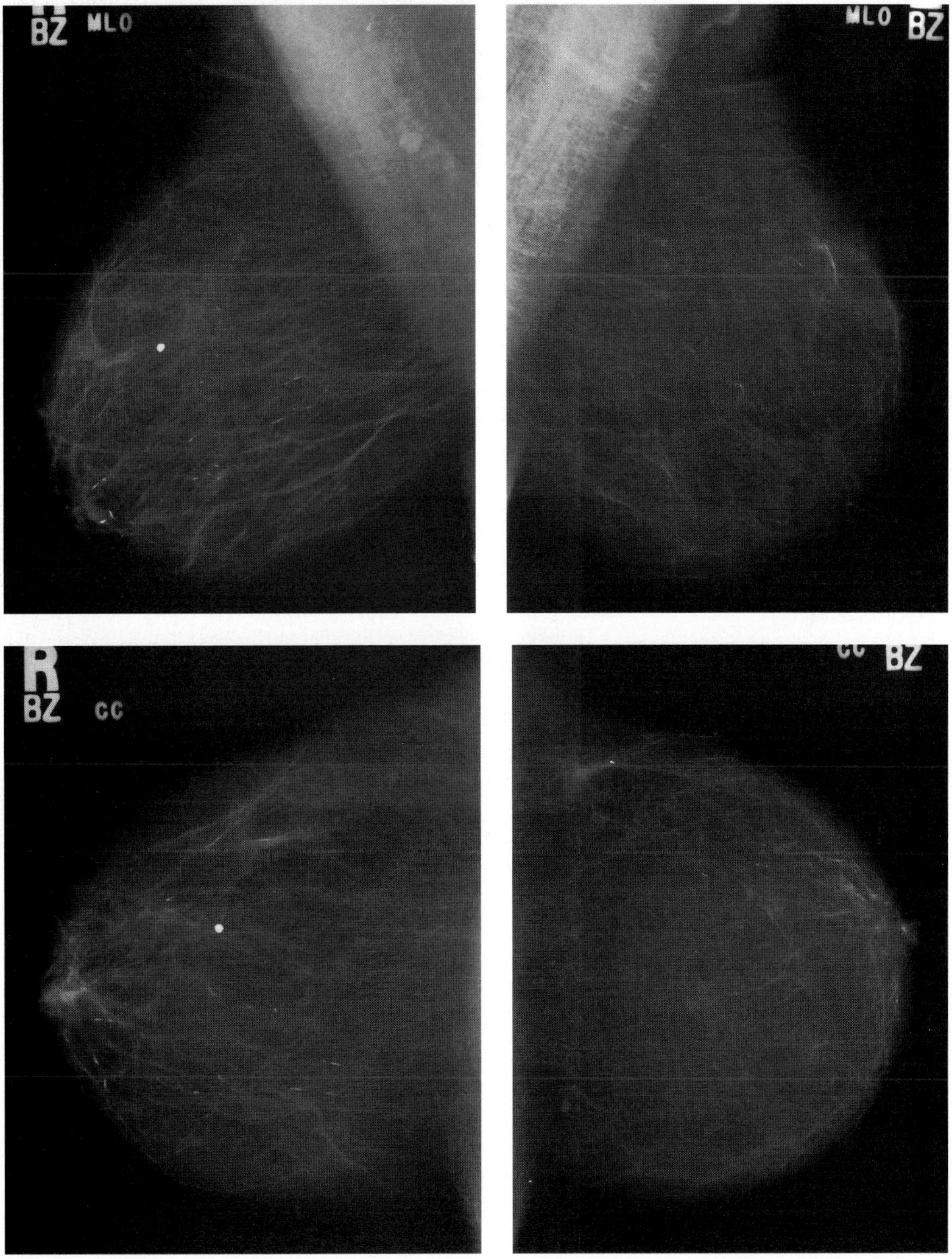

A B C D

Figure 198–1. There are benign calcifications in the right breast. Both breasts are predominantly fatty and normal in appearance. (A). Right MLO mammogram. (B). Left MLO mammogram. (C). Right CC mammogram. (D). Left CC mammogram.

Ultrasound

Frequency

- 13 MHz

Mass

- margin: ill defined
- echogenicity: hyperechoic
- retrotumoral acoustic appearance: no shadowing
- shape: irregular (Fig. 198–2)

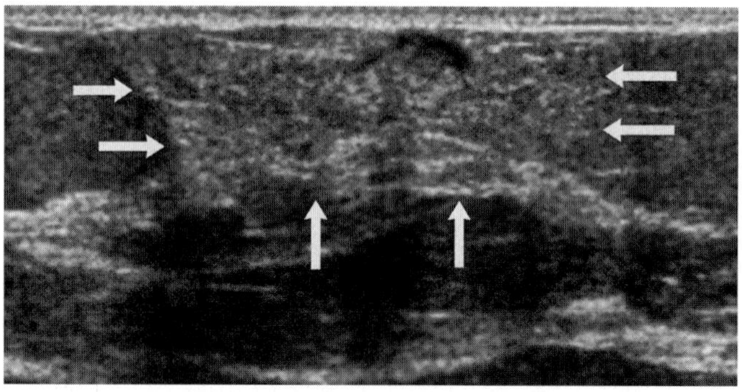

Figure 198–2. Right antiradial breast sonogram: The palpable lump corresponds to a uniformly hyperechoic area (arrows). The superficial linear hypoechogenicity corresponded to a small vessel by color Doppler.

Pathology

- fat necrosis

Management

- BI-RADS Assessment Category 3, probably benign; short-interval follow-up

Pearls and Pitfalls

Homogeneous, circumscribed hyperechoic sonographic masses are generally benign. Differential diagnosis includes fat necrosis, fibrosis, hyalinized fibroadenomas, and angiolipomas. In this clinical setting, fat necrosis is the most likely etiology for the sonographic findings. She was not biopsied. Patient returned 1 month later and palpable lump and sonographic findings had decreased greatly in size.

Suggested Readings

1. Stavros AT, Thickman D, Rapp CL, Dennis MA, Parker SH, Sisney GA. Solid breast nodules: use of sonography to distinguish between benign and malignant lesions. *Radiology* 1995;196:123–143.

Case 199

Case History

A 58-year-old woman presents with a palpable left breast lump.

Physical Examination

- left breast: 1 cm soft nodule in the upper outer quadrant
- right breast: normal exam

Mammogram

Mass

- architectural distortion (Fig. 199–1)

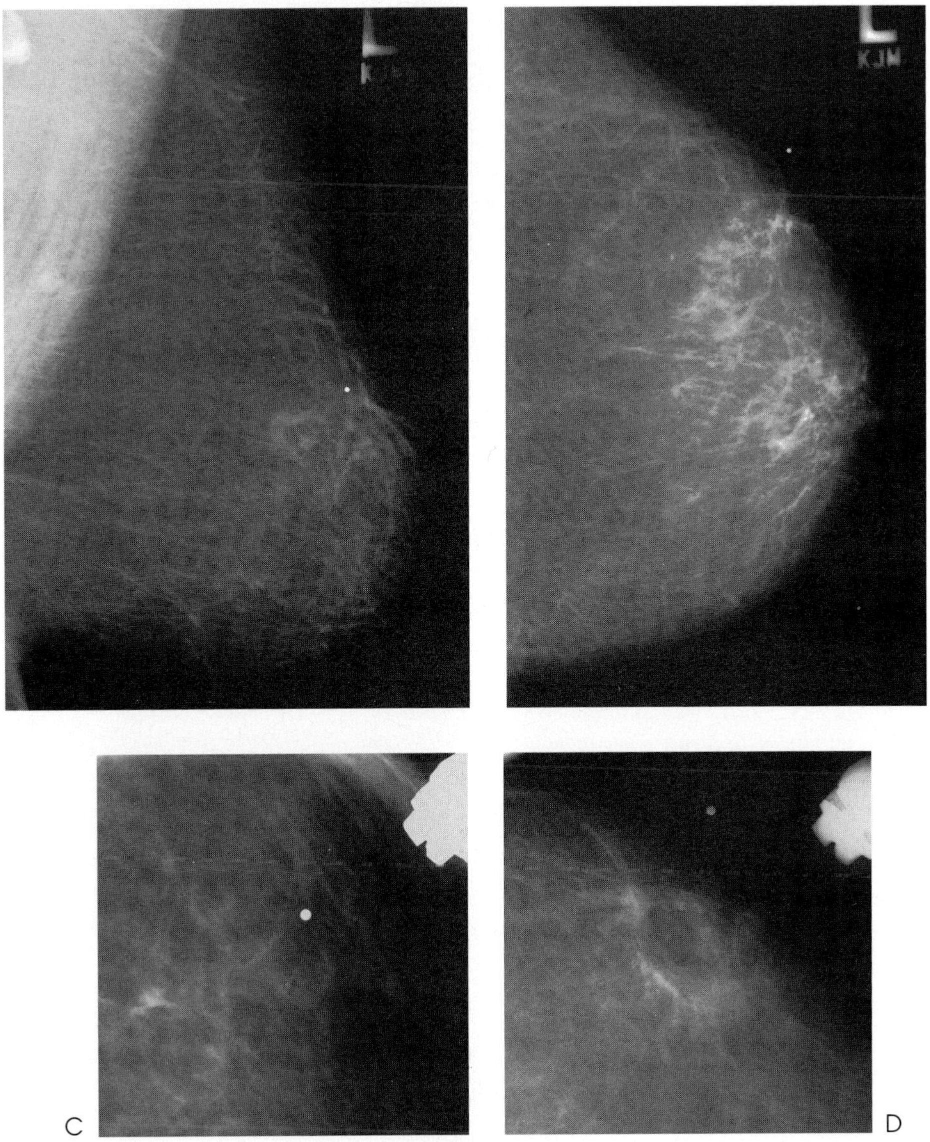

A B C D

Figure 199–1. Left breast mammograms: Although the breast is predominantly fatty in composition, no mass is associated with the radiographic marker. The marker identifies the location of a palpable lump. In the CC spot compression view, there is a subtle small area of architectural distortion associated with the radiographic marker. (A). Left MLO mammogram. (B). Left CC mammogram. (C). Left MLO spot compression mammogram. (D). Left CC spot compression mammogram.

Ultrasound

Low Frequency

Frequency

- 7 MHz

Mass

- margin: ill defined
- echogenicity: hypoechoic
- retrotumoral acoustic appearance: no shadowing
- shape: oval with large lobulations (Fig. 199–2)

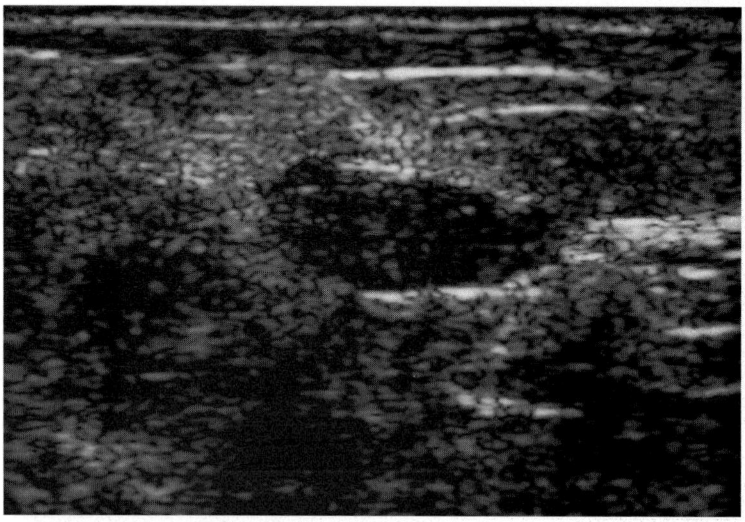

Figure 199–2. Left breast antiradial sonogram: The palpable lump corresponds to a well-defined oval hypoechoic mass without posterior acoustic shadowing. Increased echogenicity superficial to the mass may be due to architectural distortion.

High Frequency

Frequency

- 11.5 MHz (Fig. 199–3)

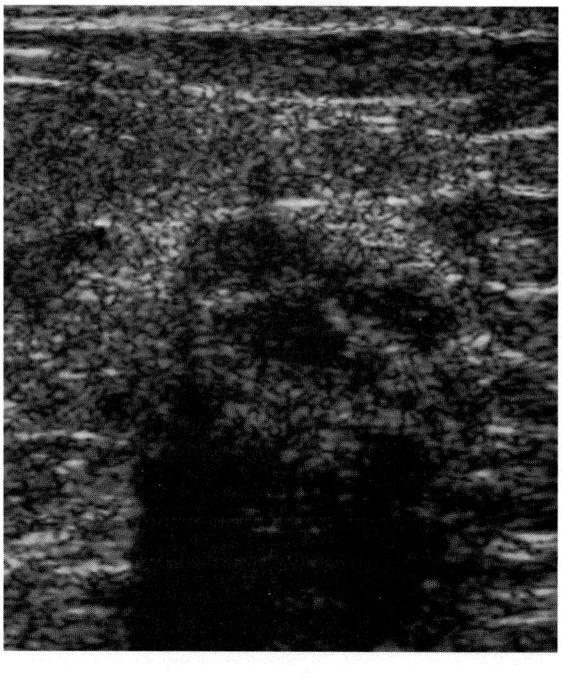

Figure 199–3. Left breast antiradial sonogram: Higher-frequency sonographic examination of the same mass as Figure 199–2 demonstrates more internal heterogeneous echogenicity compared with the lower-frequency examination. Furthermore, the higher-frequency examination demonstrates that the margin of the mass is ill defined and there is diffuse posterior acoustic shadowing.

Pathology

- infiltrating ductal carcinoma

Management

- BI-RADS Assessment Category 4, suspicious; biopsy should be considered

Pearls and Pitfalls

This case is an example that sonographic information is useful even in a predominantly fatty breast. The mammographic architectural distortion is subtle, but the sonographic exam clearly identifies a suspicious mass. This case also illustrates that high-frequency sonography provides additional diganostic information that improves diagnostic confidence. If one ignores or overlooks the anterior hyperechogenicity on the low-frequency exam, one may erroneously decide to characterize this mass as a probably benign lesion. However, the high-frequency study clearly demonstrates several malignant characteristics (i.e., ill-defined margin, heterogeneous echogenicity).

Suggested Readings

1. Stavros AT, Thickman D, Rapp CL, Dennis MA, Parker SH, Sisney GA. Solid breast nodules: use of sonography to distinguish between benign and malignant lesions. *Radiology* 1995;196:123–134.

Case 200

Case History

A 69-year-old woman presents for screening mammogram.

Physical Examination

- bilateral breast: multiple lumps

Mammogram

Calcifications (Fig. 200–1)

- type: pleomorphic/heterogeneous
- distribution: grouped/clustered

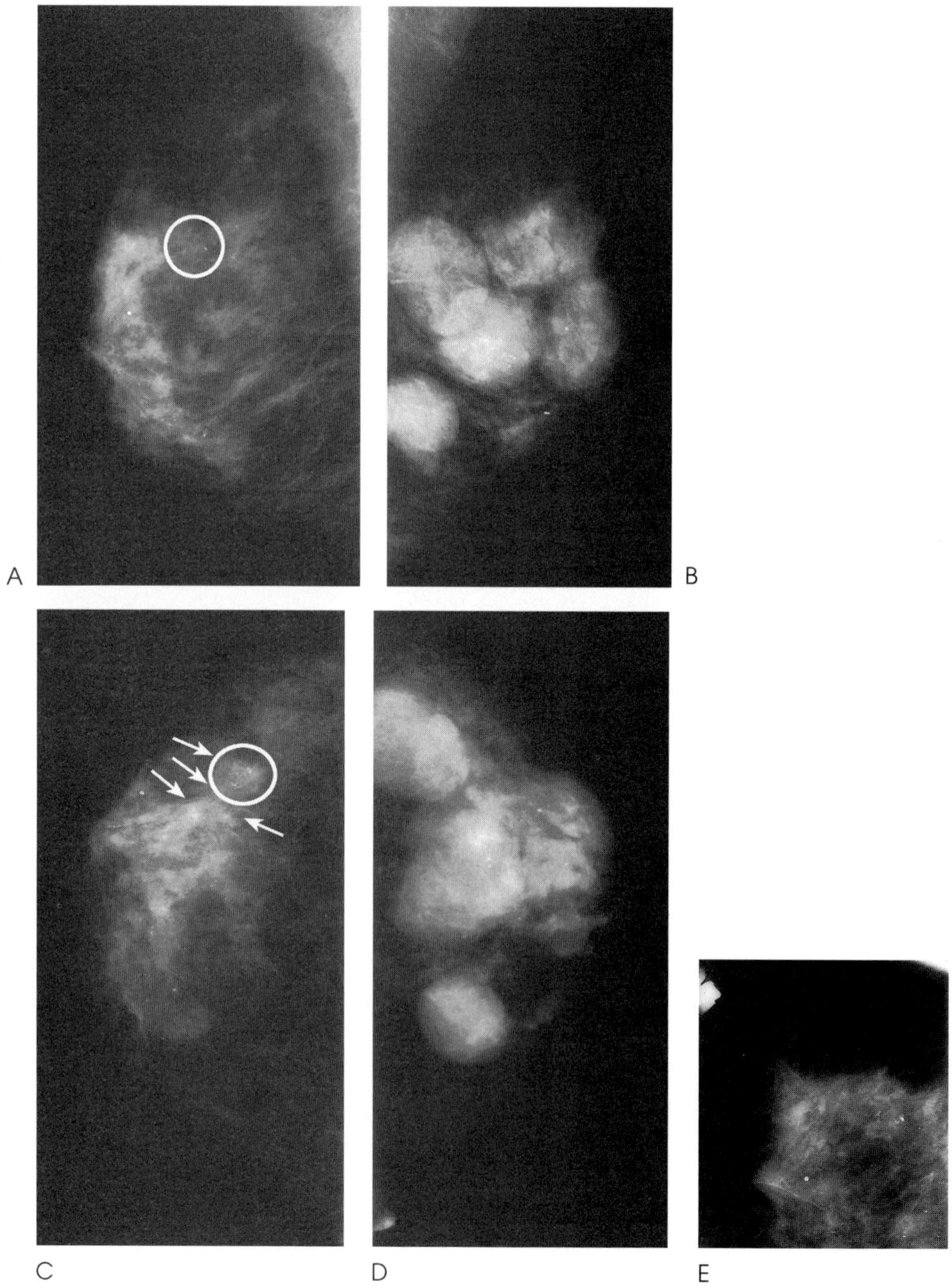

Figure 200–1. The right breast has a cluster of heterogeneous calcifications (circle) in the upper outer breast. These calcifications are associated with architectural distortion in the CC view. The left breast has multiple round and oval masses that have been stable for several years. (A). Right MLO mammogram. (B). Left MLO mammogram. (C). Right CC mammogram. (D). Left CC mammogram. (E). Right ML spot magnification mammogram.

Ultrasound

Frequency

- 12 MHz

Mass

- margin: ill defined
- echogenicity: hypoechoic
- retrotumoral acoustic appearance: posterior shadowing distal to mass
- shape: irregular (Fig. 200–2)

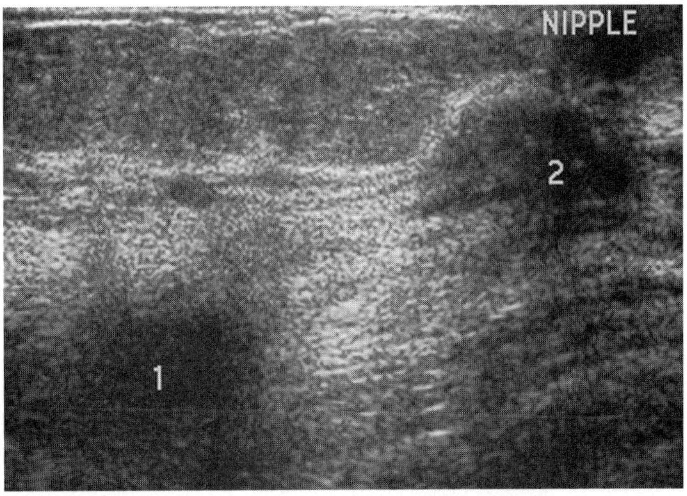

Figure 200–2. Right radial breast sonogram: Two hypoechoic irregular masses are present. The first mass (1) is in the upper outer quadrant and the second mass (2) is next to the nipple.

Pathology

- mixed ductal and lobular carcinoma
- two separate foci of mixed ductal and lobular carcinoma

Management

- BI-RADS Assessment Category 5, highly suggestive of malignancy

Pearls and Pitfalls

In this case, it was not clear if the architectural distortion was associated with the abnormal calcifications as the distortion was only visible in one view. Furthermore, the architectural distortion appeared much larger than the area of the calcifications. Sonography may be helpful when there is a mammographic imaging discrepancy. In this case, the abnormal mammographic calcifications and architectural distortion correspond to multifocal disease.

Suggested Readings

1. Baker JA, Soo MS. The evolving role of sonography in evaluating solid breast masses. *Semin Ultrasound CT MR* 2000;21:286–296.
2. Buchberger W, Niehoff A, Obrist P, DeKoekkoek-Doll, Dunser M. Clinically and mammographically occult breast lesions: detection and classification with high-resolution sonography. *Semin Ultrasound CT MR* 2000;21:325–336.

Case 201

Case History

A 45-year-old woman presents with thickening in the right breast, which she thinks might be a pulled muscle.

Physical Examination

- right breast: large, mildly tender firm area extending from 9:00 to 12:00 in the right breast
- left breast: normal exam

Mammogram

Mass (Fig. 201–1)

- margin: ill defined
- shape: oval
- density: isodense

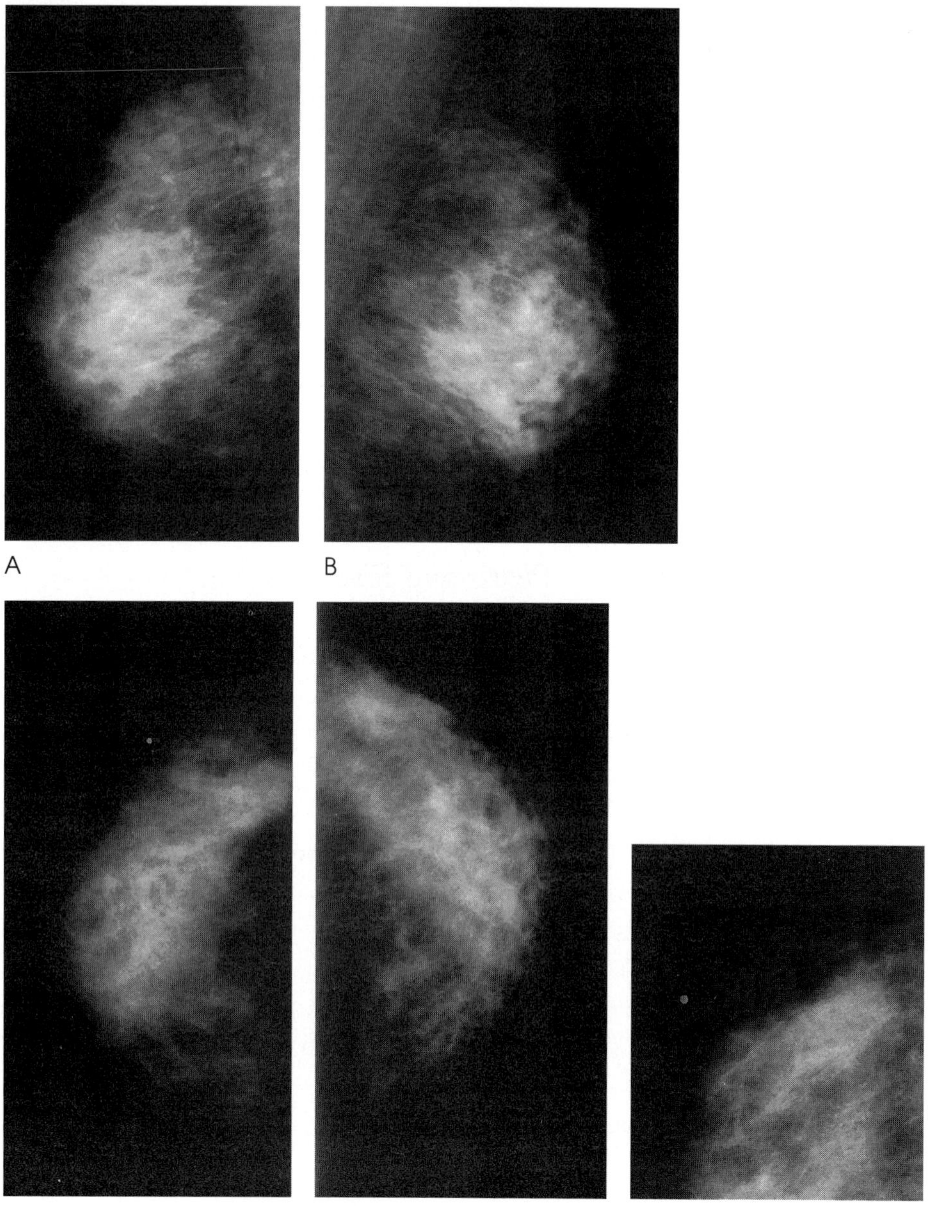

A B C D E

Figure 201–1. There is an ill-defined mass in the right upper outer quadrant. The size of the mass is difficult to determine because of the surrounding heterogeneous parenchymal density. (A). Right MLO mammogram. (B). Left MLO mammogram. (C). Right CC mammogram. (D). Left CC mammogram. (E). Right MLO spot compression mammogram.

Ultrasound

Frequency

- 10 MHz

Mass

- margin: ill defined
- echogenicity: hypoechoic
- retrotumoral acoustic appearance: extensive acoustic shadowing
- shape: irregular (Fig. 201-2)

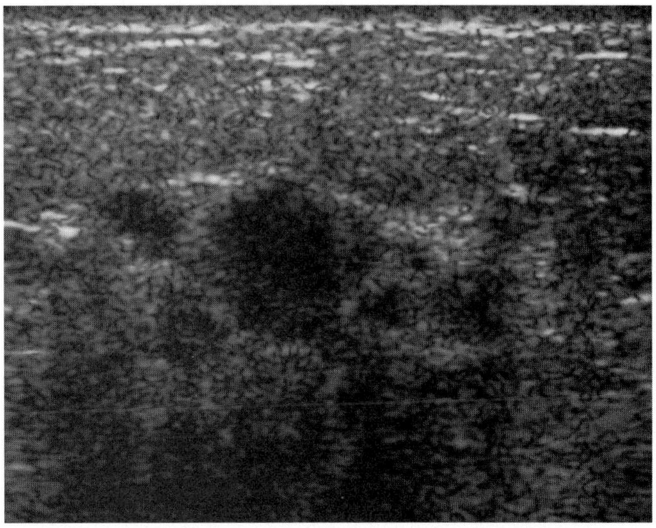

Figure 201-2. Right radial breast sonogram: In the upper outer quadrant, there are several hypoechoic, ill-defined solid nodules.

Other Modalities (Fig. 201-3)

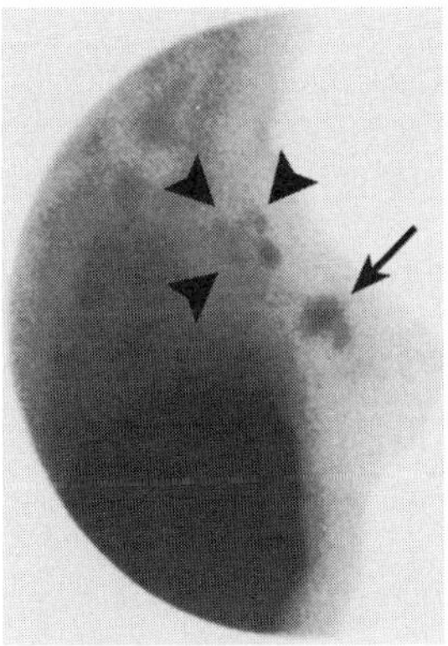

Figure 201-3. Tc-99m Sestamibi scan: The exam shows abnormal increased uptake within the breast (arrow) and in axillary lymph nodes (arrowheads).

Pathology

- infiltrating ductal carcinoma
- Stage II-B infiltrating ductal carcinoma with 9/13 nodes positive

Management

- BI-RADS Assessment Category 4, suspicious; biopsy should be considered

Pearls and Pitfalls

When the size or extent of a malignancy are not clear, ultrasound, MRI, and scintiammography can be helpful in determining the extent of tumors. In this case, scintimammography was useful as it demonstrated malignant extension into the axillary nodes.

Suggested Readings

1. Klaus AJ, Klingensmith WC, Parker SH, Stavros AT, Sutherland JD, Aldrete KD. Comparative value of 99mTc-sestamibi scintimammography and sonography in the diagnostic workup of breast masses. *AJR* 2000;174:1779–1783.
2. Palmedo H, Biersack HJ, Lastoria S, et al. Scintimammography with technetium-99 m methoxyisobutylisonitrile: results of a prospective European multi-centre trial. *European J of NM* 1998;25:375–385.
3. Waxman AD. The role of 99mTc methoxyisobutylisonitrile in imaging breast cancer. *Semin Nucl Med* 1997;27:40–54.

Case 202

Case History

A 42-year-old woman presents with a small superficial left breast lump.

Physical Examination

- left breast: a soft superficial lump at the 12:00 position
- right breast: normal exam

Ultrasound

Frequency

- 10 MHz

Mass

- margin: ill defined
- echogenicity: heterogeneous
- retrotumoral acoustic appearance: posterior shadowing distal to mass
- shape: ellipsoid (Fig. 202–1)

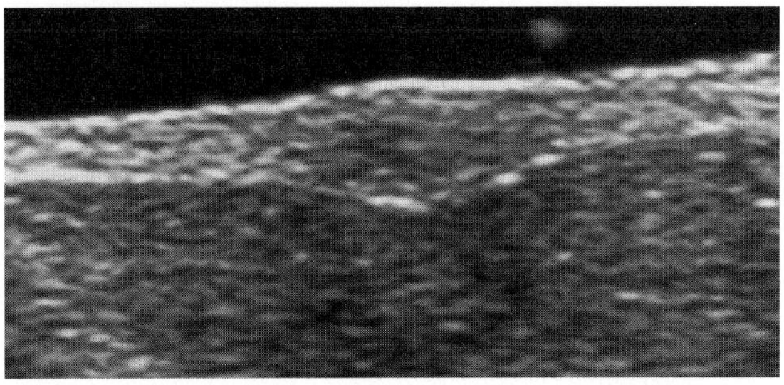

Figure 202–1. Left antiradial breast sonogram: The palpable lump corresponds to an ill-defined oval mass with heterogeneous echogenicity that is within the skin.

Pathology

- smooth muscle hamartoma

Management

- BI-RADS Assessment Category 3, probably benign; short-interval follow-up

Pearls and Pitfalls

Sonography is useful to identify superficial palpable masses. If additional mammographic imaging is needed, then a radiopaque dot may be placed over the sonographic mass and tangential mammographic views may be performed.

Suggested Readings

1. Ragsdale BD. Tumors of fatty, muscular, and osseous tissue. In: Elder D, ed. *Histolopathology of the Skin.* Philadelphia: Lippincott-Raven; 1997:933–975.

Case 203

Case History

A 40-year-old woman presents with a palpable right breast lump.

Physical Examination

- right breast: skin dimpling associated with irregular mass, which is fixed to the chest wall, at the 4:00 position in the inframammary fold
- left breast: normal exam

Mammogram

Mass (Fig. 203-1)

- margin: indistinct
- shape: focal asymmetric density
- density: high density

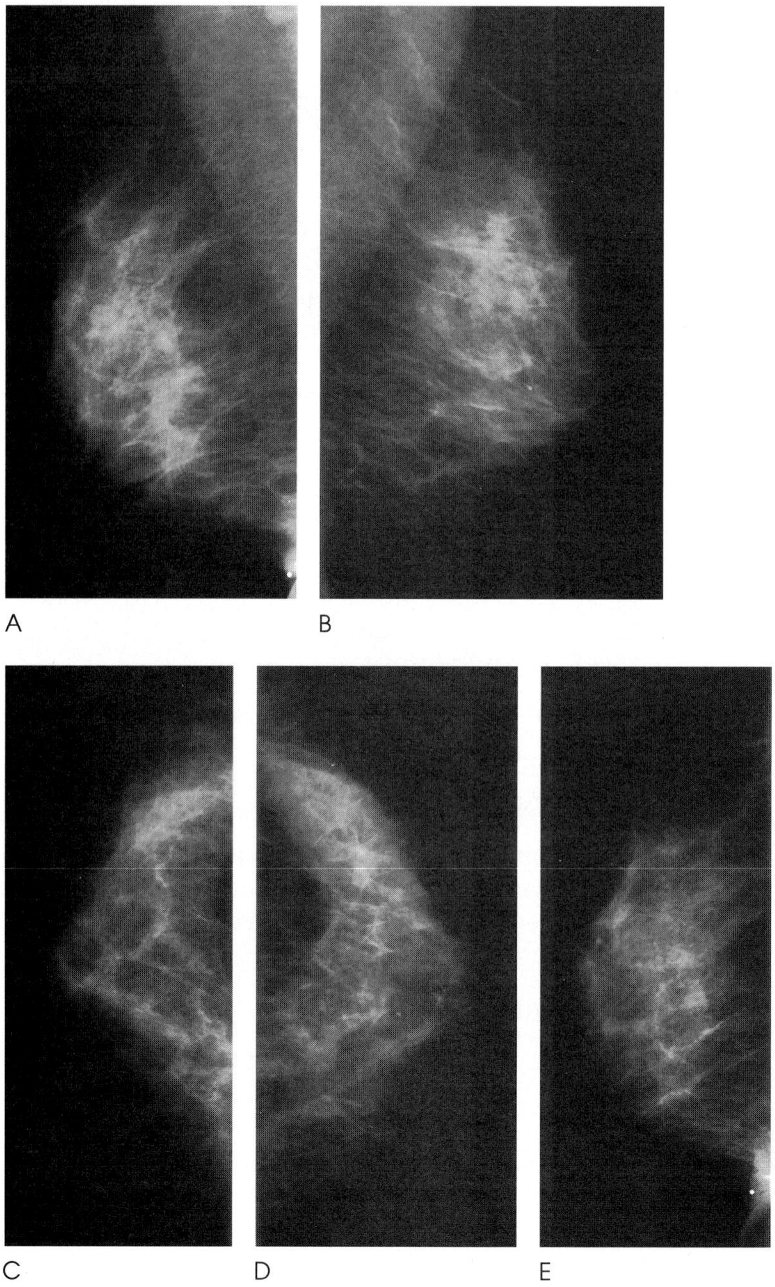

Figure 203-1. In the right inframammary fold (A,E), there is skin thickening and focal ill-defined density. (A). Right MLO mammogram. (B). Left MLO mammogram. (C). Right CC mammogram. (D). Left CC mammogram. (E). Right ML mammogram.

Ultrasound

Frequency

- 7.5 MHz

Mass

- margin: ill defined
- echogenicity: hypoechoic
- retrotumoral acoustic appearance: severe shadowing, mass completely obscured
- shape: irregular (Fig. 203–2)

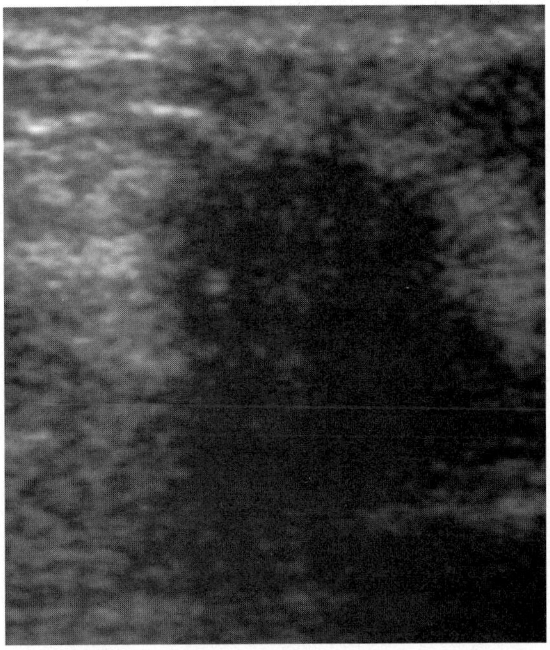

Figure 203–2. Right antiradial breast sonogram: The palpable mass corresponds to an irregular, hypoechoic, heavily shadowing mass. Superficially, there is extension of the spiculations into the skin.

Pathology

- infiltrating ductal carcinoma
- tumor infiltrated into dermis

Management

- BI-RADS Assessment Category 5, highly suggestive of malignancy

Pearls and Pitfalls

This is an example of an unusual location for tumor. When masses are in the extreme periphery of the breast (e.g., inframammary fold, peripheral axilla), they are commonly a greater challenge to image mammographically. Optimal imaging is also dependent upon the body habitus and flexibility of the patient. In these cases, sonography is useful to assist characterization of the lesion and provide guidance for biopsy.

Suggested Readings

1. American College of Radiology Committee on Quality Assurance in Mammography. *Mammography Quality Control Manual.* Reston: ACR; 1999.
2. Jackson VP. Breast sonography. In: Bassett LW, Jackson VP, Jahan R, Fu YS, Gold RH, eds. *Diagnosis of the Diseases of the Breast.* Philadelphia: WB Saunders; 1997:185–196.

Case 204

Case History

A 46-year-old woman presents with right nipple discharge.

Physical Examination

- right breast: clear discharge expressed from nipple
- left breast: normal exam, no discharge

Mammogram (Fig. 204–1)

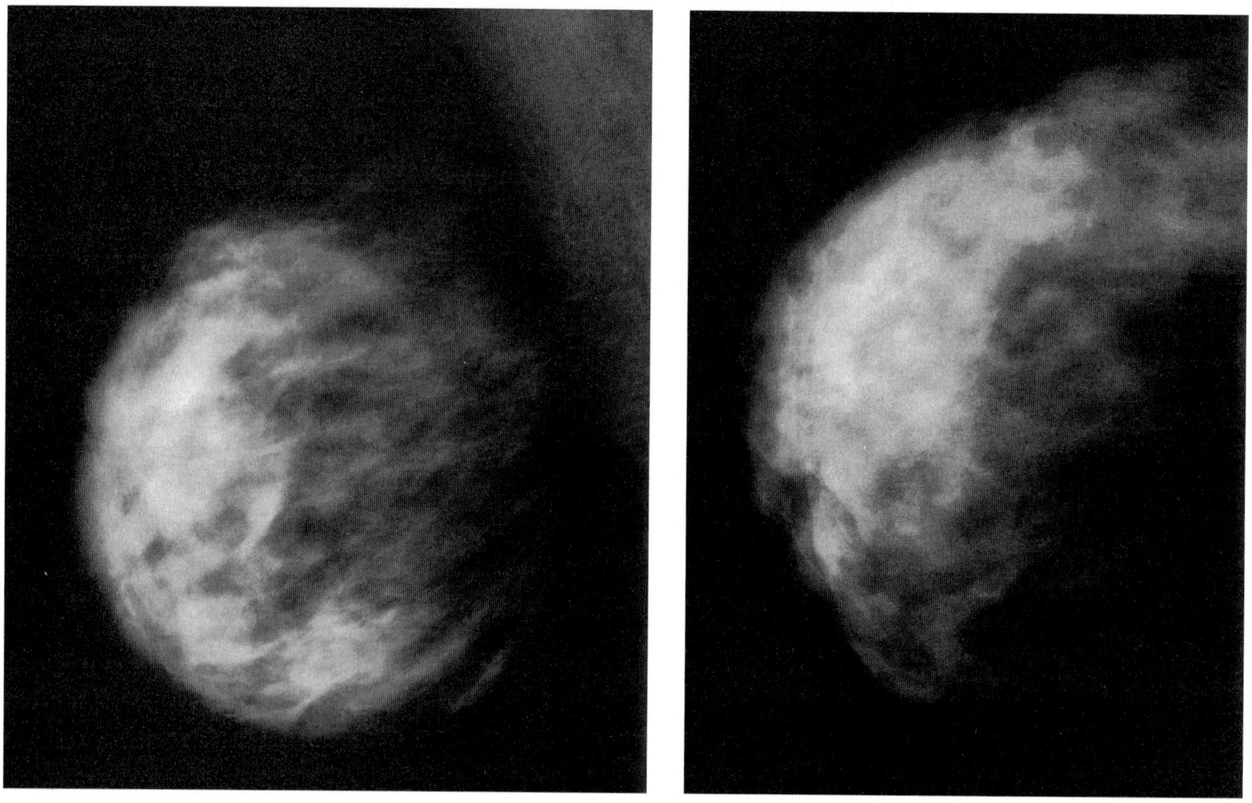

A

B

Figure 204–1. Normal heterogeneously dense right breast. (A). Right MLO mammogram. (B). Right CC mammogram.

Ultrasound

Frequency

- 13 MHz

Mass

- echogenicity: hypoechoic
- retrotumoral acoustic appearance: no shadowing
- shape: ellipsoid (Figs. 204–2 and 204–3)

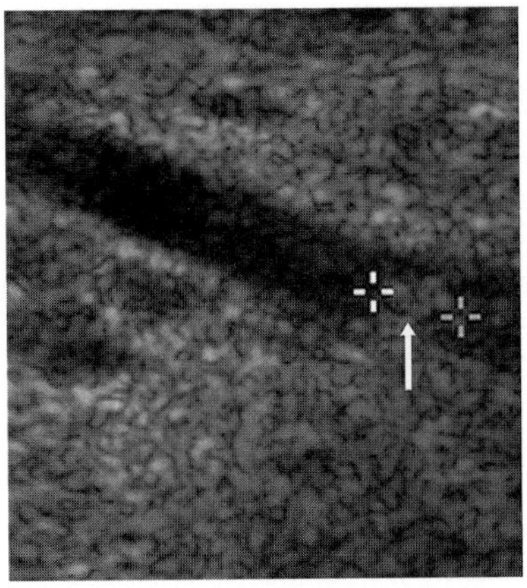

Figure 204–2. Right radial breast sonogram: At the 6:00 position of the nipple, there is a dilated duct. Within the duct is a small solid hypoechoic mass (arrow) (see Color Plate 204–2).

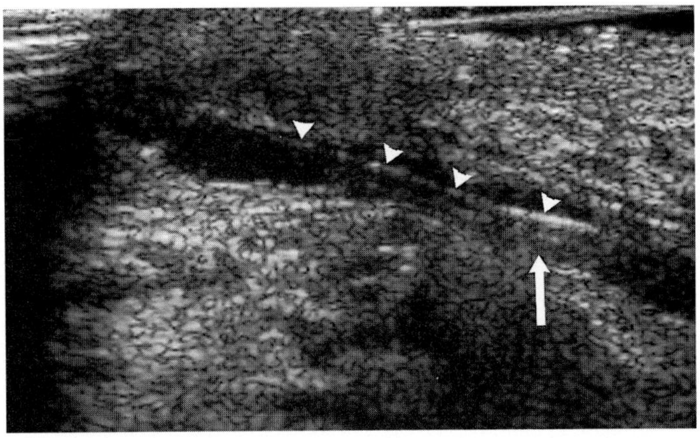

Figure 204–3. Right radial breast sonogram: Sonography was used intraoperatively to identify the dilated duct demonstrated in Figure 204–2. The surgeon inserted a wire into the nipple. With real-time sonography, the wire (arrowheads) was demonstrated within the abnormal duct touching the intraductal mass (arrow).

Pathology

- benign papilloma

Management

- BI-RADS Assessment Category 4, suspicious; biopsy should be considered

Pearls and Pitfalls

Although ductography is the usual method to evaluate ducts, high-frequency sonography may be used to systematically evaluate ducts around the nipple. The operator places one end of the transducer at the nipple and rotates the transducer around the nipple. The ducts will be demonstrated in a radial orientation so they will appear as linear anechoic fluid collections. In patients with abnormal nipple discharge, sonographic findings that suggest a focal etiology of the discharge include one or a few dilated ducts within the same quadrant, intraductal or intracystic solid mass, or a solid mass near the nipple not associated with fluid. If no ducts or masses are identified or if all the ducts are dilated, then ductography is necessary to further evaluate the ducts.

Suggested Readings

1. Sardanelli F, Imperiale A, Zandrino F, et al. Breast intraductal masses: US-guided fine-needle aspiration after galactography. *Radiology* 1997;204:143–148.

Case 205

Case History

A 71-year-old woman presents with left bloody nipple discharge.

Physical Examination

- left breast: small clear, yellow discharge from 3:00 duct; no bloody discharge observed
- right breast: normal exam

Mammogram (Figs. 205–1 and 205–2)

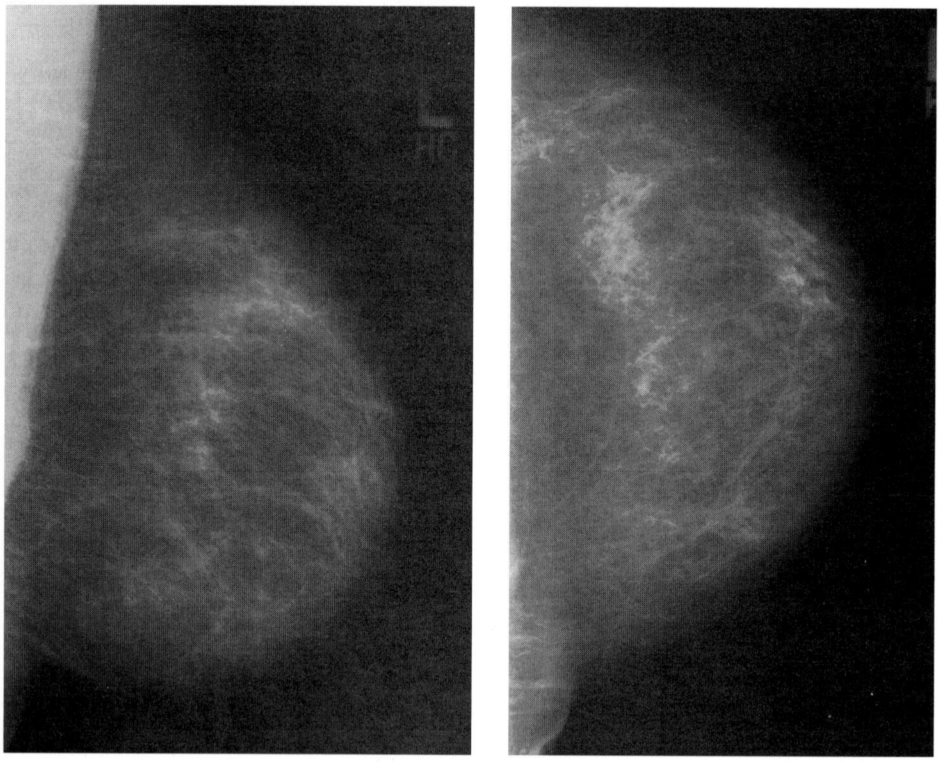

A B

Figure 205–1. Normal left breast mammogram. (A). Left MLO mammogram. (B). Left CC mammogram.

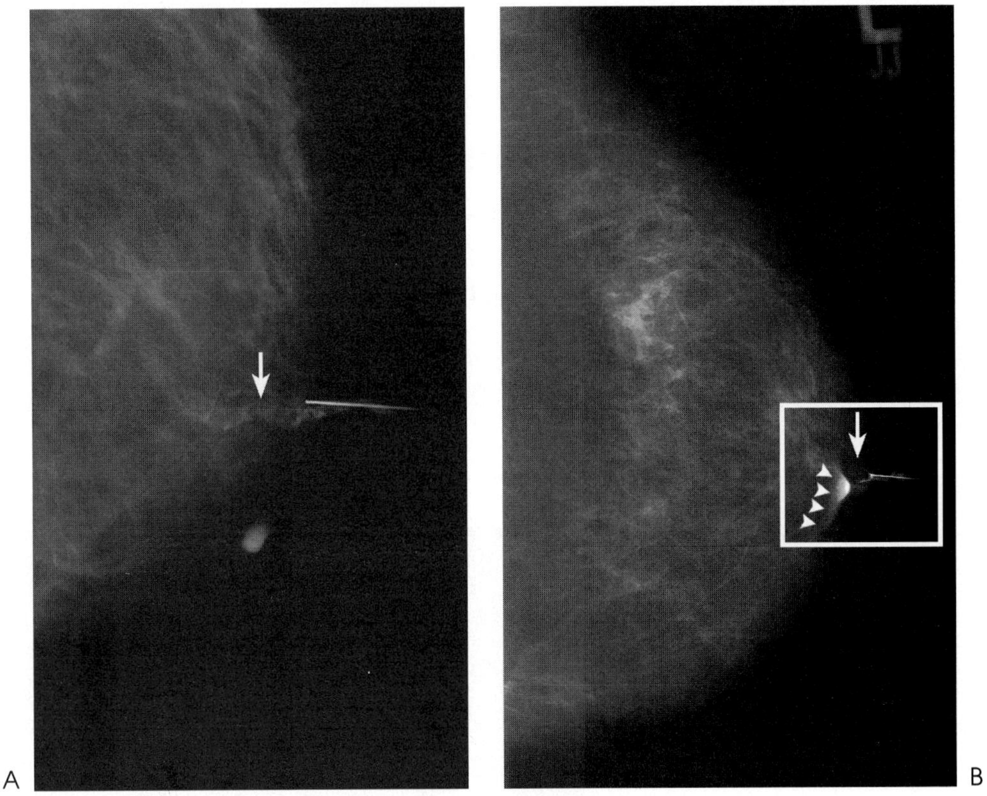

Figure 205–2. Left ductogram: Contrast is obstructed by a lobulated intraluminal mass (arrow). Because the mass obstructs the duct, contrast flows retrograde and spills outside the nipple (arrowheads). (A). Left MLO ductogram. (B). Left CC ductogram.

Pathology

- benign papilloma

Management

- BI-RADS Assessment Category 4, suspicious; biopsy should be considered

Pearls and Pitfalls

1. About 50% of women with spontaneous discharge have papillomas.
2. Causes for intraluminal masses on ductography include inspissated debris, hematoma, papilloma, malignant papillary lesions, and ductal carcinoma in situ (with or without invasion).
3. Ductography findings of papilloma include: ductal dilatation and intraductal mass. The mass may distend the duct or, occasionally, sessile papillomas may produce duct irregularity.

Suggested Readings

1. Jones M. Procedures for breast diagnosis and treatment. In: *Atlas of Breast Imaging*. Malden: Blackwell Science; 1996:188–214.
2. Kramer SC, Rieber A, Gorich J, et al. Diagnosis of papillomas of the breast: value of magnetic resonance mammography in comparison with galactography. *Eur Radiol* 2000;10:1733–1736.
3. Woods ER, Helvie MA, Ikeda DM, Mandell SH, Chapel KL, Adler DD. Solitary breast papilloma: comparison of mammographic, galactographic and pathologic findings. *AJR* 1992;159:487–491.

Case 206

Case History

A 72-year-old woman presents with left bloody nipple discharge.

Physical Examination

- left breast: bloody discharge expressed from nipple; otherwise normal exam
- right breast: no discharge; normal exam

Mammogram (Fig. 206–1)

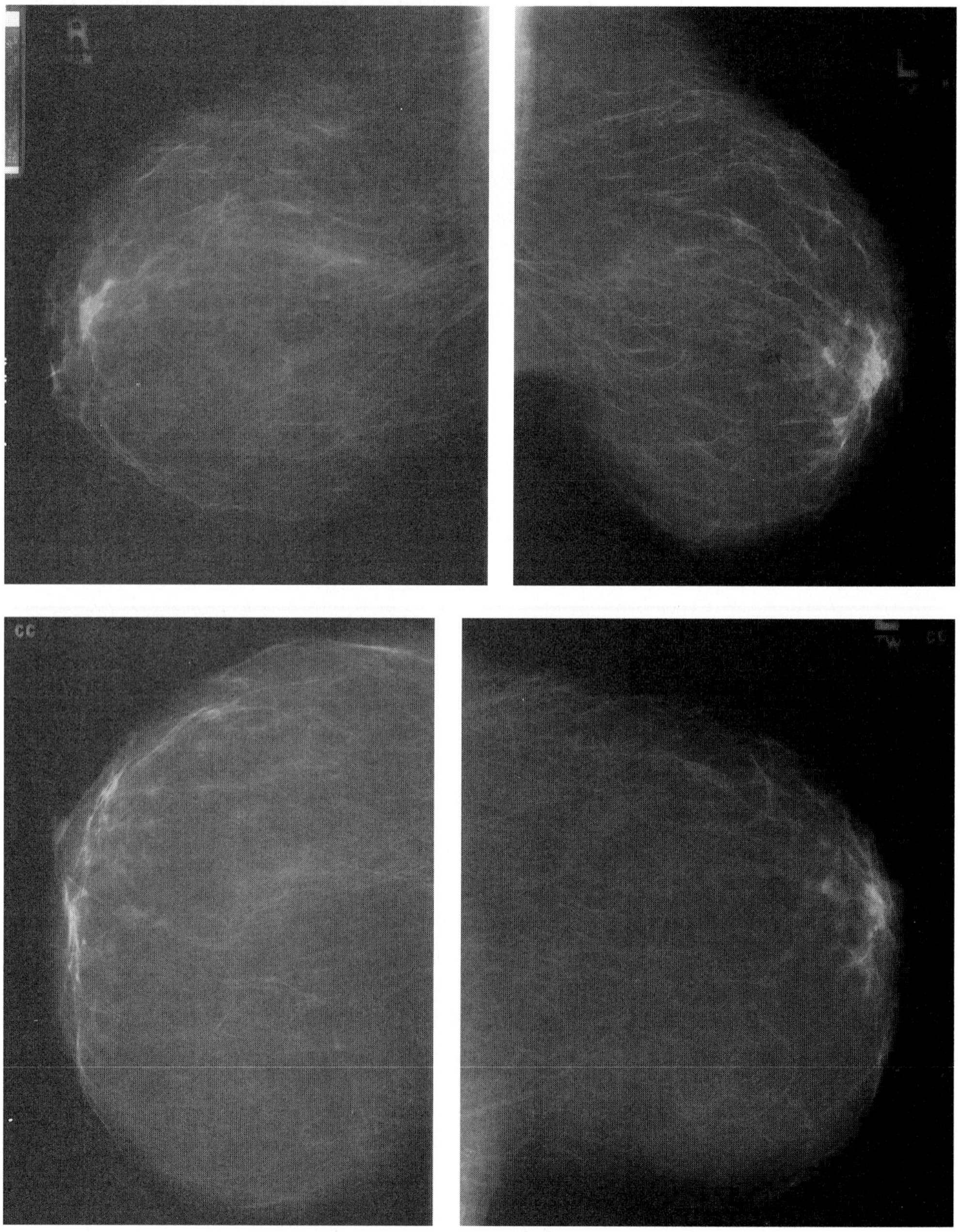

A B C D

Figure 206–1. Normal bilateral breasts that are almost entirely fat. Nipples are not in profile in both MLO views. (A). Right MLO mammogram. (B). Left MLO mammogram. (C). Right CC mammogram. (D). Left CC mammogram.

Ultrasound

Frequency

- 13 MHz

Mass

- margin: well defined
- echogenicity: hypoechoic
- retrotumoral acoustic appearance: no shadowing
- shape: ellipsoid (Fig. 206–2)

A 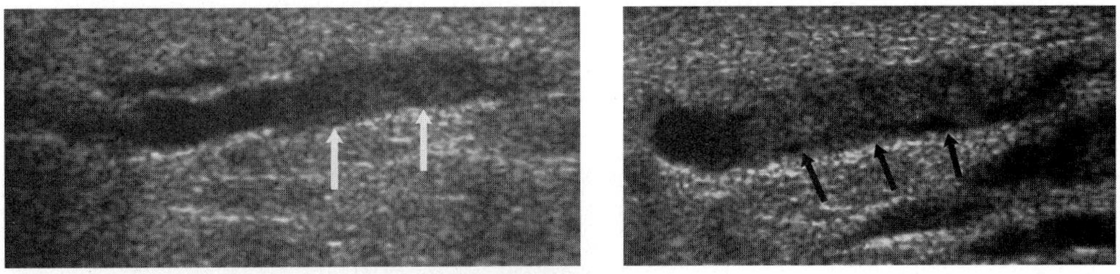 B

C 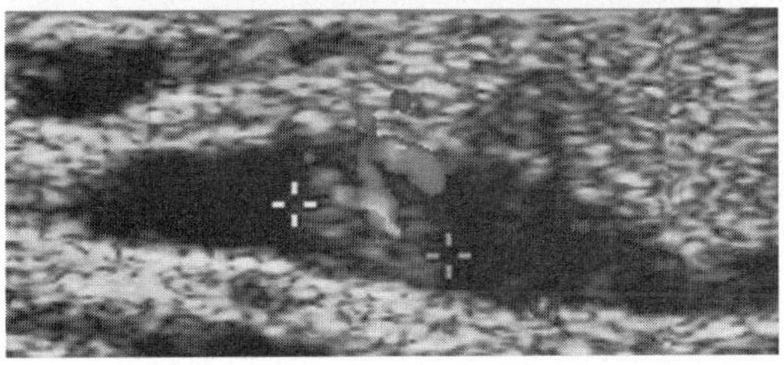

Figure 206–2. At the 4:00 position of the left breast, there is a dilated duct containing a hypoechoic sausage-shaped solid mass (arrows). (A). Left radial breast sonogram. (B). Left radial breast sonogram: close-up image of the mass (arrows). (C). Left oblique color Doppler breast sonogram: Color Doppler demonstrates vessels within the mass (see Color Plate 206–2 C).

Pathology

- ductal carcinoma in situ

Management

- BI-RADS Assessment Category 4, suspicious; biopsy should be considered

Pearls and Pitfalls

When sonography is performed for bloody discharge, dilatation of one or a few ducts in one quadrant is a serious finding. If no intraductal mass is identified and the surgeon opts for more imaging, then ductography should be performed. However, if sonographic intraductal or intracystic mass is identified, then biopsy or excision should be recommended.

Suggested Readings

1. Chung SY, Lee KW, Park KS, Lee Y, Bae SH. Breast tumors associated with nipple discharge. Correlation of findings on galactography and sonography. *Clin Imaging* 1995;19:165–171.
2. Hashimoto BE, Kramer DJ, Picozzi VJ. High detection rate of breast ductal carcinoma in situ calcifications on mammographically directed high-resolution sonography. *J Ultrasound Med* 2001;20:501–508.
3. Satake H, Shimamoto K, Sawaki A, et al. Role of ultrasonography in the detection of intraductal spread of breast cancer: correlation with pathologic findings, mammography and MR imaging. *Eur Radiol* 2000;10:1726–1732.

Case 207

Case History

An 80-year-old woman presents with left bloody discharge.

Physical Examination

- left breast: bloody discharge from duct at 5:00; otherwise normal exam
- right breast: normal exam

Mammogram (Figs. 207–1 and 207–2)

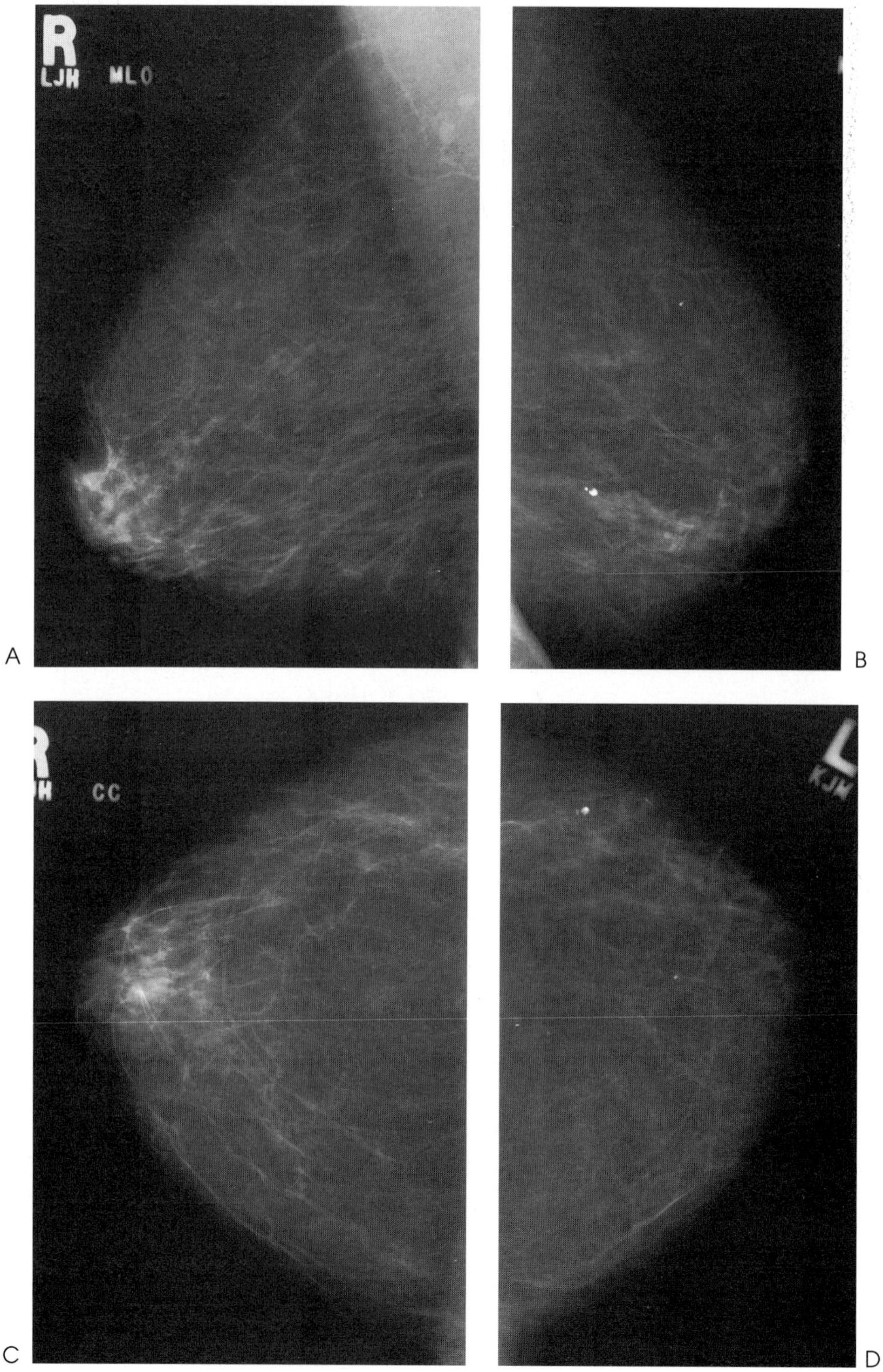

Figure 207–1. Left breast has prominent ducts in the inferior outer breast. (A). Right MLO mammogram. (B). Left lateral medial (LM) mammogram. (C). Right CC mammogram. (D). Left CC mammogram.

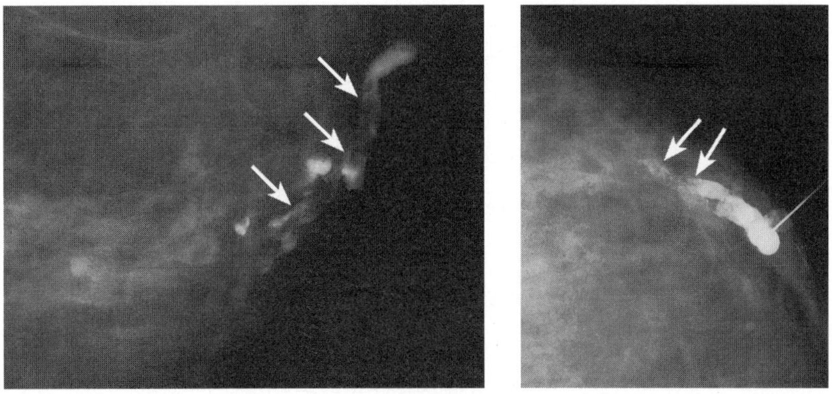

A B

Figure 207–2. Left breast ductogram: The contrast was injected into the duct at the 5:00 position. The duct contains multiple filling defects (arrows) associated with contour irregularities. (A). Left ML breast ductogram. (B). Left CC breast ductogram.

Pathology

- ductal carcinoma in situ

Management

- BI-RADS Assessment Category 4, suspicious; biopsy should be considered

Pearls and Pitfalls

1. Between 5 and 15% of intraluminal masses with ductography are due to malignancy.
2. Findings of malignancy on ductography include (1) intraluminal filling defects; (2) duct contour irregularity; (3) abrupt duct cutoff; (4) duct displaced or draped around a mass; (5) duct extravasation. Numerous intraluminal masses and extensive contour irregularity have a higher association with malignancy.

Suggested Readings

1. Cardenosa G. Ductography. In: Cardenosa G. *Breast Imaging Companion*. Philadelphia: Lippincott-Raven; 1997:372–383.
2. Dinkel HP, Trusen A, Gassel AM, et al. Predictive value of galactographic patterns for benign and malignant neoplasms of the breast in patients with nipple discharge. *Br J Radiol* 2000;73:706–714.
3. Van Zee KJ, Ortega Perez G, Minnard E, Cohen MA. Preoperative galactography increases the diagnostic yield of major duct excision for nipple discharge. *Cancer* 1998;82:1874–1880.

Case 208

Case History

An 80-year-old woman presents with left milky discharge.

Physical Examination

- left breast: milky discharge; otherwise normal exam
- right breast: normal exam

Mammogram (Fig. 208–1)

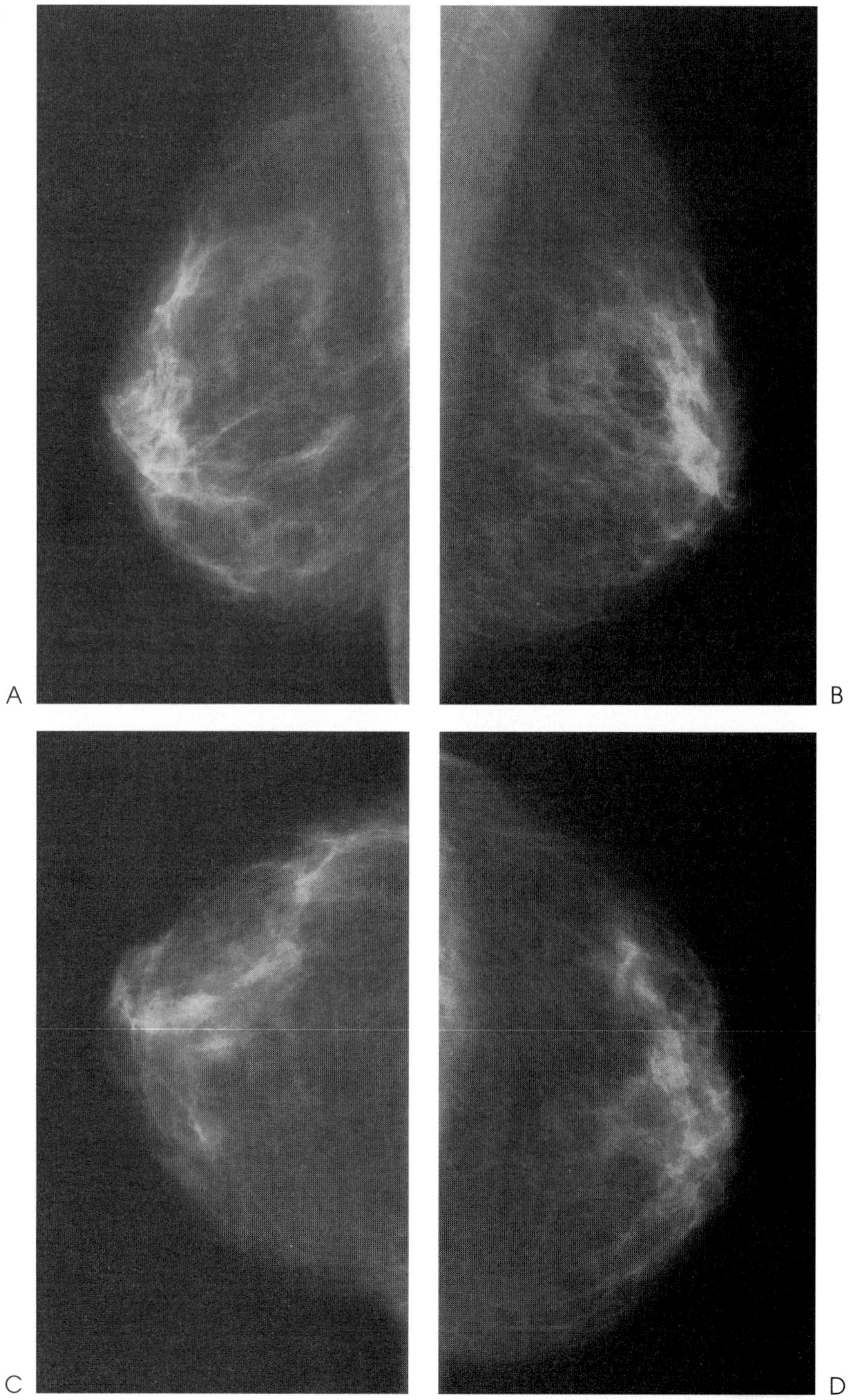

Figure 208–1. Normal bilateral mammograms with scattered fibroglandular densities. (A). Right MLO mammogram. (B). Left MLO mammogram. (C). Right CC mammogram. (D). Left CC mammogram.

Ultrasound

Frequency

- 11.5 MHz (Figs. 208-2 and 208-3)

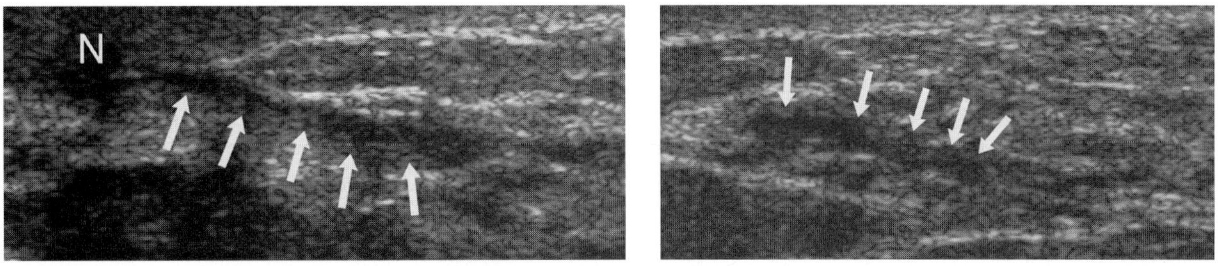

A B

Figure 208-2. There were multiple thick-walled ducts in the left upper outer quadrant, which were irregular in caliber and contour (arrows). Ducts in the other quadrants appeared normal. Nipple (N). (A). Left radial breast sonogram. (B). Left radial breast sonogram.

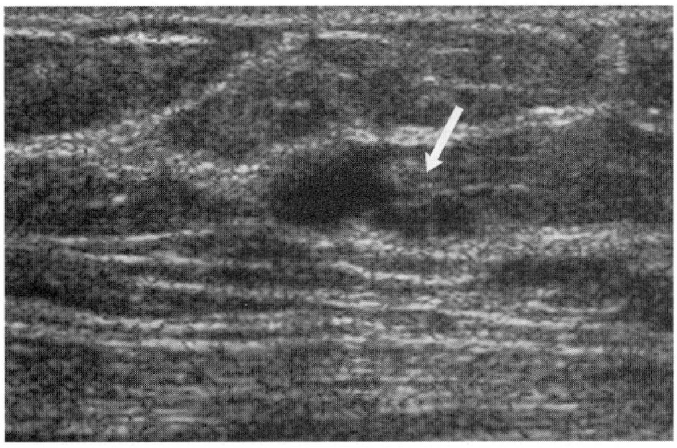

Figure 208-3. Left antiradial breast sonogram: A cross section of one abnormal duct demonstrates some asymmetric thickening on one wall (arrow).

Pathology

- ductal carcinoma in situ
- 6 cm of high-grade ductal carcinoma in situ in the left upper outer quadrant

Management

- BI-RADS Assessment Category 4, suspicious; biopsy should be considered

Pearls and Pitfalls

Sonographically, ductal carcinoma in situ may appear as (1) isolated calcifications, (2) an irregular hypoechoic mass (with or without calcifications), (3) an ill-defined hypoechoic area, or (4) abnormally focally dilated ducts. The dilated ducts may be single or multiple but are grouped together in a segment or quadrant. The ducts may contain calcifications, hypoechoic "debris," or focal masses. In this case, the malignancy appears as an irregular thickening of the ductal walls. Rarely, invasive ductal carcinoma is identified as a dilated duct.

Suggested Readings

1. Tohno D, Cosgrove DO, Sloane JP, eds. Malignant disease—primary carcinomas. In: Tohno D, Cosgrove DO, Sloane JP, eds. *Ultrasound Diagnosis of Breast Diseases.* New York: Churchill Livingston; 1994:157–180.
2. Yang WT, King W, Metreweli C. Clinically and mammographically occult invasive ductal carcinoma diagnosed by ultrasound: the focally dilated duct. *Australas Radiol* 1997;41:73–75.

Index

B

E

F

J

L

M

N

O

P

Q

R